Advances in Photodynamic Therapy

Basic, Translational, and Clinical

For a listing of recent related Artech House titles,
please turn to the back of this book.

Advances in Photodynamic Therapy

Basic, Translational, and Clinical

Michael R. Hamblin
Paweł Mróz

Editors

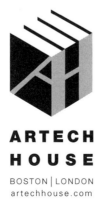

ARTECH HOUSE

BOSTON | LONDON
artechhouse.com

Library of Congress Cataloging-in-Publication Data
A catalog record for this book is available from the U.S. Library of Congress.

British Library Cataloguing in Publication Data
A catalogue record for this book is available from the British Library.

ISBN-13: 978-1-59693-277-7
ISBN-10: 1-59693-277-5

Cover design by Yekaterina Ratner

© 2008 Artech House
685 Canton Street
Norwood MA 02062

10 9 8 7 6 5 4 3 2 1

To my dearest wife Angela without whose support
this book would not have been possible.
—Michael R. Hamblin

To my wife Gosia, who lights up my world
—Paweł Mróz

Contents

CHAPTER 4
Pharmaceutical and Biological Considerations in
5-Aminolevulinic Acid in PDT   59

CHAPTER 5
Light Dosimetry and Light Sources for Photodynamic Therapy   93

CHAPTER 6
Cell Killing by Photodynamic Therapy   115

CHAPTER 12

Emerging Strategies in Photodynamic Therapy   235

CHAPTER 13

PDT and Inflammation   255

CHAPTER 22

PDT in Dermatology   419

CHAPTER 23

Role of Photodynamic Therapy (PDT) in Lung Cancer   443

CHAPTER 24

Photodynamic Therapy of the Gastrointestinal Tract Beyond the Esophagus   461

CHAPTER 29

Preface

Michael R. Hamblin and Paweł Mróz

The use of nontoxic dyes or photosensitizers (PSs) in combination with harmless visible light that is known as photodynamic therapy (PDT) has been known for over a hundred years, but is only now becoming widely used in medicine and biology. Originally developed as a tumor therapy, some of its most successful applications are for nonmalignant disease.

This book will present an up-to-date collection of the advances made in the PDT research field. It is broadly divided into three sections: basic, translational, and clinical advances. The basic advances section starts off with the historical review in Chapter 1 and then discusses the recent explosion in discovery and chemical synthesis of new PS in Chapter 2. Some guidelines on how to choose an ideal PS for a particular application are presented. The photochemistry and photophysics of PS and the two pathways known as Type I (radicals and reactive oxygen species) and Type II (singlet oxygen) photochemical processes are discussed in Chapter 3. The use of 5-aminolevulinic acid that, as a natural precursor of the heme biosynthetic pathway, stimulates accumulation of the PS protoporphyrin IX is described in Chapter 4. To carry out PDT effectively in vivo, it is necessary to ensure sufficient light reaches all the diseased tissue. This involves understanding how light travels within various tissues and the relative effects of absorption and scattering as discussed in Chapter 5.

In the translational advances section the most important factor governing the outcome of PDT (how the PS interacts with cells in the target tissue or tumor) will be discussed in Chapter 6, and the key aspect of this interaction is the subcellular localization of the PS. Examples of PSs that localize in mitochondria, lysosomes, endoplasmic reticulum, Golgi apparatus, and plasma membranes are given. Investigation of cell death pathways after illumination has proved a fruitful area of study in recent years. The necessary role of oxygen in photodynamic therapy is discussed in Chapter 7, and the resulting oxidative stress produced by the resulting reactive oxygen and their interaction with cells and tissue is covered in Chapter 8. The ability of PDT to fairly specifically target blood vessels and the vascular system (particularly of tumors) is summarized in Chapter 9. Over the years many investigators have sought to increase the ability of PSs to localize in the desired cell type or tissue by synthesizing covalent conjugates between the small PS molecules and other molecules with specific abilities to target antigens, receptors, or adhesion molecules. These studies are covered in two chapters. Chapter 10 concentrates on PS conjugates with large macromolecular vehicles such as antibodies or other proteins, while Chapter 11 covers PS conjugates with smaller molecules and conjugates that can be specifically cleaved by enzymes present at the target. Chapter 12, entitled "Emerging Strategies in PDT," covers very new approaches including nanoparticles, metronomic PDT, and two-photon PDT. Two chapters cover the interesting ability of PDT to activate the immune system, Chapter 13 mainly concentrating on the innate immune system and the induction of various kinds of inflammation by the ROS produced by PDT, while Chapter 14 covers the activation of cellular immunity after PDT and the induction of T-lymphocytes that can specifically recognize PDT-treated cancers. Chapter 15 presents some new applications of PDT in bone including possible treatments for bone cancer, osteomyelitis, and bone growth abnormalities. Chapter 16 describes a method that employs specific PSs and light to deliver drugs inside cells that would not be possible by other means is called photochemical internalization. Chapter 17 summarizes all the other modalities that have been combined with PDT to produce additive or synergistic combinations. Finally, Chapter 18 returns to the origins of PDT a hundred years ago, and discusses the abilities of PDT to destroy every kind of pathogenic microorganism including bacteria, fungi, parasites and viruses.

In the final clinical advances section we cover those applications of PDT that have been tested in at least some clinical trials, and in some cases clinical approvals have been obtained for cancer or noncancer indications. Chapter 19 covers PDT for infectious disease that is just starting to be tested clinically. PDT for cardiovascular diseases is covered in Chapter 20 where there have been clinical trials both for prevention of restenosis and for atherosclerosis.

Chapter 21 covers the use of PDT in ophthalmology, which has been a huge growth area for PDT over recent years. Likewise, the use of PDT in dermatology described in Chapter 22 has been another growth area particularly concentrating on ALA-PDT for cancer and premalignant and nonmalignant skin conditions. The role of PDT in lung cancer is discussed in Chapter 23 for both advanced and early disease. We present two chapters on clinical PDT in gastrointestinal disease. Chapter 24 concentrates on PDT for GI cancer beyond the esophagus, while Chapter 25 covers esophageal disease (both Barrett's esophagus and esophageal cancer). Likewise, we have two chapters on clinical PDT within the brain. Chapter 26 discusses PDT for detection and treatment of brain cancers (frequently highly lethal), while Chapter 27 covers the application of PDT to the nonmalignant (but difficult to treat) pituitary adenomas. The use of PDT to treat head and neck cancer (frequently recurrent after other therapies have failed) is covered in Chapter 28. Finally, the challenging application of PDT as an approach to treat disseminated cancer in the peritoneal cavity is presented in Chapter 29.

CHAPTER 1

History of PDT: The First Hundred Years

Michael R. Hamblin and Paweł Mróz

1.1 Introduction

Photodynamic therapy (PDT) can be defined as the administration of a nontoxic drug or dye known as a photosensitizer (PS) either systemically, locally, or topically to a patient bearing a lesion (frequently but not always cancer), followed after some time by the illumination of the lesion with visible light (usually long wavelength red light), which, in the presence of oxygen, leads to the generation of cytotoxic species and consequently to cell death and tissue destruction.

1.2 Early Studies with Dyes

The realization that the combination of nontoxic dyes and visible light could kill cells was first made by Oscar Raab, a medical student working with Professor Herman von Tappeiner in Munich (Figure 1.1). While investigating the effects of acridine dyes on the protozoa that cause malaria, he made the chance discovery during a thunderstorm that the combination of acridine red and light killed Infusoria, a species of paramecium [1]. He went on to show that this cytotoxic effect was greater than that of either acridine red alone, light alone, or acridine red exposed to light and then added to the paramecium. Raab associated this property of dyes (light-mediated cytotoxicity) with the optical property of fluorescence. He postulated that the effect was caused by the transfer of energy from light to the chemical, similar to the process of photosynthesis seen in plants after the absorption of light by chlorophyll. In a second paper, von Tappeiner discussed the potential future application of fluorescent substances in medicine [2]. The first report of systemic administration of a PS in humans was in 1900 by Prime, a French neurologist, who used the dye eosin (a brominated derivative of fluoroscein) orally in the treatment of epilepsy, but discovered that this treatment induced dermatitis in sun-exposed areas of skin [3]. This discovery led to the first therapeutic medical application of an interaction between a PS and light in which von Tappeiner, together with a dermatologist named Jesionek, used a combination of topically applied eosin and white light to treat skin tumors [4]. Together with Jodlbauer, von Tappeiner went on to demonstrate the requirement of oxygen in these photosensitization reactions [5] and in 1907 they introduced the term "photodynamic action" to describe this phenomenon [6].

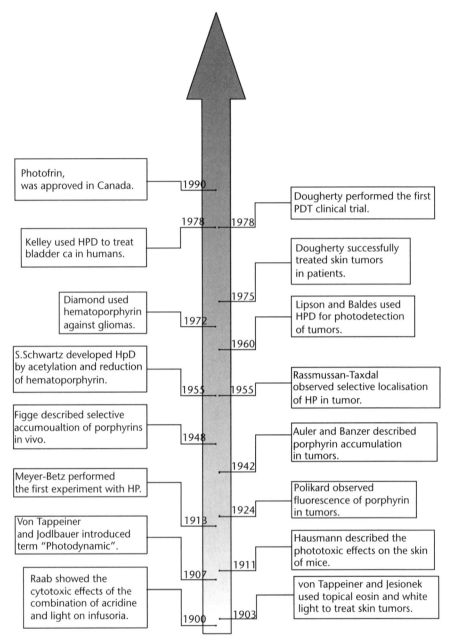

Figure 1.1   Timeline of historical milestones in development of PDT from 1900 to 1985.

1.3   Studies with Hematoporphyrin

Scherer discovered hematoporphyrin (HP) in 1841 after treating dried blood with concentrated sulfuric acid, washing the precipitate free of iron and then treating it with alcohol [7]. However, the fluorescent properties of HP were not described until 1867 [8] and the compound was named hematoporphyrin by the renowned German physiological chemist Felix Hoppe-Seyler in 1871 [9]. HP was first used as a PS by

Hausmann in 1911 in Vienna [10], who performed in vitro studies with HP and light on paramecium and on red blood cells and also described photoxic skin reactions in mice exposed to light after systemic HP administration [10]. The first case of a human undergoing photosensitization by porphyrins was during a self-experimentation carried out in 1913 by the German, Friedrich Meyer-Betz. In order to determine whether the same phototoxic effects could be induced in humans as had been seen in mice, he injected himself with 200 mg of HP and subsequently suffered prolonged pain and swelling in light-exposed areas [11]. The first report of fluorescent porphyrin localization in an experimental malignant tumor appeared in 1924 when Policard, from Lyons, France, observed characteristic red porphyrin fluorescence in a rat sarcoma illuminated with ultraviolet light from a Woods lamp [12]. In 1942, Auler and Banzer [13] from Berlin described the localization and fluorescence of exogenously administered porphyrins in experimental malignant tumors. These findings prompted Figge and Weiland in 1948 [14] to further investigate the tumor-localizing properties of porphyrins in an attempt to develop this as a method for the diagnosis and treatment of tumors. They administered a range of porphyrins, including HP, coproporphyrin, protoporphyrin, and zinc-HP, to mice with both experimentally induced and transplanted tumors and found that tumor-localized fluorescence appeared within 24 to 48 hours of administration and persisted for as long as 10 to 14 days [15]. The fluorescence was not seen in normal tissues, other than lymph nodes, omentum, fetal and placental tissue, and healing wounds.

In 1951, Manganiello and Figge [16] investigated the effects of injecting HP in three patients with head and neck malignancies, but fluorescence was not detected. This failure was attributed to the proportionately lower doses of HP given to humans (30–120 mg) as compared with those employed in previous animal experiments, and possibly also the fact that the patients had been previously irradiated. In 1955, Rassmussan-Taxdal et al. [17] gave intravenous infusions of HP hydrochloride to patients before the excision of a variety of benign and malignant lesions. Typical red fluorescence was observed in seven out of eight malignant tumors but in only one of the three benign lesions. The intensity of the tumor fluorescence increased in proportion to the administered HP dose, and with higher doses it was possible to detect a breast cancer through intact skin and a colon adenocarcinoma through the bowel wall. In 1955, Peck et al. [18] injected HP in both animals and humans to assess the potential application of inducing fluorescence in the gall bladder and the biliary tract as a potential aid in biliary surgery. In all the animals studied, red fluorescence was observed in the gall bladder and biliary tree. In three out of five human subjects, no tumor or lymphatic localization was seen following the administration of relatively low doses (30–120 mg) of HP. However, with a higher dosage (1,000 mg) one patient exhibited a bright red fluorescence of a cervical carcinoma and associated inguinal lymph nodes.

1.4   Discovery of Hematoporphyrin Derivative

The previous studies demonstrated the potential role of HP as a diagnostic agent and even as a therapeutic approach for cancers. However, a major disadvantage of this compound was the large dose necessary to produce consistent accumulation of fluorescence in the tumor, which also led to unacceptable skin phototoxicity. In 1955, Schwartz et al. [19] demonstrated that the HP preparation used in previous studies was actually an impure mixture of compounds consisting of several different porphyrins, each with different properties. He showed that, after partial purification, the more pure HP fraction obtained localized only very poorly in tumors, whereas the residue of impurities left behind had much greater affinity for the tumor tissue. Schwartz continued his experiments in an attempt to further purify this tumor-localizing fraction in the impure HP mixture. Among other procedures he tested was the treatment of crude HP with a mixture of acetic and sulfuric acids, filtering the resulting mixture and then neutralizing with sodium acetate, before redissolving the precipitate in saline to produce a substance that subsequently became known as hematopoprhyrin derivative (HpD). This preparation was found to be approximately twice as phototoxic as crude HP, having a potentially lethal effect on mice injected with a sufficient dose of the substance and subsequently exposed to light. The nature of the phototoxic reaction was similar to that previously demonstrated by Hausmann [10] with skin irritation, edema and erythema, leading to skin necrosis and death. Animals kept in the dark suffered no ill effects. The severity of the reaction was dependent on three factors: the drug dose, the duration of light exposure, and the time interval between drug administration and light exposure. Schwartz then persuaded Lipson, from the Mayo Clinic, to discontinue his work on HP and concentrate on HpD studies. Together with Baldes, Lipson further demonstrated the property of tumor localization [20] using HpD, and in the early 1960s they became interested in the potential use of HpD for tumor detection. Using tumors growing in experimental animals, they showed that HpD at much smaller doses was more effective than crude HP in tumor localization and in distinguishing malignant from normal tissues [21].

1.5 Clinical Photodection Studies with HpD

Lipson, Baldes, and Gray [22] in 1967 were the first to study the potential fluorescent localization of HpD in tumors in patients undergoing bronchoscopy or esophagoscopy for suspected malignant disease. Light of the appropriate wavelength to activate HpD fluorescence (400 nm) was produced by a filtered mercury arc lamp and transmitted via a fiber-optic cable through the endoscope to the suspicious lesion. Tissue fluorescence was observed through a filter, which excluded reflected excitation light from the mercury arc lamp. A total of 15 patients were studied, 9 undergoing bronchoscopy, 5 undergoing esophagoscopy, and 1 undergoing both procedures. HpD was given intravenously at a dose of 2 mg/kg body weight, 3 hours before endoscopy. Of these 15 patients, 14 were found to have histologically proven malignancy of which 10 were detected by HpD fluorescence. Failure to detect the other lesions was attributed to inadequate light exposure of relatively inaccessible tumors. A number of different malignant tumor types exhibited fluorescence, but the only benign lesion, an empyema, failed to demonstrate any fluorescence. Side effects caused by cutaneous photosensitization were only seen in one patient.

In a subsequent report in 1967, Lipson et al. [23] investigated 50 patients using fluorescent bronchoscopy with HpD. Of 34 malignant tumors accessible to the bronchoscope, 32 exhibited fluorescence but none of the benign lesions did so. In the same year, Gray et al. [24] studied cervical and vaginal lesions using HpD-mediated fluorescence detection. Fluorescence was demonstrated in all but one of 34 malignant lesions, but over half (13 of 23) of the benign lesions also fluoresced. Further histological review, however, revealed the presence of either carcinoma in situ or severe dysplasia in most of these lesions. In 1968, Gregorie and colleagues reported the use of HpD fluorescence in a large series of 226 patients, including 173 malignant tumors and 53 benign lesions [25]. Fluorescence was detected in 84% of adenocarcinomas, 77% of squamous carcinomas, and 62.5% of sarcomas. Squamous carcinomas had the highest fluorescence compared with either the adenocarcinomas or the sarcomas. Only 22% of the benign lesions, which included leg ulcers, postirradiation ulcers, and burns, exhibited relatively low levels of fluorescence. Although a significant difference was found between the fluorescence observed in benign and malignant lesions, they concluded that the comparatively low sensitivity and specificity of this technique limited its use in tumor detection. However, it was proposed that fluorescence detection might have a role in defining tumor margins, especially during endoscopic procedures. In 1971, Leonard and Beck reported a study of tumor detection using HpD in 40 patients with suspected head and neck tumors [26]. Red HpD fluorescence was seen in 29 patients with biopsy-proven cancer, and in 5 patients the HpD fluorescence was used to detect the extent of the lesions and determine the choice of biopsy site. Three benign tumors and four inflammatory lesions exhibited no fluorescence, but two out of four biopsies of "normal tissue" were fluorescent. This finding was ascribed to the presence of lymphoid tissue in the biopsy specimen, and the authors proposed that the affinity of HpD for lymphoid organs would lead to considerable confusion in the diagnosis of head and neck malignancies.

Despite this problem, Lipson and coworkers [27] continued to produce encouraging results using HpD fluorescence in the detection of early cancers and dysplastic changes in the uterine cervix. However, false positives consisting of squamous metaplasia, chronic cervicitis, and one case with no obvious histological abnormality were seen. Workers at the Mayo Clinic assessed the localization of HpD in cases of early-stage lung cancer [28, 29]. Successful detection of carcinoma in situ was described using a system in which violet light from a filtered mercury lamp was alternated at high frequency with white light, allowing both tumor fluorescence and normal visualization during endoscopic examinations. Similarly, in 1979, a fluorescence detection system employing a krypton ion laser was developed, with a 405-nm wavelength to excite porphyrin during endoscopy [30]. The potential application of HpD fluorescence using this system for localization of early lung cancer was demonstrated in an animal model by Hayata and Dougherty [31]. In 1982, Hayata used a similar system to study 36 patients with bronchial neoplasms and 4 with metaplasia [32]. Following HpD injection, endoscopic examination detected three of the early lesions and 33 of the more advanced lesions. Three severely dysplastic lesions were identified and one mildly atypical lesion was not fluorescent. There were three false negatives that were attributed to blood or necrotic tissue obscuring the lesions. Using HpD and filtered mercury arc lamp to study bladder tumors, in 1983 Benson et al. [33, 34] demonstrated a positive correlation between the fluorescence of the resected specimens and the presence of tumor on histological examination, including some macroscopically normal areas containing carcinoma in situ or severe dysplasia. Normal urothelium showed no fluorescence and the optimal differential fluorescence between tumor and normal tissues was seen 2 to 3 hours after HpD administration. However, in order to have any significant clinical impact, early macroscopically normal lesions need to be reliably identified. These lesions are, however, often extremely difficult to distinguish from normal tissues caused by autofluorescence. Despite the use of equipment to subtract background fluorescence, this technique has not found a practical role in everyday clinical practice [35].

1.6   Cancer Treatment with Porphyrins and Light in Animal Models

The first suggestion that the combination of the tumor-localizing and the phototoxic properties of porphyrins such as HP and HpD might be exploited to produce an effective treatment for cancer was made in 1972 in *The Lancet* by Diamond and coworkers [36] from San Francisco. These authors had originally wondered whether porphyrins might potentiate the effects of ionizing radiation (X-rays), but having found that this was not the case, went on to test the hypothesis that HP may serve as a selective photosensitizing agent to destroy cancer exposed to light. The effect of light activation of HP was studied in glioma cells in culture that were exposed to white light for 50 minutes in the presence of HP and underwent 100% cell death. When the same cell line was used to induce subcutaneous tumors in mice, a similar effect was seen with a marked reduction in tumor volume following light exposure delivered 24 hours after systemic HP administration. Tumor growth was suppressed for 10 to 20 days, but regrowth then occurred from viable areas remaining in deeper regions of the tumor. Histological examination showed coagulation necrosis in all but the deepest regions of the tumors. Neither HP alone, nor light alone produced any effect. The authors concluded that PDT offered a new approach to the treatment of brain tumors and other neoplasms resistant to other therapies.

In 1975, Dougherty and coworkers [37] at the Roswell Park Cancer Institute in Buffalo reported the first successful complete tumor cures following administration of HpD and activation with red light in the treatment of experimental tumors. Mice carrying spontaneous or implanted mammary tumors were injected with 2.5 to 5.0 mg/kg HpD and rats with implanted Walker 256 carcinosarcomas or bearing 7,12-dimethylbenz(a)anthracene (DMBA)–induced mammary tumors received 5 to 15 mg/kg HpD. Tumors were then exposed to red light from a xenon arc lamp for three 1-hour periods over 5 days. Using a definition of cure as no palpable tumor at least 2 months after the last treatment, 48% of the transplanted mouse mammary tumors were cured. Similar results were observed with the rat DMBA-induced tumors using 15 mg/kg HpD with light exposure at 24 hours. Lower doses of HpD or light failed to induce complete tumor regression, and neither drug nor light alone had any effect [37]. Toxicity studies in mice showed that exposure of the entire abdominal area to light 24 hours after HpD administration produced a typical photosensitivity reaction with 50% mortality at 24 hours. This mortality was greatly reduced when the drug-to-light interval was increased to 48 hours, but at this time the tumor–liver ratio had decreased to 0.86 and the cure rate for the same tumor was reduced to 20%, less than half that seen at 24 hours [37].

In the same year, Kelly, an urologist working at St. Mary's Hospital in London, United Kingdom, demonstrated that human bladder tumor cells transplanted into mice could be destroyed using PDT [38]. Subcutaneous tumors displayed typical red fluorescence following HpD administration, and subsequent light exposure produced ulceration and variable destruction of the tumor nodules with the majority (22 of 32) being totally or almost totally destroyed.

1.7 Early Clinical Studies with HpD and Light

A milestone in the development of PDT occurred in 1976. Following the successful treatment of animal tumors using porphyrin-based PDT described above, Kelly and Snell proceeded to the first human study of the effects of PDT using HpD in five patients with bladder cancer [39]. At cystoscopy, only limited tumor fluorescence was observed, but the resected specimens fluoresced brightly after removal. Microscopic examination of the resected specimens showed fluorescence confined to malignant and premalignant lesions, including some apparently normal areas, which were subsequently shown on histology to be dysplastic or malignant. In one patient with extensive recurrent bladder carcinoma, following failed traditional therapies, a quartz rod connected to a mercury vapor lamp was used to photoactivate HpD and induce tumor destruction. Tumor necrosis was seen in the illuminated area and there was no effect in the unilluminated areas following treatment [39].

In 1978, Dougherty reported the first large series of patients successfully treated with PDT [40]. Twenty-five patients with 113 primary or secondary skin tumors, all of which were refractory or had recurred following conventional treatment, were treated with HpD followed by exposure to red light from a xenon arc lamp at times ranging from 24 to 168 hours after injection. Ninety-eight lesions completely regressed, thirteen exhibited a partial response, and only two were resistant to treatment. The primary tumor types that responded included squamous cell carcinomas (SCC), basal cell carcinomas (BCC), and malignant melanomas, and the metastatic skin lesions arising from primary tumors of the breast, colon, and endometrium. Side effects included sunburn, erythema, edema, and in some cases skin necrosis, although these effects were reduced by increasing the time interval between HpD injection and light exposure to at least 3 days. This study demonstrated that PDT could be used successfully in the treatment of various malignant tumors even where conventional therapies had failed [40].

Since then, many more studies have been published confirming the clinical effectiveness of PDT in the treatment of a variety of tumors. The superficial location and the ease of light application make primary and secondary skin tumors ideally suited to treatment with PDT. Deeper and larger lesions may require multiple treatments, but smaller lesions are easily treated, often leaving no scarring. Complete responses were seen in 70% to 80% of BCC, 50% of malignant melanomas, 20% of SCC, and 80% of secondary tumors [41–45]. It was soon realized that PDT could be used bronchoscopically in the treatment of inoperable obstructing lung tumors refractory to radiotherapy, often with dramatic improvement in symptoms and pulmonary function [46–48]. It was also found to be useful in the treatment of early lung cancers not suitable for resection [49, 50]. The first report by Hayata et al. in 1982 [50] described a significant bronchoscopic response in the majority of patients, but only 1 patient of 14 was cured.

Following the early report from Kelly et al. describing PDT of a bladder tumor using HpD, many clinical studies have assessed the use of PDT in transitional cell carcinomas of the bladder [51]. Benson et al. [34] reported four cases of in situ carcinoma responding to PDT, and Ohi and Tsuchiya [52] published a series of 11 superficial tumors successfully treated using light delivery via a flexible cystoscope in 1983. In 1985 Haas et al. [53] reported a series of 14 patients with bladder carcinoma in situ treated with PDT. Eleven were disease free at 26 months and two of the three that subsequently relapsed were successfully retreated. In 1987, Prout et al. [54] treated 19 patients with bladder tumors of whom 9 (47%) had a complete response with 37 of 50 individual tumors eradicated. The potential of using PDT in the treatment of esophageal cancer was also realized around this time. In 1984, McCaughan et al. [55] reported the use of PDT in the treatment of seven patients with obstructing carcinoma in which all lesions responded, regardless of histological type, with good palliation in all cases. Two patients obtained relief of dysphagia for up to 11 months following treatment. The following year Hayata et al. [42] reported the effects of PDT in superficial esophageal lesions and early gastric cancer in patients who refused or were unfit for surgery. In the esophagus complete responses were seen in four cases, although three of these also received radiotherapy. Of 16 patients with early gastric cancer four were treated with PDT alone and all had a complete response. Twelve patients in this series later underwent resection, and a complete response was seen in five patients previously treated with PDT.

1.8   Explosion of Interest in PDT from 1980s Onwards

Figure 1.2 shows the total number of papers published on PDT each year from 1970 to date. After a reasonably steady total varying between 15 to 50 publications per year from 1970 to 1984, it can be seen that beginning in 1985 and continuing to the present there has been an exponential increase in the numbers of annual publications on PDT. This period covered the initial discovery of ALA-induced PPIX as a modality for PDT in 1990, the first regulatory approval for Photofrin as a treatment for bladder cancer in Canada in 1993, successive U.S. approvals for Photofrin as a palliative treatment for patients with completely or partially obstructing esophageal cancer in 1995, and the approval of Photofrin for palliation of symptoms in patients with completely or partially obstructing endobronchial nonsmall cell lung cancer in 1998. In 1999, the U.S. Food and Drug Administration (FDA) announced the approval of Levulan Kerastick (aminolevulinic acid HCl) to be used in conjunction with photodynamic therapy for treatment of actinic keratoses (precancerous skin lesions) of the face or scalp.

In 2000, Visudyne™ (verteporfin for injection, liposomal benzoporphyrin derivative monoacid ring A) PDT received approval for the treatment of the wet

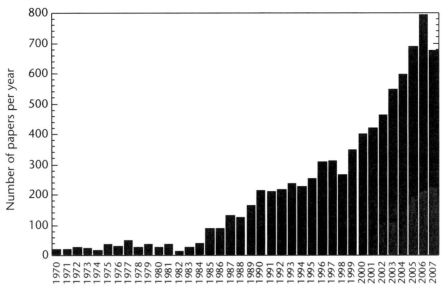

Figure 1.2   Number of papers published on PDT each year from 1970 to present.

form of age-related macular degeneration (AMD), the leading cause of blindness in people over the age of 50 in the Western world. In 2001, the FDA also approved Visudyne therapy for the treatment of occult subfoveal choroidal neovascularization (CNV) secondary to AMD. In August, 2002, Visudyne therapy for occult macular degeneration was granted marketing authorization in European countries by the European Commission (EMEA). In October 2004, QLT, Inc. reported that the drug has been approved in over 50 countries for extended indications, including occult CNV, in the European Union, Japan, Australia, and New Zealand; CNV due to pathologic myopia in the United States, Canada, and the European Union; and CNV due to presumed ocular histoplasmosis syndrome in the United States. At the end of 2001, Foscan® was approved with obligations by the EMEA (but not by the FDA) for the palliative treatment of patients with advanced head and neck squamous cell cancer. In 2003, Photofrin was approved in the United States for the ablation of high-grade dysplasia associated with Barrett's esophagus in patients who do not undergo esophagectomy.

The combination of many innovative mechanistic studies of PDT, reports of novel animal studies in which PDT is applied for hitherto untested diseases, and an increasing number of clinical trials of new and established PS, together with further regulatory approvals for new indications of PDT, all suggest that the level of interest in PDT will keep increasing for the foreseeable future.

References

[1]   Raab, O., "Uber die Wirkung fluoreszierender Stoffe auf Infusorien," *Z. Biol.*, Vol. 39, 1900, pp.524–546.

[2]   Von Tappenier, H., "Uber die Wirkung fluoreszierender Stoffe auf Infusorien nach Versuchen von O. Raab," *Muench Med. Wochenschr*, Vol. 47, 1900, p. 5.

[3]   Prime, J., Les accidentes toxiques par l'eosinate de sodium, Paris: Jouve and Boyer, 1900.

[4]   Jesionek, A., and H. von Tappenier, "Therapeutische Versuche mit fluoreszierenden Stoffen," *Muench Med. Wochneshr*, Vol. 47, 1903, pp. 2042–2044,.

[5]   Von Tappeiner, H., and A. Jodlbauer, "Uber Wirkung der photodynamischen (fluorieszierenden) Stoffe auf Protozoan und Enzyme," *Dtsch. Arch. Klin. Med.*, Vol. 80, 1904, pp. 427–487.

[6]   Von Tappeiner, H., and A. Jodlbauer, Die Sensibilisierende Wirkung fluorieszierender Substanzer. Gesammte Untersuchungen uber die photodynamische Erscheinung, Leipzig: F. C. W. Vogel, 1907.

[7]   Scherer, H. "Chemisch-physiologische untersuchungen," *Ann. Chem. Pharm.*, Vol. 40, 1841, p. 1.

[8]   Thudichum, J. L., Tenth Report of the Medical Officer of the Privy Council, London: H. M. Stationary Office, 1867.

[9]   Hoppe-Seyler, F., Med Chem Untersuchungen, Berlin: Eberhard-Karls-Universitat, 1871.

[10] Hausman, W., "Die sensibilisierende wirkung des hematoporphyrins," *Biochem. Z.*, Vol. 30, 1911, p. 276.

[11] Meyer-Betz, F., "Untersuchungen uber die Biologische (photodynamische) Wirkung des Hamatoporphyrins und anderer Derivative des Blut- und Galenfarbstoffs," *Dtsch Arch Klin Med*, Vol. 112, 1913, pp. 475–503.

[12] Policard, A., "Etudes sur les aspects offerts par des tumeurs experimentales examinees a la lumiere de Wood," C. R. Soc. Biol., Vol. 91, 1924, pp. 1423–1428.

[13] Auler, H., and G. Banzer, "Untersuchungen uber die Rolle der Porphyrine bei geschwulstkranken Menschen und Tieren," *Z. Krebsforsch*, Vol. 53, 1942, pp. 65–68.

[14] Figge, F. H., and G. S. Weiland, "The Affinity of Neoplastic Embryonic and Traumatized Tissue for Porphyrins and Metalloporphyrins," *Anat. Rec.*, Vol. 100, 1948, p. 659.

[15] Figge, F. H., G. S. Weiland, and L. O. Manganiello, "Affinity of Neoplastic, Embryonic and Traumatized Tissues for Porphyrins and Metalloporphyrins," *Proc. Soc. Exp. Biol. Med.*, Vol. 68, 1948, pp. 640–641.

[16] Manganiello, L. O., and F. H. Figge, "Cancer Detection and Therapy II. Methods of Preparation and Biological Effects of Metalloporphyrins," Bull. School Med. Univ. Maryland, Vol. 36, 1951, pp. 3–7.

[17] Rassmussan-Taxdal, D. S., G. E. Ward, and F. H. Figge, "Fluorescence of Human Lymphatic and Cancer Tissues Following High Doses of Intravenous Hematoporphyrin," *Cancer*, Vol. 8, 1955, 78–81.

[18] Peck, G. C., H. P. Mack, and W. A. Holbrook, "Use of Hematoporphyrin Fluorescence in Biliary and Cancer Surgery," *Ann. Surg.*, Vol. 21, 1955, pp. 181–188.

[19] Schwartz, S. K., K. Absolon, and H. Vermund, "Some Relationships of Porphyrins, X-Rays and Tumours," Univ. Minn. Med. Bull., 1955, Vol. 27, pp. 7–8.

[20] Lipson, R. L., and E. J. Baldes, "The Photodynamic Properties of a Particular Hematoporphyin Derivative," *Arch. Dermatol.*, Vol. 82, 1960, pp. 508.

[21] Lipson, R. L., Baldes, E. J., and Olsen, A. M., "The Use of a Derivative of Hematoporphyrin in Tumor Detection," *J. Natl. Cancer Inst.*, 1961, Vol. 26, pp. 1–11.

[22] Lipson, R. L., E. J. Baldes, and A. M. Olsen, "Hematoporphyrin Derivative: A New Aid for Endoscopic Detection of Malignant Disease," *J. Thorac. Cardiovasc. Surg.*, Vol. 42, 1961, pp. 623–629.

[23] Lipson, R. L., E. J. Baldes, and M. J. Gray, "Hematoporphyrin Derivative for Detection and Management of Cancer," *Cancer*, Vol. 20, 1967, pp. 2255–2257.

[24] Gray, M. J., R. L. Lipson, and J. V. Maeck, et al., "Use of Hematoporphyrin Derivative in Detection and Management of Cervical Cancer," *Am. J. Obstet. Gynecol.*, Vol. 99, 1967, pp. 766–771.

[25] Gregorie, H. B., Jr., E. O. Horger, and J. L. Ward, et al., "Hematoporphyrin-Derivative Fluorescence in Malignant Neoplasms," *Ann. Surg.*, Vol. 167, 1968, pp. 820–828.

[26]   Leonard, J. R., and W. L. Beck, "Hematoporphyrin Fluorescence: An Aid in Diagnosis of Malignant Neoplasms," *Laryngoscope*, Vol. 81, 1971, pp. 365–372.

[27]   Kyriazis, G. A., H. Balin, and R. L. Lipson, "Hematoporphyrin-Derivative-Fluorescence Test Colposcopy and Colpophotography in the Diagnosis of Atypical Metaplasia, Dysplasia, and Carcinoma In Situ of the Cervix Uteri," *Am. J. Obstet. Gynecol.*, Vol. 117, 1973, pp. 375–380.

[28]   Kinsey, J. H., D. A. Cortese, and D. R. Sanderson, "Detection of Hematoporphyrin Fluorescence During Fiberoptic Bronchoscopy to Localize Early Bronchogenic Carcinoma," *Mayo Clin. Proc.*, Vol. 53, 1978, pp. 594–600.

[29]   Cortese, D. A., J. H. Kinsey, and L. B. Woolner, et al., "Clinical Application of a New Endoscopic Technique for Detection of In Situ Bronchial Carcinoma," *Mayo Clin. Proc.*, Vol. 54, 1979, pp. 635–641.

[30]   Profio, A. E., D. R. Doiron, and E. G. King, "Laser Fluorescence Bronchoscope for Localization of Occult Lung Tumors," *Med. Phys.*, Vol. 6, 1979, pp. 523–525.

[31]   Hayata, Y., and T. J. Dougherty, *Laser and Hematoporphyrin Derivative in Cancer*, Tokyo: Igaku-Shoin, 1983.

[32]   Hayata, Y., H. Kato, and J. Ono, et al., "Fluorescence Fiberoptic Bronchoscopy in the Diagnosis of Early Stage Lung Cancer," *Recent Results Cancer Res.*, Vol. 82, 1982, pp. 121–130.

[33]   Benson, R. C., Jr., G. M. Farrow, and J. H. Kinsey, et al., "Detection and Localization of In Situ Carcinoma of the Bladder with Hematoporphyrin Derivative," *Mayo Clin. Proc.*, Vol. 57, 1982, pp. 548–555.

[34]   Benson, R. C., Jr., J. H. Kinsey, and D. A. Cortese, et al., "Treatment of Transitional Cell Carcinoma of the Bladder with Hematoporphyrin Derivative Phototherapy," *J. Urol.*, Vol. 130, 1983, pp. 1090–1095.

[35]   Profio, A. E., and D. R. Doiron, "Dose Measurements in Photodynamic Therapy of Cancer," *Lasers Surg. Med.*, Vol. 7, 1987, pp. 1–5.

[36]   Diamond, I., S. G. Granelli, and A. F. McDonagh, et al., "Photodynamic Therapy of Malignant Tumours," *Lancet,* Vol. 2, 1972, pp. 1175–1177.

[37]   Dougherty, T. J., G. B. Grindey, and R. Fiel, et al., "Photoradiation Therapy. II. Cure of Animal Tumors with Hematoporphyrin and Light," *J. Natl. Cancer Inst.*, Vol. 55, 1975, pp. 115–121.

[38]   Kelly, J. F., M. E. Snell, and M. C. Berenbaum, "Photodynamic Destruction of Human Bladder Carcinoma," *Br. J. Cancer*, Vol. 31, 1975, pp. 237–244.

[39]   Kelly, J. F., and M. E. Snell, "Hematoporphyrin Derivative: A Possible Aid in the Diagnosis and Therapy of Carcinoma of the Bladder," *J. Urol.*, Vol. 115, 1976, pp. 150-151, 1976.

[40]   Dougherty, T. J., J. E. Kaufman,, and A. Goldfarb, et al., "Photoradiation Therapy for the Treatment of Malignant Tumors," *Cancer Res.*, Vol. 38, 1978, pp. 2628–2635.

[41]   Dougherty, T. J., "Photosensitizers: Therapy and Detection of Malignant Tumors," *Photochem. Photobiol.*, Vol. 45, 1987, pp. 879–889.

[42]   Hayata, Y., H. Kato,, and H. Okitsu, et al., "Photodynamic Therapy with Hematoporphyrin Derivative in Cancer of the Upper Gastrointestinal Tract," *Semin. Surg. Oncol.,* Vol. 1, 1985, pp. 1–11.

[43]   Tomio, L., F. Calzavara, and P. L. Zorat, et al., "Photoradiation Therapy for Cutaneous and Subcutaneous Malignant Tumors Using Hematoporphyrin," in, D. R. Doiron and C. J. Gomer (eds.), *Porphyrin Localization and Treatment of Tumors*, New York: A. R. Liss, 1984. pp. 829–840.

[44]   Wile, A. G., J. Coffey, and M. Y. Nahabedian, et al., "Laser Photoradiation Therapy of Cancer: An Update of the Experience at the University of California, Irvine, *Lasers Surg. Med.*, Vol. 4, 1984, pp. 5–12.

[45] Wile, A. G., A. Dahlman, and R. G. Burns, et al., "Laser Photoradiation Therapy of Cancer Following Hematoporphyrin Sensitization," *Lasers Surg. Med.*, Vol. 2, 1982, pp. 163–168.

[46] Balchum, O. J., D. R. Doiron, and G. C. Huth, "Photoradiation Therapy of Endobronchial Lung Cancers Employing the Photodynamic Action of Hematoporphyrin Derivative," *Lasers. Surg. Med.*, Vol. 4, 1984, pp. 13–30.

[47] Lam, S., N. L. Muller, and R. R. Miller, et al., "Predicting the Response of Obstructive Endobronchial Tumors to Photodynamic Therapy," *Cancer*, Vol. 58, 1986, pp. 2298–2306.

[48] LoCicero, J., 3rd, M. Metzdorff, and C. Almgren, "Photodynamic Therapy in the Palliation of Late Stage Obstructing Non-Small Cell Lung Cancer," *Chest*, Vol. 98, 1990, pp. 97–100.

[49] Cortese, D. A., and J. H. Kinsey, Hematoporphyrin Derivative Phototherapy in the Treatment of Bronchogenic Carcinoma," *Chest*, Vol. 86, 1984, pp. 8–13.

[50] Hayata, Y., H. Kato, and C. Konaka, et al., "Hematoporphyrin Derivative and Laser Photoradiation in the Treatment of Lung Cancer," *Chest*, Vol. 81, 1982, pp. 269–277.

[51] Nseyo, U. O., S. L. Lundahl, and D. C. Merrill, "Whole Bladder Photodynamic Therapy: Critical Review of Present-Day Technology and Rationale for Development of Intravesical Laser Catheter and Monitoring System," *Urology*, Vol. 36, 1990, pp. 398–402.

[52] Ohi, T., and Tsuchiya, "A. Superficial Bladder Tumours," in *Lasers and Hematoporphyrin Derivative in Cancer*, Y. Hayata and T. J. Dougherty (eds.), Tokyo: Igaku-Shoin, 1983, pp. 79–84.

[53] Haas, G. P., B. P. Shumaker, and F. W. Hetzel, et al., "Phototherapy of Bladder Cancer: Dose/Effect Relationships," *J. Urol.*, Vol. 136, 1986, pp. 525–528.

[54] Prout, G. R., Jr., C. W. Lin, and R. Benson, Jr., et al., "Photodynamic Therapy with Hematoporphyrin Derivative in the Treatment of Superficial Transitional-Cell Carcinoma of the Bladder," *N. Engl. J. Med.*, Vol. 317, 1987, pp. 1251–1255.

[55] McCaughan, J. S., Jr., W. Hicks, and L. Laufman, et al., "Palliation of Esophageal Malignancy with Photoradiation Therapy," *Cancer*, Vol. 54, 1984, pp. 2905–2910.

CHAPTER 2

Photosensitizers for Photodynamic Therapy and Imaging

Manivannan Ethirajan, Courtney Saenz, Anurag Gupta, Mahabeer P. Dobhal, and Ravindra K. Pandey

2.1 Introduction

hematoporphyrin derivative (HpD)1 and its purified version Photofrin® 2 were the first photo-sensitizers investigated clinically for use in photodynamic therapy (PDT). However, these compounds are produced as a mixture of a large number of monomers, dimers and higher oligomers, show long-term skin sensitivity and phototoxicity in patients and exhibit poor long wave length absorption. To overcome with these problems, a set of second generation photosensitizers such as (chlorins, bacteriochlorins, phthalocyanines) are being developed in various laboratories for quite sometime. Some of the porphyrin-based compounds, e. g., Levulan® 3, Radachlorin® 4, Visudyne® 5, Foscan® 6 (Figure 2.1) and other sensitizers have approval by various health organizations for cancer or non-cancer indications. Radachlorin® 4 is a product of Radapharma, Russia, and absorbs at 662 nm. It has been studied as a PDT agent in Russia for various malignant tumors. The compound 5, Visudyne®, also known as verteporfin™, is a product of Novartis pharmaceuticals; the clinical studies revealed that it is very effective for age-related macular degeneration (AMD). Foscan® 6 is a chlorin-based photosensitizer (652 nm) has been approved in Europe as a PDT agent for prostate and head and neck cancer treatment. Several third generation photosensitizers are under clinical or late preclinical stages, developed on the basis of SAR/QSAR studies. Table 2.1 lists the PDT agents that are approved or under clinical trials for the treatment of cancer.

2.2 Ideal Properties of Photosensitizers

Photosensitizers (PS) are one of the key elements in PDT. After the approval of Photofrin® for PDT treatment, researchers from all over the world became actively involved in developing efficient PS. An ideal PS should fulfill the following requirements:

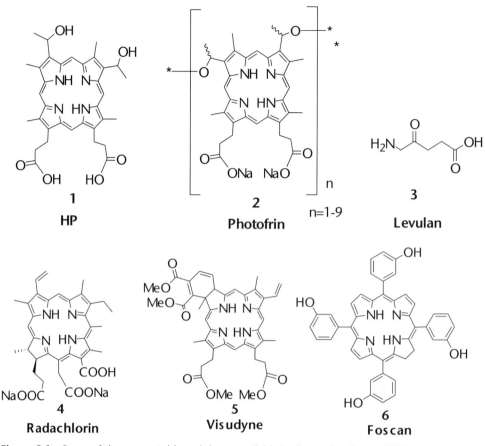

Figure 2.1   Some of the nonmetal-based drugs available in the market for the PDT.

1. It should be able to produce singlet oxygen efficiently because singlet oxygen and Type II photochemical reaction is responsible for the majority of lesions generated during PDT.

2. It should have high absorption coefficient at the long wavelength region (700 to 800 nm). Porphyrin-based PS have a strong absorption band around 400 nm called the "Soret" band, and a satellite absorption band (Q-band) between 600 and 800 nm. Only the wavelength >600 nm is useful for PDT treatment. Porphyrins, chlorins and bacteriochlorins have 22-, 20-, and 18-p electrons respectively in their aromatic rings confined to approximately the same region in space. Therefore the maximageneral exhibit long wavelength absorption in the range of porphyrins is more blue-shifted, usually around 600 nm. Chlorins' Q-band is around 630–650 nm, in chlorins it is in the range of 650–700 nm, and bacteriochlorins' maximawhereas the bacterio-chlorins the absorption falls between 700 nm and740–800 nm so that they are capable for treating larger tumors and those, which are deeply seated. However, the electronic absorption characteristic is also influenced by the nature of the substituents (electron donating or electron withdrawing) present at the peripheral position of the molecules.

Table 2.1   List of photosensitizers that Are Currently in the Market or in Clinical Trials

Photosensitizer	Basic Structure	Wavelength Absorbtion/nm	Coordinated Metal	Manufacturer
Photofrin®	Porphyrin	630	—	Axcan Pharma, Inc
Photogem®	Porphyrin	630	—	Moscow Institute of High Chemical Technologies
Hematoporphyrin IX	Porphyrin	630	—	Chongqing Huading Modern Biopharmaceutics Co.
Hemporfin®	Porphyrin	630	—	Fudan-zhangjing BioPharmaceuticals Co,
Levulan®	Aminolevulinic acid	635	—	DUSA Pharmaceuticals.
Metvix®	Aminolevulinic acid	635	—	PhotoCure USA
Visudyne®	Benzoporphyrin	689	—	Novartis Pharmaceuticals
Foscan®	Chlorin	652	—	Biolitec AG
HPPH (Photochlor*)	Chlorin	665	—	Roswell Park Cancer Institute (RPCI)
Talaforfin®	Chlorin	664	—	Light Sciences
Purpurinimide 277*	Chlorin	700	—	RPCI
idctlparBacteriopurpur inimide 605*	Bacteriochlorin	796	—	RPCI
Photrex®* Purlytin	Purpurin	664	Tin	Miravant Medical Technologies
TOOKAD®*	Bacteriochlorin	763	Palladium	Negma-Lerads and Steba Laboratories Ltd.
Lutex®*	Texaphyrin	732	Lutetium	Pharmacyclics Inc.
PC4®*	Phthalocyanine	680	Silicon	V.I. Technologies
CGP55847®	Phthalocyanine	680	Zinc	QLT Phototherapeutics
Photosense®	Phthalocyanine	670	Aluminum	General Physics Institute

*Currently under clinical trials/toxicological studies.

3. It should have no dark toxicity, minimal or absent skin photosensitivity, and should selectively accumulate in tumor tissue (preferential tumor retention, fast tumor accumulation, and rapid clearance), in order to minimize skin phototoxicity.

4. The distribution of PS is important in PDT processes and is influenced by its chemical structure. It is particularly useful if PS is amphiphilic (water soluble but containing a hydrophobic matrix), which should facilitate the crossing of cell membranes.

5. It should be stable and easy to dissolve in the injectable solvents (formulation). However, after administration, the compounds should show high tumor accumulation and rapid clearance from the system.

6. It should be chemically pure and can be obtained in a short- and high-yielding synthetic route.

Unfortunately, to date, no PS with all these ideal characteristics has been developed.

2.3 Porphyrins as Photosensitizers in PDT

Porphyrin systems in general fulfill most of the features listed above. The basic structure of porphyrin unit is consisting of four pyrrole subunits joining one another via the methylene subunits to form a tetrapyrrole macrocycle.

Because of its extensive conjugation, the porphyrin molecule is fluorescent and it can be excited by visible light to produce triplet state which has a very short lifetime singlet state. However, porphyrins as such (without exposing to light) do not exhibit any toxic effects on patients. For these reasons, several porphyrin-based compounds are currently in various stages of clinical trials as photodynamic agents.

2.3.1 Importance of Porphyrins as Photosensitizers

To achieve the desired photodynamic effect, the photosensitizer on activation with an appropriate wavelength should produce a high quantum yield of singlet oxygen. In general, porphyrin systems satisfy this demand [1]. The porphyrins and related tetrapyrrolic systems are among the most widely studied of all macrocyclic compounds [2]. In fact, in one capacity or another, these versatile molecules have influenced nearly all disciplines in chemistry. Porphyrins are 22π-electron aromatic macrocycles (Figure 2.2) that exhibit characteristic optical spectra with a strong π-π^* transition around 400 nm (Soret band) and usually four Q bands in the visible region.

In the porphyrin system, two of the peripheral double bonds in opposite pyrrolic rings are cross-conjugated and are not required to maintain aromatic character.

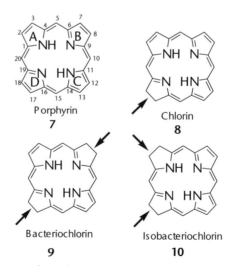

Figure 2.2 General structures of porphyrin and its analogs. Arrows indicate reduced bonds.

Thus, reduction of one or both of these cross-conjugated double bonds (to give chlorins and bacteriochlorins, respectively) maintains much of the aromaticity, but the change in symmetry results in bathochromically shifted Q bands with higher extinction coefficients. Nature uses these optical properties of the reduced porphyrins to harvest solar energy for photosynthesis with chlorophylls and bacteriochlorophylls as both antenna and reaction-center pigments [2]. The long wavelength absorption of these natural chromophores led to explorations of their use as photosensitizers in photodynamic therapy [2]. Most bacteriochlorins exhibit long-wavelength absorptions between 740 to 800 nm [3] (Figure 2.3). Similarly, naphthalocyanines also have shown absorption near 800 nm (Figure 2.4), so these compunds could also be potentially useful for treating deeply seated and highly pigmented tumors. Porphyrins or substituted porphyrins exhibit long wavelength absorption around 630 to 650 nm while the absorption of chlorins is about 660 to 710 nm, depending upon the nature of peripheral substituents.

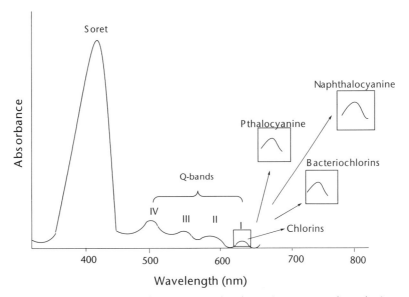

Figure 2.3 This spectrum (not in scale) represents the absorption spectra of porphyrin-type photosensitizers and location of the main peaks (longest wavelengths) for various porphyrin-type

Porphyrin	Pyro	Phthalocyanine	Purpurinimide	Bacteriopurpurinimide
630 nm	661 nm	700 nm	706 nm	790 nm

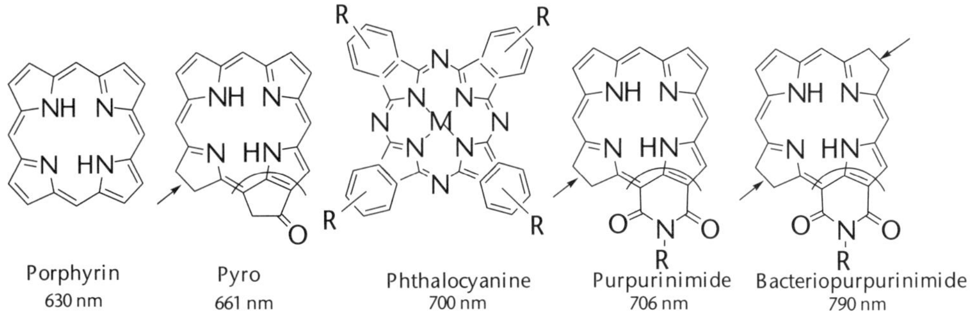

Figure 2.4 Longest wavelength absorption of various porphyrin-type structures in dichloromethane.

The energy gap between the highest occupied molecular orbit (HOMO) and the lowest unoccupied molecular orbit (LUMO) increases in this order: bacteriochlorin<isobacteriochlorin<chlorin<porphyrin [3], and as a result bacteriochlorins exhibit the longest absorption wavelength. Meanwhile, the loss of one or two double bonds causes the energy required for oxidation parallels the energy of HOMOs and decreases in this order: porphyrin>chlorin> isobacteriochlorin ≈bacteriochlorin, while reduction potentials are similar with the exception of isobacteriochlorin. Therefore, most of the naturally occurring bacteriochlorins are also the least stable analogues. In general, they were found to be extremely sensitive to oxidization, resulting in a rapid transformation into the chlorin state, which generally has a maximal absorption at or below 700 nm. Furthermore, if a laser is used to excite the bacteriochlorin in vivo, oxidation may result in the formation of new chromophore absorbing outside the laser window, reducing the photodynamic efficacy. Thus, the syntheses of stable bacteriochlorins with appropriate photochemical properties have been the aim of several porphyrin Chemists.

2.3.2   Phthalocyanines and Naphthalocyanines

The structures of phthalocyanines (Pc) and naphthalocyanine (NPc) are closely related to that of porphyrin systems except these chromophores contain four identical units of isoindole moieties linked by nitrogen atoms. The introduction of a ring system fused into a porphyrin skeleton results in a red shift of their respective long-wavelength absorption due to extended conjugation [1] (Figure 2.5).

Like Pc, the NPc possess similar structural features but the presence of an additional benzene ring attached to each isoindole units extends its conjugation and these molecules exhibit longer wavelength absorption than the corresponding Pc. This unique feature qualifies them to be attractive candidates for PDT (Figure 2.6).

2.4   Effect of Central Metal in Photosensitizing Efficacy

Porphyrins are one the best ligands in terms of thermodynamic stability and kinetic nonlability and the inner two protons (-NH) of porphyrin can be deprotonated by

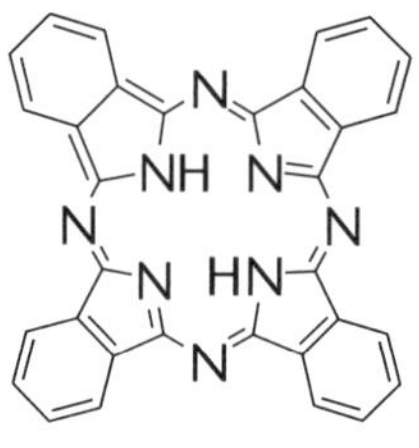

Phthalocyanine

11

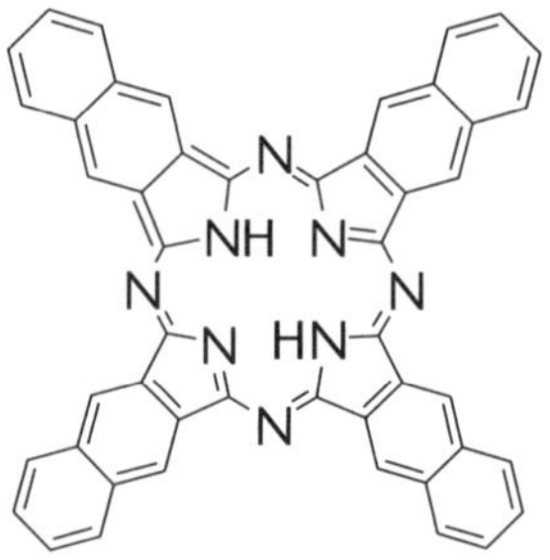

Naphthalocyanine

12

Figure 2.5   General chemical structures of Pc and NPc.

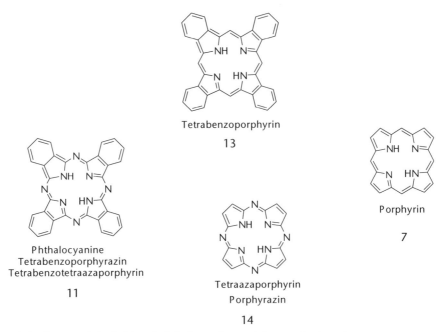

Figure 2.6   Structural similarities of phthalocyanine and the porphyrin systems.

strong alkoxide bases and forming dianionic species. Alternatively, the inner two pyrrole nitrogens can also be protonateduner acidic conditions. These four nitrogens in the inner core are capable of binding with metals and form stable metal complexes. Many of the naturally occurring porphyrins (heme, chlorophyll a and b, vitamin B12) are metal bounded and do not show any toxicity on living organisms in absence of light. It is well known that the nature of a metal atom present in the porphyrin ring can alter its photochemical and photophysical properties. Porphyrins can donate two protons giving a dianion (15) or accept two protons giving a dication (16) (Figure 2.7)

The electronic absorption spectrum of the porphyrin type compounds change when the molecule is coordinated with a metal atom. In general, the four absorption bands in the visible region of the parent porphyrin are replaceed with two absorption bands and the Soret band in general shows a strong absorption in the range of 350–420 nm (Figure 2.8). Therefore, formation of metalloporphyrins, in most cases, drastically alters its optical properties, which has a significant effect on the photostability of the compound [4]. The presence of central metal also significantly alters its singlet oxygen producing efficacy. For example, the conversion of the

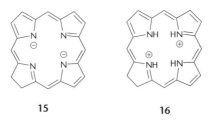

Figure 2.7   Dianionic and dicationic species of porphyrin.

mono-L-aspartyl chlorin e6 17 (MACE) to the corresponding tin(IV) complex 18 stabilized the system and increase the singlet oxygen quantum yield from 0.77 to 0.89. However, replacing the tin with zinc metal (compound 19) reduced the singlet oxygen producing efficiency (Figure 2.9).

There are several metalloporphyrins reported in the literature but mainly transition metals and group 13 and 14 metals have been investigated for the photosensitizers (such as Zn, Pd, Sn, Ru, Pt, In, Lu, Gd, and Al) [2]. It is generally observed that in porphyrin systems the presence of diamagnetic metal generally increases the lifetime of the triplet-excited state is increased and hence the triplet quantum yield of the porphyrin. Since the triplet quantum yield is directly related to the efficiency of

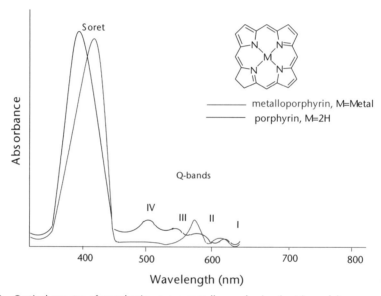

Figure 2.8 Optical spectra of porphyrin versus metalloporphyrins (not in scale).

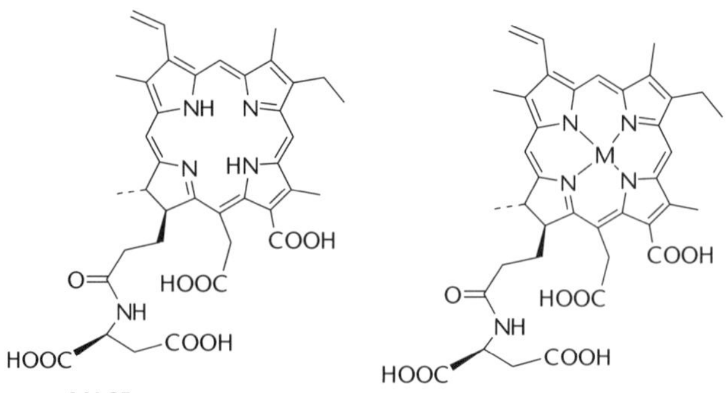

Figure 2.9 Structure of MACE and the corresponding metallated analogs.

generating singlet oxygen, the metal that generates a longer lifetime of the triplet state should be more effective photosensitizers.

So far only a limited number of porphyrin-based PS are known in the literature that do not produce singlet oxygen but are reported as effective photoactive agents. One such example is Cu(II) octaethyl benzochlorin **22** [5], which was synthesized by reacting the metal precursor **20** with POCl₃ and DMF (under the Vilsmeier reaction conditions) (Figure 2.10). The resulting product was found to be active against leukemia cells in vitro and in a rat bladder tumor model. This unusual result is rationalized based on the interactions between the iminium ion of the photosensitizer and biomolecules. Surprisingly, the corresponding metal-free analogue displayed limited tumor response only during the time between administration of the drug and PDT, which clearly indicated the potential role of central copper metal in PDT efficacy. Interestingly, the zinc analogue 23 was photoactive in murine colon carcinoma cells.

2.4.2 Metallated Photosensitizer as PDT Agents

Recently, a considerable number of metallated tetrapyrroles are being investigated such as PS and some of them are at various stages of clinical trials for cancer treatment (Table 2.1). Among the metal complexes of bacteriochlorins, the corresponding palladium analog is of particular interest. Scherz et al. [6] converted the bacteriopheophorbide a **24** into the corresponding palladium complex **25** (also called WST09 or Tookad®) by two different methodologies. In the first approach, a solution of bacteriopheophorbide a **24** and Pd-acetate in dichloromethane was added to a suspension of sodium ascorbate in methanol (Figure 2.11). In another approach, a solution of bacteriopheophorbide a **24** and Pd-acetate in chloroform was treated with methanolic 6-O-palmitoyl-L-ascorbic acid solution. Because of the importance of palladium-bacteriopheophorbide a **25** (Tookad®) [7] as a photosensitizer in PDT aspect, this particular analog has been subjected to both in vitro and in vivo, including toxicological studies. It exhibits long wavelength absorption at 763 nm and its extinction coefficient in chloroform [7] is 10^5 mol⁻¹cm⁻¹.

Vakrat et al. [8] has shown that the hydrophilic derivatives of bacteriochlorin palladium complexes generate mainly hydroxyl radical and a small amount of sin-

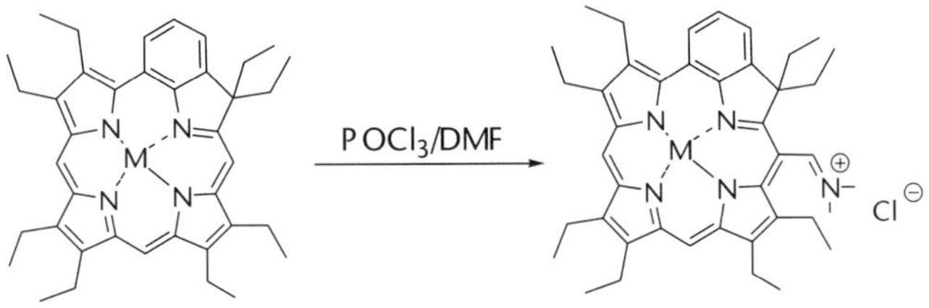

$$\text{P OCl}_3/\text{DMF}$$

20, M= Cu

21 M Z

22, M= Cu

23 M= Zn

Figure 2.10 Structure of metallated benzochlorins.

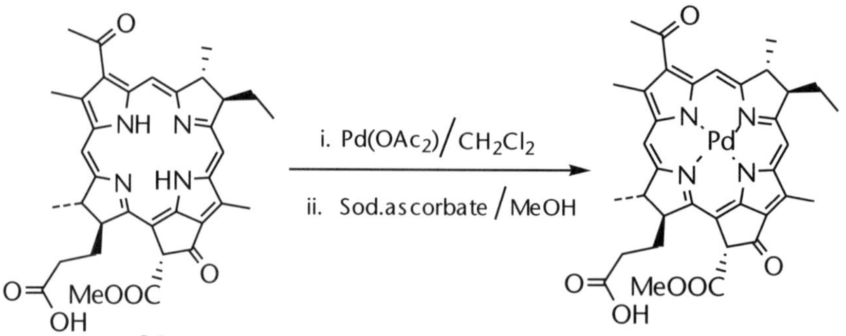

Figure 2.11 Synthesis of TOOKAD®.

glet oxygen. The photocytotoxicity of this derivative in cell cultures was 10 times lower (LD_{50} = 300 nM) than that of the hydrophobic one (LD_{50} = 10–20 nM). Koudinova et al. [7] investigated the utility of Pd-bacteriopheophorbide a (Tookad®) as the photosensitizer to treat small cell carcinoma of the prostate (SCCP), the relatively rare but most aggressive variant of prostate cancer. It is believed that the Tookad® targeted the tumor vasculature leading to inflammation, hypoxia, necrosis, and tumor eradication. The experiment was performed as i.v. administration of Tookad® and immediate illumination from a xenon light source or a diode laser. Tookad® cleared rapidly from the circulation within a few hours and did not accumulate in tissues. It was reported that subcutaneous tumors exhibited complete healing within 28 to 40 days, reaching an overall long-term cure rate of 69%, followed for 90 days after PDT.

The toxicity of Tookad® was investigated by Chen et al. [9] in normal canine prostate and PDT was performed by irradiating the surgically exposed prostate, bladder, and colon. All animals recovered well without urethral complications and it was concluded that at therapeutic PDT levels, there was no structural or functional urethral damage and hence Tookad® PDT appears to be a promising candidate for prostate cancer patients. In another experiment, Tremblay et al. [10] studied the endobronchial phototoxicity of Tookad®. Fourteen pairs of large White-Landrace male piglets were given intravenous Tookad® followed by laser light illumination of the left mainstem bronchus. Different settings for light dose (fluence), fluence rate (FR), drug dose (D), and drug-light interval (DLI) were applied to each pair. It was concluded that within the specific ranges of light dose (fluence), fluence rate, drug dose, and drug-light interval, the normal bronchus could be preserved during PDT with Tookad®.

Miravant Medical Technologies developed a photosensitizer marketed under the name of Purlytin® (29), a tin metallated chlorin derivative which exhibits 20 to 30 nm red-shift in its electronic absorption spectrum when compare to its non-metallated parent compound [1, 11]. During the clinical trials Puryltin has shown good efficacy for patients with cutaneous metastatic breast cancer and Kaposi's sarcoma. Unfortunately, it also produced high skin phototoxicity, which limits its application as a photosensitizer in PDT (Figures 2.12 and 2.13).

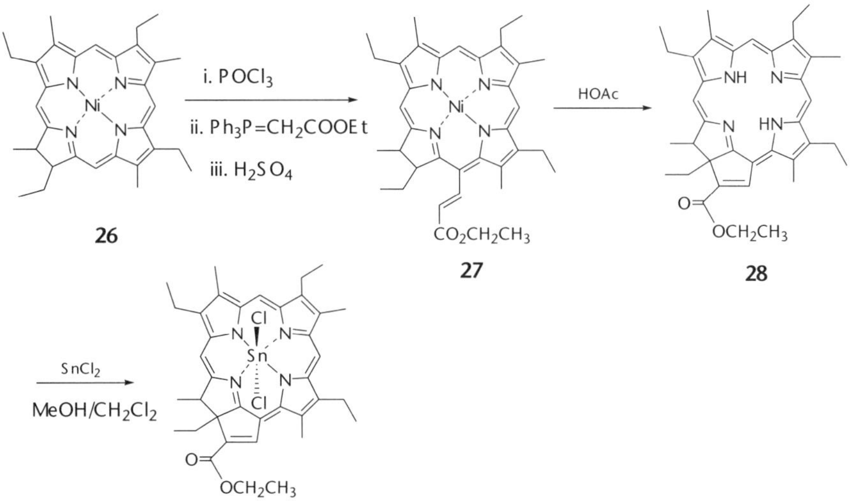

Figure 2.12 Synthesis of Purlytin.

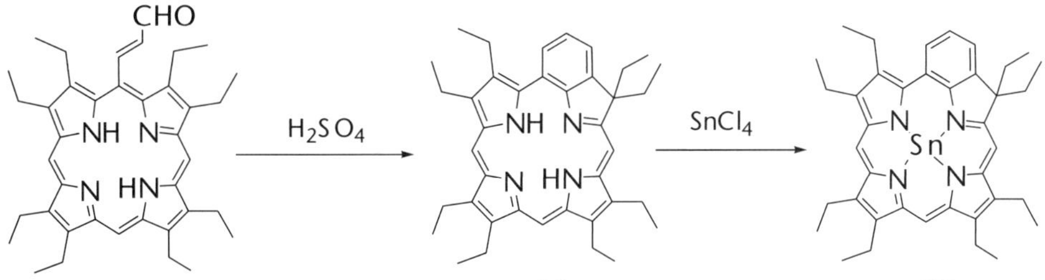

Figure 2.13 Synthesis of tin benzochlorin derivative **32**

The tin (IV) metallated benzochlorin analog **32** was prepared by an acid cata-lyzed cyclization and it displayed significantly enhanced phototoxicity photoproperties against murine leukemia L1210 cells in vitro and transplanted urothelial cell carcinoma in rats than the corresponding nonmetallated sulfonated analogue [12].

Meerovich et al. showed that the bachteriochlorophyllide-serine (Bchl-ser) derivative **33** is an effective infrared photosensitizer for PDT and fluorescent diag-nostic agent (Figure 2.14). These authors have further shown that the Bchl-ser does not only have a high value of accumulation in the tumor tissues but also exhibited significant inhibition of tumor growth. Unfortunately, this compound was not stable under in vivo PDT conditions [13] which limited its application (Figure 2.15).

A series of water soluble porphyrin-based photosensitizers have also been devel-oped by introducing polar functionalities at the mesopositions of the tetrapyrrolic system. Substituting the pyridinium groups at the meso position of the tetrapyrrolic

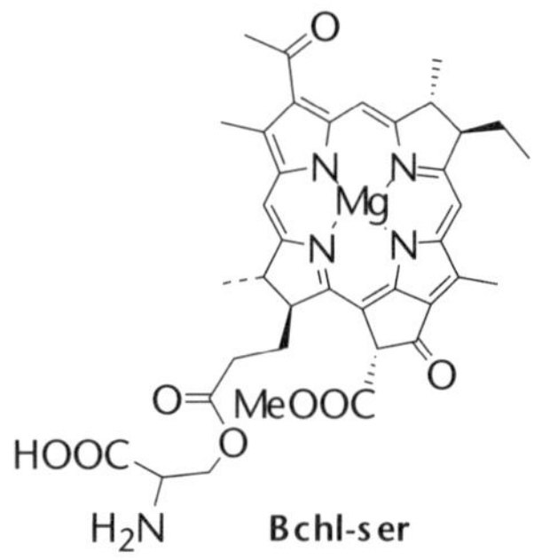

Figure 2.14 Structure of Bchl-Ser **33**.

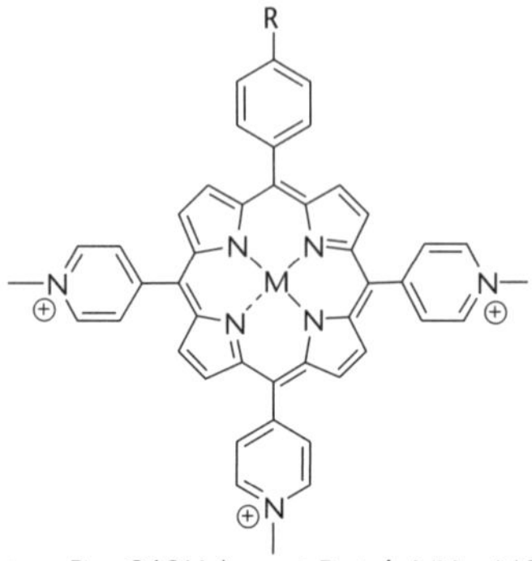

34, M= Mn , R = C(CH$_3$)$_3$ or t-Butyl, NH$_2$, NO$_2$ or OH

35, M= Ni ,   R = C(CH$_3$)$_3$ or t-Butyl, NH$_2$, NO$_2$ or OH

Figure 2.15 Structure of water-soluble metalloporphyrins.

system (34) increased its solubility in water and produced significant PDT efficacy. However replacing the central manganese metal with nickel **35**, diminshed its photo-dynamic activity. In a series of sulfonated porphyrins, disulfonated porphyrin analogue **36** (Figure 2.16) showed improved photosensitizing activity compared to corresponding its symmetrically di, tri, and tetra substituted derivatives [14]. However, at higher doses these compounds were found to produce neurotoxicity in mice.

Ishizumi et al. synthesized (Au-NPe6) by incorporating the gold atom in the center core of NPe6 **37** (Talaporfin® which is currently under clinical trials for endobronchial lung cancer and cutaneous malignancies [15]), and demonstrated that the compound 38 (Figure 2.17) is capable of accumulating in the tumor tissues at a higher concentration and the gold atom was still intact with the ligand even after it is incorporated in tumors tissues [16].

Nakae et al. [17] have reported the synthesis of a series of Gallium metallated porphyrins with variable lipophilicity and evaluated their tumor localizing property on Syrian golden hamsters bearing tumors. A direct correlation between overall lipophilicity and tumor efficacy was observed and the photosensitizer bearing two decyl side chain (43) was found to be the most effective (Figure 2.18).

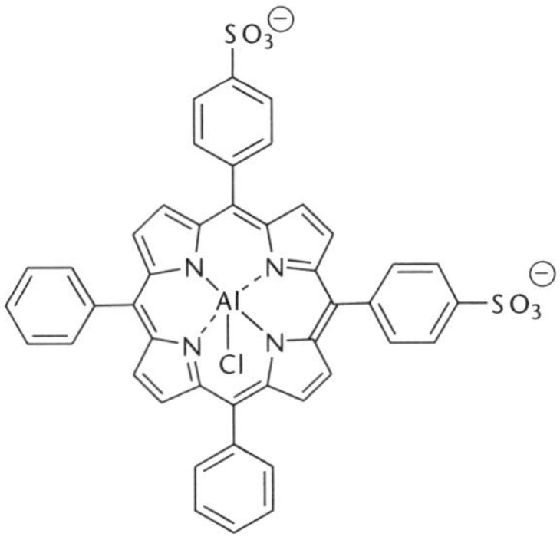

36

Figure 2.16   Structure of di-sulfonated porphyrin **36**.

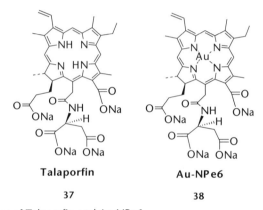

Talaporfin   Au-NPe6

37   **38**

Figure 2.17   Structures of Talaporfin and Au-NPe6.

Narula et al. [18] demonstrated that the utility of radiolabeled Indium (and Gallium) coproporphyrin derivative **44** (^{111}In and ^{67}Ga) over the corresponding Technetium (Tc-99m) analog with a shorter half-life than ^{111}In- and ^{67}Ga- nuclides (Figure 2.19) in imaging of atheromatous plaque in animal models, which make them attractive candidates for detecting unstable plaques.

Pandey and coworkers have recently reported the synthesis and biological activity of a series of metallated photosensitizers, including the In(III) HPPH methyl ester **46**. The Indium complex was found to be more photostable than the corresponding free base HPPH (**45**), with higher singlet oxygen producing ability. Interestingly, the insertion of Indium to HPPH did not alter its intracellular localization property and both analogues were found to localize in mitochondria. However, the presence of Indium made a significant improvement (8–10 fold) in PDT efficacy (Color plate 1). (Figure 2.20).

This approach was then extended to 9,10-dioxo pyropheophorbide series a **48–51** [20] and two interesting observations were noted: (1) the introduction of

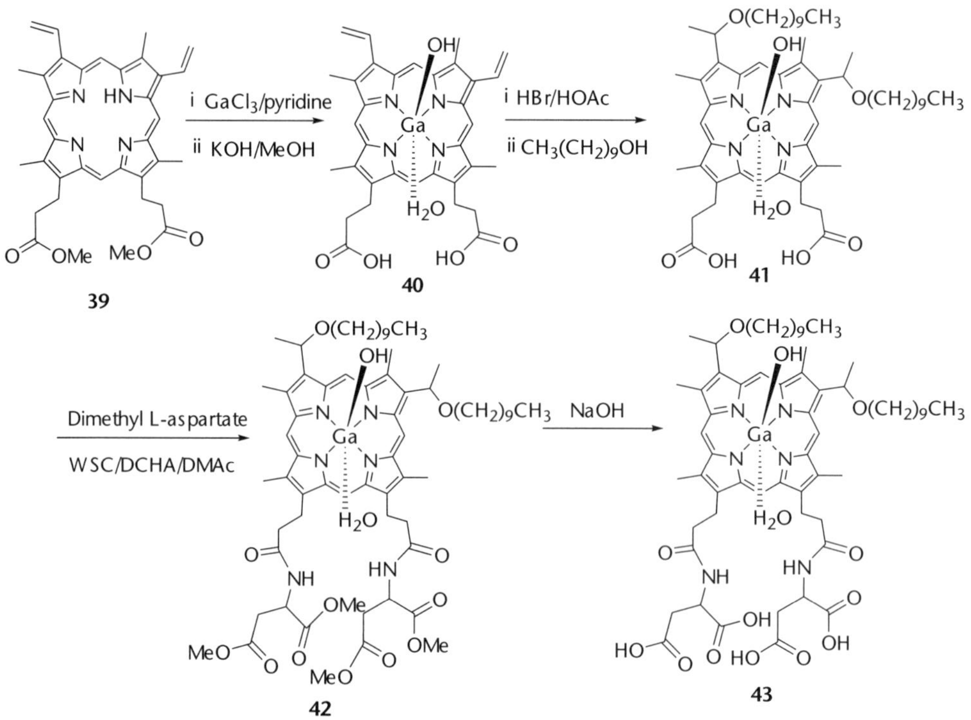

Figure 2.18 Synthesis of Ga-porphyrin complex **43**.

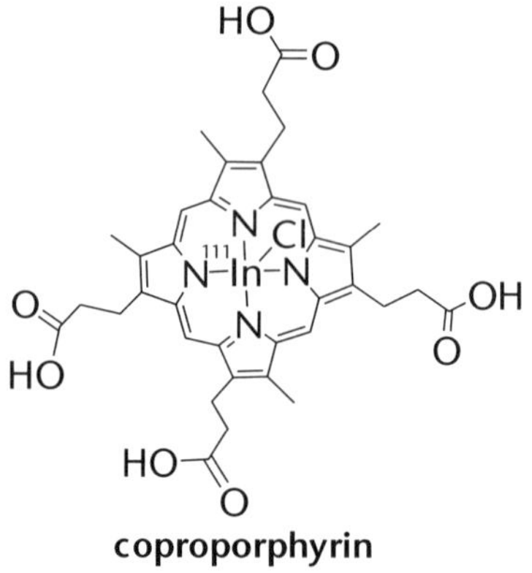

Figure 2.19 Structure of Indium metallated coproporphyrin.

another keto group in the isocyclic ring reduced the photosensitizing efficacy, and (2) the insertion of Indium as a central metal enhanced the efficacy of the parent molecule. However, the In(III) complex of the dioxo-analogs (**52–55**) was found to be less effective (Figure 2.21) than In(III)HPPH methyl ester **46**. This study suggested that the position of the ketogroup in isocyclic ring of the HPPH moiety plays a remarkable role in PDT efficacy.

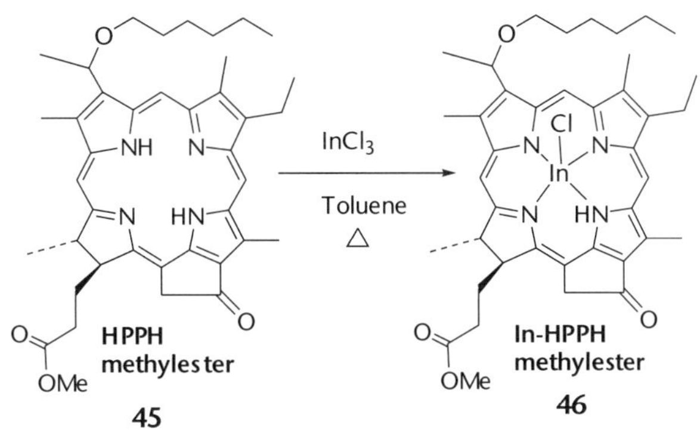

Figure 2.20 Synthesis of Indium derivative of HPPH.

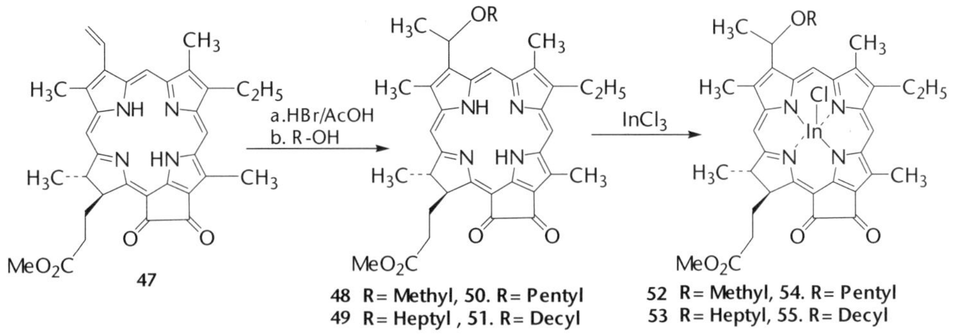

Figure 2.21 Synthesis of Indium derivative of HPPH-methyl ester.

2.4.3 PBR Binding Affinity of Metallated Porphyrins: Chlorins and Their PDT Efficacy

The peripheral benzodiazepine receptor (PBR) is an 18 KDA protein of the outer mitochondrial membrane. It is involved in numerous functions including steroid biosynthesis, cell proliferation, and calcium channel modulations. Another intriguing aspect of PBR is its association with PDT. Verma et al. [22] were the first to study the binding affinity of certain porphyrins to the PBR with prominent correlation with photosensitizing efficacy (Figure 2.22).

To investigate the utility of metallated and free-base analogs as fluorescent probes for PBR, a series of metallated pyropheophorbide-a analogs were synthesized. Some of these analogs, including the In(III)HPPH, showed significant binding to PBR. However, no direct correlation between PK11195 (PBR probe) and PDT efficacy was observed (see Figures 2.23 and 2.24). Compared to HPPH, the In(III)HPPH showed significant enhancement in vitro (Figure 2.24) and in vivo PDT efficacy (Figure 2.25) with no difference in site of localization (Figure 2.24). As can be seen from the results summarized in Figure 2.25, compared to HPPH methyl ester 45 (please note that there is no difference between the PDT efficacy of HPPH and HPPH methyl ester. In vivo, the enzyme esterases convert the methyl ester functionality to the corresponding carboxylic acid), the In(III) HPPH 46 produced

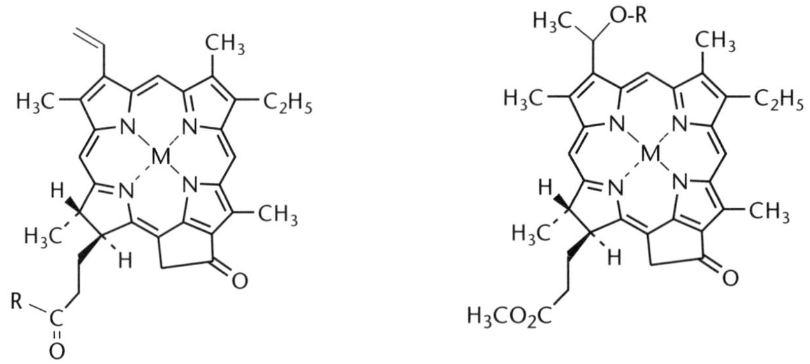

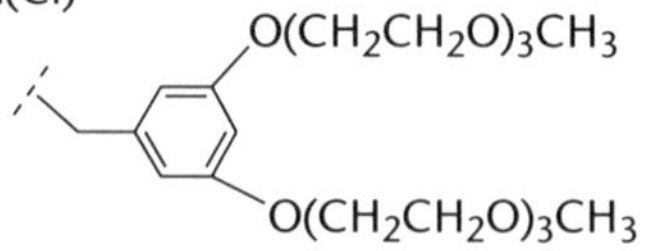

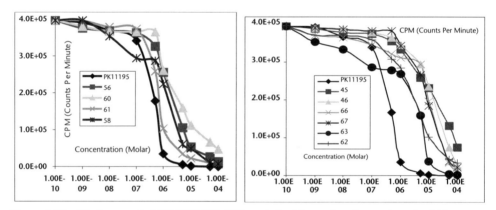

Figure 2.22 Pyropheophorbide-a analogs investigated for PBR binding affinity.

56. M = 2H, R = OMe
57. M = 2H, R = OH
58. M = In(Cl), R = Ome
59. M = In(Cl), R = OH
60. M = Zn, R = OMe
61. M = Ni, R = OMe
62. M = In(Cl), R = N(CH$_2$COOH)$_2$
63. M = In(Cl), R = NH-CH(COOH)CH$_2$(COOH)

45. M = 2H, R = Hexyl
46. M = In(Cl), R = hexyl
66. M = In(Cl), R = (CH$_2$CH$_2$O)$_3$CH$_3$
67. M = In(Cl)

Figure 2.23 Displacement of 3H-PK11195 (PBR probe) with a series of pyropheophorbide-a analogs.

8-fold enhancement in PDT efficacy. For example, at a drug dose of 0.4 mmol/kg, compound 45 gave 60% long-term tumor response (6/10 mice were tumor free on day 90, where as only 0.05 mmol/kg of In(III)HPPH methyl ester 46 was required for similar tumor response). Interestingly, insertion of central metal did not make any difference in site of localization and both compounds localized in the mitochondria [80].

2.4.4 Metallated Phthalocyanines and Naphthalocyanines

The problems encountered with Photofrin [1, 23] and other porphyrin-based photosensitizers especially those associated with skin phototoxicity led to the

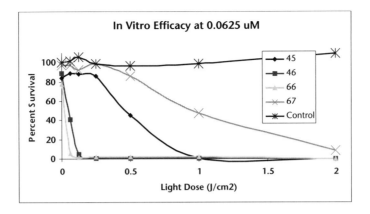

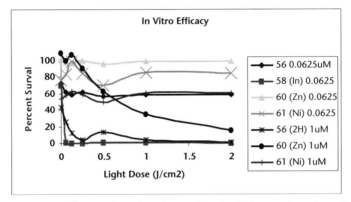

Figure 2.24 In vitro PDT efficacy of a series of pyropheophorbide-a analogs (metallated versus nonmetallated).

CGP 55847

68

Figure 2.25 Structure of Zn metallated Pc.

development of another series of PDT agents which possess basic structure of phthalocyanine (Pc) and naphthalocyanine (Npc) system. These compounds are effective generators of singlet oxygen having strong absorption bands in the range of 650 to 800 nm. Most of these compounds were hydrophobic, with benefit of relatively higher uptake in tumor than healthy tissue. However, the overall lipophilicity of the molecules could easily be altered [1, 24].

Pc and NPc are an extended version of porphyrin s ystem and exhibit a unique structure in which each pyrrole moiety is fused with a benzene ring and therefore it has an extended conjugation and hence these molecules absorb at longer wavelengths with respect to porphyrin system. This unique quality makes it as a better candidate for the photosensitizers and hence the treatment of deeply seated tumors and highly pigmented tumors is feasible. This unique characteristic may have an advantage in developing improved PDT agents with higher tissue penetration ability. Besides, these chromophores exhibit weak absorption bands in the range of 400–600 nm which could minimize the skin phototoxicity, a major drawback associated with most of the porphyrin-based compounds. In addition, both Pc and Npc are excellent singlet oxygen generators and are also capable of forming metal complexes with metals; interestingly, chelation of metal atom might increase its singlet oxygen efficiency to nearly 100%.

Recently a novel phthalocyanine-based photosensitizer, Zinc phthalocyanine **68** (CGP55847) [25], was developed by Ciba-Geigy (Figure 2.25), is undergoing clinical trials phase I and II against squamous cell carcinomas of the upper aerodigestive tract (Figure 2.26).

Photosense® (69) is another Pc derivative containing aluminum as a central metal. It was developed in Russia and has entered clinical trials against skin, breast, GI, and lung malignancies and neovascularization of the eye [26]. To decrease the hydrophobic nature of Pc, the sulfonic acid groups are introduced at the benzene moieties which makes it more hydrophilic in nature and hence better bioavailable.

Li et al. [27] have also reported an efficient synthesis of synthesized silicon metallated Pc, SiPc-BOA **72** by reacting of **70** with acid chloride **71** in presence of base. This axially substituted Pc **72** (Figure 2.27) is reconstituted with low-density lipoprotein (LDL) to afford high payload nanoparticles, at the same time retaining the size of the native LDL. The results indicate that LDL-SiPc-BOA was an effective PDT agent for LDLR-overexpressing hepatoblastoma G2 (HepG2) tumor cells.

The photosensitizer names PC4 **73** is a silicon-based metallophthalocyanine (Figure 2.28) developed by Vitex, USA, and is currently under clinical trials against breast, human colon, and ovarian cancers [28]. The corresponding Npc molecules have an additional benzene ring fused on the periphery of the each isoindole subunit; because of this extended conjugation, they possess more red-shifted absorptions (740–780 nm) than the Pc (Figure 2.29).

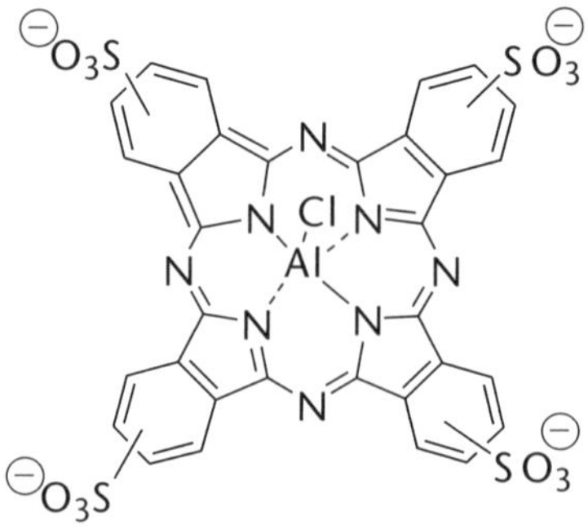

Photosense

69

Figure 2.26 Structure of Photosense.

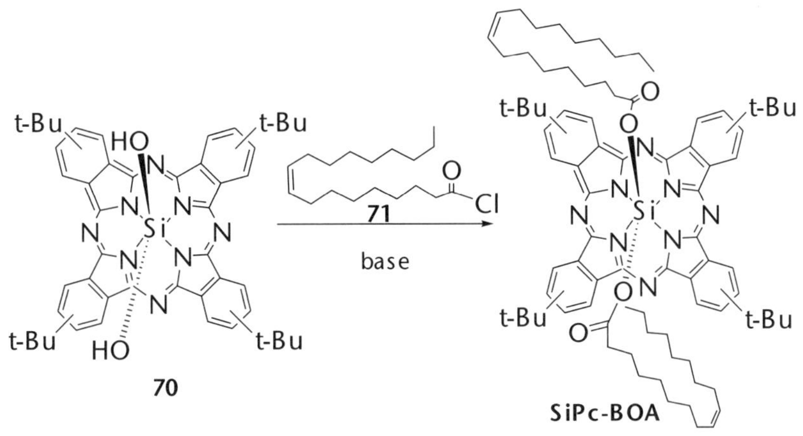

Figure 2.27 Synthesis of SiPc-BOA.

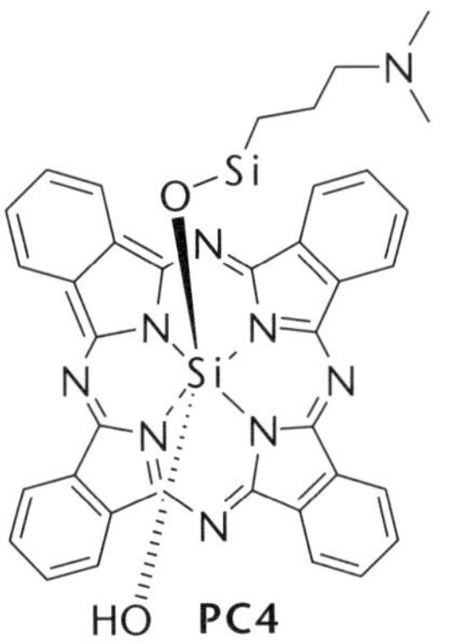

Figure 2.28 Structure of PC4.

This characteristic feature makes these compounds good candidates as photo-sensitizers for the treatment of highly pigmented melanomas and deeply seated tumors [29].

Kenney and his group [30] have reported the synthesis and biological efficacy of a series of silicon coordinated NPcs with various long chain axial ligands.

A Aluminum coordinated naphthalosulfobenzoporphyrin 81 (Al-NSBP) signifi-cant photosensitizing efficacy in showed a   BALB/c mice analog produced limited efficacy, while corresponding mono- sulfonated [31].

bis(tri-n-hexyl silyloxy silicon 2,3-naphthalocyanine 82 (SiNc) displayed the optimal photoactive property against the ocular melanoma in pigmented rabbits (Figure 2.31). It selectively destroyed the localized tumor without affecting the adja-cent normal tissue and did not show any exudative retinal detachments [32].

Most of the second generation PS in general are known to accumulate in tumor mainly via the passive diffusion mechanism. The hydrophobic nature of these photosensitizers made it extremely difficult to formulate most of these compounds.

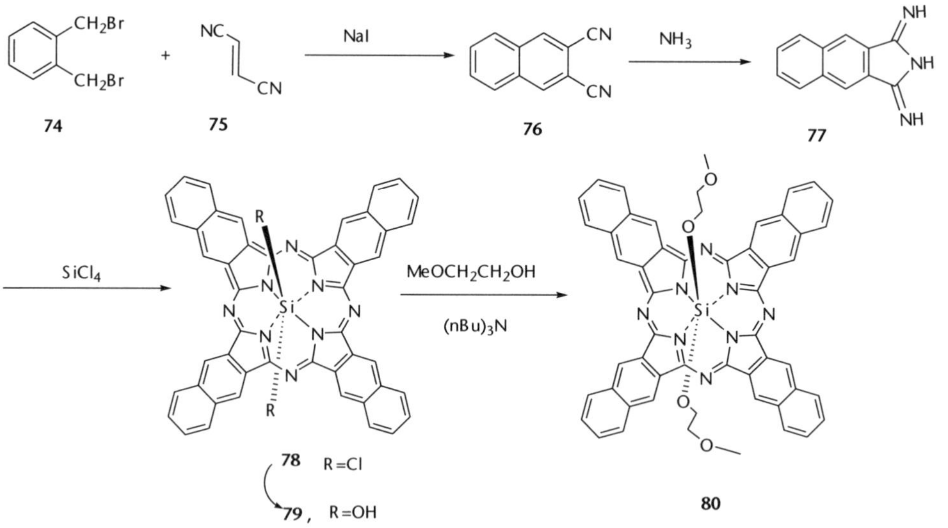

Figure 2.29 Synthesis of Silicon Naphthalocyanine derivative 80.

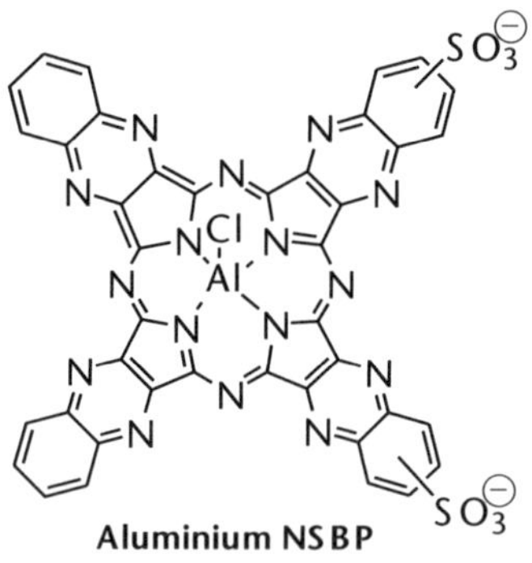

Aluminium NSBP

81

Figure 2.30 Structure of Al-NSBP.

The insertion of metal in general increases the PDT efficacy. But at higher doses these compounds also produce dark toxicity, which could also limit their application in PDT. Most of the porphyrin analogs have the tendency to aggregate in solution, leading to photo-inactivity due to enhanced rate of excited singlet states deactivation by internal conversion to the ground state. Recently, bulky axial ligands have been introduced in Pc and NPc in order to reduce their tendency to aggregate, favoring the formation of monomeric and photoactive forms of the sensitizer. It is also observed that the presence of detergents have minimized the formation of the aggregation [1, 33].

2.4.5 Expanded Metalloporphyrins

Texaphyrins are aromatic macrocycles but containing tripyrrolic units linked by nitrogen atoms, as shown in Figure 2.32. These "expanded" penta-aza heterocycle

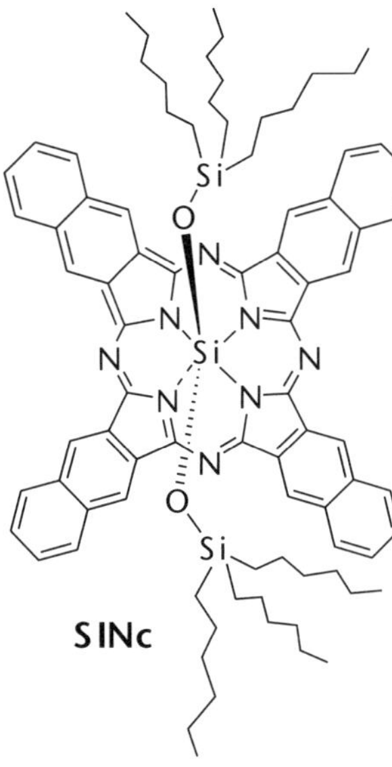

Figure 2.31 Structure of SINc.

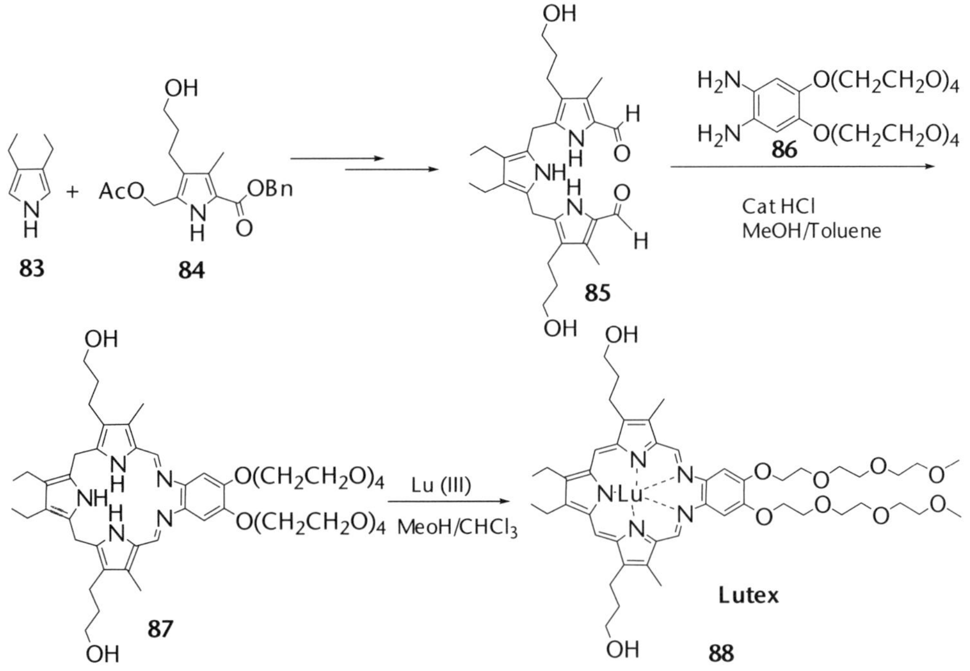

Figure 2.32 Synthesis of PDT agent Lutex®.

are also called porphyrazines and resemble porphyrins and other naturally occurring tetrapyrrolic prosthetic compounds. Similar to tetrapyrrolic macrocycle, these are colored compounds and have a 22π electron system. Therefore, it exhibits longer wavelength absorption >700 nm, depending on the nature of the substituents present at the peripheral positions. Moreover, it has five coordinating nitrogen atoms within the central core that is roughly 20% larger than the porphyrin, which enables it to accommodate a variety of metals other than porphyrin [1, 2].

A well-known metal complex of texaphyrin (Lutex) is currently being developed by Pharmacyclics, USA. In the structure of Lutex 88 [34] Lutetium metal is coordinated with the texaphyrin core structure in which one of the pyrrole subunits is replaced by diaza derivative of benzene, as shown in Figure 2.32. Because of its penta-aza core, it showed strong absorption between 730 and 770 nm. This penetration by light range of wavelength coincides with the or optimal region for the tissue penetration by light and hence if effective, these compounds could be better agents for patients suffering from large tumors. It is also been proved to cure breast cancer and malignant melanomas and currenlty is undergoing phase II clinical trials (Figure 2.33).

It leads to observed that the incorporation of diamagnetic metals leads to higher triplet quantum yields and more efficient generation of singlet oxygen. For example, zinc and cadmium metallated texaphyrins have shown very high triplet quantum yields but the corresponding paramagnetic derivatives (Mn, Sm, and Eu) did not produce any detectable amount of triplet quantum yields. Among the series of metal analogs the zinc metallated compound 89 showed very high photoactivity and exhibited very high single oxygen quantum yield. Similarly, peripherally substituted metallated compounds **90** and **91** also demonstrated significant PDT efficacy [35].

2.5 Problems Associated with Porphyrin-Based Photosensitizers

Porphyrins and metalloporphyrins tend to form molecular assemblies (aggregates) by spontaneous self-association in aqueous solution. Among various aggregates reported in the literature, two types known as H-aggregates and J-aggregates are important. H-aggregates are those in which the dipole moment of the monomers is perpendicular to the line connecting to the centers (i.e., face-to-face arrangement). In the case of J-aggregates, the dipole moment of the monomers is parallel to the line connecting to the centers (i.e., side-by-side arrangement). Several factors are known to trigger these aggregations, for example, structure of porphyrin and its substituents, pH and ionic strength of the medium, and the nature of the surfactant present in the medium and other electrostatic interactions (H-bonding, Van der Waals, hydrophobic and hydrophilic interactions, axial coordination, and other weak

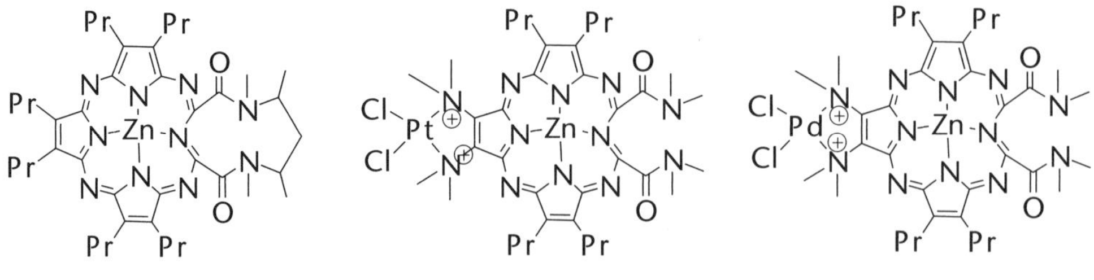

89   **90**   **91**

Figure 2.33 Structure of metallated expanded porphyrins.

intermolecular interactions). Mainly π-π lateral interactions play a crucial role in controlling these aggregations in solution. Dimerization or aggregation of porphyrins significantlylowered the quantum yield of singlet oxygen and in addition it increased the production of H_2O_2 via super oxide (O_2^-) species. It is believed that in vivo, most of the porphyrins are in disaggregated forms; however, certain metal compounds (e.g., In) sitting at the top of the molecule tends to have less aggregation. Therefore, such compounds might be more effective candidates for photodynamic therapy [4].

2.6   Importance of Bifunctional Agents (Imaging and PDT)

The PDT group at Roswell Park Cancer Institute has recently shown the applicability of porphyrin-based compounds in developing multimodality agents (PET/PDT, MRI/PDT, Optical Imaging/PDT) which can be used for both tumor imaging, tumor metastasis and phototherapy. In recent years PET has become an attractive tool for tumor imaging [36]. In this approach, a positron-emitting radioisotope is injected into the host body at nontherapeutic doses. During the imaging procedure, a positron is emitted by an unstable isotope and collides with an electron. The positron and electron annihilate each other and the excess energy due to the annihilation results in the release of two gamma particles in the opposite directions. The two gamma particles are detected using a ring of detectors—coincidence counting. After detection of the gamma rays, 3-D images can be reconstructed to show the location(s) and concentration of the radioisotope/radiolabeled tracers. Therefore, for developing an agent for imaging and therapy and also to investigate the tumor metastasis it will be advantageous to have a radionuclide with longer half-life. Such bifunctional agents could be useful for both imaging and therapy (Figure 2.34). The

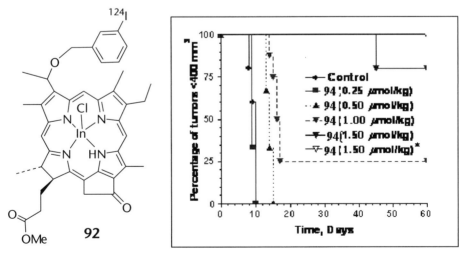

Figure 2.34   The in vivo photosensitizing efficacy of PS 92 at variable concentrations. C3H mice (5 mice/group) bearing RIF tumors were exposed to a laser light (665 nm, 135 J/cm², 75 mW/cm²) for 30 min at 24 h postinjection; * (665 nm, 128 J/cm², 14 mW/cm² for 2.5h at 24 h postinjection). Mice that did not show any tumor regrowth were considered to be cured (tumor was flat).

in vivo efficacy of 92 was investigated in C3H mice bearing RIF tumors (4–5 mm in diameter) at variable drug doses (0.5, 1.0 and 1.5 mmol/kg). The tumors were then exposed with light (665 nm, 135J/cm^2, 75mW/cm^2, 30 min) at 24h post injection. From the results summarized in Figure 2.35, it can be seen that at higher concentration the photosensitizer was quite effective and the results are summarized in Figure 2.35.

In 2005 the PDT group at Roswell Park Cancer Insititute and University of Buffalo group [37] in a joint project showed the utility of a certain ^{124}I labeled photosensitizer as effective tumor imaging (PET) and PDT agent (Color Plate 2) which produced improved tumor contrast over the ^{18}F (FDG). In general, most of the porphyrin-based photosensitizers take 24 to 48h for optimal uptake in tumors (Figure 2.34). Therefore for developing useful bifunctional agents (e. g. ^{124}I = 4 days) than 18F (half-life = 4 days) in this respect, is a suitable candidate for designing tumor imaging by positron emission tomography110 min). On the basis of the results obtained so far, photosensitizer 92 looks a promising for tumor imaging with and without PDT, a radionuclide with longer half-life.

In a similar study, Nakijama and coworkers have shown the utility of Gallium metallated porphyrin (95) for tumor imaging. In their approach, the DTPA side chain attached to compound 94, was labeled with ^{111}In and evaluated for tumor scintigraphy [38]. The results indicated that, compared to the free base analog 98, the corresponding Gallium complex produced significantly higher accumulation in animal tumor models (Figure 2.35).

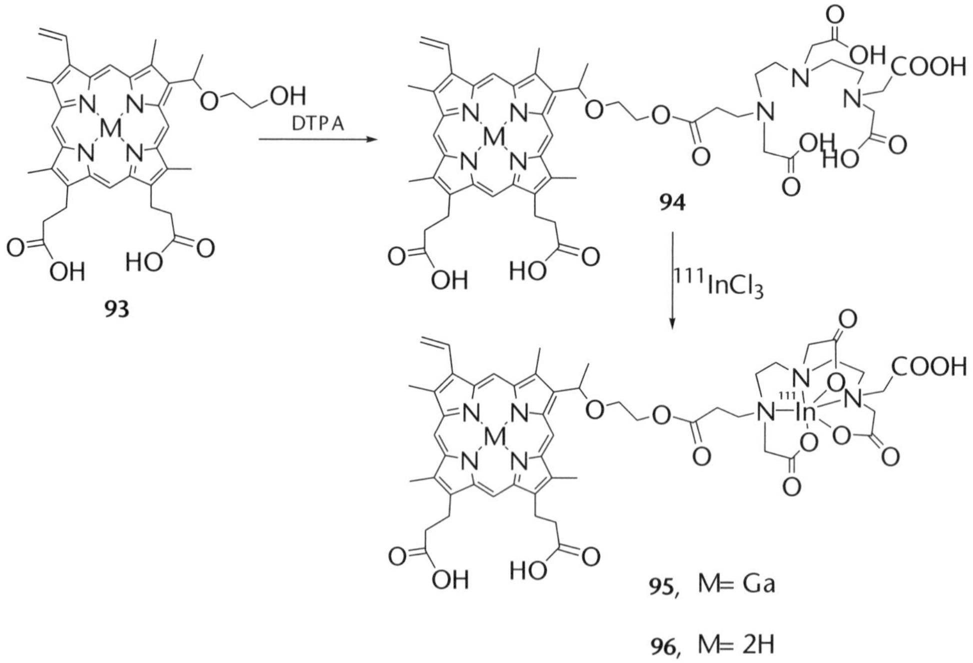

Figure 2.35 Synthesis of bifunctional agent **97**.

2.7 Conclusions

In recent years photodynamic therapy has made numerous significant advances. Due to the efforts of chemists, biologists, and physicists, the development of new photosensitizers has essentially eliminated the problem of prolonged cutaneous phototoxicity. The long-wavelength photosensitizers (>700 nm) developed in various laboratories should also solve the problem of the depth of light penetration into tissue. However, photosensitizers are only one of the key ingredients of PDT. Therefore, in order to optimize PDT it is of fundamental importance to maximize the utility of in vivo singlet oxygen produced by exposing the tumors (containing photosensitizers) and adjust the light dosimetry accordingly. In this respect, metallated photosensitizers (>650 nm) could play an enormous role due to their simple synthesis, high singlet oxygen production, and stability. Insertion of an appropriate central metal in a photosensitizer with appropriate functionality provides enormous opportunities for developing multifunctional agents. Thus a single molecule can be used for nuclear imaging (PET/SPECT) and phototherapy. At the PDT Center of Roswell Park Cancer Institute, we have been investigating the utility of this approach by determining the utility of certain photosensitizers for a "see and treat" approach, which is currently being extended by developing certain multifunctional metallated photosensitizers with and without target-specific moieties.

The applications of PDT are also expanding for many noncancerous conditions. The areas currently being investigated are prevention of restenosis after balloon angioplasty for cardiac artery disease, treatment of rheumatoid arthritis, and for a number of infectious diseases. The understanding of pharmacokinetic and pharmacodynamic characteristics of known or new compounds will certainly help chemists to synthesize improved PDT/imaging agents.

Acknowledgments

The financial support from the NIH (CA55791, CA109914B, and CA114053A) and the Oncologic Foundation of Buffalo is gratefully acknowledged. A partial support from the shared resources of the RPCI support grant (P30CA16056) is also appreciated. Dr. M. P. Dobhal is thankful to Dr. N. K. Jain, Vice-Chancellor, University of Rajasthan, Jaipur, India, for the study-leave award.

References

[1] Pandey, R. K., et al., "Nature: a Rich Source for Developing Multifunctional Agents. Tumor-Imaging and Photodynamic Therapy," *Laser Surg. Med.*, Vol. 38, No. 5, 2006, pp. 445–467.

[2] Pandey, R. K., and G. Zheng, "Porphyrins as Photosensitizers in Photodynamic Therapy," in *The Porphyrin Handbook*, K. M. Kadish, K. M. Smith, and R. Guilard, (eds.), Vol. 6, pp. 157–230, Boston: Academic Press, 2000.

[3] Stratis-Cullum, D. N., et al., "Spectroscopic Data of Biologically and Medically Relevant Species and Samples," in *Biomedical Photonics Handbook*, pp. 65-1-65-136, T. Vo-Dinh, (ed.) New York: CRC Press,, 2003.

[4] Ali, H., and J. E. Van Lier, "Metal Complexes as Photo- and Radiosensitizers," *Chem. Rev.*, Vol. 99, No. 9, 1999, pp. 2379–2450.

[5] Selman, S. H., et al., "Copper Benzochlorin, a Novel Photosensitizer for Photodynamic Therapy: Effects on a Transplantable Urothelial Tumor," *Photochem. Photobiol.*, Vol. 57, No. 4, 1993, pp. 681–685.

[6] Scherz, A., et al., U.S. Patent No. US 6,569,846 B1, "Palladium-Substituted Bacteriochlorophyll Derivatives and Use Thereof," 2003.

[7] Koudinova, N. V., et al, "Effects of Pd-bacteriopheophorbide (TOOKAD)-Mediated Photodynamic Therapy on Canine Prostate Pretreated with Ionizing Radiation," *Int. J. Cancer*, 2003, Vol. 104, No. 6, pp. 782–731.

[8] Vakrat, Y., et al., "Bacteriochlorophyll Derivatives: Phototoxicity, Hydrophobicity & Oxygen Radicals Production," *Free Radical Biol. Med.*, Vol. 27, 1999, Suppl. 1, S129.

[9] Chen, Q., et al., "Preclinical Studies in Normal Canine Prostate of a Novel Palladium-Bacteriopheophorbide (WST09) Photosensitizer for Photodynamic Therapy of Prostate Cancers," *Photochem. Photobiol.*, Vol. 76, 2002, pp. 438–445.

[10] Tremblay, A., et al., "Endobronchial Phototoxicity of WST 09 (Tookad®), a New Fast-Acting Photosensitizer for Photodynamic Therapy: Preclinical Study in the Pig," *Photochem. Photobiol.*, Vol. 78, No. 2, 2003, pp. 124–130.

[11] Morgan, A. R., et al., "New Photosensitizers for Photodynamic Therapy: Combined Effect of Metallopurpurin Derivatives and Light on Transplantable Bladder Tumors," *Cancer Res.*, Vol. 48, No. 1, 1988, pp. 194–198.

[12] Garbo, G. M., et al., "In Vivo and In Vitro Photodynamic Studies with Benzochlorin Iminium Salts Delivered by Lipid Emulsions," *Photochem. Photobiol.*, Vol. 68, No. 4, 1998, pp. 561–568.

[13] Meerovich, I. G., et al., "Fluorescent and Photodynamic Properties of Infrared Photosensitizer Bachteriochlorophyllide-Serine," *Proc. SPIE*, Vol. 5449, 2004, pp. 247–256.

[14] Ding, L., et al., "Anti-Human Immunodeficiency Virus Effects of Metalloporphyrins-Ellipticine Complexes," *Biochem. Pharm.*, Vol. 44, No. 8, 1992, pp.1675–1679.

[15] Detty, M. R., S. L. Gibson, and S. J. Wagner, "Current Clinical and Preclinical Photosensitizers for Use in Photodynamic Therapy," *J. Med. Chem.*, Vol. 47, No. 16, 2004, pp. 3897–3915.

[16] Ishizumi, T., et al., "Spectrometric Characteristics and Tumor-affinity of a Novel Photosensitizer: Mono-L-aspartyl Aurochlorin e6," *Photodiagnosis and Photodynamic Therapy*, Vol. 1, No. 4, 2004, pp. 295–301.

[17] Nakae, Y., et al., "Convenient Screening Method Using Albumin For The Tumor Localizing Property of Ga-Porphyrin Complexes," *J. Photochem. Photobiol A*, Vol. 172, No. 1, 2005, pp. 55–61.

[18] Kulkarni, P. V., D. Jain, and J. Narula, "Radio Indium and Gallium Labeled Porphyrins for Medical Imaging," in *Application of Accelerators in Research and Industry—16th International Conference*, Vol. CP576, J. L. Duggan and I. L. Morgan, (eds.), pp. 837–840, 2001.

[19] Chen, Y., et al., —unpublished results.

[20] Rosenfield, A., et al., "Photosensitizers Derived from 132-Oxo-Methyl Pyropheophorbide-a: Enhanced Effect of Indium (III) as a Central Metal in In Vitro and In Vivo Photosensitizing Efficacy," *Photochem. Photobiol.*, Vol. 82, No. 3, 2006, pp. 626–634.

[21] Chen, Y., et al., "Methyl Pyropheophorbide-a Analogs: Potential Fluorescent Probes for the Peripheral-Type Benzodiazepine Receptor. Effect of Central Metal in Photosensitizing Efficacy," *J. Med. Chem.*, Vol. 48, No. 11, 2005, pp. 3692–3695.

[22] Verma, A., and S. H. Snyder, "Characterization of Porphyrin Interactions with Peripheral Type Benzodiazepine Receptors, Molecular Pharmacology," *Mol. Pharmacol.*, Vol. 34, No. 6, 1988, pp. 800–805.

[23] Jori, G., "Tumour Photosensitizers: Approaches to Enhance the Selectivity and Efficiency of Photodynamic Therapy," *J. Photochem. Photobiol. B: Biol.*, Vol. 36, No. 2, 1996, pp. 87–93.

[24] Rosenthal, I., "Phthalocyanines as Photodynamic Sensitizers," *Photochem. Photobiol.*, Vol. 53, No. 6, 1991, pp 859–870.

[25] Love, W. G., et al., "Liposome-Mediated Delivery of Photosensitizers: Localization of Zinc (II)-Phthalocyanine within Implanted Tumors After Intravenous Administration," *Photochem. Photobiol.*, Vol. 63, 1996, pp. 656–661.

[26] Avetisov, S. E., et al., "The First Results of Phase IIA of Clinical Studies of Photodynamic Therapy for Subretinal Neovascular Membranes with Photosense," *Vestn. Oftalmol.*, Vol. 121, 2005, pp. 6–9.

[27] Li, H., et al., "High Payload Delivery of Optical Imaging and Photodynamic Therapy Agents to Tumors Using Phthalocyanine Reconstituted Low-density Lipoprotein Nanoparticles," *J. Biomedical Optics*, Vol. 10, No. 4, 2005, pp. 041203-1-7.

[28] Miller, J. D., et al., "Photodynamic Therapy with the Phthalocyanine Photosensitizer Pc 4: The Case Experience with Preclinical Mechanistic and Early Clinical-Translational Studies," *Toxicol. Appl. Pharmacol.*, Vol. 224, 2007, pp. 290–299.

[29] Lo, P. -C., et al., "Photodynamic Effects of a Novel Series of Silicon(IV) Phthalocyanines Against Human Colon Adenocarcinoma Cells," *Photodiagnosis Photodynamic Ther.*, Vol. 4, No. 2, 2007, pp. 117–123.

[30] Zuk, M. M., et al., "Effect of Delivery System on the Pharmacokinetics and Tissue Distribution of Bis(Di-isobutyl Octadecylsiloxy)Silicon 2,3-Naphthaocyanine (isoBOSNIC), a Photosensitizer for Tumor Therapy," *Photochem. Photobiol.*, Vol. 63, No. 1, 1996, pp. 132–140.

[31] Margaron, P., et al, "Photodynamic Properties of Naphthosulfobenzoporphyrazins, Novel Asymmetric, Amphiphilic Phthalocyanine Derivatives," *J. Photochem, Photobiol. B-Biol.* Vol. 14, No. 3, 1992, pp. 187–199.

[32] Hill, R. A., et al., "Photodynamic Therapy of Ocular Melanoma with Bis Silicon 2,3-Naphthalocyanine in a Rabbit Model," *Invest. Ophthamol. Vis. Sci*, Vol. 36, No. 12, 1995, pp. 2476–2481.

[33] Haglili, Y. -V., et al., "The Microenvironment Effect on the Generation of Reactive Oxygen Species by Pd-bacteriopheophorbide," *J. Am. Chem. Soc.*, Vol. 127, No. 17, 2005, pp. 6487–6497.

[34] Sessler, J. L., et al., "Texaphyrins: Synthesis and Applications," *Acc. Chem. Res.*, Vol. 27, No. 2, 1994, pp. 43–50.

[35] Garrido-Montalban, A., et al., "Studies on Seco-Porphyrazines: A Case Study on Serendipity," *Dalton Trans.*, Vol. 11, No. 2003, pp. 2093–2102.

[36] Berger, A., "How Does It Work? Positron Emission Tomography," *BMJ*, Vol. 326, No. 7404, 2003, pp. 1449.

[37] Pandey, S. K., et al., "Multimodality Agents for Tumor Imaging (PET, Fluorescence) and Photodynamic Therapy. A Possible 'See and Treat' Approach," *J. Med. Chem.*, Vol. 48, No. 20, 2005, pp. 6286–6295.

[38] Nakajima, S; et al., "[111]In-labeled Mn Metalloporphyrin for Tumor Imaging," *Nucl. Med. Biol.*, Vol. 20, No. 2, 1993, pp. 231–237.

CHAPTER 3

Photophysics and Photochemistry in Photodynamic Therapy

Robert W. Redmond

3.1 Introduction

Photodynamic therapy (PDT) is dependent on the activation of a photosensitizing dye in tissue with light to generate a reactive excited state, from which photochemical processes are initiated that are ultimately deleterious to the diseased cells and tissue that are targeted for eradication. The term "photodynamic" is often taken as the action produced by light activation with specific reference to three essential components of the process: light, photosensitizer, and oxygen. Although the basic photophysics and photochemistry of photosensitizers has been studied in great detail over the last few decades, there remains substantial questions regarding the exact mechanisms that operate in cells and in vivo under therapeutic conditions. This chapter will cover the basic photophysics and photochemistry of photodynamic dyes, the impact that the local environment can exert in determining the primary mechanisms that take place in biological systems, and the secondary processes that must be considered in the context of the overall mechanism of the photodynamic process.

3.2 Electronic Excitation and Excited States

To initiate a photodynamic process the dye must absorb at the wavelength of the illuminating light, an expression of the first law of photochemistry. In addition, the photons must be of sufficient energy to produce *electronic* excitation of the molecule. This requires energy in the ultraviolet (UV), visible (VIS), or very near infrared (NIR) spectral region. Shorter wavelength (higher energy) radiation is ionizing and longer wavelength light excites molecular vibration but is insufficient for electronic excitation. For application in tissue, where penetration depth is a consideration, UV and blue light have less application other than for superficial treatments, and in general it is dyes that extend to the red and NIR that are preferred due to the lack of native competitive absorbers in the tissue in this "optical window." However, it should be noted that the process cannot be pushed too far into the infrared due to the energetics of the process. Lower energy infrared light can penetrate deeper in tissue but the photons are not sufficiently energetic to produce the electronic excitation required for photodynamic action.

Dye excitation and the photophysical processes that result are best understood with reference to a simplified Jablonski energy level diagram, shown in Figure 3.1. The actual absorption of a photon (hv) is a very rapid event, occurring on the order of 10^{-15} s and electronic excitation occurs before any change in the relative position of the atoms in the molecule (vibration), the so-called Franck-Condon effect. Excitation occurs to discreet energy levels in the excited state of the molecule and is rapidly followed by vibrational relaxation (VR) as the excited molecule equilibrates its geometry to the lowest energy configuration. Quantum mechanical selection rules determine that the excitation process is highly allowed when there is no change in the overall spin multiplicity of the molecule. Molecules exist in the most favorable energetic ground state where, typically, electrons (designated with spin +1/2 and −1/2) are paired such that the sum (S) of all spin quantum numbers is zero. The spin multiplicity (Ms) is given by 2S+1 and for a typical organic molecule the resultant Ms of 1 denotes a singlet state. For photodynamic sensitizers the absorption of a photon produces an excited singlet state (S_1). If higher energy photons are used the excitation process may generate a higher excited state (S_2), but in general a rapid relaxation occurs between singlet states via a process called internal conversion (IC) to the lowest excited singlet state (S_1), as shown in Figure 3.1. Thus, the lowest vibrational and electronic excited state (S_1, v=0) is relevant for photosensitizer photophysics and it is from this state that fluorescence is initiated (Kasha's rule).

The lowest excited singlet state (S_1) is considerably longer-lived than the upper excited states due to the larger separation in energy that exists between it and the ground state (S_0) than among the upper excited singlet states (the "energy gap" law), such that even though the relaxation from S_1 to S_0 is allowed on the basis of spin multiplicity, the probability of nonradiative relaxation by internal conversion is reduced due to the large energy gap between the states. A competing relaxation pathway that comes into play in photodynamic agents is a change in spin of an

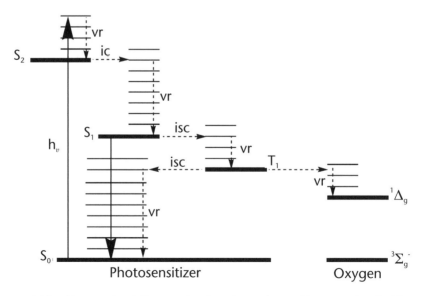

Figure 3.1 Jablonski energy level diagram showing electronic transitions associated with photodynamic agents.

excited electron to generate a "triplet" state where the two unpaired electrons are now of the same spin, the sum of the overall spin is 1, and the resultant spin multiplicity is 3. This is the opposite of the S_1-S_0 process in that the transition is disfavored on the basis of spin multiplicity but much more favored on account of the much smaller energy gap between the S_1 and T_1 states. The lowest triplet state produced (T_1) is the most important state in the photodynamic effect.

3.3 Rates of Excited State Processes

It is clear from the simplified description given above that there are two electronic excited states that are of interest to PDT. The S_1 state is primarily of interest, not for any chemical reason but for the fact that a minor proportion of S_1 states are deactivated by radiative relaxation to the ground state, whereby a photon of light is emitted that corresponds to the S_1-S_0 energy gap. Radiative relaxation between states of the same mulitiplicity is formally designated "fluorescence." The commonly used photosensitizers in PDT and in experimental studies have appreciable fluorescence and this property is a very useful tool for imaging tumors, determining drug pharmacokinetics, and evaluating dosimetry of PDT. The relaxation rate of the S_1 state is determined by the sum of all the rate constants for the processes that contribute—radiative relaxation to the ground S_0 state (fluorescence), nonradiative relaxation to S_0 (internal conversion), and nonradiative intersystem crossing (ISC) to the T_1 state. From the energy level diagram shown in Figure 3.1 the overall rate of decay of the S_1 state is given by the sum of $k_f + k_{ic} + k_{isc}$, the rate constants for the processes of fluorescence emission, internal conversion to S_0, and intersystem crossing to T_1, respectively. The reciprocal of this value is the lifetime (τ_s) of the S_1 state.

$$\tau_s = \frac{1}{k_f + k_{ic} + k_{isc}} \tag{3.1}$$

The quantum yield of formation (Φ) of any of these processes can be defined as the ratio of the number of molecules undergoing the process to the number of molecules that absorb a photon. In terms of kinetics it is defined as the rate constant for the process divided by the sum of rate constants for all the processes that deactivate the excited molecule. For example, in the absence of other reaction pathways, the quantum yield of fluorescence (Φ_f) is given by:

$$\Phi_f = \frac{k_f}{k_f + k_{ic} + k_{isc}} \tag{3.2}$$

The sum of the quantum yields for fluorescence (Φ_f), internal conversion (Φ_{ic}) and intersytem crossing (Φ_{isc}) is typically unity in simple solutions. For most photodynamic agents the energy gap between S_1 and S_0 states is large, the gap between S1 and T1 states is small and as a result the internal conversion process is negligible so that intersystem crossing predominates $\Phi_{isc} > \Phi_f > \Phi_{ic}$ and $\Phi_f + \Phi_{isc} \approx 1$.

The S_1 lifetime of PDT photosensitizers is typically on the order of 1 to 15 ns. The lifetime of the T_1 state is orders of magnitude longer due to the fact that its deactivation to the S_0 ground state involves both a spin flip and a large T_1-S_0 energy gap with the result that the inherent triplet lifetime in the absence of any interactions with other molecules is typically hundreds of microseconds or longer. The large difference in S_1 and T_1 lifetime has a major influence on the probability of bimolecular reaction from these two states. For an excited state reaction to occur with another species in a fluid medium, the rate is the product of the bimolecular rate constant, k_r (in $M^{-1}s^{-1}$) and the molar concentration of the reactant involved. For typical S_1 and T_1 lifetimes of 10 ns and 100 μs, respectively, the concentration of reactant required to interact with 50% of the excited states would be 10^{-2} M for S_1 but only 10^{-6} M for T_1, assuming a maximum bimolecular rate constant approaching the diffusion rate of $\sim 10^{10}$ $M^{-1}s^{-1}$. Thus, it is much more likely that the T_1 state is involved in bimolecular reactions, from a purely kinetic point of view, although the heterogeneous nature of cells and tissue may alter this simplified view.

3.4   Two Photon Excitation

The above discussion is based on the normal photodynamic situation of one-photon absorption process using low intensity illumination. However, there are approaches to photosensitizer activation that involve other excitation strategies that are worth mentioning. Two-photon fluorescence microscopy is widely used in biology for imaging purposes. The process depends on simultaneous (nonresonant) two-photon absorption to generate the fluorescent excited state. The requirement for simultaneous absorption means that two photons must arrive in the vicinity of the absorbing chromophore within a very short time for excitation to occur. This and the fact that two-photon absorption cross-sections are quite low contributes to the requirement for very high light intensity. In practice, this is achieved by tightly focusing a very short pulse of laser light in a small volume of a sample to achieve sufficient intensity for two-photon absorption to occur. Although the initial excited states reached by this mechanism are slightly different than that produced in the normal one-photon process, deactivation typically brings the molecule back to the same S_1 state before initiating fluorescence, intersystem crossing, and so forth, as shown in Figure 3.2. In terms of fluorescence microscopy, there is a benefit in that high-resolution images can be obtained with greater depth of penetration and less problems of out-of-plane photobleaching and induced photochemistry in the sample as a whole, as effects are confined to the small 3-D volume where the light intensity is sufficient to pump the two-photon absorption process.

As the combined energy of two photons is absorbed in the process, the wavelength of light used is longer (less energy) than for the analogous one-photon process, allowing the laser wavelength to be red-shifted to the NIR region where penetration of light into tissue is greater. Attempts have been made to adopt this excitation mode for PDT to achieve greater depth of penetration of light and subsequent photodynamic action in tissue, but this comes at the cost of the far greater expense for the high-intensity, short-pulsed laser sources required and a rastering method to sweep the excitation spot through the target tissue volume [1].

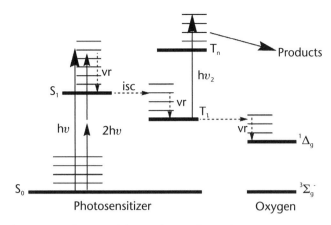

Figure 3.2   Simultaneous and sequential two-photon absorption processes.

Sequential (resonant) two-photon absorption has also been investigated experimentally for photodynamic purposes [2]. In this approach the intensity and wavelength are chosen to maximize a two-step process where an excited state is produced and then further excited within its lifetime by absorption of a second photon to an upper excited state (e.g., T_1 to T_n). The intensity required for this approach is far lower than that of the nonresonant approach and the purpose is different, in that more energetic states are accessed from which novel photochemical processes may occur that generate other reactive products, such as free radicals, that lead to cell killing. In essence the latter approach is also a means to increase depth of penetration if one considers the states accessed to be those accessed by a one-photon absorption of shorter wavelength UV light. However, it also requires pulsed laser sources to optimally pump the excitation to the upper excited state.

3.5   Singlet Oxygen Generation

Finally, the discussion of photosensitizer behavior comes to the generation of singlet molecular oxygen $^1\Delta_g$, the mediator of photodynamic damage in living systems. Molecular oxygen is atypical in that it has two unpaired electrons in the ground state and therefore the lowest electronic state is a triplet state ($^3O_2$, or more formally, $^3\Sigma_g^-$). The lowest excited state is a singlet state ($^1\Delta_g$) that lies at an energy (E_Δ) of 94.1 kJ mol^{-1} above the ground state and due to the difference in spin multiplicity between these states the direct excitation of the $^3\Sigma_g^-$ to $^1\Delta_g$ transition is highly improbable. However, $^1\Delta_g$ can be formed in high efficiency via an energy transfer mechanism involving photosensitizer excited states. Energy transfer occurs through collisions between molecules and in simplified terms the probability for transfer occurring depends on a number of factors including the excited state lifetime, reactant concentrations, spin multiplicity of reactant, and product states and the energetics of the states involved. For the typical system of an excited state donor (*D) transferring energy to an acceptor (A), the energy of the excited acceptor state (*A) should be lower than the donor (*D) and the concentration of A should be high enough such that the product, k_r [A], is greater than the unimolecular rate constant, k′ , for deactivation of *D in absence of A. Additionally, the transfer should comply with the Wigner spin conservation rules.

$$*D + A \xrightarrow{ET} D + *A \qquad (3.3)$$

There are actually two possible pathways for $^1\Delta_g$ production from excited photosensitizers [3]. The first is an oxygen-enhanced intersystem crossing from the S_1 state to generate the T_1 state, which can occur only if the S_1–T_1 energy difference is greater than the energy of $^1\Delta_g$, as shown in case B in Figure 3.3. Spin conservation is obeyed in this reaction with singlet + triplet reactants leading to singlet + triplet products.

$$S_1 + 3\sum_g^- \xrightarrow{isc} T_1 + {}^1\Delta_g \qquad (3.4)$$

Reaction 4 constitutes only a partial deactivation of the photosensitizer, as the product is the lower excited T_1 state. However, even if the S_1–T_1 energy difference is greater than the energy of $^1\Delta_g$ the process may not occur when there is a higher triplet level (e.g.,T_2) that lies below S_1 in energy. In such a case, shown in case C in Figure 3.3, intersystem crossing can occur to the T_2 state followed by rapid internal conversion to T_1 without generation of $^1\Delta_g$. Where the S_1–T_1 energy difference is less than E_Δ (case A) the only route to formation of $^1\Delta_g$ is by the more common energy transfer pathway, deactivating the T_1 state to ground state with concomitant formation of $^1\Delta_g$, as shown in reaction 5. In terms of spin conservation there is no conflict with this process either as triplet + triplet reactants give rise to singlet + singlet products. The situations of singlet + singlet reactants leading singlet + triplet products or triplet + triplet reactants giving singlet + triplet products would not obey spin conservation rules.

$$T_1 + {}^3\sum_g^- \xrightarrow{ET} S_0 + {}^1\Delta_g \qquad (3.5)$$

For case B in Figure 3.3, where $\Delta E\,(S_1\text{-}T_1) > E_\Delta$ and $E(S_1) < E(T_2)$, there is obviously a possibility to generate two molecules of $^1\Delta_g$ per photon absorbed. Unfortunately for PDT, this is not usually the case for typical photodynamic agents.

Oxygen quenching of excited states is a complex process. The quenching of the T_1 state by oxygen has both energetic and charge transfer contributions that control the value of the rate constant and the quantum yield of $^1\Delta_g$ formation for a given photosensitizer [3]. The rate constant has a maximum of 4/9 of the diffusion controlled rate due to the fact that only four of the nine possible intermediate complexes formed have multiplicities (singlet or triplet) that can lead to product formation and the value is typically $\sim 2 \times 10^9$ M^{-1} s^{-1} for most photosensitizers in water. Given that the concentration of oxygen in air saturated water is 2.85×10^{-4} M and a typical T_1 lifetime is $\sim 100\,\mu$s ($k_d = 10^4$s^{-1}), the bimolecular reaction of the T_1 state with oxygen ($k_{obs} \sim 6 \times 10^5$ s^{-1}) accounts for almost 100% of the T_1 deactivation under these conditions. However, the quantum yield of $^1\Delta_g$ formation (Φ_Δ) does not necessarily equate to the Φ_{isc} value. Under conditions where all T_1 states are quenched by oxygen the Φ_Δ value is = Φ_{isc} and is better defined by

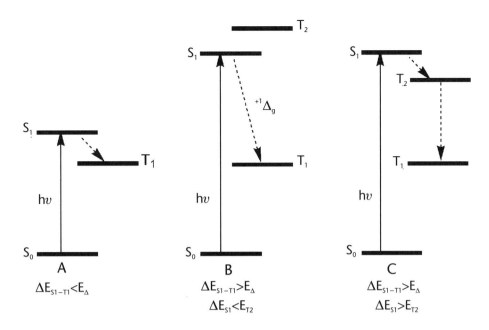

Figure 3.3   Energy level diagram for $^1\Delta_g$ sensitization for different singlet and triplet energy configurations.

$$\Phi_\Delta = S_\Delta \, x \Phi_{isc} \tag{3.6}$$

where S_Δ denotes the fraction of oxygen quenching interactions with T_1 that lead to $^1\Delta_g$ formation. For the majority of photosensitizers of relevance to therapeutic and experimental PDT the Φ_{isc} values are > 0.5 and S_Δ values approach unity [4]. The measured yield of $^1\Delta_g$ formation also depends on oxygen concentration and this is of vital importance in PDT. A more full relationship that takes this into consideration can be expressed as

$$\Phi_\Delta = S_\Delta \, x \Phi_{isc} \, x \, \frac{k_q [O_2]}{k_q [O_2] + k_d} \tag{3.7}$$

Singlet oxygen is a metastable, electronically excited state and its lifetime (τ_Δ) is solvent-dependent as it relaxes by electronic to vibrational energy transfer with its environment, with the rate determined by the extent of overlap in energies between the states involved. The shortest lifetime is exhibited in pure water, where $\tau_\Delta = 4\,\mu s$ and can be as long as in the millisecond regime in polyhalogeno-carbons such as Freon. Biological systems such as cells and tissue are heterogeneous, consisting of domains that differ in environment and the predominant biomolecules present. However, the lifetime will be ultimately limited by water as the major overall cellular component and the diffusion range of the excited $^1\Delta_g$ formed is severely limited [5]. An interesting aspect of the solvent-dependent τ_Δ value has been the use of heavy water (D2O) as a means to confirm the involvement of $^1\Delta_g$ in the photodynamic mechanism, the effect being increased due to the >10-fold longer lifetime in D2O.

As discussed in a subsequent section this effect may not be realized in biological systems, even when $^1\Delta_g$ is intimately involved.

3.6   Type I and Type II Photochemistry

Photodynamic action has traditionally been discussed in terms of Type I and Type II mechanisms. The typical Type II reaction, described above, involves energy transfer from excited state photosensitizer to oxygen to form $^1\Delta_g$. However, the Type II reaction formally indicates only an initial interaction of the excited photosensitizer with oxygen [6]. Although there are some claims that direct electron transfer to oxygen can also occur to form the superoxide anion radical (O_2^-), there are more likely secondary pathways to account for the production of this species, discussed later.

The Type I mechanism is differentiated by the primary interaction of the excited photosensitizer taking place with a molecule other than oxygen [6]. It is often referred to as a "radical" mechanism but we will discuss later the involvement of secondary radical species under conditions where the initial reaction is of a Type II nature, so this is somewhat of a misnomer. In reality, the Type I mechanism covers electron transfer, atom (e.g., hydrogen) abstraction, photoadditions, and various other bimolecular photochemical reactions.

The actual mechanism(s) that operates in a biological system will depend on the local environment experienced by the photosensitizer. Specifically, the pathways taken depend on the rate constant for inherent deactivation of the photosensitizer excited state (k_d) and the various bimolecular rate constants for reaction with oxygen (k_q), and a variety of potential reactants $(k_R$-$k_Z)$ and the respective concentrations of these species; that is:

$$-\frac{d[^*PS]}{dt} = k_d + k_q\left[O_2\right] + k_R[R] + k_S[S] + k_T[T] + \cdots k_Z[Z] \tag{3.8}$$

Under normal air atmosphere the $^1\Delta_g$ pathway predominates in simple solution for most photosensitizers, due to the high value of both kq and [O2], Given that $^1\Delta_g$ is the primary reactive oxygen species formed from excitation of photodynamic agents, we should consider its fate in biological systems. As discussed previously, the lifetime of $^1\Delta_g$ is solvent-dependent and shortest (4 μs) in water. Within this short lifetime reaction with various substrates is possible. Singlet oxygen is an electrophile and its reactions fall into a few broad categories. Singlet oxygen undergoes the "ene" reaction where it adds to double bond systems and also forms endoperoxide species on insertion into ring systems via a 2+4 Diels-Alder cycloaddition reaction, as shown in Figure 3.4.

The major biomolecules that are substrates for $^1\Delta_g$ include cholesterol and unsaturated lipids, proteins, and nucleic acid bases. All of these alterations have the potential to disrupt cellular function and lead to cell death. Addition of $^1\Delta_g$ to unsaturated lipids directly forms hydroperoxides [7] that can lead to further chain lipid peroxidation reactions. Similarly, formation of protein peroxides [8] also disrupts structure and function and these species are attracting attention in biology. Oxidation of nucleic acid bases favors the purines, especially guanine, eventually forming the mutagenic product, 8-oxo-7,8 dihydro-guanosine (8-oxo-dG) [9].

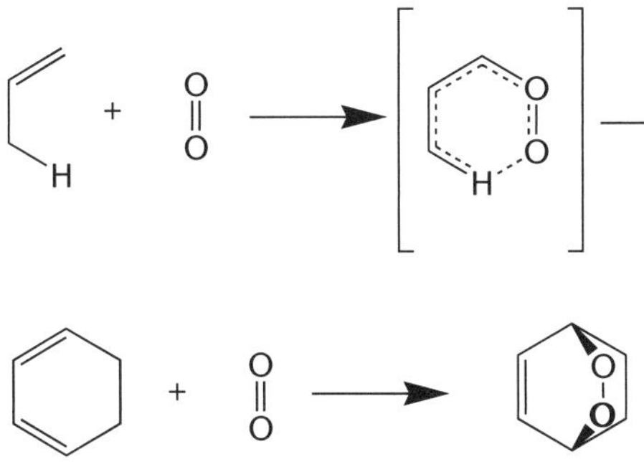

"ene" reaction

endoperoxide

Figure 3.4 Electrophilic reactions of singlet oxygen.

3.7 Spectroscopic Methods to Determine Reaction Mechanisms

Photochemical mechanisms of photodynamic agents can be measured using a variety of spectroscopic, chemical, and biological methods. The behavior of both the precursor excited states and $^1\Delta_g$ itself can be probed using spectroscopic techniques. Both absorption and emission spectroscopy can be useful in studying the photophysics and photochemistry of photosensitizers. The behavior of the S1 state of photosensitizers can be studied by detection of the fluorescence emitted by this state. Although the S1 state is probably not directly involved in photodynamic reactions, it can give valuable information on the environment of the photosensitizer in biological systems. It can also provide information on photosensitizer aggregation, which tends to decrease fluorescence (and intersystem crossing) by providing a more accessible channel for nonradiative relaxation to the ground state [10]. The tetrapyrrole-based photosensitizers that are used as PDT agents (porphyrins, chlorins, phthalocyanines, etc.) are prone to aggregation, and sensitizer fluorescence in tissue can be more useful as a guide to photodynamic activity than absorption given that aggregation tends to quench fluorescence (and has less of an effect on absorbance) and the fluorescent monomer is also the species generating $^1\Delta_g$.

For mechanistic purposes, it is generally more relevant to study the T_1 state as it is more likely to be involved in bimolecular chemical reactions due to its longer lifetime.

The T1 state transfers energy to oxygen to form singlet oxygen ($^1\Delta_g$). Thus, one could follow the behavior of either of these species to obtain mechanistic information. Technically, direct detection of $^1\Delta_g$ is more difficult. The energy level diagrams for the ground and lowest excited states of oxygen are shown in Figure 3.5.

There are two spectroscopic methods for detection of $^1\Delta_g$, based on the transitions shown in Figure 3.5. The first approach is to detect the low-intensity phosphorescence emission that accompanies the relaxation of the $^1\Delta_g$ state to the ground state. The second approach is to measure the absorption corresponding to the $^1\Delta_g$ to $^1\sum_g^+$ transition. The higher lying excited state, $^1\sum_g^+$, at an energy of 157 $kJ\,mol^{-1}$ can also be accessed following energy transfer from sufficiently energetic T_1 states higher, but this state rapidly deactivates by internal conversion to the $^1\Delta_g$ state, from which reactions occur. Absorption of 1.91 μm IR light corresponding to the energy difference between $^1\Delta_g$ and $^1\sum_g^+$ promotes this allowed transition and

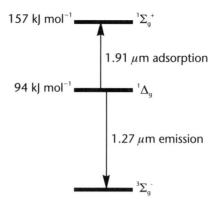

Figure 3.5 Energy level diagram for the lowest excited states of oxygen.

can be used to follow the time-dependent formation and decay of $^1\Delta_g$, even under microscopy conditions [11].

Of the two approaches, the most prevalent technique used for $^1\Delta_g$ is the direct phosphorescence emission in the near IR with a maximum at 1,270 nm. This is a weak but detectable emission in homogeneous solutions of photosensitizer in different solvents lacking chemical reactivity with $^1\Delta_g$, but becomes more challenging in biological systems due to the fact that the lifetime depends on the environment, predominantly water, where emission is weakest and shortest-lived (4 μs) and may be further reduced by reactions with biomolecules in the environment. The direct detection of $^1\Delta_g$ in cells has proven somewhat controversial. Emission has been measured in cells and tissue using sensitive detection approaches but the question remains whether the emission is actually cellular or extracellular in origin. Where time-resolved approaches have been utilized there are also conflicting estimates for the lifetime of $^1\Delta_g$ in cells. Using approaches with isolated cell constituents Kanofsky estimated the lifetime (on the basis of reactions with cellular constituents) to be less than 250 ns. In later experiments the first convincing detection of cellular $^1\Delta_g$ was by Wilson's group where a lifetime of 600 ns was estimated [12]. However, Ogilby's group has also shown convincing data in recent years using microscopic approaches to $^1\Delta_g$ measurement in cells that the lifetime may be much greater, approaching the solvent-determined limit [13, 14]. This latter observation is puzzling given that $^1\Delta_g$ is an oxidizing species and induces oxidative damage in cells and tissue via reaction with biomolecules, but the results of Ogilby's group suggest that most of the $^1\Delta_g$ is deactivated by solvent collision rather than reaction with the cell constituents.

The measurement of $^1\Delta_g$ in cells does not provide a large amount of mechanistic information, other than confirming the involvement of $^1\Delta_g$ at some stage in the process, as only a portion of the $^1\Delta_g$ produced is actually detected and the fraction may be small and represent the least relevant in terms of generating chemical change and biological responses (e.g., if arising from $^1\Delta_g$ that is produced by extracellular photosensitizer or has diffused out of cells after generation). The detection of emission from $^1\Delta_g$ in tissue, irrespective of its microscopic source, may be very useful for dosimetry and mechanistic purposes in PDT. In an approach termed singlet oxygen luminescence dosimetry (SOLD), the continuous monitoring of luminescence from the treated volume can determine relative levels of $^1\Delta_g$ generation and highlight adverse factors such as high-dose-rate-induced oxygen depletion and photobleaching of the photodynamic dye in the tissue [15].

In terms of elucidating mechanisms an argument can be made that is of greater value to monitor the behavior of the triplet state of the photosensitizer as this is the immediate precursor to $^1\Delta_g$. In addition, one monitors the strong absorption of excited state photosensitizer species rather than the weak IR phosphorescence emission from $^1\Delta_g$. This is achieved by transient absorption spectroscopy where a short laser pulse is used to excite a significant population of photosensitizer ground states to S_1, from which the T_1 state is heavily populated within 10 ns by intersystem crossing. The T_1 state can be easily followed by its absorption properties, which differ from the ground state. The loss of the T_1 species, by relaxation to the ground state, by reaction with oxygen to produce $^1\Delta_g$ or by direct reaction with other species can be readily measured using this technique and aid in determining primary photochemical mechanisms of photodynamic sensitizers, and in some cases to probe the immediate environment of the subcellular location of photosensitizer [16].

3.8 Influence of Biological Environment

Before discussing possible alternative mechanisms one must also consider the cellular milieu. Unlike the homogeneous solutions often used to determine fundamental photochemical behavior, the nature of cells and tissue is highly heterogeneous and this complicates the interpretation of photosensitizer behavior. This is easily understood in a very simplistic representation of cells as compartments of different physicochemical nature (e.g., aqueous-based cytosol versus lipophilic cell membranes). The cellular heterogeneity also affects the localization of the photosensitizer itself and rather than being isotropically distributed within the cell its localization will depend on its own physicochemical properties (charge, hydrophobicity, etc.) and how they match with different cellular locales. Some photosensitizers are known to localize in cell membranes, some in cytoplasm, and others are more organelle-specific for lysosome, mitochondria, nucleus, and so forth [17]. A photosensitizer that localizes in cell membranes may be reactive with unsaturated lipids or proteins that are not encountered by a photosensitizer that localizes in the cytosol. In addition to the heterogeneity in potential reactive substrates for excited photosensitizer, the concentrations of photosensitizer and substrates must be considered in terms of local concentration, rather than overall bulk concentration. For a photosensitizer that specifically localizes to the cell membrane, the local concentration of the photosensitizer can be orders of magnitude higher than that based on bulk volume and this can have a great influence on reaction mechanisms. It should be noted that oxygen, as an uncharged small molecule, is free to diffuse throughout the biological environment and is not constricted by such compartmentalization arguments.

In cellular systems the complex heterogeneity makes reaction mechanisms difficult to predict. In the simplest situation under normal atmosphere where there are few possibilities for direct reaction of T_1 with other substrates, the nonradiative deactivation of the T_1 state (reaction 9) will be dominated by energy transfer to oxygen to form $^1\Delta_g$, shown in reaction 10, as discussed above.

$$PS(T_1) \xrightarrow{k_d} PS(S_0) \tag{3.9}$$

$$PS(T_1) + O_2 \xrightarrow{k_d} PS(S_0) + ^1\Delta_g \tag{3.10}$$

This ideal photodynamic situation, where $^1\Delta_g$ is generated in high yield and no other competitive reactions occur, can be altered in the cellular environment. One practical problem that can arise in PDT is when the light is delivered at sufficiently high fluence rate to the target tissue such that the generation of $^1\Delta_g$ and its subsequent reaction in cells and tissue consumes oxygen at a rate that exceeds its replenishment from vascular supply. This photochemical oxygen depletion has been recognized as a problem in therapeutic scenarios and can be avoided simply by reducing the irradiance of the illuminating light. When only reactions 9 and 10 are in operation the effect of photochemical oxygen depletion is simply a reduction in the photodynamic effect, as less $^1\Delta_g$ is generated per photon absorbed. However, when other reactions are possible the distribution of reactivity may change as reaction 10 reduces in importance. Some other possible reactions can be considered below. If the photosensitizer localizes specifically to a compartment or organelle of the cell then its local concentration can be high enough such that the excited T_1 state can react with a neighboring ground state photosensitizer molecule. One possible reaction that has been observed for photosensitizers in cells is electron transfer, shown in reaction 11 below to form a radical ion pair [16].

$$PS(T_1) + PS(S_0) \xrightarrow{k_{et}} PS^{\cdot+} + PS^{\cdot-} \tag{3.11}$$

Photosensitizer radical cations (PS+) are relatively unreactive species but the semireduced radical (PS-) is capable of secondary electron transfer to other compounds, including oxygen, to form the superoxide anion radical, $O_2^{\cdot-}$, which could also contribute to downstream oxidation reactions.

$$PS^{\cdot-} + O_2 \xrightarrow{k_{et}} PS(S_0) + O_2^{-} \tag{3.12}$$

Reaction 12 is a far more probable reaction than direct electron transfer from the T_1 state to oxygen to form $O_2^{\cdot-}$. which cannot compete with energy transfer to form $^1\Delta_g$. Formation of $O_2^{\cdot-}$ by direct photosensitized electron transfer has been implicated in many photodynamic studies. but is probably erroneously assigned as reaction 12 is a more probable source for $O_2^{\cdot-}$.

The above reactions consider only processes that involve photosensitizer and oxygen. However, there are many other possible reactants in the cell that could react with the excited state photosensitizer, particularly proteins. Although unsaturated lipids are potential reactants for $^1\Delta_g$ and many free radicals that can initiate chain lipid peroxidation, they are unlikely targets for direct reaction with excited state photosensitizer. The hydrogen abstraction reaction that can take place between free radicals and unsaturated lipids is unlikely to occur for T_1 states of photosensitizer for a number of reasons. Such reactions occur from higher energy T_1 states that have

$n\pi^*$ configuration. Promotion of an electron to this type of excited state results in a more localized electron density on the heteroatom (O, N. S, etc.) and they are therefore free radical-like in nature.

$$PS + LH \xrightarrow{\ k_{abs}\ } PS^{\cdot}H + L\cdot \tag{3.13}$$

However, photodynamic agents are much lower in energy and have $\pi\pi^*$ configuration, where the electrons are delocalized in the excited state, the state is less radical in nature and hydrogen atom transfer is unlikely. However, electron transfer reactions are possible and both oxidative and reductive electron transfer reactions can occur.

$$PS + \left(T_1\right) + R \xrightarrow{\ k_{ox}\ } PS^{\cdot+} + R^{\cdot-} \tag{3.14}$$

$$PS + \left(T_1\right) + R \xrightarrow{\ k_{red}\ } PS^{\cdot-} + R^{+} \tag{3.15}$$

Thus, the distribution of the reaction pathways of the T_1 state depends on the relative rate constants for each reaction and the (local) concentration of the reactants. The overall rates of reaction of PS (T_1), and formation of products like $PS^{\cdot-}$ and $PS^{\cdot+}$ can be determined using transient absorption spectroscopy as these species have different absorption spectra that can be used as "fingerprints" for their involvement, as shown in Figure 3.6. Typical rate constants for each of the above processes can be considered to evaluate reaction probabilities under different conditions. The example chosen is rose bengal for which widespread data is available [18–20].

Reaction	PS products	Rate constant
^{3}RB	RB	$6.6 \times 10^4 \ \mathrm{s^{-1}}$
^{3}RB + O_2	RB, $^1\Delta_g$	$1.6 \times 10^9 \ \mathrm{M^{-1}s^{-1}}$
^{3}RB + RB	RB$^+$, RB$^-$	$7.6 \times 10^8 \ \mathrm{M^{-1}s^{-1}}$
^{3}RB + guanine	RB$^-$	$5.5 \times 10^7 \ \mathrm{M^{-1}s^{-1}}$
^{3}RB + NADH	RB$^-$	$4.9 \times 10^8 \ \mathrm{M^{-1}s^{-1}}$
PS (T_1) + ascorbate	RB$^-$	$2.4 \times 10^8 \ \mathrm{M^{-1}s^{-1}}$
PS$^-$+O_2	RB, O_2^-	$1.5 \times 10^8 \ \mathrm{M^{-1}s^{-1}}$

It should be noted that oxygen is highly critical regardless of the pathway followed. In analogy to radiation chemistry, oxygen is required to "fix" the oxidative damage. For example, the generation of a radical ion, $R^{\cdot-}$, is unlikely to lead to damage in the absence of oxygen to form $O2^-$. Oxygen is also required for chain lipid peroxidation where peroxyl radicals, formed by reaction of oxygen with the lipid radicals, are essential to propagate the chain [21]. Given that the presence of oxygen is required for relevant chemical damage, the most preferential route for the types of molecules used as photosensitizers in photodynamic applications will always be via $^1\Delta_g$ formation and a depletion of oxygen reduces the photodynamic effect.

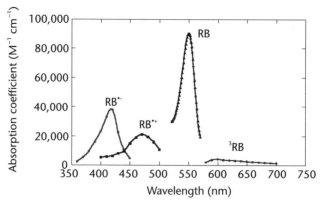

Figure 3.6 Absorption spectra of ground state RB, the excited triplet state (3RB), and semireduced (RB-) and semioxidized (RB+) radicals.

3.9 Rate Constants and Biological Reality

One must always exercise caution when using rate constants measured for simple bimolecular reactions in solution to postulate mechanistic pathways in biological samples. The influence of local concentrations of reactants was discussed above. For example, a hydrophobic photosensitizer that is localized in a membrane compartment will experience a very high local concentration of lipid and although the oxygen concentration may be higher in the lipid environment, its diffusion coefficient in the membrane may be smaller than water. To complicate matters, the $^1\Delta_g$ generated in the membrane may also encounter a very high local concentration of reactive lipids and proteins that drives reactions to occur, despite relatively low rate constants for bimolecular reaction in solution. Another obvious complication is when the photosensitizer is precomplexed to a potential reactant when activation occurs. Photodynamic agents that bind to DNA or proteins are good examples of this situation. Precomplexation via hydrophobic or ionic interactions places both species in close proximity such that diffusion is not required for encounter to occur and even kinetically improbable reactions can occur. Not only can complexation favor a particular reaction path, but it can also inhibit others. Such an example is the binding of various photodynamic agents to globular proteins where the binding site may protect the photosensitizer from encounter with other reactants, even oxygen. Benzoporphyrin derivative monoacid ring A (BPDMA) binds strongly to serum albumin resulting in a 10x longer triplet state than seen in solution on the absence of the protein [10].

3.10 Secondary Reactive Oxygen Species (ROS)

The above reactions have been considered in terms of primary reactions that occur from the photosensitizer excited states. However in considering the overall mechanism of cellular oxidation that results from photodynamic treatment one should also consider the secondary processes that occur after the illumination ceases. Research into photodynamic action in cells and tissue has focused on either the primary photoprocesses of the photosensitizer or on a variety of ultimate end points, such as cell death. The intermediary aspects of photodynamic action have received less attention and we will focus here on $^1\Delta_g$ and secondary reactive oxygen species (ROS), pathways of formation, and their relative contribution to overall cellular oxidation processes.

The maximum lifetime of $^1\Delta_g$ in cells is limited to a few microseconds at most, which severely limits the range of diffusion to react with possible substrate molecules to a few hundreds of nanometers, which is small in scale to cellular dimensions [5]. As mentioned previously, the lifetime of $^1\Delta_g$ is lengthened by an order of magnitude when H_2O is replaced by deuterated water (D_2O). In many model systems, a variety of chemical and biological outcomes are enhanced to a similar extent but this may not necessarily be the case in biological systems due to kinetic considerations. Replacement of H_2O with D_2O in cells will only lead to enhanced response if the lifetime of $^1\Delta_g$ is not already limited by reaction with cellular components. For example, if the shorter lifetimes mentioned above are indeed accurate for intracellular $^1\Delta_g$, the sum of the rate constants for reaction dominate the solvent-induced relaxation and extension of the latter rate constant will have negligible effect. Should the response be due to $^1\Delta_g$ escaping extracellularly before reaction, then a D_2O effect may indeed be observed. Thus, one must be careful in interpreting the effects of D_2O in biological systems.

In addition we must also be careful in attributing all photodynamic effects to the reactions of $^1\Delta_g$ in situations where this species is either detected via its phosphorescence emission or implicated by a positive D_2O effect. If this were the case all reactions would immediately cease a few microseconds after the activating light is turned off. There are various pathways to generation of secondary ROS that could have postillumination effects in photodynamic situations. From a purely chemical point of view there are products of the initial reactions of $^1\Delta_g$ that can initiate further oxidation reactions. These include membrane lipid hydroperoxides (LOOH) that are relatively unstable and can be broken down to form free radicals that cause further chain peroxidation that can seriously impact the cell. Photosensitizers that selectively act at various organelle locations can also lead to delayed biological responses that generate ROS. Mitochondrial damage can lead to a loss of function and an uncoupling of electron transport in oxidative phosphorylation, and the leakage of electrons can generate $O2^-$ and then hydrogen peroxide (H_2O_2) in the presence of the antioxidant enzyme superoxide dismutase (SOD). Primary photodynamic reactions often lead to an increase in intracellular calcium (Ca^{2+}) levels, an important signaling event. Other oxidative pathways that can be initiated include activation of phospholipase A2, lipoxygenase (LOX) and cyclooxygenase (COX) enzymes in response to membrane oxidation and Ca2+ increases, and these pathways can increase the peroxide burden in the cell and overall oxidative stress [21]. A further enzymatic process that can contribute to delayed oxidative damage is the activation of NADPH oxidase (NOX). This membrane-localized enzyme accepts an electron from an intracellular flavin donor and ultimately transfers the electron to molecular oxygen to form $O2^-$, which can also be converted to H_2O_2 by reaction with protons [22].

These secondary processes that generate other oxidative agents can extend the spatial and temporal range of photodynamic action in cells and tissue [5]. The diffusion distance of an ROS is inversely proportional to its lifetime in a given environment, with that latter dependent on its reactivity, unless it is an excited state like $^1\Delta_g$ with an inherent lifetime limit. In terms of reactivity of ROS, the highly reactive hydroxyl radical (HO·) and other -oxyl radicals (RO·) will not travel far from their site of generation whereas less reactive species like lipid hydroperoxides (LOOH), hydrogen peroxide (H_2O_2), peroxyl radicals (ROO·), and carbon-centered radicals (R·) can have effects at more distant sites and delayed in time with respect to their shorter-lived relatives. To further complicate matters, many of these species are interconvertible (e.g., the dismutation of the fairly unreactive $O2^-$ generates H_2O_2, which is also relatively unreactive but can be converted in a metal-catalyzed reaction to highly reactive HO· [21]).

Thus, less reactive, secondary ROS have the potential to spread oxidative damage in biological damage on a spatial and temporal scale. The scale of these effects in both dimensions can be seen on the oxidative stress produced in cell populations generated by photodynamic treatment.

Figure 3.7 shows the time-dependent increase in ROS generation measured following photodynamic treatment of cells containing the $^1\Delta_g$ photosensitizer, deuteroporphyrin (DP) using a derivative of the general oxidative stress probe dichloro-dihydro-fluorescein (DCF), which becomes fluorescent on intracellular oxidation. From this figure it can be appreciated that ROS generation continues for a long time following cessation of photodynamic treatment. This oxidation cannot be due to postillumination generation of $^1\Delta_g$. Thus, secondary routes to ROS generation occur in the treated cells that contribute to the overall cellular response to photodynamic treatment. Depending on the dose provided, the relative contribution of primary ($^1\Delta_g$) and secondary ROS to cellular responses may vary, with the former contributing more under high PDT dose conditions.

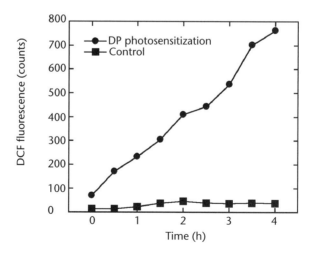

Figure 3.7 Delayed production of ROS, measured from intracellular DCF fluorescence following photosensitization of EMT6 murine sarcoma cells with 0.5 μM DP.

The situation is also complicated in the spatial dimension by secondary ROS processes. The maximum lifetime of $^1\Delta_g$ in a water-based biological environment of 4 μs, corresponds to a 2-D diffusion distance of 125 nm, which is small on the overall dimension of the cell. Thus, reactions of primary $^1\Delta_g$ are restricted to a small volume surrounding the photosensitizer location in the cell [5]. However, the observed effects of photodynamic treatment are cellwide. For example, DNA damage and mutagenesis is observed following treatment with nonnuclear photosensitizers where direct reaction of $^1\Delta_g$ with DNA is unlikely on the basis of diffusion distance [17, 23]. Similarly, mitochondrial photosensitization by $^1\Delta_g$ results in delayed oxidative stress via electron leakage from the respiratory chain.

The generation of secondary ROS leading to establishment of oxidative stress at the spatial level of the cell can also lead to effects at the extracellular level. The so-called bystander effect describes the generation of effects in cells that were not exposed to a primary insult, in this case a photodynamic treatment, but are in proximity to cells that were [24]. Such effects are often similar to those experienced in the targeted cells and can involve oxidative chemistry. Obviously, the mediation of bystander effects by the short-lived primary species, $^1\Delta_g$, cannot operate in this situation and longer-lived and less reactive species are required. Given the extracellular route and diffusion length required, less reactive secondary ROS such as H2O2 or LOOH products may be possible candidates for mediating bystander responses in cell populations and in tissue subjected to photodynamic treatment.

References

[1]   Khurana, M., et al., "Quantitative In Vitro Demonstration of Two-Photon Photodynamic Therapy Using Photofrin((R)) and Visudyne((R))," *Photochem. Photobiol.*, Vol. 83, 2007, pp. 1441–1448.

[2]   Smith, G., et al., "An Efficient Oxygen Independent Two-Photon Photosensitization Mechanism," *Photochem. Photobiol.*, Vol. 59, 1994, pp. 135–139.

[3]   Schmidt, R., "Photosensitized Generation of Singlet Oxygen," *Photochem. Photobiol.*, Vol. 82, 2006, pp. 1161–1177.

[4]   Redmond, R. W., and J. N. Gamlin, "A Compilation of Singlet Oxygen Yields from Biologically Relevant Molecules," *Photochem. Photobiol.*, Vol. 70, 1999, pp. 391–475.

[5]   Redmond, R. W., and I. E. Kochevar, "Spatially Resolved Cellular Responses to Singlet Oxygen," *Photochem. Photobiol.*, Vol. 82, 2006, pp. 1178–1186.

[6]   Foote, C. S., "Definition of Type I and Type II Photosensitized Oxidation," *Photochem Photobiol*, Vol. 54, 1991, pp. 659.

[7]   Girotti, A. W., "Photosensitized Oxidation of Membrane Lipids: Reaction Pathways, Cytotoxic Effects, and Cytoprotective Mechanisms," *J. Photochem. Photobiol. B*, Vol. 63, 2001, pp. 103–113.

[8]   Davies, M. J., "Singlet Oxygen-Mediated Damage to Proteins and Its Consequences," *Biochem. Biophys. Res. Commun.*, Vol. 305, 2003, pp. 761–770.

[9]   Cadet, J., et al., "Singlet Oxygen Oxidation of Isolated and Cellular DNA: Product Formation and Mechanistic Insights," *Photochem. Photobiol.*, Vol. 82, 2006, pp. 1219–1225.

[10] Aveline, B. M., T., Hasan, and R. W. Redmond, "The Effects of Aggregation, Protein Binding and Cellular Incorporation on the Photophysical Properties of Benzoporphyrin Derivative Monoacid Ring A (BPDMA)," *J. Photochem. Photobiol. B*, Vol. 30, 1995, pp. 161–169.

[11] Andersen, L. K., and P. R. Ogilby, "Time-Resolved Detection of Singlet Oxygen in a Transmission Microscope," *Photochem. Photobiol.*, Vol. 73, 2001, pp. 489–492.

[12] Niedre, M., M. S. Patterson, and B. C. Wilson, "Direct Near-Infrared Luminescence Detection of Singlet Oxygen Generated by Photodynamic Therapy in Cells In Vitro and Tissues In Vivo," *Photochem. Photobiol.*, Vol. 75, 2002, pp. 382–391.

[13] Skovsen, E., et al., "Lifetime and Diffusion of Singlet Oxygen in a Cell," *J. Phys. Chem. B*, Vol. 109, 2005, pp. 8570–8573.

[14] Zebger, I., et al., "Direct Optical Detection of Singlet Oxygen from a Single Cell," *Photochem. Photobiol.*, Vol. 79, 2004, pp. 319–322.

[15] Jarvi, M. T., et al., "Singlet Oxygen Luminescence Dosimetry (SOLD) for Photodynamic Therapy: Current Status, Challenges and Future Prospects," *Photochem. Photobiol.*, Vol. 82, 2006, pp. 1198–1210.

[16] Aveline, B. M., R. M. Sattler, and R. W. Redmond, "Environmental Effects on Cellular Photosensitization: Correlation of Phototoxicity Mechanism with Transient Absorption Spectroscopy Measurements," *Photochem. Photobiol.*, Vol. 68, 1998, pp. 51–62.

[17] Oleinick, N. L., and H. H. Evans, "The Photobiology of Photodynamic Therapy: Cellular Targets and Mechanisms," *Radiat. Res.*, Vol. 150, 1998, pp. S146–156.

[18] Lambert, C. R., and I. E. Kochevar, "Does Rose Bengal Triplet Generate Superoxide Anion?," *J. Am. Chem. Soc.*, Vol. 118, 1996, pp. 3297–3298.

[19] Lambert, C. R., and I. E. Kochevar, "Electron Transfer Quenching of the Rose Bengal Triplet State," *Photochem. Photobiol.*, Vol. 66, 1997, pp. 15–25.

[20] Lee, P. C., and M. A. Rodgers, "Laser Flash Photokinetic Studies of Rose Bengal Sensitized Photodynamic Interactions of Nucleotides and DNA," *Photochem. Photobiol.*, Vol. 45, 1987, pp. 79–86.

[21] Halliwell, B., and J. M. C. Gutteridge, Free Radicals in Biology and Medicine, Third Edition, New York: Oxford University Press, 2007.

[22] Bedard, K., and K. H. Krause, "The NOX Family of ROS-Generating NADPH Oxidases: Physiology and Pathophysiology," *Physiol. Rev.*, Vol. 87, 2007, pp. 245–313.

[23] Ouedraogo, G. D., and R. W. Redmond, "Secondary Reactive Oxygen Species Extend the Range of Photosensitization Effects in Cells: DNA Damage Produced Via Initial Membrane Photosensitization," *Photochem. Photobiol.*, Vol. 77, 2003, pp. 192–203.

[24] Dahle, J., et al., "Bystander Effects in Cell Death Induced by Photodynamic Treatment UVA Radiation and Inhibitors of ATP Synthesis," *Photochem. Photobiol.*, Vol. 73, 2001, pp. 378–387.

CHAPTER 4

Pharmaceutical and Biological Considerations in 5-Aminolevulinic Acid in PDT

Norbert Lange

4.1 Introduction

The fundamental building block of most red-absorbing, naturally occurring photosensitizers (see Chapter 1) is 5-aminolevulinic acid (5-ALA). Mammals, plants, and bacteria assemble this low molecular compound to produce porphyrins, chlorins, and (iso-) bacteriochlorins, respectively. These "pigments of life," as termed appropriately by Alan R. Battersby, a pioneer in the chemistry of living systems [1], fulfill essential biological functions such as oxygen transport (heme), electron transport, phase II metabolism (cytochrome c), and photosynthesis [2]. Despite relatively large amounts of these tetrapyrrols produced daily, naturally occurring photosensitization is relatively rare. Nature has provided us (and other organisms) with powerful protection mechanisms by (1) introducing metal ions into the central nucleus of the porphyrinic structure (one has to take into account that first-generation photosensitizers in PDT have been prepared by primary removal of the central metal ion, iron, or magnesium in the cases of heme and chlorophyll a, respectively) and (2) tightly controlling the enzyme-mediated formation of 5-ALA itself.

However, sometimes these control mechanisms run out-of-control and signs of skin photosensitization can be observed. One commonly cited example is porphyria cutanea tarda [3, 4]. This disease is characterized by an increased activity of 5-ALA synthase and porphobilinogen deaminase (see below). Besides increased skin photosensitivity, clinical signs of this disease are red fluorescent urine and marked fluorescence in the teeth. The reason for the phenomena is a flaw in the body's heme-making machinery that suddenly provides excess substrates for heme biosynthesis. This, in turn, leads to the accumulation of protoporphyrin IX, (PpIX) the penultimate precursor of heme (see Figure 4.1).

In contrast to all other intermediates in heme biosynthesis, PpIX is a decent photosensitizer that is inactivated by the incorporation of ferrous iron. Therefore, one could deduce that providing excess 5-ALA (or other heme precursors) leads to the temporary accumulation of photosensitizers and should be suitable for photodynamic purposes. Indeed, exposing plants to exogenous 5-ALA has been shown to result in the overproduction of endogenous photosensitizers, and has

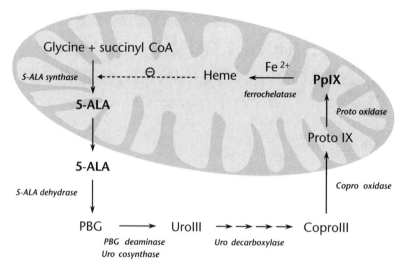

Figure 4.1 Heme biosynthetic pathway in mammals. 5-ALA synthase catalyzes the condensation of glycine and succinyl CoA into one molecule of 5-ALA. This is followed by the asymmetric condensation of two 5-ALA molecules by 5-ALA dehydrase into one molecule of porphobilinogen (PBG). An enzymatic cascade then converts four molecules of PBG into a tetrapyrrole ring that undergoes decarboxylations and oxidations, leading to the formation of PpIX. Ferrochelatase inserts a ferrous iron (Fe^{2+}) into PpIX to produce heme. The formation of 5-ALA is tightly controlled via a negative feedback mechanism exerted by heme on the expression of 5-ALA synthase. UroIII = uroporphyrinogen III, CoproIII = coproporphyrinogen III, Proto IX = protoporphyrinogen IX.

therefore been used for herbicidal purposes in agriculture but without commercial success [5]. However, the intermittent accumulation of PpIX due to metabolic alterations in heme biosynthesis in mammalian cells can be used for photodynamic and photodiagnostic purposes.

Following preliminary investigations by Malik and Lugaci [6] on 5-ALA-mediated photodynamic inactivation of erythroleukaemic cells, Kennedy et al. suggested the use of 5-ALA for the treatment of superficial skin disorders [7, 8]. Their initial setup was simple and efficient. A cream containing 20% (w/w) of 5-ALA was applied to 80 lesions of basal cell carcinomas for 3 to 6 h. Then, the lesions were irradiated using a 500W lamp equipped with a 600-nm long-pass filter. This led to clearance in 90% of all cases. The simplicity, as well as the marked selectivity of PpIX generation in neoplastic tissue following administration of 5-ALA, has made this compound the most studied agent in PDT (besides this, the fact that 5-ALA is a naturally occurring compound might also have contributed to this phenomenon.). Indeed, 5-ALA-mediated PDT can be considered one of the most selective treatments of neoplastic tissue. Dermatology is probably the medical field in which topical 5-ALA-PDT has been the most employed. However, the potential use of 5-ALA-mediated PDT goes far beyond dermatologic applications. This approach has been also assessed in gynecology, urology, gastroenterology, and pulmonology for the treatment of malignant conditions such as brain, vulval, vaginal, bladder, or aerodigestive tumors, as well as early-stage lung cancer [9–18] (see Figure 4.2). Furthermore, the fluorescent properties of PpIX have also been exploited for the fluorescence diagnosis of conditions that require histological surveillance but are barely visible. Thus, targeted biopsies or resections have shown advantages in the case of malignant glioma [9], carcinoma in situ (CIS) of the bladder, and early-stage lung carcinoma [10], as well as in a premalignant condition called Barrett's esophagus [11, 12]. However, more recently, 5-ALA-mediated PDT has been proposed in other therapeutic (e.g., rheumatology, bacterial inactivation) and cosmetic areas (skin rejuvenation, acne treatment, and hair removal) [13, 14].

The purpose of this chapter is to provide the reader with the fundamentals of 5-ALA-mediated PDT and photodiagnosis. The relevant clinical indications will be discussed elsewhere in this book. Following an introduction into heme biosynthesis, the main factors that potentially lead to the selective PpIX accumulation in neoplastic tissue upon exogenous administration of 5-ALA will be described. After the description of the biopharmaceutical as well as pharmaceutical properties of 5-ALA, concepts that have been shown to improve this treatment strategy will be presented.

4.2 Heme Biosynthesis

The chemical structure of PpIX, the photosensitizer used in 5-ALA-mediated PDT, was first disclosed in 1934 [15, 16]. However, its building blocks were still essentially unknown at that time. Years later, Shemin and Rittenberg were able to provide experimental evidence that glycine is one of the early compounds in heme biosynthesis [17]. By swallowing 66 grams of [^{15}N] glycine over three days, the ^{15}N content in Shemin's heme rose quickly to a maximum. Indeed, in most mammalian tissues (exceptions are red blood cells that lack a nucleus and most of their mitochondria, as well as the lens of the human eye), heme is generated in eight distinct steps (see Figure 4.1). Four of these enzymatically controlled reactions take place in the mitochondria and the other four in the cytoplasm. In the first step, which takes place in the inner mitochondrial membrane, 5-ALA is formed by the condensation of glycine and succinyl CoA (in plants and microorganisms, the initial step is the use of glutamic acid to assemble 5-ALA) Based on daily excretion of heme-related compounds, one can calculate that more than 200 mg of 5-ALA are produced daily in an adult human body. This step is catalyzed by the folic acid-containing enzyme 5-ALA synthase (5-ALA-S, E.C. 2.3.1.37, the enzyme classification numbers have been included to make it easier to get more detailed information on the corresponding enzyme in online databases such as http://www.brenda.uni-koeln.de/) in six consecutive reaction steps. In mammalian cells, two different genes control the expression of two isoforms of this enzyme, 5-ALA S1 and 5-ALA S2 [18, 19]. While the expression of the latter is specific to erythroid cells, the expression of the former is ubiquitous. The activity of this housekeeping isoform, 5-ALA S1, can be directly inhibited by heme in nonerythroid cells [20]. However, the suppression of 5-ALA S1 transcription, thereby decreasing 5-ALA S1 mRNA half-life and blocking the transport of 5-ALA S1's precursor protein have been identified as the main negative feedback mechanism to control the formation of excess 5-ALA and consequent accumulation of PpIX in normal cells [21–23].

Following their translocation into the cytosol, two molecules of 5-ALA are then condensed nonsymmetrically to give porphobilinogen with the participation of

5-ALA dehydrase (5-ALA-D; E.C. 4.2.1.24; even without any further enzyme-catalyzed action, this tetrapyrrolic key compound in heme biosynthesis will form different fluorescent porphyrins, although in much lower yields). The activity of 5-ALA-D is Zn^{2+}-dependent and can be inhibited by numerous metal ions. Increased accumulation of 5-ALA in the blood and the urine are clinical symptoms of lead poisoning [24, 25].

In a third step, through a concerted action of two enzymes, PBG-D deaminase (E.C. 4.3.1.8) and Uroporphyrinogen III cosynthase (E.C: 4.2.1.75), the characteristic tetrapyrrolic skeleton is formed. First, PBG-D assembles four identical PBG molecules in a head-to-tail manner. Then, under the action of uroporphyrinogen III cosynthase, asymmetrically substituted uroporphyrinogen III is produced (in principle, 15 isomers are possible using four asymmetrically substituted PBG molecules. PpIX was the ninth isomer in Fischer's list of possible porphyrins resulting from heme biosynthesis). Without this intervention, hydroxybilane would be released leading to the formation of uroporphyrinogen I. However, the cosynthase enables the formation of an asymmetric molecule in which the methyl substituents in ring D are inverted with respect to rings A, B, and C.

After the formation of the fundamental tetrapyrrolic skeleton, uroporphyrinogen III is further processed through a couple of enzymatic oxidations. First, all of the acetic acid side chains are decarboxylated by uroporphyrinogen III decarboxylase (E.C. 4.1.1.37) to form methyl groups leading to coproporphyrinogen III. This last is then translocated into the intramitochondrial membrane space. This process seems to be tightly controlled by the action of the peripheral benzodiazipin receptor (PBR) located at the outer mitochondrial membrane [26]. Coproporphyrinogen oxidase (E.C. 1.3.3.3), loosely bound to the inner mitochondrial membrane, mediates the decarboxylation and oxidation of the two propionate substituents on rings A and B, respectively. This strongly oxygen-dependent process results in the formation of the 18Π electron system that causes the characteristic absorption and emission spectra of porphyrins. Up to this point, the synthetic pathway of porphyrins is identical in plants and mammals. However, at this point in plants, magnesium is inserted into the tetrapyrrolic nucleus; in mammals, ferrous iron is used under the influence of the enzyme ferrochelatase (E.C. 4.99.1.1) during the final phase of heme assembly (in cephalopoda, such as sepia and octopus, Cu^{2+} is inserted instead of Fe^{2+}, causing the blue appearance of blood in these animals).

4.3 Selective PpIX Formation in Neoplastic Tissue

In most organisms, to prevent excess porphyrin production, 5-ALA biosynthesis is tightly controlled by several mechanisms, including the negative feedback control mentioned in the previous section. However, exogenously administered 5-ALA bypasses this regulatory step, thus leading to the temporarily increased production of heme and its precursors. The formation of each of these intermediates is preliminarily limited by the activity of the respective enzyme and the substrate concentration within the cell and its intimate surrounding. Although temporarily increased PpIX formation subsequent to 5-ALA exposure can be observed in nearly all nucleated cells, PpIX accumulation seems to take place predominantly in neoplastic cells. In terms of tumor-to-normal tissue (T/N) ratio of formed PpIX, 5-ALA-mediated PDT can be considered one of the most selective cancer treatments available today. Contrasts from 10:1 up to 90:1 have been reported depending on the pathologic condition, applied drug dose, and time post-administration [27].

Since the first reports of 5-ALA-induced PpIX, many investigations have been carried out to determine the main mechanisms that underlie this extraordinary selectivity. Even though our current knowledge of heme biosynthesis is still limited, from a strictly formal kinetic point of view, the slowest step between the uptake of 5-ALA and formation of PpIX must be faster than the transformation of PpIX into heme to attain an accumulation of the photoactive compound. Furthermore, this mechanism has to be prominent in diseased tissue as compared to the healthy counterpart. Table 4.1 lists potential factors that might lead to the preferential accumulation of PpIX in neoplastic tissue. Most likely, the observed tumor selectivity of 5-ALA-mediated PpIX cannot be attributed to one sole factor, but to a complex interaction of several factors that might, furthermore, vary based on the type of disease, its stage and grade, its location, and the route of administration.

4.3.1   Heme Biosynthesis and Altered PpIX Formation

Until today, most studies related to selective 5-ALA-induced PpIX accumulation in neoplastic cells have been carried out with respect to alterations in heme biosynthesis. Gibson et al. have determined the uptake of ^{14}C 5-ALA in two human and two rodent tumor cell lines [28, 29]. Since no significantly different uptake rates have been observed, the authors have attributed differences in PpIX formation to metabolic alterations such as increased PBG-D activity in some cell lines. Also, others have found increased activity of "PpIX-preceding" enzymes in tumoral cell lines. Comparing the profiles of enzymatic activity in rat hepatic tumor cells to their nor-

Table 4.1   Factors Affecting Selective PpIX Accumulation

Global Factor	Specific Factor
Altered metabolic turnover in heme biosynthesis	Enhanced activity of pre-PpIX enzymes
	Decreased activity of post-PpIX enzymes
	Benzodiazepine receptor expression
Altered cellular properties of neoplasms	5-ALA uptake
	Confluence
	Proliferation
	Differentiation
	Mitochondrial content
	Cell density
	Iron pool/transferrin receptor
Environmental factors	pH
	Temperature
	Lymphatic drainage
	Tissular pressure
	Vascularization
	Tissue integrity

mal counterparts of epithelial origin, Kondo et al. found increased PBG-S activity and decreased ferrochelatase activity in neoplastic cells [30]. Navone et al. have reported that the activities of 5-ALA-D, PBG-D, as well as uroporphyrinogen III decarboxylase were higher in biopsies obtained from mouse and human breast cancer as compared to normal mammary tissue, resulting in 20 times higher levels of PpIX in the neoplastic tissue [31–33]. Such findings are in agreement with other reports in the literature. High PBG-D activities were found in malignant cells, non-malignant cells, and fast-replicating cells from regenerating liver [34–36]. Increased PBG-D activity and decreased ferrochelatase activity was also revealed for malignant and precancerous esophageal tissue as compared to the normal esophageal wall [37, 38]. However, the ratio of these activities does not appear to correlate with the degree of PpIX accumulation [37]. Furthermore, Hilf et al. succeeded in transfecting human breast cancer MCF-7 and mesothelioma H-MESO-1 cells with plasmid vectors encoding for PBG-D [39]. By this procedure, PBG-D activity was increased by a factor of 2.5 and 4, respectively, as compared to the wild-type counterparts. However, no statistically significant different PpIX accumulation was observed upon exogenous exposure to 5-ALA.

In studies on three different bladder cancer cell lines and one normal, immortalized bladder cell line carried out by Krieg and coworkers, PBG-D activity seemed to play only a minor role with respect to differences in PpX formation [40]. In these studies, PpIX formation correlated better with ferrochelatase activity and iron availability. However, the lower differentiated cell line still showed increased PBG-D activity in parallel with reduced ferrochelatase activity. These results are in agreement with a later study of the same group on human colonic cells [41]. The group chose three colon carcinoma (CaCo2, HT29, SW480) and stromal fibroblasts to mimic important aspects of malignant mucosa of the GI tract. This group, which found that tumor-specific PPIX accumulation is strongly influenced, observed differences in activity between the PPIX-producing PBGD and the PPIX-converting ferrochelatase when compared to fibroblasts.

The involvement of the proteasome, another factor that might influence enzymatic activities related to heme biosynthesis, has been badly neglected so far. This large, multiprotein construct situated in the cytoplasm and nucleus is responsible for endogenous protein degradation. The proteasome-mediated ubiquitin-dependent proteolysis is a housekeeping mechanism that turns off specific protein functions at the right time, in the right place, and in a nonreversible manner [42]. When it malfunctions, the altered degradation of cell regulators by this proteolytic machinery may well contribute to the unchecked proliferation in neoplastic cells. Recently, Malik and coworkers have addressed the question of whether decreased proteasome activity can explain the increased PpIX accumulation in neoplastic tissue [43, 44]. They found that the inhibition of proteasome activity by clasto lactacastin B-lactome or hemin indeed decreased the specific degradation of PBG-D. Furthermore, inhibition of 5-ALA-D, which not only has a role in heme biosynthesis but also regulates the activity of the proteasome, decreased the intracellular PBG-D pool and in turn reduced the sensitivity of challenged cells to 5-ALA PDT. However, no studies specifically focusing on the degradation [26] of PBG-D in neoplastic tissue have been reported in the literature. Therefore, the further elucidation of proteasome-related mechanisms with respect to 5-ALA-induced PpIX accumulation might be necessary in the future.

Once the cytoplasmatic assembly of coproporphyrinogen is finished, this complex has to cross the mitochondrial membrane to be converted into PpIX and subsequently into heme. Most likely, several recognition sites are involved in this translocation. Recently, the benzodiazepin receptor (PBR) has been identified as a key element in this transport [26]. PBR has been shown to bind with high affinity to PpIX and other porphyrin-like molecules, [26, 45, 46]. It is abundantly expressed on the outer mitochondrial membrane in neoplastic cells from the colon, brain, ovary, and liver. These cells are known for their predominant accumulation of PpIX subsequent to administration of 5-ALA [47–51].

The role of PBR in 5-ALA-induced PpIX accumulation in ARA 2J cells was recently addressed by Mesenholler et al [26]. In their experiments, inhibition of PBR by 1-(2-chlorophenyl)-N-methyl-N-(1-methylpropyl)-3-isoquinolinecarboxamide, dipyridamole, or 7-(dimethylcarbamoloxy)-6-phenylpyrrolo-[2,1-d]benzothiazepine as competitive ligands to PBR resulted in a significant decrease in PpIX formation.

Therefore, the abundant expression of PBR and its high affinity for PpIX may well explain an increased PpIX accumulation in neoplastic cells, even in the absence of alterations of the activity of enzymes in heme biosynthesis. In addition to these factors directly related to heme biosynthesis, other factors might additively or synergistically be involved in the 5-ALA-mediated PpIX formation in neoplastic cells.

4.3.2 Characteristics of Neoplastic Cells and Altered PpIX Formation

The introduction of ferrous iron into the porphyrinic nucleus of PpIX leads to the ultimate formation of photoinactive heme. As two key players are involved in this step, not only the activity of ferrochelatase (see above), but also the availability of iron has to be taken into account.

Proteins containing iron control many metabolic processes involved in energy balance and DNA synthesis in cells. Therefore, iron is crucial to maintain cell survival. Furthermore, it is essential in the expression and regulation of signals that control cell cycle progression [52–54]. In the plasma of vertebrates, two atoms of Fe(II) are bound with high affinity by serum transferrin (Tf). The affinity of Tf for iron declines as a function of decreasing pH (see below). A majority of cells in an organism acquire iron from Tf. Following binding of iron-laden Tf to the transferrin receptor I, iron is acquired by receptor-mediated endocytosis. Then, the escalating acidification in the endosomal/lysosomal milieu to a pH of about 5.5 triggers the release of iron from Tf. Iron is then transported through the endosomal membrane to enter a poorly defined "intracellular iron pool." From this pool, iron can be used or stored in ferritin for later use. There is some experimental evidence for lower iron concentrations in neoplastic tissue as compared to normal tissue. These observations were predominantly attributed to low extracellular pH values, leading to the premature release of iron from Tf [55–58]. Furthermore, in some cases, macrophage-induced withdrawal of iron has been discussed to be a part of host defense mechanisms against unwanted cell proliferation [58]. In general, iron uptake mechanisms seem not to differ between normal and neoplastic cells. However, it has been demonstrated that neoplastic cells, dispose of higher TfR1 levels and take up iron faster [59–65]. These findings have led to the use of iron chelators as anticancer agents due to the apparently greater affinity of cancer cells for this essential element [66, 67]. However, the higher total iron concentration on neoplastic cells does not necessarily mean a higher availability for ferrochelatase-mediated incorporation into PpIX. Studies in reticulocytes of rodent origin have demonstrated that ferritin-bound iron is only poorly incorporated into heme biosynthesis [68–71]. Furthermore, due to the increased nucleic size and, thus, decreased extranuclear volume in neoplastic cells, it is more likely that iron is directly delivered to the nucleus for mitosis rather than to the mitochondria to maintain heme synthesis [72]. Finally, others have found no correlation between expression of TfR1 and PpIX formation following incubation with 5-ALA in cells of neoplastic origin [35, 54].

The growing state of cells is another factor that potentially influences iron availability. Independently, Moan and coworkers and Krieg and coworkers observed an increase in PpIX formation with increasing cell density, from subconfluency to confluency; this increase was characterized by a decreasing iron pool [73]. These observations are in agreement with the findings of Pourzand et al. [74]. In their experiments, normal human skin fibroblast variations in the free-iron pool strongly correlated with the PpIX accumulation following exposure to 5-ALA. Furthermore, confluent cells were less susceptible than subconfluent cells to removal of freely available iron by EDTA.

Due to the location of PpIX synthesis, the total mitochondrial content could also influence the sensitivity of cells to exposure to 5-ALA. Gibson et al. have measured the PpIX formation and the mitochondrial content in different cell lines and established a good correlation between these parameters [75]. More recently, however, the PpIX formation in central and peripheral arteries could not be correlated with the mitochondrial content following systemic administration of 5-ALA to rats [76].

Differences in 5-ALA uptake between neoplastic and normal cells have also been discussed to explain the preferential accumulation of PpIX in the former ones. Predominately due to their high metabolic turnover, neoplastic cells often display increased need for nutrients, such as amino acids. For most substances, the uptake is accomplished by endocytosis or active transporter systems. Transporter systems for amino acids are often abundantly expressed in neoplastic cells [77, 78]. Furthermore, in order to keep pace with the increased demand for amino acids, expression of transporter isoforms, absent in normal cells, has been reported. Therefore, due to the high similarity of 5-ALA with some amino acids, an educated guess might be that 5-ALA is at least in part recognized by such amino acid transporters. Thus, the cellular uptake of 5-ALA could be favored in neoplastic cells and consequently explain the preferential accumulation of PpIX.

Recently, contributions from biochemistry and molecular biology have improved our knowledge of 5-ALA uptake mechanisms. They have been specifically studied in cells originating from the biliary duct, colon, choroids plexus, brain synaptosomes, and intestinal tissue. Uptake mechanisms seem to vary based upon the characteristics of the particular cell line and its origin. Cells from a human extrahepatic carcinoma selectively transport 5-ALA through the action of intestinal transport peptide transporter 1 (PEPT1) in a pH-dependent manner [79]. Furthermore, structurally related compounds such as γ-aminobutyric acid (GABA), glycine, or L-glutamic acid did not compete with the active transport of 5-ALA. However, other compounds such as dipeptides or cefadroxil strongly inhibited the uptake of 5-ALA [80]. In contrast, β-amino acids, taurine, and GABA competitively inhibited the transport of 5-ALA in cells derived from human adenocarcinoma. Furthermore, transporters of {insert math symbol here} -alanine played a major role in this context [80]. These studies are in agreement with Langer et al., who show the involvement of glycine in amelanotic carcinomas [81].

Studies performed in WiDr adenocarcinoma cells have shown increased PpIX formation with increasing 5-ALA doses up to a concentration of about 1 mM [80]. Then, a plateau was reached. The subsequently deduced Michaelis-Menten constant of about 10 mM permits the assumption that, in these cells, transmembrane transport is not the rate-limiting step in 5-ALA-mediated PpIX synthesis. This is in agreement with Krieg et al. who, after metabolic characterization of different cell lines, concluded that PpIX buildup cannot be explained by differences in 5-ALA uptake [41]. With respect to PpIX formation, a minor role of different uptake rates between normal and neoplastic cells is further supported by the observation that the transport of more lipophilic 5-ALA esters such as hexylaminolevulinate (see below) is not inhibited by 5-ALA's transport inhibitors, but shows identical or increased selectivity in vivo [82–84].

4.3.3 Tumor Environment and Morphology and Altered Heme Biosynthesis

In recent years, our knowledge with respect to the genomic and proteomic alterations that lead to microscopic and macroscopic changes in established and developing tumors has substantially increased [85, 86]. Macroscopic manifestations of such environmental changes include increased angiogenic activity, interstitial pressure, and temperature. Furthermore, alterations in proteolytic activity and tissue architecture as well as changes in pH, hypoxia, expression of cytokines, and tumor-associated proteins can be observed in the microenvironment of tumors.

5-ALA-PDT has been extensively used in dermatology (see Chapter 23). After topical administration, drugs are generally retained in and on the skin surface for a certain amount of time. Compounds of higher molecular weight than 500 daltons have inherently low permeability through the skin [87]. The top layer of the epidermis, the stratum corneum (SC), is composed of dead cells. It is a few microns thick and functions as the main protection against influences of the environment. Due to its composition of approximately 40% protein, 40% water, and 20% lipids, the SC is rather impermeable. Small molecules can cross this outermost layer via passive diffusion, through transcellular, intercellular, or appendageal pathways. While diffusion through the viable epidermal layers into the blood circulation is only limited for very lipophilic and high molecular weight compounds, the penetration through the SC represents the rate-limiting step for most drugs following topical administration [88]. The loss or alteration in the integrity of the skin's barrier function associated with the clinical signs of skin cancer, actinic keratosis, or psoriasis facilitates 5-ALA penetration into the lesion and increases the generation of PpIX. On the other hand, 5-ALA's relatively high hydrophilicity may prevent its penetration into hyperkeratotic lesions and favor its efflux from deep nodular lesions into the local microcirculation [89–92].

In transgenic mice with rapidly growing hyperplasia, dysplasia, and cancer, the integrity of the SC and other epidermal layers changes dramatically as compared to the corresponding wild-type phenotype [93]. Furthermore, UV light-induced alterations of the skin integrity considerably increase PpIX formation [94, 95]. This loss and subsequent increased uptake of 5-ALA following topical administration can be reasonably simulated by tape-stripping to remove the SC from the skin of nude mice and increase the uptake of 5-ALA and the formation of PpIX by a factor of three [96, 97]. Furthermore, an increased systemic uptake has been observed. In 2002, Tsai et al. showed in vivo that PpIX formation increases as a function of the skin's barrier disruption according to an E_{max} model [93].

Investigations of 5-ALA in other organs show an extraordinarily selective PpIX buildup in neoplastic tissue. Tissue morphology plays an important role as in urology, where tumor-to-normal tissue ratios between 8 and 2,410 have been reported for PpIX accumulation [98]. It has been shown that 5-ALA-mediated fluorescence diagnosis is particularly useful for the detection of carcinoma in situ (CIS) of the bladder. McKenny et al. have shown that although CIS often shows normal urothelial thickness, it shows loss of tissue polarity and crowding of denuded urothelium [99]. Mitotic features associated with disorganized architecture and cellular dyscohesion can be observed in CIS by histopathological examination [100]. Scanning electron microscopy of transitional cell carcinomas revealed rounded cells with pleomorphic microvilli [101, 102]. Hyperplasic lesions, responsible for false positives in 5-ALA-mediated photodiagnosis of bladder cancer, show similar tissue characteristics.

Another example of tissue alterations associated with disease is glioblastomas. Healthy human [103] brain is well protected against environmental fluctuations in the blood by the blood-brain-barrier (BBB) and the blood cerebrospinal fluid barrier. The exchange of nutrients between the blood and the brain is tightly controlled by transporter systems and receptors located at the luminal and antiluminal membranes. However, the formation of disorganized neovascularization associated with the increased angiogenic activity in brain tumors often leads to the disruption of the BBB. Indeed, 5-ALA-mediated fluorescence detection to delineate malignant tissue during brain surgery has been shown to significantly prolong patient survival due to improved tumor resection [104]. In experimental animal models, 5-ALA-mediated PDT has been tested for the treatment of glioblastoma [105–110]. Preferential accumulation with tumor-to-normal brain ratios of approximately 6:1 was found. A significantly higher uptake of 5-ALA in tumor tissue in a rat C6 glioma model was reported by Obwegeser et al. [110]. The highest tumor-to-normal tissue ratio of 1.8:1 for 5-ALA was reported about 15 minutes after systemic administration. However, it should be pointed out that, as for metabolic alterations, the loss of tissue integrity and biological barrier function can probably not fully explain the preferential PpIX accumulation in brain, bladder, and skin cancer.

Besides its role in perfusion-related remodeling of tissue, angiogenesis is often associated with regional hyperthermia [103]. The increase in regional temperature was in 2003 confirmed by thermographic methods in human breast cancer [111]. These studies revealed a correlation between microvessel density and the temperature. In addition to its diagnostic use in breast cancer screening, thermography has been proposed for other medical indications such as neurology, vascular disorders, rheumatic disease, and skin cancer, all of which are indications for known selective PpIX formation [112]. In a recent thermographic study on the detection of bladder cancer, temperature differences ranging from $0.5°\,C–1.6°\,C$ were observed between tumoral and healthy urothelium [113]. A slightly enhanced temperature will further boost the production of PpIX upon administration of 5-ALA [80, 114–120]. It has been shown that the PGB-D-catalyzed dimerization of 5-ALA is two times higher at $45°\,C$ as compared to $37°\,C$ [121]. Moan et al. have calculated the activation energies for the uptake of 5-ALA, the formation of porphobilinogen and PpIX in vitro, to be 42 kJ/mol, 71 kJ/mol, and 54 kJ/mol, respectively [118]. In normal human and mouse skin, the uptake of 5-ALA was found to be independent from the temperature and the activation energy for PpIX formation in vivo was calculated to be 71 kJ/mol. Assuming that the Arrhenius equation applies an increase in temperature of $1.6°\,C$ will lead to a nearly threefold increase in the rate of PpIX formation at body temperature.

Larger tumors have been shown to differ significantly with respect to their environmental pH [121]. Microregions of larger tumors and small tumor nodules often reside in an acidic environment. This can be attributed to the increased production of lactic acid in cells present at distances $>200\,\mu$m from a functional blood supply. In response to the subsequent hypoxia, cells are forced to maintain their energy balance through anaerobic glycolysis. Although several authors reported optimal PpIX formation at physiological pH in cell culture [122–125], the influence of the pH is less pronounced in intact tissue [126]. However, the low extracellular pH in tumors can potentially influence the pharmacokinetic profile of PpIX itself. Since protonated PpIX is more lipophilic than unprotonated, it will bind more strongly to lipid membranes and, thus, display reduced clearance [127]. Furthermore, lipophilic forms of protonated PpIX are more likely to form aggregates [128, 129]. Their elimination from the tissue is further dominated by (1) an adequate lymphatic drainage, and (2) the presence of macrophages. Thus, the reduced lymphatic drainage could contribute to a poor elimination of formed PpIX.

4.4   Pharmaceutical and Biopharmaceutical Considerations

In and of itself, the outstanding selectivity of 5-ALA to induce PpIX in neoplastic tissue does not automatically make this a potent drug candidate for PDT treatments. Other parameters have to be considered in order to "get the right drug to the right place at the right dose and at the right time." If one considers that 5-ALA represents the discovery of a lead structure or a "hit" in the curriculum of a R&D process, the following steps will include preformulation studies, stability testing, structure optimization, and characterization and determination of the pharmacokinetic and metabolic profile.

4.4.1   On the Pharmacokinetics of 5-ALA

In pharmaceutical sciences, the term "pharmacodynamics" is a description of "what the drug does to the body." This was handled in more or less detail in the previous section of this chapter. On the other hand, the term "pharmacokinetics" refers to "what the body does to the drug." In pharmacokinetics, the fate of the drug is followed from its administration, distribution, and metabolism until elimination. According to Kennedy [130], 39% of all failures in clinical development resulted from problems with respect to poor pharmacokinetic properties of a given compound. This might also be the reason for 5-ALA's "failure"* to gain general acceptance in a wide medical community despite its outstanding selectivity.

With a molecular weight of 167 Da, 5-ALA can be classified as a low molecular weight compound. It has two pKa values of 4.05 and 8.3, for the carboxylic and amine functions, respectively (see Figure 4.2) [122].

At physiological pH, more than 90% of 5-ALA is present as a zwitterion. Due to its low molecular weight and double charge, 5-ALA is rather water-soluble, displaying an octanol-water partition coefficient of 0.03 [122]. Compounds characterized by such physicochemical properties show only limited capacities to reach and finally enter target cells in appropriate amounts.

5-ALA has been applied by the most common routes of drug administration: oral, parenteral, and topical. Given orally or intravenously, 5-ALA is eliminated from the human body with a half-life of 45 and 50 minutes, respectively [131–133]. As expected from the unfavorable physicochemical properties, 5-ALA's poor bioavailability is further underlined by its small volume of distribution of 8.3L. A large proportion (>65%) of 5-ALA is excreted unchanged in the urine or trapped by the first-pass metabolism. Since the clinical success of PDT relies on the local concentration of 5-ALA to induce therapeutically relevant doses of PpIX at the target site, rather high doses of 5-ALA have to be applied to warrant the desired therapeutic outcome. To cause more than 90% cell death, the threshold for such levels has been evaluated in cell culture studies to be between 0.01 and 0.17 mg/ml [124, 134–136]. However, 5-ALA administered at high doses has been shown to lead to significant side effects, including nausea, vomiting, and transient abnormalities in liver function. Furthermore, significant decreases in systolic and diastolic blood and pulmonary pressure have been reported [137, 138]. Fortunately, in most clinically

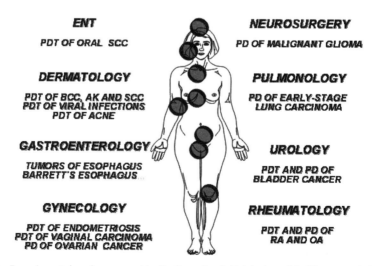

Figure 4.2 Experimental and approved indications for 5-ALA-induced PpIX accumulation.

relevant indications for the use of 5-ALA, the treatment is limited to areas that are easily accessible to local irradiation, either directly or through endoscopic means. Therefore, 5-ALA-mediated PDT has been primarily assessed clinically for (non-) neoplastic lesions of the skin, lungs, oral cavity, gastrointestinal tract, bladder, and female reproductive tract. In consequence, topical routes are suitable in view of the superficial nature of these epithelial lesions.

In order to exert a therapeutic effect after topical administration, 5-ALA first has to be released from its vehicle, then transported from its administration site to the adjacent compartment and deeper tissue layers and finally taken up into the intracellular space. The principal transport mechanisms for this process include: (1) active transport, (2) facilitated diffusion, (3) filtration, and (4) passive diffusion via para- or transcellular pathways. Key parameters that dominate the crossing across mostly lipophilic biological barriers are molecular size and shape as well as solubility, polarity, charge, and lipophilicity.

The tissue penetration of 5-ALA following topical administration has been the subject of numerous studies. However, most of these have used the fluorescence of PpIX as an indirect measure to assess 5-ALA's penetration depth. Furthermore, most studies vary widely with respect to administration conditions and pharmaceutical formulation, making exact comparison difficult. In a report by Wennberg et al., concentrations of 5-ALA up to 0.5 mg/ml were found in basal cell carcinomas at a depth of 0.5 mm, while no 5-ALA was found in normal tissue at this depth [139]. However, they established no depth concentration profiles using a microdialysis technique. Liquid scintillation spectrometry of radiolabeled 5-ALA is another technique to determine the penetration depth of this compound following topical application. In xenograft mouse models, penetration depths of as much as 5 mm into the tumor were reported [140]. However, the majority of 5-ALA was found in the outer 2 mm. At this depth, 5-ALA concentrations as high as 20 mg/ml in human BCCs were reported by McLoone et al. and Ahmadi et al. [141, 142]. The importance of the stratum corneum for 5-ALA diffusion into the target tissue is supported by the observation by Johnson et al. that 5-ALA is only achieving penetration depths of 100–150 μm through intact porcine skin [143]. In tissues in which major penetration barriers are absent (e.g., vagina) diffusion of 5-ALA as far as 6 mm can be observed [144]. 5-ALA-mediated PDT seems to be limited by the amount of drug that can penetrate into the interstitial space of the target tissue and subsequently enter the target cell.

4.4.2   Pharmaceutical Concepts in 5-ALA-Mediated PDT

Attempts to improve the bioavailability of 5-ALA or its capacity to induce PpIX can be subdivided into four main categories (see Table 4.2).

4.4.2.1   Means to Enhance 5-ALA Penetration

The simplest approach to enhance the penetration depth of a therapeutic compound after topical administration is the addition of penetration enhancers such as dimethyl sulfoxide (DMSO) to the corresponding formulation. DMSO is an extensively studied solvent used in transdermal drug delivery. Besides its action on

Table 4.2 Concepts and Rationale for Controlled Drug Delivery of 5-Aminolevulinic Acid (ALA)

Method		Rational
Chemical enhancement	DMSO	Enhanced penetration/cell differentiation
	Glycolic acid	Enhanced penetration
	EDTA	Iron chelation
	Desfferioxamine	
	CP94	
Vehicle formulation	Lotion, film, ointment,ge	Improved release
	Liposomes	Penetration enhancementIImproved release
	Nanoparticles	Improved delivery
Physical method	Iontophoresis	Enhanced penetration
	Erbium:YAG laser	Disruption of SC
	Tape-stripping	Disruption of SC
	Temperature	Enhanced enzymatic activity
	Ultrasound	Disruption of SC/enhanced penetation
	Microdermoabrasion	Disruption of SC/enhanced penetation
Chemical modification	5-ALA derivatives	Enhanced penetration
		Increased uptake
		Selective cleavage

tissular lipids and proteins, it has been shown to activate various enzymes in heme biosynthesis, in particular 5-ALAS and PBG-D, through stimulation of differentiation [145–148] and may act synergistically on the generation of PpIX. Typically, 2% to 20% of DMSO is added to the formulations intended for topical use [140, 149–151]. Early in the research on 5-ALA-mediated PDT, Malik et al. found significantly increased accumulation on mouse skin using 2% (w/w) of DMSO as compared to 5-ALA alone [152]. More recently, de Rosa et al [151] showed that the addition of DMSO significantly increased the flux of 5-ALA across mouse skin in vitro. In vivo, a 2.5-fold increase of PpIX formation was observed when 20% of DMSO was added to an oil-in-water emulsion as compared to the control formulation lacking DMSO. Glycerol monooleate, a lipid penetration enhancer, considerably increased the in vitro permeation and retention of 5-ALA [153]. A 40% increase in PpIX accumulation was observed in excised pig bladder mucosa when DMSO was added to a solution containing 180 mM 5-ALA [154]. No beneficial effect was observed when 5-ALA was encapsulated into lipid carriers such as liposomes [140, 155–157].

Modulation of the transport and dissolution of ionic drugs through the skin can also be achieved by a modality termed as "ion pairing." Ion pairs are neutral species formed through electrostatic interactions between oppositely charged ions. Without altering the skin's barrier function of chemical structure of the drug, the thus-formed more lipophilic ion pair shows increased solubility in lipophilic barriers. Recently, the effect of lipophilic counter-ions on the permeation of 5-ALA in combination with phloretin and 6-ketocholestanol was tested in porcine skin [158]. The latter combination was found to increase the diffusion of 5-ALA by a factor of 1.7. Addition of cetylpyridinium chloride further doubled the penetration of 5-ALA. In another study, other lipophilic salts of 5-ALA derivatives increased the porphyrin formation in vitro and in vivo [159].

4.4.2.2   Adjuvants to Alter Heme Biosynthesis

Besides increasing the intracellular production of PpIX, circumventing its conversion into heme is another means to increase the formation of photoactive porphyrins. This is typically done by the removal of ferrous iron through the action of iron chelators. 1,10-Phenanthroline (an iron chelator) has been shown to increase 5-ALA-mediated PpIX formation in vitro [160]. Mouse tumors responded better to 5-ALA PDT when this modulator was added. Ethylenediamine-tetraacetic acid (EDTA), desferrioxamine, or 3-hydroxypyridine-4-ones (HPOs) have also been tested [152, 161–170]. A significant increase of PpIX fluorescence intensity in mouse skin after addition of EDTA was reported independently by Malik et al. and de Rosa et al. [151, 152]. While EDTA is a broadband chelator for a multitude of metallic ions, DFO is a clinically approved chelator specific for iron. At equal concentrations, DFO has been shown to be superior to EDTA with respect to PpIX formation in vitro [161]. Up to a 44-fold increase in PpIX formation was observed in V79 Chinese hamster lung fibroblast when DFO was added to 5-ALA-containing solution. In agreement with Peng et al., Orenstein and coworkers found a positive impact on nodular BCC when EDTA and DMSO were given along with 5-ALA [162, 163]. However, the cure rates of superficial BCC were only minimally affected by these agents. Marti et al. and Chang et al. observed that PpIX accumulation can be doubled in urothelial mucosa after topical administration of 5-ALA solutions containing DFO and HPO, respectively [154, 164]. However, the role of iron-chelating agents in improving clinical outcome has yet to be discussed, since potential undesired collateral damage due to increased accumulation in normal cells must be considered.

4.4.2.3   Physical Means to Enhance 5-ALA Penetration

As the most important barrier of the skin is the SC, simple removal of this barrier will enhance the penetration of drugs into the epidermis. This can be achieved by various techniques including curettage, tape-stripping, dermabrasion, and delipidation. In accordance with a semiquantitative study of van den Akker et al., de Rosa et al. showed a significantly increased penetration of PpIX buildup and 5-ALA penetration following tape-stripping [97, 165, 166]. More sophisticated means to alter the skin's barrier function, such as laser-mediated ablation, have also been investigated. Depending on the fluence rate, Shen et al. observed a 1.7 to 4.9 times higher PpIX fluorescence intensity in experimental animal models pretreated with an Er-YAG laser as compared to untreated controls [167]. Using a single light pulse of a Q-switched ruby laser, Lee et al. showed a nearly 7 times increase of 5-ALA delivery [168, 169]. Less spectacular, but apparently as efficient, is the application of vacuum to the treatment site prior to the application of topical drugs such as 5-fluorouracil or 5-ALA [169].

Ultrasound has been shown to significantly enhance the transdermal delivery of therapeutic agents. Ma et al. demonstrated a 45% increase in the accumulation of PpIX when ultrasound was applied to a xenograft mouse model prior to application of 5-ALA [170]. In accordance with these studies, significantly accelerated PpIX formation was observed in an experimental hamster model of oral neoplasms with low-frequency ultrasound [171]. Another physical means to control the delivery of compounds through biological barriers is iontophoresis [172]. This method facilitates the transport of ionic species by the application of an electronic current. In most cases, the iontophoresis-mediated transport across the skin is directly proportional to the magnitude of the current. Iontophoresis mostly functions through two distinct mechanisms. While in (i) electromigration, the applied potential causes movement between the charged compound and the respective electrode. In (ii) electroosmosis, the convective solvent flow from the anode to the cathode enhances the transport of cations and neutral polar compounds. Although apparently less effective than laser-mediated drug delivery of 5-ALA [173], significant delivery at physiological pH can be achieved by this method. Rodes et al. have studied the iontophoresis of 5-ALA to normal human skin [174]. PpIX formation as well as the phototoxic effect were directly correlated to the applied current. Later, Lopez et al. examined the iontophoresis of 5-ALA as a function of pH in porcine skin [175–177]. At physiological pH, 5-ALA delivery was shown to be a linear function of the applied concentration between 1 and 100 mM. In this pH range, the principal transport mechanism was electroosmosis. The gradual decrease in pH shifted the transport mechanism towards electromigration without altering the total amount of 5-ALA delivered to the skin. In an attempt to optimize 5-ALA iontophoresis, reduction of the NaCl concentration in the anode led to a 3- to 4-fold increase in 5-ALA flux. Transport of 5-ALA across the skin and the amount delivered into the skin (SC and [epidermis + dermis]) were ~4-fold greater with iontophoresis relative to the passive application of a DMSO formulation. Interestingly, the transfollicular route seems to be of particular importance, as shown by the preferential accumulation of PpIX in pilosebaceous units [178]. Since the application of an aqueous solution for iontophoresis has to be considered as suboptimal in clinical practice, Merclin et al. have used a hydrogel containing 5-ALA, without losing the increase of 5-ALA delivery to the skin [179].

4.4.2.4 Chemical Modification

In improving the delivery of 5-ALA, the most important breakthrough has recently been made by chemical modification. This approach aims at modulating the physicochemical properties of a drug by covalent modification, resulting in improved bioavailability and pharmacological properties. Such compounds have been designed to serve several purposes (e.g., to decrease unwanted toxicity and to overcome problems with pharmacokinetics, such as too slow or too fast absorption and clearance, as well as poor bioavailability). The principles of this methodology as applied to 5-ALA PDT and photodiagnosis have been recently reviewed in detail by Fotinos et al. [180].

The limiting factor for the delivery of substances into or through the skin is the epidermis. Applied topically, the drug has to partition between the predominant aqueous phase of biological fluids and lipid biomembranes. Since all the constituents of the skin range widely in polarity, the drug should have an appropriate balance between hydrophilic and lipophilic properties, which will allow it to diffuse in and out of these media.

The octanol/water partition coefficient P, and more specifically, its logarithm (log P) are commonly used to describe the lipophilic properties of a compound. Although no general rule can be applied to all drug molecules, some general considerations can be made. For instance, within a homologous series of molecules, drug absorption usually increases with lipophilicity and then reaches a maximum value, where it plateaus for a few units of log P, and thereafter steadily decreases, resulting in a parabolic relationship between log P and drug penetration. In general, molecules with log P values below 0 (i.e., hydrophilic) have good water-solubility but poor permeability through lipid layers, whereas drugs with log P values far higher than 3 tend to be absorbed in lipophilic media.

As mentioned above, the greatest disadvantage accompanying the topical administration of 5-ALA, especially with respect to its poor bioavailability, can be ascribed to the physicochemical properties of this hydrophilic, zwitterionic molecule. Due to these unfavorable properties, high doses and long application times are often necessary to induce sufficient amounts of PpIX in target tissue.

The simplest way to improve the physicochemical properties of 5-ALA is the chemical transformation of the highly polar carboxyl functionality into a more lipophilic ester group. Figure 4.3 shows how the reaction of 5-ALA with an alcohol, in the presence of a coupling agent, accomplishes this simple transformation.

Lipophilicity is one of the key parameters in the bioavailability of 5-ALA derivatives and can be easily varied (e.g., in the case of n-alkyl esters) by modifying the alkyl chain length. An additional advantage of using this esterification approach is that it leaves the amine functionality unmodified and free to become protonated at physiological pH. This is a key aspect since this positive charge in the N-terminal end of the molecule imparts good water solubility and attraction forces to negatively charged tissue. Although most clinical, as well as preclinical, work has been carried out on 5-ALA alkyl esters, some more sophisticated derivatives have been tested predominantly in cell cultures [181–185].

Uehlinger and coworkers [122] determined the log P values for a homologous series of 5-ALA alkylesters. In agreement with de Rosa et al. [151], they found a negative log P value for 5-ALA (~–1.5), and, except for the ALA methyl ester (MAL), which has a log P value of –0.9, all other derivatives were found to be lipophilic in nature. Thus, it was shown that, by simple esterification, the P values of ALA derivatives can be varied by more than four orders of magnitude (ALA versus ALA octylester (OAL)) (see Figure 4.4).

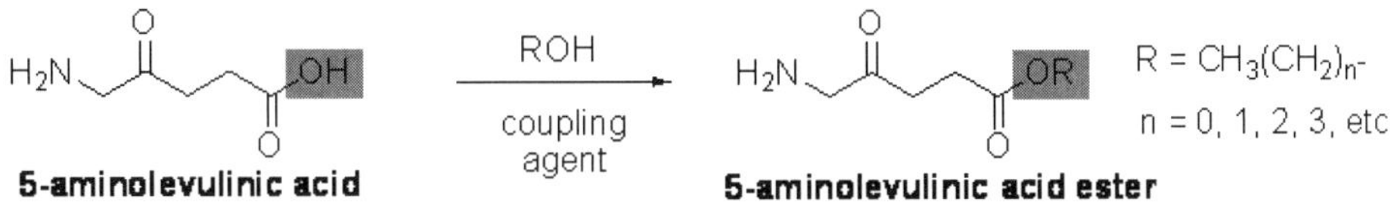

Figure 4.3   5-Aminolevulinic acid derivatization from a highly polar carboxylic acid to a lipophilic ester.

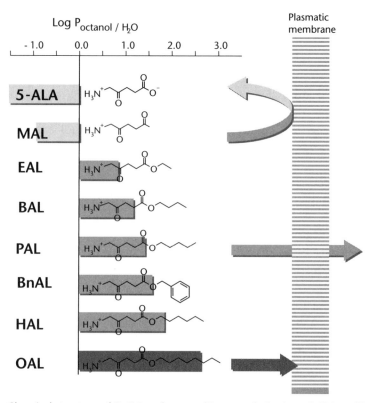

Figure 4.4 Chemical structure of 5-ALA and some of its ester derivatives. 5-ALA and its methyl ester (MAL) have a negative log Poctanol/H₂O and therefore cannot cross a biological membrane by passive diffusion. 5-ALA octyl ester (OAL), the most lipophilic 5-ALA ester studied, has a high affinity for lipid environment and is therefore trapped within the biological membranes. The derivatives with an intermediate lipophilicity, namely 5-ALA ethyl (EAL), butyl (BAL), pentyl (PAL), benzyl (BnAL) and hexyl (HAL) esters, are more appropriate to cross biological membranes by passive diffusion.

However, in order to display an optimum flux across the SC and other biological barriers, the drug must have a balanced water and lipid solubility. This relationship can be described by Fick's first law of diffusion $(dQ/dt=J_{drug}=(P \cdot D/h) \cdot \Delta c \cdot A)$, where dQ/dt is the amount of drug diffused per unit time, J_{drug} the drug flux, P the partition coefficient, D the diffusion coefficient, h the path length of the barrier, and A the treated (skin) surface area. In order to enhance drug delivery, these parameters must be manipulated in order to optimize the system for a particular application. The ability of 5-ALA esters to induce a higher formation of porphyrins following typical administration in vivo remains a controversial subject. Often, the role and effect of the vehicle used has not been taken into account (cream versus ointment versus emulsion, etc.) such that unambiguous conclusions cannot be reached. While for urology applications an aqueous solution seems to be ideal with respect to the improved delivery of HAL to the urothelium, for other purposes the partition coefficient between the tissue and the delivery vehicle also has to be considered. A too highly lipophilic vehicle, such as an oily cream, will retain lipophilic compounds, reducing their flux into the tissue.

To illustrate, topical administration of 5-ALA pentyl ester failed to induce higher amounts of porphyrins in the epidermis of mice with normal skin and skin altered by UV light irradiation. Although higher amounts of porphyrins were found in the SC relative to 5-ALA, no difference was noted in the dysplastic layers of the epidermis [94, 97]. In a more recent study using HAL applied to normal mice in a lipophilic vehicle, 5-ALA induced higher porphyrin formation than HAL over a 0.5% to 40% (w/w) concentration range, after short application times. Only after 24 hours of continuous application did HAL show slightly higher fluorescence intensities [97]. These results have been confirmed with nude mice following exposure to 5-ALA, MAL, HAL, and OAL [186].

So far, the only derivatives that have successfully improved porphyrin formation upon topical skin application in vivo are 5-ALA ethyl and propyl esters [187]. MAL application and subsequent irradiation has also resulted in greater tumor growth inhibition than 5-ALA [188]. In addition, in human AK in vivo, the biodistribution of porphyrins after topical application of 5-ALA and MAL has been compared [189]. Although porphyrin formation was found to be more efficient when using 5-ALA, the selectivity for diseased tissue was greater for its derivative.

When comparing 5-ALA with its long-chain esters after topical application, one finds a significantly longer lag time before the onset of the porphyrin signal with the 5-ALA derivatives. This can be partly explained by the "reservoir function" of the SC for the lipophilic derivatives, which slows their penetration to the target tissue. Removing the SC by tape-stripping often leads to essentially identical levels of fluorescence induced by 5-ALA and HAL, emphasizing the important role of the SC's barrier and reservoir function. de Rosa et al. exposed explanted mouse skin to aqueous solutions containing 5-ALA and 5-ALA esters and determined the accumulated amount of the drug in the SC and the epidermis [166, 190]. After 6 hours of application, significantly more HAL and OAL were retained in the viable epidermis, in the viable dermis, and in the SC, as compared to 5-ALA, indicating that hydrophilic vehicles could positively influence the delivery of lipophilic 5-ALA derivatives to the skin. Recently, we have shown that the formulation of HAL in hydrogels largely improved the release of the drug and the formation of porphyrins in nude mice as compared to the same compound formulated in a cream [191, 192]. In general, the use of an aqueous solution of lipophilic 5-ALA derivatives results in a more homogenous distribution of both porphyrins as well as their precursors in vitro and in vivo. Foster et al. used three-dimensional cell cultures to show that after exposure to HAL solutions, porphyrin fluorescence was equally distributed within their multicellular tumor spheroids [193]. Marti et al. showed porphyrin fluorescence was more homogenously distributed and reached deeper cell layers when using HAL as compared to 5-ALA [154, 194].

There are indications that 5-ALA enters cells via active transport mechanisms such as the PEPT1 transporter, and were identified as possible transporter systems for the uptake of 5-ALA into rat pancreatoma cells [195]. Additionally, Döring et al. [196] have identified the PEPT2 transporter system for the transmembrane transport of 5-ALA into the epithelial cells of kidneys. In spite of evident resemblance between the chemical structure of 5-ALA and γ-aminobutyric acid (GABA), it was determined that 5-ALA but not GABA competes with the active uptake of PEPT1 and PEPT2 into the cell. Furthermore, some derivatives of 5-ALA such as the hexyl ester derivative have shown higher affinity to the PEPT2, but not to the PEPT1, transporter than 5-ALA itself [197]. However, in a human adenocarcinoma cell line (WiDr), GABA and other structurally related compounds such as taurine and γ-alanine, which are transported by the BETA transporter system, effectively inhibited the uptake of 5-ALA [80]. Furthermore, other amino acids, in particular those with polar, uncharged groups, were found to interfere with the uptake mechanism of ALA. In contrast to 5-ALA, the transport of MAL was only slightly influenced by β-alanine, while no inhibition was reported for the even more lipophilic HAL [80], suggesting that a passive diffusion mechanism or endocytosis across the cell membrane becomes increasingly more dominant for the more lipophilic ALA esters. The assumption of passive membrane diffusion is further supported by Whitaker's observation [195] that the PEPT1 transporter system actively carries 5-ALA but not 5-ALA esters through cellular membranes. Nevertheless, there is a possibility that other transporter systems are involved in carrying ALA esters across the membrane; for instance, nonpolar amino acids were found to inhibit the uptake of MAL by about 60% [82].

At this time, two ALA derivatives are being clinically evaluated. In dermatology, where poor penetration of 5-ALA through the SC has limited its application for the treatment of nodular BCCs and SCCs, MAL was recently granted marketing authorization for the photodynamic treatment of AK and nodular BCC across Europe and Australia [198–200]. Although this compound is predominantly used for therapeutic purposes, it is increasingly used for detection purposes in dermatology [14].

The second derivative, HAL, obtained approval from 26 European countries for the improved detection of bladder cancer lesions, a fact that changed patient management in a significant number of cases. This compound was earlier found to be suitable for the fluorescence photodetection of human bladder carcinoma in situ (CIS) [83, 201, 202].

From the large variety of 5-ALA esters, the choice of HAL is based on preclinical studies using excised pig bladder mucosa [154], which was used for (pro)drug screening. The authors selected HAL for its water-urine solubility and porphyrin-formation efficacy at low doses compared to ALA. It was determined that HAL induces porphyrin formation faster and in higher amounts than does ALA itself; thus, more than a twofold PpIX formation rate at a concentration nearly 50 times lower was observed with this ester. Furthermore, as demonstrated by fluorescence microscopy, the drug penetrates deeper and more homogeneously across the entire urothelium, which is promising with respect to the phototherapeutic treatment of urothelial lesions.

The initial clinical study [84] compared the abilities of HAL versus 5-ALA to induce porphyrins in tumors and early cancerous disease with respect to the precursor concentration, its pharmacokinetics, and its selectivity. Quantitative measurements of the fluorescence intensities in papillary tumors were used to evaluate the optimal conditions. Color plate 3 demonstrates the advantageous use of HAL-induced fluorescence for the diagnosis of early-stage urothelial neoplasm.

The preliminary data reported in this pilot study indicates a high sensitivity and specificity of this method as compared with traditional histopathological analysis, and a clear advantage over 5-ALA installation at more than 20-fold lower drug doses. These promising results were also obtained with instillation periods as short as 30 minutes [203]. The reduction of the instillation time drastically increases patient comfort, makes outpatient treatment and examination in private urology offices feasible, and helps to reduce the costs of hospitalization. Moreover, fluorescence microscopy biopsies of papillary tumors have shown that porphyrin fluorescence was more homogeneously distributed and found in deeper tissue layers after instillation with HAL as compared with 5-ALA [194]. Hence, one may also expect HAL to be the superior drug for PDT. After completing a phase II trial [83], the subsequent phase III trial revealed that HAL cystoscopy enabled the identifcation of 28% more patients suffering from carcinoma in situ than conventional inspection using white light [202]. Furthermore, when using fluorescence, more papillary lesions were seen compared to standard cystoscopy. Thus, this new technique might lead to more complete resection and thus lower recurrence rates [202, 204]. The following phase III study showed that the improved tumor detection using HAL fluorescence cystoscopy resulted in a different patient management of 21% of the patients [204]. Recent phase III trials performed in the United States confirmed this general trend in the improvement of bladder cancer detection when using HAL [205].

Due to significant improvements in dermatology and urology with these compounds, they are also expected to be well-suited for other medical applications where porphyrin-mediated PDT and PD have shown promising results. However, history has shown that a particular compound must be carefully adapted to the specific clinical requirements with respect to its lipophilicity and porphyrin formation ability. Therefore, it is important to find valid preclinical tests to predict whether or not 5-ALA derivatives are useful for a particular indication. Furthermore, physiological parameters have to be taken into account. For instance, the intravenous or oral administration of simple 5-ALA alkyl esters will not have any advantages over 5-ALA, since these are quickly degraded in human serum and under the strongly acidic environment of the stomach.

Degradation of 5-ALA esters may be an advantage for some applications, such as PDT and PD of Barrett's esophagus. In this particular case, topical application might be preferable to systemic application. The extremely fast uptake of long-chain 5-ALA esters could be sufficient to provide high prodrug doses to the mucosa during passage of liquid solutions. Since these esters can be administered at lower doses than 5-ALA to induce higher fluorescence intensities, side effects associated with oral 5-ALA administration (>60 mg/kg), such as nausea and hypertension, can be greatly reduced. Besides PD and PDT of Barrett's esophagus, fluorescence-mediated PD of early human lung cancer seems to be another potential application of 5-ALA derivatives. The physicochemical properties of lipophilic prodrugs might also be favorable for the PD of neoplasms in the respiratory tract for several reasons. Although these compounds have not been shown to be superior to 5-ALA with respect to the rate of porphyrin formation in excised paranasal sheep mucosa, they can be applied at significantly lower doses [126]. Furthermore, it is important to consider that the main protective mechanism of the lungs is based on the evacuation of foreign material through a constant flow of mucus. This mucus, which is produced by goblet cells, submucosal glands, and epithelial cells, consists of two different layers. The upper (highly lipophilic) layer, which determines viscoelastic properties of the mucus, contains macromolecules, which are in part polymerized.

This layer is supported by another layer, which consists of water and ions. Thus, in contrast to 5-ALA, 5-ALA esters are very soluble in both mucus layers, as well as in surfactant-containing solutions used in their formulation, all of which might help improve the spatial drug distribution throughout the organ after inhalation.

Most drug delivery strategies for 5-ALA can also be adapted to the more lipophilic derivatives. These strategies have been recently reviewed by Donnelly et al. and Lopez et al. [206, 207]. However, care should be taken with respect to the hydrophilicity of the delivery vehicle, as shown recently by Collaud et al. [191, 192].

4.5 Conclusions

The introduction of 5-ALA and its lipophilic derivatives is a promising approach in biomedical optics. PDT with 5-ALA is one of the most selective modalities in the treatment of neoplastic disease. Although considerable information revealing the mechanisms underlying this specific selectivity has been collected, our knowledge about this process is far from complete. From the above considerations, it seems clear that several factors are responsible for the selective accumulation of PpIX.

Since most of the enzymatic parameters in heme biosynthesis are known from the literature and are readily available from public databases (see e.g., BRENDA database), kinetic simulations of the entire biosynthesis based on standard or reversible Michaelis-Menten kinetics might be helpful.

Elucidation of heme biosynthesis in neoplastic cells will not just be important for the development of more potent treatment strategies using 5-ALA or its derivatives. Describing the major mechanisms for the selectivity of 5-ALA-induced PpIX formation would provide new starting points for the development of new and more selective drugs outside the field of biomedical optics (e.g., for chemotherapeutic purposes), targeting this specific deficiency in neoplastic cells. One might, for instance, consider developing antisense drugs that specifically target the mRNA encoding for overexpressed enzymes in heme biosynthesis. Furthermore, if lack of iron is the major point, one could imagine the development of a drug that changes in therapeutic efficacy in the presence or absence of ferrous iron.

5-ALA derivatives have proven to improve substantially the local bioavailability of 5-ALA in vitro and in vivo. Depending on the respective derivatives, drug doses as small as two orders of magnitude lower than 5-ALA are necessary to achieve similar or sometimes even better therapeutic results. In some cases, 5-ALA n-alkyl esters have induced porphyrins more selectively in the target tissue. In other cases, the increased production of porphyrins led to a substantial shortening of the drug-light-interval. The superiority of 5-ALA esters over 5-ALA has been recently underlined by the approval of Metvix® for the treatment of AK in Europe and Australia and Hexvix® for the improved diagnosis of bladder cancer.

However, the huge opportunities remain largely unexplored in underlying 5-ALA derivative-related research with respect to compounds that show enhanced activity following systemic administration. Therefore, the treatment or diagnosis of some life-threatening diseases such as brain tumors, breast cancer, or ovarian cancer can only be achieved with simple 5-ALA derivatives. In the future, it might be favorable for researchers working in the field to adopt lessons learned from rational prodrug design to 5-ALA derivatives in order to further increase the impact of this research area.

References

[1]   Battersby, AR. Tetrapyrroles: the pigments of life. Nat. Prod. Rep., 2000, 17, 507–526

[2]   Beri, R., and Chandra, R., "Chemistry and biology of heme. Effect of metal salts, organometals, and metalloporphyrins on heme synthesis and catabolism, with special reference to clinical implications and interactions with cytochrome P-450," *Drug Metab Rev*, Vol. 25, 1993, pp. 49–152.

[3]   Mascaro, J. M., "Porphyria cutanea tarda: clinical manifestations," *Curr Probl Dermatol*, Vol. 20, 1991, pp. 79–90.

[4]   Mascaro, J. M., et al., "New aspects of porphyrias," *Curr Probl Dermatol*, Vol. 13, 1985, pp. 11–32.

[5]   Askira, Y., Rubin, B., and Rabinowitch, H. D., "Differential response to the herbicidal activity of delta-aminolevulinic acid in plants with high and low SOD activity," *Free Radic Res Commun*, Vol. 12–13 Pt 2, 1991, pp. 837–843.

[6]   Malik, Z., and Lugaci, H., "Destruction of erythroleukaemic cells by photoactivation of endogenous porphyrins," *Br J Cancer*, Vol. 56, 1987, pp. 589–595.

[7]   Kennedy, J. C., Pottier, R. H., and Pross, D. C., "Photodynamic therapy with endogenous protoporphyrin IX: basic principles and present clinical experience," *J Photochem Photobiol B*, Vol. 6, 1990, pp. 143–148.

[8]   Kennedy, J. C., and Pottier, R. H., "Endogenous protoporphyrin IX, a clinically useful photosensitizer for photodynamic therapy," *J Photochem Photobiol B*, Vol. 14, 1992, pp. 275–292.

[9]   Stummer, W., et al., "Fluorescence-guided resections of malignant gliomas—an overview," *Acta Neurochir Suppl*, Vol. 88, 2003, pp. 9–12.

[10] Jichlinski, P., and Leisinger, H. J., "Fluorescence cystoscopy in the management of bladder cancer: a help for the urologist!," *Urol Int*, Vol. 74, 2005, pp. 97–101.

[11] Stepinac, T., et al., "Endoscopic fluorescence detection of intraepithelial neoplasia in Barrett's esophagus after oral administration of aminolevulinic acid," *Endoscopy*, Vol. 35, 2003, pp. 663–668.

[12] Eisendrath, P., and Van Laethem, J. L., "Endoscopic fluorescence detection of low and high grade dysplasia in Barrett's oesophagus using systemic or local 5-aminolaevulinic acid sensitization," *Gastrointest Endosc*, Vol. 55, 2002, pp. 297–298.

[13] Szeimies, R. M., Landthaler, M., and Karrer, S., "Non-oncologic indications for ALA-PDT," *J Dermatolog Treat*, Vol. 13 Suppl 1, 2002, pp. S13–18.

[14] Fritsch, C., and Ruzicka, T., "Fluorescence diagnosis and photodynamic therapy in dermatology from experimental state to clinic standard methods," *J Environ Pathol Toxicol Oncol*, Vol. 25, 2006, pp. 425–439.

[15] Fischer, H., *Orth H. Chemie des Pyrrols, Vol. 2*. Leipzig: Akademischer Verlag, 1937.

[16] Fischer, H., *Orth H. Chemie des Pyrrols, Vol. 1*. Leipzig: Akademischer Verlag, 1934.

[17] Shemin, D., "An illustration of the use of isotopes: the biosynthesis of porphyrins," *Bioessays*, Vol. 10, 1989, pp. 30–35.

[18] Cotter, P. D., et al., "Assignment of the human housekeeping delta-aminolevulinate synthase gene (ALAS1) to chromosome band 3p21.1 by PCR analysis of somatic cell hybrids," *Cytogenet Cell Genet*, Vol. 69, 1995, pp. 207–208.

[19] Cox, T. C., et al., "Erythroid 5-aminolevulinate synthase is located on the X chromosome," *Am J Hum Genet*, Vol. 46, 1990, pp. 107–111.

[20] Sinclair, P. R., and Granick, S., "Heme control on the synthesis of delta-aminolevulinic acid synthetase in cultured chick embryo liver cells," *Ann N Y Acad Sci*, Vol. 244, 1975, pp. 509–520.

[21] Tyrrell, D. L., and Marks, G. S., "Drug-induced porphyrin biosynthesis. V. Effect of protohemin on the transcriptional and post-transcriptional phases of -aminolevulinic acid synthetase induction," *Biochem Pharmacol*, Vol. 21, 1972, pp. 2077–2093.

[22] Kikuchi, G., and Hayashi, N., "Regulation by heme of synthesis and intracellular translocation of delta-aminolevulinate synthase in the liver," *Mol Cell Biochem*, Vol. 37, 1981, pp. 27–41.

[23] Hamilton, J. W., et al., "Heme regulates hepatic 5-aminolevulinate synthase mRNA expression by decreasing mRNA half-life and not by altering its rate of transcription," *Arch Biochem Biophys*, Vol. 289, 1991, pp. 387–392.

[24] Tomokuni, K., and Ogata, M., "Relationship between lead concentration in blood and biological response for porphyrin metabolism in workers occupationally exposed to lead," *Arch Toxicol*, Vol. 35, 1976, pp. 239–246.

[25] Tomokuni, K., and Kawanishi, T., "Relationship between activation of delta-aminolevulinic acid dehydratase by heating and blood lead level," *Arch Toxicol*, Vol. 34, 1975, pp. 253–258.

[26] Mesenholler, M., and Matthews, E. K., "A key role for the mitochondrial benzodiazepine receptor in cellular photosensitisation with delta-aminolaevulinic acid," *Eur J Pharmacol*, Vol. 406, 2000, pp. 171–180.

[27] Abels, C., et al., "In vivo kinetics and spectra of 5-aminolaevulinic acid-induced fluorescence in an amelanotic melanoma of the hamster," *Br J Cancer*, Vol. 70, 1994, pp. 826–833.

[28] Gibson, S. L., et al., "A regulatory role for porphobilinogen deaminase (PBGD) in delta-aminolaevulinic acid (delta-ALA)-induced photosensitization?" *Br J Cancer*, Vol. 77, 1998, pp. 235–243.

[29] Gibson, S. L., et al., "Time-dependent intracellular accumulation of delta-aminolevulinic acid, induction of porphyrin synthesis and subsequent phototoxicity," *Photochem Photobiol*, Vol. 65, 1997, pp. 416–421.

[30] Kondo, M., et al., "Heme-biosynthetic enzyme activities and porphyrin accumulation in normal liver and hepatoma cell lines of rat," *Cell Biol Toxicol*, Vol. 9, 1993, pp. 95–105.

[31] Navone, N. M., et al., "Rhodanese and ALA-S in mammary tumor and liver from normal and tumor-bearing mice," *Comp Biochem Physiol B*, Vol. 102, 1992, pp. 83–85.

[32] Navone, N. M., et al., "Mouse mammary carcinoma delta-aminolevulinate dehydratase," *Comp Biochem Physiol B*, Vol. 96, 1990, pp. 729–731.

[33] Navone, N. M., et al., "Heme biosynthesis in human breast cancer—mimetic "in vitro" studies and some heme enzymic activity levels," *Int J Biochem*, Vol. 22, 1990, pp. 1407–1411.

[34] Mamet, R., et al., "Regulation of heme synthesis in the regenerating rat liver," *Biochem Med Metab Biol*, Vol. 43, 1990, pp. 263–270.

[35] Schoenfeld, N., et al., "The heme biosynthetic pathway in lymphocytes of patients with malignant lymphoproliferative disorders," *Cancer Lett*, Vol. 43, 1988, pp. 43–48.

[36] Schoenfeld, N., et al., "The heme biosynthetic pathway in the regenerating rat liver. The relation between enzymes of heme synthesis and growth," *Eur J Biochem*, Vol. 166, 1987, pp. 663–666.

[37] Hinnen, P., et al., "Porphyrin biosynthesis in human Barrett's oesophagus and adenocarcinoma after ingestion of 5-aminolaevulinic acid," *Br J Cancer*, Vol. 83, 2000, pp. 539–543.

[38] Hinnen, P., et al., "Biochemical basis of 5-aminolaevulinic acid-induced protoporphyrin IX accumulation: a study in patients with (pre)malignant lesions of the oesophagus," *Br J Cancer*, Vol. 78, 1998, pp. 679–682.

[39] Hilf, R., Havens, J. J., and Gibson, S. L., "Effect of delta-aminolevulinic acid on protoporphyrin IX accumulation in tumor cells transfected with plasmids containing porphobilinogen deaminase DNA," *Photochem Photobiol*, Vol. 70, 1999, pp. 334–340.

[40] Krieg, R. C., et al., "Cell-type specific protoporphyrin IX metabolism in human bladder cancer in vitro," *Photochem Photobiol*, Vol. 72, 2000, pp. 226–233.

[41] Krieg, R. C., et al., "Metabolic characterization of tumor cell-specific protoporphyrin IX accumulation after exposure to 5-aminolevulinic acid in human colonic cells," *Photochem Photobiol*, Vol. 76, 2002, pp. 518–525.

[42] Adams, J., "Development of the proteasome inhibitor PS-341," *Oncologist*, Vol. 7, 2002, pp. 9–16.

[43] Grinblat, B., Pour, N., and Malik, Z., "Regulation of porphyrin synthesis and photodynamic therapy in heavy metal intoxication," *J Environ Pathol Toxicol Oncol*, Vol. 25, 2006, pp. 145–158.

[44] Grunberg-Etkovitz, N., et al., "Proteasomal degradation regulates expression of porphobilinogen deaminase (PBGD) mutants of acute intermittent porphyria," *Biochim Biophys Acta*, Vol. 1762, 2006, pp. 819–827.

[45] Verma, A. F., S.L.; Hirsch, D.J.; Song, S.Y.; Dillahey, L.F.; Williams, J.R.; Snyder, S.H. , "Photodynamic tumor therapy: Mitochondrial benzodiazepine receptors as a therapeutic target.," *Molec. Med.*, Vol. 4, 1998, pp. 40–45.

[46] Wendler, G., et al., "Protoporphyrin IX binding and transport by recombinant mouse PBR," *Biochem Biophys Res Commun*, Vol. 311, 2003, pp. 847–852.

[47] Katz, Y., Eitan, A., and Gavish, M., "Increase in peripheral benzodiazepine binding sites in colonic adenocarcinoma," *Oncology*, Vol. 47, 1990, pp. 139–142.

[48] Cornu, P., et al., "Increase in omega 3 (peripheral-type benzodiazepine) binding site densities in different types of human brain tumours. A quantitative autoradiography study," *Acta Neurochir (Wien)*, Vol. 119, 1992, pp. 146–152.

[49] Hardwick, M., et al., "Peripheral-type benzodiazepine receptor (PBR) in human breast cancer: correlation of breast cancer cell aggressive phenotype with PBR expression, nuclear localization, and PBR-mediated cell proliferation and nuclear transport of cholesterol," *Cancer Res*, Vol. 59, 1999, pp. 831–842.

[50] Katz, Y., et al., "Increased density of peripheral benzodiazepine-binding sites in ovarian carcinomas as compared with benign ovarian tumours and normal ovaries," *Clin Sci (Lond)*, Vol. 78, 1990, pp. 155–158.

[51] Batra, S., and Iosif, C. S., "Elevated concentrations of mitochondrial peripheral benzodiazepine receptors in ovarian tumors," *Int J Oncol*, Vol. 12, 1998, pp. 1295–1298.

[52] Brodie, C., et al., "Neuroblastoma sensitivity to growth inhibition by deferrioxamine: evidence for a block in G1 phase of the cell cycle," *Cancer Res*, Vol. 53, 1993, pp. 3968–3975.

[53] Darnell, G., and Richardson, D. R., "The potential of iron chelators of the pyridoxal isonicotinoyl hydrazone class as effective antiproliferative agents III: the effect of the ligands on molecular targets involved in proliferation," *Blood*, Vol. 94, 1999, pp. 781–792.

[54] Gao, J., Lovejoy, D., and Richardson, D. R., "Effect of iron chelators with potent anti-proliferative activity on the expression of molecules involved in cell cycle progression and growth," *Redox Rep*, Vol. 4, 1999, pp. 311–312.

[55] Rostkowska-Nadolska, B., Pospiech, L., and Bochnia, M., "Content of trace elements in serum of patients with carcinoma of the larynx," *Arch Immunol Ther Exp (Warsz)*, Vol. 47, 1999, pp. 321–325.

[56] Stout, D. L., and Becker, F. F., "Heme synthesis in normal mouse liver and mouse liver tumors," *Cancer Res*, Vol. 50, 1990, pp. 2337–2340.

[57] Stout, D. L., and Becker, F. F., "Heme enzyme patterns in genetically and chemically induced mouse liver tumors," *Cancer Res*, Vol. 46, 1986, pp. 2756–2759.

[58] Weinberg, E. D., "The role of iron in cancer," *Eur J Cancer Prev*, Vol. 5, 1996, pp. 19–36.

[59] Munro, H. N., and Linder, M. C., "Ferritin: structure, biosynthesis, and role in iron metabolism," *Physiol Rev*, Vol. 58, 1978, pp. 317–396.

[60] Larrick, J. W., and Cresswell, P., "Modulation of cell surface iron transferrin receptors by cellular density and state of activation," *J Supramol Struct*, Vol. 11, 1979, pp. 579–586.

[61] Pascale, R. M., et al., "Transferrin and transferrin receptor gene expression and iron uptake in hepatocellular carcinoma in the rat," *Hepatology*, Vol. 27, 1998, pp. 452–461.

[62] Richardson, D. R., and Baker, E., "The effect of desferrioxamine and ferric ammonium citrate on the uptake of iron by the membrane iron-binding component of human melanoma cells," *Biochim Biophys Acta*, Vol. 1103, 1992, pp. 275–280.

[63] Richardson, D. R., and Baker, E., "The release of iron and transferrin from the human melanoma cell," *Biochim Biophys Acta*, Vol. 1091, 1991, pp. 294–302.

[64] Richardson, D. R., and Baker, E., "The uptake of iron and transferrin by the human malignant melanoma cell," *Biochim Biophys Acta*, Vol. 1053, 1990, pp. 1–12.

[65] Trinder, D., Zak, O., and Aisen, P., "Transferrin receptor-independent uptake of differic transferrin by human hepatoma cells with antisense inhibition of receptor expression," *Hepatology*, Vol. 23, 1996, pp. 1512–1520.

[66] Richardson, D. R., "Therapeutic potential of iron chelators in cancer therapy," *Adv Exp Med Biol*, Vol. 509, 2002, pp. 231–249.

[67] Lovejoy, D. B., and Richardson, D. R., "Iron chelators as anti-neoplastic agents: current developments and promise of the PIH class of chelators," *Curr Med Chem*, Vol. 10, 2003, pp. 1035–1049.

[68] Ponka, P., and Lok, C. N., "The transferrin receptor: role in health and disease," *Int J Biochem Cell Biol*, Vol. 31, 1999, pp. 1111–1137.

[69] Ponka, P., and Richardson, D. R., "Can ferritin provide iron for hemoglobin synthesis?" *Blood*, Vol. 89, 1997, pp. 2611–2613.

[70] Richardson, D. R., Ponka, P., and Vyoral, D., "Distribution of iron in reticulocytes after inhibition of heme synthesis with succinylacetone: examination of the intermediates involved in iron metabolism," *Blood*, Vol. 87, 1996, pp. 3477–3488.

[71] Ponka, P., Schulman, H. M., and Wilczynska, A., "Ferric pyridoxal isonicotinoyl hydrazone can provide iron for heme synthesis in reticulocytes," *Biochim Biophys Acta*, Vol. 718, 1982, pp. 151–156.

[72] Johnson, S., "Do mitochondria regulate cellular iron homeostasis through citric acid and haem production? Implications for cancer and other diseases," *Med Hypotheses*, Vol. 60, 2003, pp. 106–111.

[73] Moan, J., et al., "Protoporphyrin IX accumulation in cells treated with 5-aminolevulinic acid: dependence on cell density, cell size and cell cycle," *Int J Cancer*, Vol. 75, 1998, pp. 134–139.

[74] Pourzand, C., et al., "The iron regulatory protein can determine the effectiveness of 5-aminolevulinic acid in inducing protoporphyrin IX in human primary skin fibroblasts," *J Invest Dermatol*, Vol. 112, 1999, pp. 419–425.

[75] Gibson, S. L., et al., "Relationship of delta-aminolevulinic acid-induced protoporphyrin IX levels to mitochondrial content in neoplastic cells in vitro," *Biochim Biophys Res Commun*, Vol. 265, 1999, pp. 315–321.

[76] Gabeler, E. E., et al., "Aminolaevulinic acid-induced protoporphyrin IX pharmacokinetics in central and peripheral arteries of the rat," *Photochem Photobiol*, Vol. 78, 2003, pp. 82–87.

[77] McGivan, J. D., "Rat hepatoma cells express novel transport systems for glutamine and glutamate in addition to those present in normal rat hepatocytes," *Biochem J*, Vol. 330 (Pt 1), 1998, pp. 255–260.

[78] Dudeck, K. L., et al., "Evidence for inherent differences in the system A carrier from normal and transformed liver tissue. Differential inactivation and substrate protection in membrane vesicles and reconstituted proteoliposomes," *J Biol Chem*, Vol. 262, 1987, pp. 12565–12569.

[79] Neumann, J., and Brandsch, M., "Delta-aminolevulinic acid transport in cancer cells of the human extrahepatic biliary duct," *J Pharmacol Exp Ther*, Vol. 305, 2003, pp. 219–224.

[80] Rud, E., et al., "5-aminolevulinic acid, but not 5-aminolevulinic acid esters, is transported into adenocarcinoma cells by system BETA transporters," *Photochem Photobiol*, Vol. 71, 2000, pp. 640–647.

[81] Langer, S., et al., "Active and higher intracellular uptake of 5-aminolevulinic acid in tumors may be inhibited by glycine," *J Invest Dermatol*, Vol. 112, 1999, pp. 723–728.

[82] Gederaas, O. A., et al., "5-Aminolaevulinic acid methyl ester transport on amino acid carriers in a human colon adenocarcinoma cell line," *Photochem Photobiol*, Vol. 73, 2001, pp. 164–169.

[83] Jichlinski, P., et al., "Hexyl aminolevulinate fluorescence cystoscopy: new diagnostic tool for photodiagnosis of superficial bladder cancer—a multicenter study," *J Urol*, Vol. 170, 2003, pp. 226–229.

[84] Lange, N., et al., "Photodetection of early human bladder cancer based on the fluorescence of 5-aminolaevulinic acid hexylester-induced protoporphyrin IX: a pilot study," *Br J Cancer*, Vol. 80, 1999, pp. 185–193.

[85] Hanahan, D., and Weinberg, R. A., "The hallmarks of cancer," *Cell*, Vol. 100, 2000, pp. 57–70.

[86] Fidler, I. J., "The organ microenvironment and cancer metastasis," *Differentiation*, Vol. 70, 2002, pp. 498–505.

[87] Govil, S. K. Transdermal drug delivery systems. In: P. Tyle (ed.), *Drug Delivery Devices*, New York: Marcel Dekker, 1988.

[88] Saldanha, G., Fletcher, A., and Slater, D. N., "Basal cell carcinoma: a dermatopathological and molecular biological update," *Br J Dermatol*, Vol. 148, 2003, pp. 195–202.

[89] Cairnduff, F., et al., "Superficial photodynamic therapy with topical 5-aminolaevulinic acid for superficial primary and secondary skin cancer," *Br J Cancer*, Vol. 69, 1994, pp. 605–608.

[90] Dijkstra, A. T., et al., "Photodynamic therapy with violet light and topical 6-aminolaevulinic acid in the treatment of actinic keratosis, Bowen's disease and basal cell carcinoma," *J Eur Acad Dermatol Venereol*, Vol. 15, 2001, pp. 550–554.

[91] Morton, C. A., et al., "Photodynamic therapy for basal cell carcinoma: effect of tumor thickness and duration of photosensitizer application on response," *Arch Dermatol*, Vol. 134, 1998, pp. 248–249.

[92] Moan, J., Ma, L. W., and Iani, V., "On the pharmacokinetics of topically applied 5-aminolevulinic acid and two of its esters," *Int J Cancer*, Vol. 92, 2001, pp. 139–143.

[93] Tsai, J. C., et al., "In vitro/in vivo correlations between transdermal delivery of 5-aminolaevulinic acid and cutaneous protoporphyrin IX accumulation and effect of formulation," *Br J Dermatol*, Vol. 146, 2002, pp. 853–862.

[94] van den Akker, J. T., et al., "Protoporphyrin IX fluorescence kinetics and localization after topical application of ALA pentyl ester and ALA on hairless mouse skin with UVB-induced early skin cancer," *Photochem Photobiol*, Vol. 72, 2000, pp. 399–406.

[95] van den Akker, J. T., et al., "Chronic UVB exposure enhances in vitro percutaneous penetration of 5-aminulevulinic acid in hairless mouse skin," *Lasers Surg Med*, Vol. 34, 2004, pp. 141–145.

[96] van den Akker, J. T., et al., "Systemic component of protoporphyrin IX production in nude mouse skin upon topical application of aminolevulinic acid depends on the application conditions," *Photochem Photobiol*, Vol. 75, 2002, pp. 172–177.

[97] van den Akker, J. T., et al., "Topical application of 5-aminolevulinic acid hexyl ester and 5-aminolevulinic acid to normal nude mouse skin: differences in protoporphyrin IX fluorescence kinetics and the role of the stratum corneum," *Photochem Photobiol*, Vol. 72, 2000, pp. 681–689.

[98] Jichlinski, P., and Leisinger, H. J., "Photodynamic therapy in superficial bladder cancer: past, present and future," *Urol Res*, Vol. 29, 2001, pp. 396–405.

[99]   McKenney, J. K., et al., "Morphologic expressions of urothelial carcinoma in situ: a detailed evaluation of its histologic patterns with emphasis on carcinoma in situ with microinvasion," *Am J Surg Pathol*, Vol. 25, 2001, pp. 356–362.

[100] Milord, R. A., Lecksell, K., and Epstein, J. I., "An objective morphologic parameter to aid in the diagnosis of flat urothelial carcinoma in situ," *Hum Pathol*, Vol. 32, 2001, pp. 997–1002.

[101] Herd, M. E., and Williams, G., "Scanning electron microscopy in early human bladder neoplasia," *Histopathology*, Vol. 8, 1984, pp. 611–618.

[102] Newman, J., and Hicks, R. M., "Diffuse neoplastic change in urothelium from tumour-bearing human lower urinary tract," *Scan Electron Microsc*, 1981, pp. 1–10.

[103] Joseph, L. P., "Breast cancer detection," *Science*, Vol. 284, 1999, pp. 743.

[104] Stummer, W., et al., "Fluorescence-guided resection of glioblastoma multiforme by using 5-aminolevulinic acid-induced porphyrins: a prospective study in 52 consecutive patients," *J Neurosurg*, Vol. 93, 2000, pp. 1003–1013.

[105] Bogaards, A., et al., "Fluorescence image-guided brain tumour resection with adjuvant metronomic photodynamic therapy: pre-clinical model and technology development," *Photochem Photobiol Sci*, Vol. 4, 2005, pp. 438–442.

[106] Bogaards, A., et al., "Increased brain tumor resection using fluorescence image guidance in a preclinical model," *Lasers Surg Med*, Vol. 35, 2004, pp. 181–190.

[107] Lilge, L., Portnoy, M., and Wilson, B. C., "Apoptosis induced in vivo by photodynamic therapy in normal brain and intracranial tumour tissue," *Br J Cancer*, Vol. 83, 2000, pp. 1110–1117.

[108] Stummer, W., et al., "In vitro and in vivo porphyrin accumulation by C6 glioma cells after exposure to 5-aminolevulinic acid," *J Photochem Photobiol B*, Vol. 45, 1998, pp. 160–169.

[109] Stummer, W., et al., "Technical principles for protoporphyrin-IX-fluorescence guided microsurgical resection of malignant glioma tissue," *Acta Neurochir (Wien)*, Vol. 140, 1998, pp. 995–1000.

[110] Obwegeser, A., Jakober, R., and Kostron, H., "Uptake and kinetics of 14C-labelled meta-tetrahydroxyphenylchlorin and 5-aminolaevulinic acid in the C6 rat glioma model," *Br J Cancer*, Vol. 78, 1998, pp. 733–738.

[111] Yahara, T., et al., "Relationship between microvessel density and thermographic hot areas in breast cancer," *Surg Today*, Vol. 33, 2003, pp. 243–248.

[112] Jones, B. F., "A reappraisal of the use of infrared thermal image analysis in medicine," *IEEE Trans Med Imaging*, Vol. 17, 1998, pp. 1019–1027.

[113] Stefanadis, C., et al., "Increased temperature of malignant urinary bladder tumors in vivo: the application of a new method based on a catheter technique," *J Clin Oncol*, Vol. 19, 2001, pp. 676–681.

[114] Kinoshita, M., and Hynynen, K., "Mechanism of porphyrin-induced sonodynamic effect: possible role of hyperthermia," *Radiat Res*, Vol. 165, 2006, pp. 299–306.

[115] Juzeniene, A., et al., "The influence of temperature on photodynamic cell killing in vitro with 5-aminolevulinic acid," *J Photochem Photobiol B*, Vol. 84, 2006, pp. 161–166.

[116] Hirschberg, H., et al., "Enhanced cytotoxic effects of 5-aminolevulinic acid-mediated photodynamic therapy by concurrent hyperthermia in glioma spheroids," *J Neurooncol*, Vol. 70, 2004, pp. 289–299.

[117] Juzeniene, A., et al., "Temperature effect on accumulation of protoporphyrin IX after topical application of 5-aminolevulinic acid and its methylester and hexylester derivatives in normal mouse skin," *Photochem Photobiol*, Vol. 76, 2002, pp. 452–456.

[118] Moan, J., et al., "The temperature dependence of protoporphyrin IX production in cells and tissues," *Photochem Photobiol*, Vol. 70, 1999, pp. 669–673.

[119] Juzenas, P., et al., "Uptake of topically applied 5-aminolevulinic acid and production of protoporphyrin IX in normal mouse skin: dependence on skin temperature," *Photochem Photobiol*, Vol. 69, 1999, pp. 478–481.

[120] van den Akker, J. T., et al., "Effect of elevating the skin temperature during topical ALA application on in vitro ALA penetration through mouse skin and in vivo PpIX production in human skin," *Photochem Photobiol Sci*, Vol. 3, 2004, pp. 263–267.

[121] Anderson, P. M., and Desnick, R. J., "Purification and properties of delta-aminolevulinate dehydrase from human erythrocytes," *J Biol Chem*, Vol. 254, 1979, pp. 6924–6930.

[122] Uehlinger, P., et al., "5-Aminolevulinic acid and its derivatives: physical chemical properties and protoporphyrin IX formation in cultured cells," *J Photochem Photobiol B*, Vol. 54, 2000, pp. 72–80.

[123] Krammer, B., and Uberriegler, K., "In-vitro investigation of ALA-induced protoporphyrin IX," *J Photochem Photobiol B*, Vol. 36, 1996, pp. 121–126.

[124] Fuchs, C., et al., "H-dependent formation of 5-aminolaevulinic acid-induced protoporphyrin IX in fibrosarcoma cells," *J Photochem Photobiol B*, Vol. 40, 1997, pp. 49–54.

[125] Bech, O., Berg, K., and Moan, J., "The pH dependency of protoporphyrin IX formation in cells incubated with 5-aminolevulinic acid," *Cancer Lett*, Vol. 113, 1997, pp. 25–29.

[126] Lange, N., et al., "Routine experimental system for defining conditions used in photodynamic therapy and fluorescence photodetection of (non-) neoplastic epithelia," *J Biomed Opt*, Vol. 6, 2001, pp. 151–159.

[127] Friberg, E. G., et al., "pH effects on the cellular uptake of four photosensitizing drugs evaluated for use in photodynamic therapy of cancer," *Cancer Lett*, Vol. 195, 2003, pp. 73–80.

[128] Moan, J., Smedshammer, L., and Christensen, T., "Photodynamic effects on human cells exposed to light in the presence of hematoporphyrin. pH effects," *Cancer Lett*, Vol. 9, 1980, pp. 327–332.

[129] Moan, J., et al., "Photosensitizing efficiencies, tumor- and cellular uptake of different photosensitizing drugs relevant for photodynamic therapy of cancer," *Photochem Photobiol*, Vol. 46, 1987, pp. 713–721.

[130] Kennedy, T., "Managing the drug discovery/development interface," *Drug Discovery Today*, Vol. 2, 1997, pp. 436–444.

[131] Dalton, J. T., et al., "Clinical pharmacokinetics of 5-aminolevulinic acid in healthy volunteers and patients at high risk for recurrent bladder cancer," *J Pharmacol Exp Ther*, Vol. 301, 2002, pp. 507–512.

[132] Dalton, J. T., et al., "Pharmacokinetics of aminolevulinic acid after intravesical administration to dogs," *Pharm Res*, Vol. 16, 1999, pp. 288–295.

[133] Dalton, J. T., Meyer, M. C., and Golub, A. L., "Pharmacokinetics of aminolevulinic acid after oral and intravenous administration in dogs," *Drug Metab Dispos*, Vol. 27, 1999, pp. 432–435.

[134] Moan, J., et al., "Photobleaching of protoporphyrin IX in cells incubated with 5-aminolevulinic acid," *Int J Cancer*, Vol. 70, 1997, pp. 90–97.

[135] Eleouet, S., et al., "In vitro fluorescence, toxicity and phototoxicity induced by delta-aminolevulinic acid (ALA) or ALA-esters," *Photochem Photobiol*, Vol. 71, 2000, pp. 447–454.

[136] Xiang, W., et al., "Photodynamic effects induced by aminolevulinic acid esters on human cervical carcinoma cells in culture," *Photochem Photobiol*, Vol. 74, 2001, pp. 617–623.

[137] Waidelich, R., et al., "Clinical experience with 5-aminolevulinic acid and photodynamic therapy for refractory superficial bladder cancer," *J Urol*, Vol. 165, 2001, pp. 1904–1907.

[138] Waidelich, R., et al., "Early clinical experience with 5-aminolevulinic acid for the photodynamic therapy of upper tract urothelial tumors," *J Urol*, Vol. 159, 1998, pp. 401–404.

[139] Wennberg, A. M., et al., "Delta-aminolevulinic acid in superficial basal cell carcinomas and normal skin-a microdialysis and perfusion study," *Clin Exp Dermatol*, Vol. 25, 2000, pp. 317–322.

[140] Casas, A., et al., "The influence of the vehicle on the synthesis of porphyrins after topical application of 5-aminolaevulinic acid. Implications in cutaneous photodynamic sensitization," *Br J Dermatol*, Vol. 143, 2000, pp. 564–572.

[141] McLoone, N., R. F. Donnelly, P. A. McCarron, M. Walsh and K. McKenna, "Aminolevulinic acid penetration into nodular basal cell carcinomas: influence of different concentrations and application times on amounts of ala delivered via a bioadhesive patch," *Clin. Photodyn*, Vol. 1, 2004, pp. 5–6.

[142] Ahmadi, S., et al., "Evaluation of the penetration of 5-aminolevulinic acid through basal cell carcinoma: a pilot study," *Exp Dermatol*, Vol. 13, 2004, pp. 445–451.

[143] Johnson, P. G., Hui, S. W., and Oseroff, A. R., "Electrically enhanced percutaneous delivery of delta-aminolevulinic acid using electric pulses and a DC potential," *Photochem Photobiol*, Vol. 75, 2002, pp. 534–540.

[144] Donnelly, R. F., P. A. McCarron, A. D. Woolfson, A. Zawislak and J. H. Price, "Autoradiographic imaging of 5-aminolevulinic acid penetration through vaginal tissue," *Clin. Photodyn*, Vol. 1, 2004, pp. 6–7.

[145] Schoenfeld, N., et al., "Protoporphyrin biosynthesis in melanoma B16 cells stimulated by 5-aminolevulinic acid and chemical inducers: characterization of photodynamic inactivation," *Int J Cancer*, Vol. 56, 1994, pp. 106–112.

[146] Fujita, H., et al., "Sequential activation of genes for heme pathway enzymes during erythroid differentiation of mouse Friend virus-transformed erythroleukemia cells," *Biochim Biophys Acta*, Vol. 1090, 1991, pp. 311–316.

[147] Malik, Z., Lugaci, H., and Hanania, J., "Stimulation of Friend erythroleukemic cell cytodifferentiation by 5-amino levulinic acid; porphyrins, cell size, segregation of sialoglycoproteins, and nuclear translocation," *Exp Hematol*, Vol. 16, 1988, pp. 330–335.

[148] Beaumont, C., et al., "Effects of succinylacetone on dimethylsulfoxide-mediated induction of heme pathway enzymes in mouse friend virus-transformed erythroleukemia cells," *Exp Cell Res*, Vol. 154, 1984, pp. 474–484.

[149] Bugaj, A., et al., "The effect of skin permeation enhancers on the formation of porphyrins in mouse skin during topical application of the methyl ester of 5-aminolevulinic acid," *J Photochem Photobiol B*, Vol. 83, 2006, pp. 94–97.

[150] Soler, A. M., et al., "Photodynamic therapy of superficial basal cell carcinoma with 5-aminolevulinic acid with dimethylsulfoxide and ethylendiaminetetraacetic acid: a comparison of two light sources," *Photochem Photobiol*, Vol. 71, 2000, pp. 724–729.

[151] De Rosa, F. S., et al., "A vehicle for photodynamic therapy of skin cancer: influence of dimethylsulphoxide on 5-aminolevulinic acid in vitro cutaneous permeation and in vivo protoporphyrin IX accumulation determined by confocal microscopy," *J Control Release*, Vol. 65, 2000, pp. 359–366.

[152] Malik, Z., et al., "Topical application of 5-aminolevulinic acid, DMSO and EDTA: protoporphyrin IX accumulation in skin and tumours of mice," *J Photochem Photobiol B*, Vol. 28, 1995, pp. 213–218.

[153] Steluti, R., et al., "Topical glycerol monooleate/propylene glycol formulations enhance 5-aminolevulinic acid in vitro skin delivery and in vivo protophorphyrin IX accumulation in hairless mouse skin," *Eur J Pharm Biopharm*, Vol. 60, 2005, pp. 439–444.

[154] Marti, A., et al., "Optimisation of the formation and distribution of protoporphyrin IX in the urothelium: an in vitro approach," *J Urol*, Vol. 162, 1999, pp. 546–552.

[155] Kosobe, T., et al., "Size and surface charge effect of 5-aminolevulinic acid-containing liposomes on photodynamic therapy for cultivated cancer cells," *Drug Dev Ind Pharm*, Vol. 31, 2005, pp. 623–629.

[156] Casas, A., and Batlle, A., "Aminolevulinic acid derivatives and liposome delivery as strategies for improving 5-aminolevulinic acid-mediated photodynamic therapy," *Curr Med Chem*, Vol. 13, 2006, pp. 1157–1168.

[157] Casas, A., et al., "ALA and ALA hexyl ester in free and liposomal formulations for the photosensitisation of tumour organ cultures," *Br J Cancer*, Vol. 86, 2002, pp. 837–842.

[158] Auner, B. G., Valenta, C., and Hadgraft, J., "Influence of lipophilic counter-ions in combination with phloretin and 6-ketocholestanol on the skin permeation of 5-aminolevulinic acid," *Int J Pharm*, Vol. 255, 2003, pp. 109–116.

[159] Godal, A., et al., "New derivatives of 5-aminolevulinic acid for photodynamic therapy: chemical synthesis and porphyrin production in in vitro and in vivo biological systems," *J Environ Pathol Toxicol Oncol*, Vol. 25, 2006, pp. 109–126.

[160] Rebeiz, N., et al., "Photodestruction of tumor cells by induction of endogenous accumulation of protoporphyrin IX: enhancement by 1,10-phenanthroline," *Photochem Photobiol*, Vol. 55, 1992, pp. 431–435.

[161] Berg, K., et al., "The influence of iron chelators on the accumulation of protoporphyrin IX in 5-aminolaevulinic acid-treated cells," *Br J Cancer*, Vol. 74, 1996, pp. 688–697.

[162] Peng, Q., et al., "Distribution of 5-aminolevulinic acid-induced porphyrins in noduloulcerative basal cell carcinoma," *Photochem Photobiol*, Vol. 62, 1995, pp. 906–913.

[163] Orenstein, A., Kostenich, G., and Malik, Z., "The kinetics of protoporphyrin fluorescence during ALA-PDT in human malignant skin tumors," *Cancer Lett*, Vol. 120, 1997, pp. 229–234.

[164] Chang, S., Chern, I., and Bown, S. G., "Photodynamic therapy of rat bladder and urethra: evaluation of urinary and reproductive function after inducing protoporphyrin IX with 5-aminolaevulinic acid," *BJU Int*, Vol. 85, 2000, pp. 747–753.

[165] van den Akker, J. T., et al., "Comparative in vitro percutaneous penetration of 5-aminolevulinic acid and two of its esters through excised hairless mouse skin," *Lasers Surg Med*, Vol. 33, 2003, pp. 173–181.

[166] De Rosa, F. S., et al., "In vitro metabolism of 5-ALA esters derivatives in hairless mice skin homogenate and in vivo PpIX accumulation studies," *Pharm Res*, Vol. 21, 2004, pp. 2247–2252.

[167] Shen, S. C., et al., "In vitro percutaneous absorption and in vivo protoporphyrin IX accumulation in skin and tumors after topical 5-aminolevulinic acid application with enhancement using an erbium:YAG laser," *J Pharm Sci*, Vol. 95, 2006, pp. 929–938.

[168] Britton, J. E., et al., "Investigation of the use of the pulsed dye laser in the treatment of Bowen's disease using 5-aminolaevulinic acid phototherapy," *Br J Dermatol*, Vol. 153, 2005, pp. 780–784.

[169] Lee, W. R., et al., "Microdermabrasion as a novel tool to enhance drug delivery via the skin: an animal study," *Dermatol Surg*, Vol. 32, 2006, pp. 1013–1022.

[170] Ma, L., et al., "Production of protoporphyrin IX induced by 5-aminolevulinic acid in transplanted human colon adenocarcinoma of nude mice can be increased by ultrasound," *Int J Cancer*, Vol. 78, 1998, pp. 464–469.

[171] Charoenbanpachon, S., et al., "Acceleration of ALA-induced PpIX fluorescence development in the oral mucosa," *Lasers Surg Med*, Vol. 32, 2003, pp. 185–188.

[172] Kalia, Y. N., et al., "Iontophoretic drug delivery," *Adv Drug Deliv Rev*, Vol. 56, 2004, pp. 619–658.

[173] Fang, J. Y., et al., "Enhancement of topical 5-aminolaevulinic acid delivery by erbium:YAG laser and microdermabrasion: a comparison with iontophoresis and electroporation," *Br J Dermatol*, Vol. 151, 2004, pp. 132–140.

[174] Rhodes, L. E., et al., "Iontophoretic delivery of ALA provides a quantitative model for ALA pharmacokinetics and PpIX phototoxicity in human skin," *J Invest Dermatol*, Vol. 108, 1997, pp. 87–91.

[175] Lopez, R. F., et al., "Iontophoretic delivery of 5-aminolevulinic acid (ALA): effect of pH," *Pharm Res*, Vol. 18, 2001, pp. 311–315.

[176] Lopez, R. F., et al., "Enhanced delivery of 5-aminolevulinic acid esters by iontophoresis in vitro," *Photochem Photobiol*, Vol. 77, 2003, pp. 304–308.

[177] Lopez, R. F., et al., "Optimization of aminolevulinic acid delivery by iontophoresis," *J Control Release*, Vol. 88, 2003, pp. 65–70.

[178] Han, I., et al., "Expression pattern and intensity of protoporphyrin IX induced by liposomal 5-aminolevulinic acid in rat pilosebaceous unit throughout hair cycle," *Arch Dermatol Res*, Vol. 297, 2005, pp. 210–217.

[179] Merclin, N., Bramer, T., and Edsman, K., "Iontophoretic delivery of 5-aminolevulinic acid and its methyl ester using a carbopol gel as vehicle," *J Control Release*, Vol. 98, 2004, pp. 57–65.

[180] Fotinos, N., et al., "5-Aminolevulinic acid derivatives in photomedicine: Characteristics, application and perspectives," *Photochem Photobiol*, Vol. 82, 2006, pp. 994–1015.

[181] Schneider, R., et al., "Recent improvements in the use of synthetic peptides for a selective photodynamic therapy," *Anticancer Agents Med Chem*, Vol. 6, 2006, pp. 469–488.

[182] Berger, Y., et al., "Evaluation of dipeptide-derivatives of 5-aminolevulinic acid as precursors for photosensitizers in photodynamic therapy," *Bioorg Med Chem*, Vol. 11, 2003, pp. 1343–1351.

[183] Di Venosa, G. M., et al., "Investigation of a novel dendritic derivative of 5-aminolaevulinic acid for photodynamic therapy," *Int J Biochem Cell Biol*, Vol. 38, 2006, pp. 82–91.

[184] Battah, S., et al., "Enhanced porphyrin accumulation using dendritic derivatives of 5-aminolaevulinic acid for photodynamic therapy: an in vitro study," *Int J Biochem Cell Biol*, Vol. 38, 2006, pp. 1382–1392.

[185] Battah, S. H., et al., "Synthesis and biological studies of 5-aminolevulinic acid-containing dendrimers for photodynamic therapy," *Bioconjug Chem*, Vol. 12, 2001, pp. 980–988.

[186] Juzeniene, A., et al., "Topical application of 5-aminolevulinic acid and its methylester, hexylester and octylester derivatives: considerations for dosimetry in mouse skin model," *Photochem Photobiol*, Vol. 76, 2002, pp. 329–334.

[187] Peng, Q., et al., "Build-up of esterified aminolevulinic-acid-derivative-induced porphyrin fluorescence in normal mouse skin," *J Photochem Photobiol B*, Vol. 34, 1996, pp. 95–96.

[188] Peng, Q., et al., "5-Aminolevulinic acid-based photodynamic therapy: principles and experimental research," *Photochem Photobiol*, Vol. 65, 1997, pp. 235–251.

[189] Fritsch, C., et al., "Preferential relative porphyrin enrichment in solar keratoses upon topical application of delta-aminolevulinic acid methylester," *Photochem Photobiol*, Vol. 68, 1998, pp. 218–221.

[190] De Rosa, F. S., et al., "In vitro skin permeation and retention of 5-aminolevulinic acid ester derivatives for photodynamic therapy," *J Control Release*, Vol. 89, 2003, pp. 261–269.

[191] Collaud, S., et al., "Thermosetting gel for the delivery of 5-aminolevulinic acid esters to the cervix," *J Pharm Sci*, Vol., 2007.

[192] Collaud, S., et al., "Clinical evaluation of bioadhesive hydrogels for topical delivery of hexylaminolevulinate to Barrett's esophagus," *J Control Release*, Vol., 2007.

[193] Bigelow, C. E., et al., "ALA- and ALA-hexylester-induced protoporphyrin IX fluorescence and distribution in multicell tumour spheroids," *Br J Cancer*, Vol. 85, 2001, pp. 727–734.

[194] Marti, A., et al., "Comparison of aminolevulinic acid and hexylester aminolevulinate induced protoporphyrin IX distribution in human bladder cancer," *J Urol*, Vol. 170, 2003, pp. 428–432.

[195] Whitaker, C. J., et al., "Photosensitization of pancreatic tumour cells by delta-aminolaevulinic acid esters," *Anticancer Drug Des*, Vol. 15, 2000, pp. 161–170.

[196] Doring, F., et al., "Delta-aminolevulinic acid transport by intestinal and renal peptide transporters and its physiological and clinical implications," *J Clin Invest*, Vol. 101, 1998, pp. 2761–2767.

[197] Rodriguez, L., et al., "Study of the mechanisms of uptake of 5-aminolevulinic acid derivatives by PEPT1 and PEPT2 transporters as a tool to improve photodynamic therapy of tumours," *Int J Biochem Cell Biol*, Vol. 38, 2006, pp. 1530–1539.

[198] Morton, C. A., "Methyl aminolevulinate (Metvix) photodynamic therapy—practical pearls," *J Dermatolog Treat*, Vol. 14 Suppl 3, 2003, pp. 23–26.

[199] Freeman, M., et al., "A comparison of photodynamic therapy using topical methyl aminolevulinate (Metvix) with single cycle cryotherapy in patients with actinic keratosis: a prospective, randomized study," *J Dermatolog Treat*, Vol. 14, 2003, pp. 99–106.

[200] Foley, P., "Clinical efficacy of methyl aminolevulinate (Metvix) photodynamic therapy," J Dermatolog Treat, Vol. 14 Suppl 3, 2003, pp. 15–22.

[201] Witjes, J. A., Moonen, P. M., and van der Heijden, A. G., "Comparison of hexaminolevulinate based flexible and rigid fluorescence cystoscopy with rigid white light cystoscopy in bladder cancer: results of a prospective Phase II study," *Eur Urol*, Vol. 47, 2005, pp. 319–322.

[202] Schmidbauer, J., et al., "Improved detection of urothelial carcinoma in situ with hexaminolevulinate fluorescence cystoscopy," *J Urol*, Vol. 171, 2004, pp. 135–138.

[203] Witjes, J. A., and Douglass, J., "The role of hexaminolevulinate fluorescence cystoscopy in bladder cancer," *Nat Clin Pract Urol*, Vol. 4, 2007, pp. 542–549.

[204] Jocham, D., et al., "Improved detection and treatment of bladder cancer using hexaminolevulinate imaging: a prospective, phase III multicenter study," *J Urol*, Vol. 174, 2005, pp. 862–866; discussion 866.

[205] Fradet, Y., et al., "A comparison of hexaminolevulinate fluorescence cystoscopy and white light cystoscopy for the detection of carcinoma in situ in patients with bladder cancer: a phase III, multicenter study," *J Urol*, Vol. 178, 2007, pp. 68–73; discussion 73.

[206] Donnelly, R. F., McCarron, P. A., and Woolfson, A. D., "Drug delivery of aminolevulinic acid from topical formulations intended for photodynamic therapy," *Photochem Photobiol*, Vol. 81, 2005, pp. 750–767.

[207] Lopez, R. F., et al., "Photodynamic therapy of skin cancer: controlled drug delivery of 5-ALA and its esters," *Adv Drug Deliv Rev*, Vol. 56, 2004, pp. 77–94.

CHAPTER 5

Light Dosimetry and Light Sources for Photodynamic Therapy

Robert A. Weersink and Lothar Lilge

5.1 Introduction

Photodynamic therapy has evolved from a therapy used for primarily superficial lesions to one that is now being investigated clinically to treat large tissue volumes. Much of this evolution is due to developments in light sources and delivery methods for PDT. PDT dosimetry concepts have also evolved, with generally accepted dosimetry models based on a threshold model of action mediated by explicit input parameters. Specific treatment planning and dosimetry concepts, however, are differentiated by the treatment site and geometry. Our goal in this chapter is to bring the light dosimetry planning under a general framework, basing the treatment planning and delivery principles on those that have been developed for the mature field of radiation therapy. Intimately tied to light dosimetry is the mode of light delivery, and thus we explore the current state of light delivery technology.

In radiation oncology dose is defined either on physical or radiobiological parameters, the former using energy-based parameters and the latter considering the intrinsic biological response of the tissue along with other mitigating circumstances such as the oxygen enhancing factor [1]. A similar situation applies to PDT, where dose can be defined in relation to either physical or biological parameters. The former is commonly based on the photochemical reactants at the heart of PDT: photons, photosensitizer, and oxygen. The latter is based on the cytotoxic load leading to the biological response. The biological PDT dose can be directly quantified by the cytotoxic quantity, singlet oxygen, but currently measuring this clinically with adequate spatial resolution is unfeasible. Response monitoring is preferable to measurements of either the inputs or the cytotoxic quantity, since it enables patient-specific control of the therapy. However, PDT is commonly delivered as an acute treatment within a short period, whereas, biological effects do not manifest themselves during the treatment with the exceptions of vascular changes [2, 3] and early signs of edema. Instead, biological response may be linked to the consumption of any one of the PDT reactants, leading to dosimetry models based on photobleaching of the photosensitizer [4, 5], or oxygen consumption [6, 7]. Various models of tissue response based on explicit physical parameters have been developed, such as the critical fluence [8], effective dose model [9, 10], or the photodynamic threshold model [11, 12]. In all physical parameter models, the consumption of photons or the light gradient stands apart as the only reactant that can be controlled (within the limit imposed through tissue optics) by the medical physicist and clinical oncologist during treatment planning and PDT delivery. Active control of the other reactants is more difficult but not impossible, such as the use of hyperbaric oxygen chambers demonstrated preclinically [13] and clinically [14] and molecular targeting of the photosensitizer [15, 16].

PDT dose response models using all reactant concentrations can in principle be developed, but in practice, this is limited by available means to quantify all parameters with sufficient spatial resolution. Further, not all reactants are equally weighted when determining the treatment effect. For example, in the 1-D case, the treatment depth is given by

$$z_{th} \approx \frac{1}{\mu_{eff}} \ln\left(\frac{[Drug]S_o}{D_{th}}\right) \tag{5.1}$$

with D_{th} being the minimum dose required to achieve tissue necrosis. Hence the treatment depth, z_{th}, is logarithmically dependent on drug concentration, [Drug], and source power, S_o, and inversely related to the tissue attenuation μ_{eff}. This latter relationship will vary depending on the light delivery geometry. The relation of the treatment depth to molecular oxygen is highly nonlinear, possibly in a binary fashion as suggested by the photodynamic threshold model [12]. Further, oxygen is typically in excess at the start of the treatment, with its rate of consumption determined by the rate of light or photon delivery (i.e., if oxygen is depleted too rapidly, the PDT reaction is limited). For our discussion, we will not include these effects here.

The photochemical reaction leading to the cytotoxic substance is a quantum effect and thus depends on the photon density rather than the power density. However, power meters are more common than photon meters, and thus in practice light dosimetry is defined in terms of power and energy densities. This practice also coincides with units used to describe the maximum permissible exposure of tissues, in particular skin.

This chapter will provide brief introductions of dosimetry and planning concepts, light propagation models, solutions thereof for the different treatment geometries, applicable light sources, and light sensing devices. The chapter will conclude with a preview of novel light sources and fluence rate detection approaches.

5.1.1   Tissue Optical Properties and Light Propagation in Tissue

The shaping of the light intensity throughout the intended treatment volume is currently the simplest method of providing treatment delivery optimization for individual patients. The imagination of the physicist and oncologist towards achieving the perfect outcome is restricted by the fact that tissue acts as a low-pass filter for light propagation, leading to a rapid attenuation of the photon density and elimination of spatial/temporal intensity modulations created at the source. This is less prevalent at longer wavelengths, where μ_{eff} is lower, which drives the constant search for photosensitizers absorbing beyond the red visible spectrum. Thus, the tissue optical properties become paramount for clinically relevant light dosimetry. However, in treating sites that are superficial or within body cavities, the intended target is typically quite shallow, so differences in optical properties have only a minor effect on the light penetration through the treatment volume and thus have little effect on treatment outcome.

Light or photon transport in tissue is governed by Maxwell's equations. However, tissue is a dielectric material, with conductivity and permittivity changes on the micron length scale that renders their applicability inefficient [17, 18]. The more common approach is the use of solutions of the diffusion equation, as an approximation to transport theory [19, 20], adapted to the particular treatment geometry, such as surface exposures, spherical cavities, or solid tissue. From a physics perspective these different solutions of the diffusion equation are based on accommodating tissue boundaries and refractive index mismatches within the framework of energy conservation in transport theory. Independent of the actual geometry, the prediction of the actual fluence rate in the tissue is to a large extent determined by the tissue optical properties. Accurate measurements of the optical properties is more important for treatments of large tissue volumes as compared to surfaces, since small changes in optical properties can dramatically affect the fluence rate far from a source (see (5.1)). Measuring μ_{eff} can be made with simple attenuation measurements but accurate separation of μ_a and μ_s' is facilitated by measurements that are independent of the absolute powers (for instance, time or frequency domain measurements) since effects such as blood pooling immediately surrounding a source or dose fiber can make it difficult to precisely and accurately measure in vivo.

Numerous methods have been developed to measure optical properties for accessible tissue surfaces. Spatially resolved diffuse reflectance [21], time- or frequency-domain [22] or spectroscopy techniques (in which constituent concentrations are used as a constraint in fitting the measured reflectance spectra) [23, 24] all provide estimates based on analytical calculations. Increasingly sophisticated techniques now enable optical tomographic [25, 26] estimates of the subsurface optical properties with ~1-mm spatial resolution in bulk tissue.

In contrast, only a limited number of light power density measurements are clinically feasible for interstitial measurements, and so, light distribution in the remainder of the treatment volume needs to be modeled numerically or analytically. Commonly, volume averaged optical property values are used with spatial variations in the tissue optical properties ignored due to limitations in the ability to accurately measure the spatial variations.

For interstitial sites, several methods to determine the tissue optical properties have been derived. Zhu [27, 28] proposed a spatially resolved technique in which sources and probes are moved within catheters. It can be used to measure differences in the optical properties throughout the organ [29, 30], but is quite time-consuming. This could be overcome when using multisensory fiber probes as proposed by Pomeleau-Dalcourt et al. [31]. Weersink et al. [32] proposed a technique in which the multiple sources implanted within the tissue were switched on individually and measurements made at several points in the tissue. This provides a large data set of measurements at different source-detector separations, with analysis inherently assuming homogeneous tissue, as the large tissue volumes sampled effectively masking heterogeneities. Chin et al. [33] uses directional sensitive radiance probes, which permits quantifying heterogeneities within the tissue through spatially localized relative measurements. A frequency domain based technique in phantoms proved to be very accurate [34], but again it assumes homogeneous optical properties in the tissue. The time-resolved analogue was presented by Anderson-Engels et al. [35], which proved equally accurate in clinical testing of normal prostate, but required the same assumptions.

5.2 Light Dosimetry

5.2.1 Dosimetry Definitions and Concepts

The first step in defining the PDT dose prescription is to define the target. Following the conventions of radiation therapy, the gross tumor volume (GTV) is the visible tumor, including that seen in standard clinical imaging. This represents only part of the tumor, since invisible microscopic disease spreads from the bulk tumor mass. Adding this margin of tissue to the GTV gives an estimate of the clinical treatment volume (CTV). Judging the extent of this spread is based on clinical experience, but since this is subjective, the general rule is to be generous in assigning the size of the CTV. In external beam radiation therapy (EBRT), further uncertainty in the actual position of the target volume arises from variations in patient position between imaging and (repeat) treatment sessions, and because of organ motion, effects of lesser importance for PDT. These uncertainties are incorporated into the planning target volume (PTV). While organ motion is of less importance in PDT, the PTV nevertheless provides a good target to plan PDT delivery. The volume of tissue and organs surrounding the PTV is defined as the organs at risk (OAR) volume, with that portion of the OAR volume falling within the planning zone referred to as the planning organ at risk volume (PRV).

To assess the light dose to be received by the tissue, the most intuitive approach is to simply match the minimum light isodose contours that produce damage with the boundary of the PTV. For complex geometries, however, this approach becomes difficult to visualize, and hence to optimize. The light dose received by the PTV and any OAR can be visualized with cumulative dose volume histograms (DVH) that transform a complex 3-D visualization problem into a single 1-D plot (see Figure 5.1). In a DVH the vertical axis represents the percent of total tissue volume that has received a dose greater than any specified dose on the horizontal axis. While dose in EBRT represents cumulative dose, for PDT dosimetry, we refer to the dose in $(\mu g/g)^*J/cm^2$. If the drug concentration is constant throughout the tissue, then the cumulative dose can be described in terms of light dose only as shown in Figure 5.1.

The DVH enables the planner to objectively evaluate different dose prescriptions, not only for the PTV but also for surrounding OARs. Qualitative dose prescriptions naturally follow from the DVHs and can be given in 2 ways: D_{90}, which is the minimum light dose that covers 90% of the PTV, and V_{100}, which is the fractional volume of the PTV that receives at least 100% of the prescription dose.

In conjunction with DVHs as a visual tool, numerical optimization tools can also be used to assess treatment plans. Dose optimization considers two criteria: (1) that at least the threshold dose is delivered to the entire PTV, and (2) that the dose delivered to OARs is lower than the threshold dose, if treatment effect of parts of this organ has a negative clinical outcome. This can be summarized by the minimization of the following generalized function:

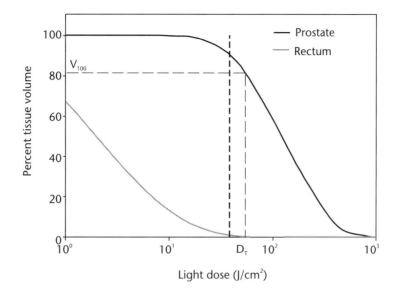

Figure 5.1 Example of a dose volume histogram (DVH) for PDT treatment of the prostate, and a neighboring organ at risk, the rectum. The threshold dose, D_T, and the dose received by 90% of the PTV, D_{90}, are shown along the x-axis. V_{100} is the percentage of treated volume that received D_T. In the example given, $V_{100} = 80\%$ for the prostate, and <5% for the rectum.

$$F = \sum_{j=1}^{M} w_j^{PTV} f(D_P, D_T) + \sum_{j=1}^{N} w_j^{OAR} f(D_O, D_T) \tag{5.2}$$

where the PTV and OAR are described by M and N voxels in the first and second terms on the right, respectively. Here $f(D_P, D_T)$ describes the relationship of the delivered PDT dose, D_P to the threshold PDT dose, D_T. If $D_P > D_T$ then $f(D_P, D_T) = 0$ and there is no increased cost in the minimization function. However, if $D_P < D_T$, then $f(D_P, D_T) > 0$, indicating an undesirable dose prescription. The function can be simply set to 1 or change in relation to $D_T - D_P$ [36]. Undesirable high doses, such as doses resulting in thermal effects, can also be considered by defining a maximum permissible dose. Unlike radiation therapy, however, there is no requirement to have a uniform dose throughout the PTV. PDT is essentially ablative, with complete response observed at doses greater than the threshold dose, and unaffected tissue in regions where the dose is less than this threshold. Thus overdosing within the PTV is permissible, since once the damage has been achieved, any extra dose has no added effect.

For the OARs, the dosing considerations are reversed. If $D_O > D_T$ there is an increased cost to the minimization function (i.e., $f(D_O, D_T) > 0$. If $D_O < D_T$, $f = 0$). The threshold dose can be different for each organ or tissue structure, depending on its sensitivity to PDT [37].

The effect of the dose delivered to each voxel, j, is weighted in the above equation using the "importance factors," w_j. In the instance of the OARs, the magnitude is proportional to the clinical impact of damage. If clinical outcome is not impacted, either by function or cosmetics, treatment of the OAR is "not important," and has no effect on the optimization of the treatment plan, and the dose to the OAR can be higher than the threshold dose. Conversely, if there is a clinical impact, the clinician may need to weigh the importance of possibly undertreating the PTV ($D_P < D_T$) with possibly overtreating the OAR ($D_O > D_T$). The relative magnitudes of the importance factors guide this balancing act.

To minimize (5.2) and optimize the dose prescription, the parameter space for planning light delivery in PDT includes essentially the same parameters as in EBRT, but with different physical implementations. These parameters include: (1) the number of sources (equivalent to the number of beams in radiation physics), (2) types of sources (equivalent to wedge or attenuators), and (3) intensity per source (equivalent to beam intensities). It is noteworthy that in EBRT there is the option of adjusting the dose rate distribution on the fly by using multileaf collimators, for which no technological equivalent exists in PDT treatment planning. For treating tissue volumes, the more analogous radiation therapy regime may be high-dose brachytherapy, in which dose implants are inserted into the tissue for a limited period of time with dose modulated by their dwell time at each position.

While PDT treatment planning is only now really beginning to explicitly use these concepts, they were understood and implemented in its initial clinical realization. We now present several representative examples of different clinical applications that highlight light geometry, required light propagation models, and the relevant planning concepts.

5.2.2 Flat Surfaces: The Collimated Beam

All currently approved and commonly applied applications of PDT are associated with treatment of flat or shallow lesions at a surface, such as actinic keratoses [38], a premalignant lesion of squamous cell carcinoma, other skin cancers, in particular basal cell carcinoma [39], and Bowen's disease. Various shallow nondermatological diseases are also approved for PDT, such as the wet form of age-related macular degeneration (AMD) [40], Barrett's esophagus [41], and viral inactivation [42].

In treating these superficial malignancies, it has been observed that normal tissue healed well following PDT [43–45], and the clinical importance of overtreating the surrounding normal tissue was negligible [46]. Hence, using the framework in Section 5.2.1, $w^{OAR} = 0$, and planning only consists of ensuring adequate dose is delivered to the malignancy or the PTV.

A single collimated beam of homogeneous intensity and large diameter is used to treat these conditions. An aperture may be used to confine the illumination to the PTV. Light propagation follows (5.1), but for treatment situations represented by tissue volumes of limited depth, $d \sim (3\mu_{eff})^{-1}$, with large extended sources of a diameter multiple times μ_{eff}^{-1} the effects of light propagation can be ignored since the fluence rate will not change sufficiently passing through the PTV to affect treatment outcome. To derive dose metrics that were independent of the photosensitizer and the particular organ surface comprising the target area, Moseley [9] also included the tissue's intrinsic sensitivity into his dosimetry model.

5.2.3 Cavities

In treatments of cavities such as the esophagus or the bladder, the same collimated beam equations apply, since the target also comprises a large extended surface. The key difference between surfaces and cavities lies in the need to consider the diffuse reflected light in the latter case as it will add to the irradiance at other locations within the cavity. The magnitude of this exposure enhancement is determined by the integrating sphere effect [47, 48] and depends on the tissue's albedo, $a = \mu'_s / (\mu_a + \mu'_s)$. The integrating sphere enhancement can result in a surface power density being up to 3.6 times the anticipated intensity based on geometrical considerations alone [49]. As the effect of the albedo determines the reflectance, the fluence rate at the hollow tissue sphere's surface is directly affected and real-time quantification of the irradiance on the cavity surface is paramount [50]. Van Stavern also demonstrated that this light confinement effect within the cavity can be enhanced through a scattering liquid of low scattering power [48].

The planning concepts for cavities must provide greater consideration of the clinical effect of overtreating surrounding tissue than the simple superficial lesion case, as sensitive tissue layers with $w^{OAR} > 0$ can be found at depths larger than one ore two penetration depths. For example, in the treatment of esophageal cancer, Photofrin-PDT using red light resulted in damage to the muscularis layer, leading to esophageal strictures [51]. With nonzero w^{OAR} the optimization of the PDT treatment necessitates that the dose to the underlying tissue, D_{OAR}, be reduced below the threshold dose. This was achieved using two strategies following from (5.1). One was to reduce the light dose to the muscularis by using green light, which has a higher μ_{eff} than red light [46, 52]. The other strategy was to use 5-ALA-Induced PPIX with selective uptake ([Drug]) in the CTV or dysplastic tissue [53]. Optimization of the therapies was based on empirical comparisons of clinical outcomes with the delivered light and drug doses rather than an analysis of light received by the tissue and drug dose parameters within the tissue. These empirical comparisons should provide the basis for a more rigorous model that can be used in treatment planning.

5.2.4 Tissue Volumes and Interstitial Light Delivery

Consistent with the concept that PDT should be a minimally invasive therapy, the common solution for delivering light to deep tissue volumes is to insert optical fibers coupled to lasers into the middle of the tissue volume. While isotropic point sources have been used in the bladder [54] and in interstitial thermal therapy [55], their use for interstitial PDT light delivery has not been reported. Instead, flat [56] or cylindrical diffusing fibers have been used for bulk tissue PDT, predominantly for brain [57, 58] and prostate [59, 60]. Current commercially available cylindrical diffusers (CeramOptec, Biolitec, Medlight, and ARTPhotonics, to name but a few) are designed to have a uniform delivery profile both along their long axis and their circumference. Another option is to use interstitial light emitting diodes, (LightSciences Oncology) which have a sufficiently small diameter (1.2–1.5 mm) that they can be safely placed deep into tissue without causing significant trauma.

The number and size of the chosen sources is determined by the shape, size, and effective tissue attenuation (μ_{eff}) of the PTV. Unless the volume is small and has a shape that can be matched perfectly by the emitting profile from a single point or cylindrical source, more than one light source will be needed to achieve sufficient coverage for a successful treatment. Analytical solutions to the diffusion equation are used to calculate the light distribution from multiple sources. The description of light fluence an isotropic light is well known:

$$\Phi(r) = \frac{3S_0 \mu_{eff}^2}{4\pi r \mu_a} e^{-\mu_{eff} r} \tag{5.3}$$

with S_0 representing the total power emitting from the source. Analytical descriptions of the fluence rate distribution from cylindrical sources in homogeneous media have been based on the integration of point sources over a known length [61] or conservation of energy [62, 63]. Today, however, it is just as easy computationally to describe the source as a sum of individual point sources [30, 32]. Consider a fiber of length l that is centered a distance r from the detector. The distance from each point on the fiber to the detector is then $r' = \sqrt{r^2 + l^2}$, and the fluence rate at the detector point becomes

$$\Phi(r') = \frac{3S_0 \mu_{eff}^2}{4\pi \mu_a} \sum_{1/2}^{1/2} \frac{1}{r'} e^{-\mu_{eff} r'} \tag{5.4}$$

This function can also be used to calculate the fluence rate of nonuniform cylindrical sources, as discussed below in the source section.

To describe the light distribution in a more complex geometry, such as multiple confined organs with heterogeneous optical properties, finite element methods can be used to solve the diffusion equation [36, 64] similar to techniques used in diffuse optical tomography. Such calculations can also be used to plan and optimize light dose prescriptions [36, 59, 64]. Initial light dosimetry planning aimed for a uniform light dose throughout the PTV, similar to the requirement in radiation medicine that radiation dose, should be uniform throughout the clinical treatment volume. PDT, however, is essentially ablative, and so the current trend in PDT planning is to ensure that the entire volume receives at least the threshold dose, with little regard for overdosing inside the target volume, as described by (5.2).

The most prevalent example of PDT in treating deep large tissue volumes is the prostate since it has percutaneous accessibility for sources and probes, a simple organ geometry, and imaging and delivery technologies that can be borrowed from other another treatment modality (i.e., brachytherapy).

Since prostate cancer is considered a multifocal disease, the PTV is the entire prostate plus permissible margins. Two critical structures are in the vicinity of the prostate, the urethra and the rectum. Each provides an example of how to include the OARs into the optimization process. Since urethral catheterization can be set in place until the urethra heals following the procedure, overtreatment of the urethra is not considered clinically significant, hence its weighting factor, w_j^{OAR}, is small. Further, our experience [65, 66] with TOOKAD suggests that the collagen tissue lining of the urethra is less sensitive to vascular mediated PDT than the prostate tissue (i.e., D_{th} for the urethra is greater than D_{th} for the prostate). Overtreatment of the rectum, however, may have greater clinical significance, since it is possible to induce a rectal fistula. Hence, the weighting factors for the rectum, w_j^{OAR}, will be higher than those for the urethra. Our early indication is that the rectum may be more sensitive to PDT than the prostate tissue when assuming equal optical properties and photosensitizing drug concentration. Hence the threshold dose is lower for the rectum than for the prostate. Since clinical testing of PDT for the prostate is in its early stages, the values of the weighting factors still need to be determined, and may depend on the photosensitizer and modality of damage (i.e., vascular vs cellular). It has taken radiation physics the better part of one century to measure and calculate analogous values for the clinical treatment of cancer using ionizing radiation. Thus for PDT to achieve widespread clinical deployment and success, PDT physicists need to intelligently design clinical trials such that these optimization factors can be accurately derived from measurements on a representative cross section of patients.

Monitoring of light received by the tissue is crucial in the treatment of large tissue volumes, since small variations in tissue optical properties significantly impact the light distribution. Monitoring is required to confirm that the actual fluence rate matches the planned fluence rate and to ensure that the dose received by all OARs is lower than critical thresholds. Appropriate medical imaging (such as MRI or ultrasound) is necessary to verify the positions of sources and any dosimetry fibers. Since only a selected number of detection positions are available, assessment of the light delivery requires that the distances between sources and detectors be accurately determined in situ. It is assumed here that a good match between calculated and measured fluence rates at these selected points can be used to indicate acceptable fluence rate throughout the organ [32, 35]. The number of inserted fibers can be reduced by using all source fibers also as detector fibers [36, 56], with light delivered sequentially. If the light dose measurements sufficiently encompass the dimensions of the entire tissue volume [29, 31], it should be possible to estimate the heterogeneous optical property distribution within the volume [30, 36, 67]. The role of online light monitoring is still evolving, in particular for adjusting the planned treatment based on the measured optical properties through renormalization of the optical power delivery [68].

Interstitially placed fluence rate sensors need to exhibit a good isotropic response [69], since the radiance distribution will not be isotropic in cases where the sensor is close to sources, interfaces with changing optical properties and local strong absorbers, such as larger blood vessels. The two most commonly used optical sensor probes achieve an isotropic response either due to strong light scattering in the fiber tip [70] or due to the inherently isotropic emission of fluorescence in organic dye [31, 71] or ruby [72] based probes. To achieve an isotropic response the scattering tip probes need a minimum size so that photons can undergo sufficient scattering events within it to lose all information of their original direction in the tissue prior to being captured at the distal end of the fiber. Typically this required probes of at least 1 mm in diameter. Conversely, fluorescence is inherently isotropic so there are no physical size limits for fluorescent fluence rate sensors. The largest disadvantage of organic fluorophore based fluence rate sensors is their exposure dependent responsivity due to photobleaching, but it was shown that for single PDT treatments this effect is negligible. For any type of fluence rate probe, scattering, or fluorescing, sensitive detection optoelectronics are required as the probe responsivity is in the range of 10^{-5} to $10^{-7} cm^{-1}$, which results in nW to be detected by small diameter probes at the edge of the PTV. A PDT treatment plan will also need to consider minimizing the number of monitoring fibers and determining the most informative locations of these fluence rate sensors.

5.3 Light Sources and Delivery

5.3.1 Current Technologies

Laser and nonlaser light sources have been reviewed previously by Brancaleon and Moseley [73], with an emphasis on topical applications of the skin and oral cavity. Lasers have predominantly been used for PDT, with the emission wavelength chosen to match the peak of the drug absorption band. Clinical light source needs were historically only satisfied by argon or KTP pumped dye lasers tuned to match the peak drug absorption band while providing sufficient overall energy within a reasonable treatment time. Wavelength tuning ability was one of the main advantageous of these lasers as multiple photosensitizers could be investigated without incurring the exorbitant costs of separate devices for each study. The typical bandwidth of dye lasers is <1 nm, and if the laser is correctly aligned to emit at the center-wavelength of the photosensitizer, it results in optimum activation of the photosensitizer from a photon delivery standpoint. For interstitial and cavity PDT applications, a significant advantage of lasers is the ease of coupling the optical power, with acceptable losses, into small diameter optical fibers. Dye lasers, with their excellent beam profiles, are well suited for this purpose. Conversely, however, an Achilles' heel of single high-power laser use for interstitial PDT is the need to split the available optical power into various implanted fibers, often at significant losses. Static [74, 75] and variable splitters [64] have been designed for this purpose but with only limited clinical impact.

The introduction of semiconductor-based diode lasers has significantly reduced the role of argon or KTP pumped dye lasers in clinical PDT. Today's preferential use of semiconductor diode lasers is primarily due to their lower costs, operation on standard 15A- to 25A electrical circuits, their ease of use due to the absence of liquid dyes and liquid cooling requirements, and the ability to theoretically match their absorption peak to any particular photosensitizer. Despite different beam divergence rates along the two perpendicular axes, the power from a diode laser can still be efficiently coupled into small diameter optical fibers. Currently, high-power laser diode bars emitting beyond 650 nm can be obtained for approximately $1,000 per watt optical output (which does not include the required diode drivers and cooling electronics). This reduction in cost enables compact multichannel laser systems (Ceramoptic, VGen). Diode lasers for PDT applications are based on AlGaInP/GaAs (635–700 nm) or AlInGaAsP/GaAs (780–1,000 nm) materials. Both provide a standard tolerance in the peak wavelength of ±3- up to 800-nm emission wavelength. Commercially available laser systems typically come with SMA or similar optical fiber connectors and predetermined coupling optics for a particular fiber core diameter and numerical aperture. The high power needed for PDT applications requires 1-D diode laser bars, with their larger spot sizes, exaggerated beam divergence compromising efficient coupling of light into small diameter (<250 μm) optical fibers. Hence, almost all commercially available optical fibers for PDT are based on 600-μm core diameter fibers with a numerical aperture of 0.36 as they are compatible with most diode laser systems.

When using diode lasers, one needs to be keenly aware that the emission wavelength is temperature-dependent, with the extent of this shift also depending on the base material; typical values are 0.18 nm/°C for red diode lasers and 0.28 nm/°C for

NIR devices emitting below 800 nm. Hence, the photoactivation efficacy for nominally similar lasers can vary for photosensitizers with a narrow excitation bands such as the Phthalocyanines [76] when temperature control is not implemented. Approved medical lasers have a much narrower tolerance in the wavelength, controlling the wavelength by adjusting the operating temperature of the diode.

Diode lasers are quoted with operating life times of several thousand hours, so an often underappreciated temperature affect is the halving of lifetime for each 10 °C temperature increase in the housing above room temperature.

A historical alternative to lasers for topical PDT are bright incandescent or halogen light sources equipped with optical filters to select an appropriate wavelength band providing up to 300 mW/cm^2 [77]. Today their use has reduced significantly and can mostly be found only in in vitro or preclinical studies. This is partially due to the poor intensity profile from the sources, and the short lifetime of the filters caused by exposure to intense heat.

In many applications light emitting diodes (LEDs) offer a cheap alternative to lasers, with more uniform light delivery distribution. LEDs are especially useful for superficial indications and offer the possibility of performing PDT in an ambulatory setting with multiple patients being treated simultaneously. There are already several commercial suppliers of LED devices for PDT (Omnilux Light Therapy, StockerYale Inc., LightScience Oncology, Biospec, Photocure). However, as Moseley [78] pointed out, there are currently no requirements for the manufacturers to validate indicated delivered dose traceable to national measurements standards and the spatial distribution of the radiant energy does not need to be disclosed. As such it is up to the user to verify these measures for appropriate PDT dosimetry. Conversely, motivated by the rather simple assembly of these devices, many academic investigators have chosen to assemble these sources themselves [79].

LEDs have been used clinically primarily for skin and oral mucosa treatments of both malignant [80] and nonmalignant [81, 82] disease. In malignant cases, only tumor thicknesses of <3 mm are considered for treatment, with the employed irradiance in the range of 30 to 100 mW/cm^2. Preclinical applications at other sites have been reported, but work is plagued by the heat generated in these devices and the need for sterilization in particular when considering implantation in vivo. The conversion of electrical energy to optical energy is only 20% for LEDs, and considering the maximum permissible thermal power delivered to the tissue must be less than 100 mW/cm^2, light delivery can take up to 2 hours for implanted LEDs or those in direct contact with the tissue.

To compare the PDT response of LEDs to that of lasers, the spectral overlap of the source emission with the drug excitation spectrum must be calculated; that is:

$$E = \int_{\lambda_1}^{\lambda_2} L(\lambda) \otimes \varepsilon(\lambda) d\lambda \qquad (5.5)$$

where E is the total photon energy required for activation of the drug, $L(\lambda)$ is the LED spectrum, and $\varepsilon(\lambda)$ is the excitation spectrum of the drug. A poor match between the LED and the drug spectra can significantly increase the total energy required for the treatment. In one example, using LEDs centered at 677 nm instead of a laser at 630 nm required more than 3.5 times the energy for the same effective treatment [83]. Treatments using the same energy for both laser and LED sources resulted in lower treatment depths for PDT using LEDs [84], a result directly attributed to the differences in the source-drug spectral overlap for the laser and LED sources.

A new LED approach is to use flexible organic LEDs (OLEDs). OLEDs are primarily being developed for small displays [85, 86] since they offer high light output and less electrical power than liquid crystal displays. Organic dyes are used as the emissive element, providing a broader wavelength tuning range than inorganic LEDs. Their diffuse light delivery, along with their flexibility, make them ideal for treating superficial wounds, since the plane of illumination can be matched to the topography of the surface. Longer treatment times are required (up to 3 hours) because of their lower powers. However, for some indications this may be a benefit since it reduces pain and allows reoxygenation. OLEDs have been packaged as a "light bandage" with the light source stuck to the treatment site, and the small power supply placed in the patient's pocket [87].

5.3.2 Light Delivery Devices

Optical fiber delivery technology developed parallel to new clinical targets. This was driven by the need to match clinical and photonics requirements at these sites. Starting with simple cut end fibers the efforts quickly branched into developing and testing side firing and diffusing tip fibers, and also special applicators for cavities such as the uterus and the esophagus. The forces driving these fiber and applicator developments are the need to increase the treatable volume per inserted fiber and to conform the fiber and applicator's emission profiles to the PTV. Whitehurst et al. [88] used diffusion theory and determined that a single flat cut optical fiber can treat only 0.05 to 0.72 cm^3 at 630 nm, thus requiring an interfiber spacing of 12 mm to provide adequate overlap within the PTV to achieve necrosis. Alternatively, a 3-cm long cylindrical diffuser can treat 6.25 to 22 cm^3 and permit an interfiber separation of 25 mm.

The use of isotropic point sources [89] is currently primarily limited to the bladder [90] as their power handling abilities are insufficient for larger tissue volumes. Further, if introduced without a protective catheter, the small scattering tip at the distal end of the optical fiber sometimes becomes detached on removal due to the friction created by the surrounding tissue. Isotropic point sources are based on the placement of a highly light scattering object at the distal end of an optical fiber. These are typically small spheres of ultrahigh density polyurethane or similar material. They can also be created by using UV activatible adhesive doped with TiO$_2$ particles. As an alternative Hudson et al. [91] proposed the use of dental paste with 27% barium sulphate powder. The isotropic emission quality of these devices is directly related to the number of scattering events photons undergo within this scattering tip, which often require sphere diameters on the order of 1 mm [92, 93].

Cylindrical emitting fibers were introduced in the early 1990s [94] and typically comprise plastic or gel based diffusers attached to a multimode optical fiber. The plastic or gel contained light scattering materials or were themselves light scattering [45, 95]. The exponentially reduced power within the diffuser as a function of its length requires a reciprocal increase of the scattering power as function of diffuser length. This is sometimes approximated through the use of short gel segments with different TiO_2 doping. Homemade and commercially obtained diffusers still do not have to meet any particular manufacturing standards, which often requires the user to perform their own quality assessments using goniometer-type devices [96] or video-based analysis systems [97]. While good-quality products will have little power emission variation in the longitudinal and azimuth direction, most do not approximate Lambertian emission in the polar plane due to the highly forward Mie scattering nature of the TiO_2 particles inside the gel and the requirement of low concentration to enable sufficient power delivery, both resulting in single scattering events, to couple photons from the core into the tissue.

Cylindrical diffusers have become the standard source for interstitial PDT, with new development including reducing the diameter so there is less impact on the traversed tissue, developing longer emitters for new indications such as cardiovascular disease [98], and shaping the emission profile along [99] or around the diffuser. These developments are currently accelerating given by the move towards achieving conformal PDT delivery, requiring more sources of varying length and emission profiles. [32, 59, 100] Additional advances in diffuser technology are aimed towards assuring flexibility to increase the clinical targets, such as the bile duct or to conform to the organ as in the case for nasopharyngeal carcinomas [101].

Emission-shaped optical fibers were developed with an eye on conformal PDT treatment planning, for improved matching of the light distribution to the PTV's shape in those cases where photosensitizer uptake is not sufficiently tumor-specific (see Figure 5.2).

To achieve emission shaping from the diffuser, a two-step process is employed. First, the scattering power of the core is modified along the length as required, to redistribute core light propagation modes into cladding modes. It is from these cladding modes that photons are coupled into the tissue using a TiO_2 doped buffer

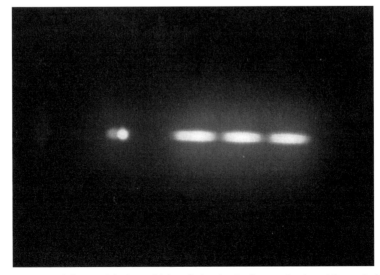

Figure 5.2   A 12-cm diffuser with sinusoidal emission in the long axis placed 2 mm below the surface of a 1% Intralipid phantom. The emission on the left of the image stems from light emitted at the distal end of the emitter. (Picture courtesy of Walsh Medical.)

[99]. This two-step process results in each point of the buffer surface approximating the emission properties of a Lambertian emitter in the azimuth and polar planes. Modulation of the scattering of core modes into the cladding is achieved by excimer laser induced damage at the core-cladding interface.

While on average more robust than isotropic point emitters (from the perspective of catastrophic failure), the emission properties of all cylindrical diffusers are subject to damage of the diffuser core due to mechanical stress. Most optical fibers, in particular for interstitial, intracavity, or intravascular applications are designed and sold as single-use articles. The effects on the fiber emission profile of resterilization and mechanical damage from handling is unclear; hot spots in the emission profiles have been reported, likely due to mechanical damage [8].

Organ conforming delivery has been reported for the cervix and the brain. In the former, the device conforms to the triangular shape of the cervix whereas the latter conforms the soft brain to the shape of the delivery device. Photodynamic ablation of the endometrium was investigated as an outpatient treatment of dysfunctional uterine bleeding. In this light delivery device, three flexible cylindrical light diffusers [102] were embedded in a cervix-shaped balloon. The resulting fluence rate measurements identified good exposure of the endometrium in the uterus, although there was inadequate light delivery in locations to which the probe did not conform, such as the endomyometrial junction and the myometrium.

Balloon irradiators for intracranial PDT were proposed by Muller and Wilson [103] and comprised an inflatable balloon filled with a 0.1% Intralipid suspension acting as a photon scattering medium. The result is a spatial randomization of the photon density on the balloon surface when the light source was placed at its center and with the brain cavity collapsed equally around the balloon. Thus, PDT dosimetry considerations assumed a 1-D fluence rate distribution into the tissue depth, similar to PDT of the bladder as described by van Stavern et al. [48].

Selm et al. [104] proposed a flexible textile that would conform to complex body surface topologies, containing plastic optical fibers for light delivery. All individual plastic optical fibers are combined at one location into a fiber bundle for light coupling. These devices are modeled on the biliblanket introduced in the early 1990s [105] for light therapy of premature babies but suffer from the same low-power transmission rates of only 40% to 50%. As compared to the biliblanket, which are operated at low power densities, the significant light loss in the textile diffuser results in a substantial temperature increase: for 1 W coupled into an 11 cm^2 blanket, temperature rises to above 40° C in less than one minute. The diffusing properties of the textile-based diffuser and the biliblanket are given by the light leakage from the plastic fibers at its bends as they are woven into the textile material. While the blanket or textile diffuser have homogenous emission on a macroscopic level, they show significant variations on a microscopic level since the separation of the optical fibers is of the same order of magnitude as the penetration depth of light in tissue. Thus fluence rate variations that can affect PDT dosimetry are still possible.

Fiber lasers have been demonstrated for thermal and ablative applications in medicine [106], but have not found entry into PDT since they do not cover the spectral range required for most photosensitizers. It is reasonable to anticipate that these limitations will be overcome in the near future. For example, in 2003 IPG Photonics presented a single-mode output from a fiber laser tunable between 770 and 780 nm and thus close to the required activation wavelength of TOOKAD. The main advantage of fiber lasers is the small core size of the fiber (typically less than 50 μm), which will allow for insertion of much smaller fibers reaching for example into the bile duct via endoscope, or the lactic ducts of the breast noninvasively. Additionally, if interstitial placement of source fibers is required one can envision using French 3 or smaller catheters or 26-gauge angiocatheters for diffuser placement and protection. Fiber lasers get their high power density and excellent power efficiency with up to 10% conversion of electrical to optical coupled power, inside a small diameter core doped optical fiber through longitudinal pumping of the active material in the fiber core, as originally proposed by Stone and Burrus [107]. It took another three decades for materials emitting in the far red to appear and be successfully demonstrated in fiber lasers. The fiber laser by IPG Photonics provides a power level of 5 to 30W well within the range required for most PDT applications. As with all fiber lasers, this device operates in quasi-continuous mode with the pulse frequency adjusted between 10 and 20 MHz, while the pulse duration is 2 to 3 ns. The influence of these short pulse durations on the efficacy of PDT may warrant some investigation, since it is conceivable that with pulse durations shorter than most triplet state lifetimes, the efficacy of pumping of the photosensitizer into the triplet state will be affected. Kawauchi et al. [108] demonstrated better in vitro growth inhibition for a 5-μsec pulse of very low repetition rates compared to cw exposure. The use of single mode fibers with cross section areas of tens of μm^2 will ultimately limit further power gains as the silica damage threshold is around 5 W/μm^2. For the near future, the introduction of fiber lasers will reduce the capital equipment cost for interstitial PDT similar to the cost reduction provided by LEDs for superficial PDT.

5.4 Summary

The requirements for PDT light dosimetry measurements and treatment planning have evolved with the available light delivery technologies, and these developments have opened up new clinical applications of PDT. Today, the use of LEDs, either inorganic or organic, has led to methods in treating superficial sites with sources that conform to the surface topography, and with light delivered at low fluence rates over an extended period of time. Lasers coupled to fibers with intensity-modulated profiles have resulted in clinical trials of PDT for bulk tissue volumes, which will only be accelerated with new developments in fiber lasers. The promise of conformal light delivery that these technologies provide can only be properly achieved with simultaneous developments in PDT treatment planning.

References

[1]   Halliwell, B., and Aruoma, O. I.: "DNA damage by oxygen-derived species—its Mechanism and Measurement in Mammalian Systems." *FEBS Lett.*, Vol 281, No 1–2, 1991, pp. 9–19.

[2]   Xiang, L. Z., et al.: "Real-time optoacoustic monitoring of vascular damage during photodynamic therapy treatment of tumor." *J. Biomed. Opt.*, Vol 12, No 1, 2007, pp. 014001.

[3] Gross, S., et al.: "Monitoring photodynamic therapy of solid tumors online by BOLD-contrast MRI." Vol 9, No 10, 2003, pp. 1327–1331.

[4] Georgakoudi, I., Nichols, M. G., and Foster, T. H.: "The mechanism of photofrin(R) photobleaching and its consequences for photodynamic dosimetry." *Photochem. Photobiol.*, Vol 65, No 1, 1997, pp. 135–144.

[5] Kunz, L., and MacRobert, A. J.: "Intracellular photobleaching of 5,10,15,20-tetrakis(m-hydroxyphenyl) chlorin (Foscan((R))) exhibits a complex dependence on oxygen level and fluence rate." *Photochem. Photobiol.*, Vol 75, No 1, 2002, pp. 28–35.

[6] Foster, T. H., et al.: "Oxygen-Consumption and Diffusion Effects in Photodynamic Therapy." *Radiat. Res.*, Vol 126, No 3, 1991, pp. 296–303.

[7] Nichols, M. G., and Foster, T. H.: "Oxygen Diffusion and Reaction-Kinetics in the Photodynamic Therapy of Multicell Tumor Spheroids." *Phys. Med. Biol.*, Vol 39, No 12, 1994, pp. 2161–2181.

[8] Jankun, J., et al.: "Optical characteristics of the canine prostate at 665 NM sensitized with tin etiopurpurin dichloride: Need for real-time monitoring of photodynamic therapy." *J. Urol.*, Vol 172, No 2, 2004, pp. 739–743.

[9] Moseley, H.: "Total effective fluence: A useful concept in photodynamic therapy." *Lasers Med. Sci.*, Vol 11, No 2, 1996, pp. 139–143.

[10] Sheng, C., et al.: "Photobleaching-based dosimetry predicts deposited dose in ALA-PpIX PDT of rodent esophagus." *Photochem. Photobiol.*, Vol 83, No 3, 2007, pp. 738–748.

[11] Lilge, L., and Wilson, B. C.: "Photodynamic therapy of intracranial tissues: A preclinical comparative study of four different photosensitizers." *J. Clin. Laser Med. Sur.*, Vol 16, No 2, 1998, pp. 81–91.

[12] Farrell, T. J., et al.: "Comparison of the in vivo photodynamic threshold dose for photofrin, mono—and tetrasulfonated aluminum phthalocyanine using a rat liver model." *Photochem. Photobiol.*, Vol 68, No 3, 1998, pp. 394–399.

[13] Chen, Q., et al.: "Improvement of tumor response by manipulation of tumor oxygenation during photodynamic therapy." *Photochem. Photobiol.*, Vol 76, No 2, 2002, pp. 197–203.

[14] Maier, A., et al.: "Hyperbaric oxygen and photodynamic therapy in the treatment of advanced carcinoma of the cardia and the esophagus." *Lasers Surg. Med.*, Vol 26, No 3, 2000, pp. 308–315.

[15] Shao, N., et al.: "Integrated molecular targeting of IGF1R and HER2 surface receptors and destruction of breast cancer cells using single wall carbon nanotubes." *Nanotechnology*, Vol 18, No 31, 2007.

[16] Demidova, T. N., and Hamblin, M. R.: "Photodynamic therapy targeted to pathogens." *Int. J. Immunopathol. Pharmacol.*, Vol 17, No 3, 2004, pp. 245–254.

[17] Liu, C. G., Capjack, C., and Rozmus, W.: "3-D simulation of light scattering from biological cells and cell differentiation." *J. Biomed. Opt.*, Vol 10, No 1, 2005.

[18] Tseng, S. H., et al.: "Pseudospectral time domain simulations of multiple light scattering in three-dimensional macroscopic random media." *Radio Sci.*, Vol 41, No 4, 2006.

[19] Wang, L. H., Jacques, S. L., and Zheng, L. Q.: "Mcml—Monte-Carlo Modeling of Light Transport in Multilayered Tissues." *Comput. Meth. Programs Biomed.*, Vol 47, No 2, 1995, pp. 131–146.

[20] Pogue, B. W., and Patterson, M. S.: "Frequency-Domain Optical-Absorption Spectroscopy of Finite Tissue Volumes Using Diffusion-Theory." *Phys. Med. Biol.*, Vol 39, No 7, 1994, pp. 1157–1180.

[21] Farrell, T. J., Patterson, M. S., and Wilson, B.: "A Diffusion-Theory Model of Spatially Resolved, Steady-State Diffuse Reflectance for the Noninvasive Determination of Tissue Optical-Properties Invivo." *Med. Phys.*, Vol 19, No 4, 1992, pp. 879–888.

[22] Patterson, M. S., et al.: "Frequency-Domain Reflectance for the Determination of the Scattering and Absorption Properties of Tissue." *Appl. Optics*, Vol 30, No 31, 1991, pp. 4474–4476.

[23] Quaresima, V., Matcher, S. J., and Ferrari, M.: "Identification and quantification of intrinsic optical contrast for near-infrared mammography." *Photochem. Photobiol.*, Vol 67, No 1, 1998, pp. 4–14.

[24] Durduran, T., et al.: "Bulk optical properties of healthy female breast tissue." *Phys. Med. Biol.*, Vol 47, No 16, 2002, pp. 2847–2861.

[25] Boas, D. A., et al.: "Imaging the body with diffuse optical tomography." *IEEE Signal Process. Mag.*, Vol 18, No 6, 2001, pp. 57–75.

[26] Ripoll, J., and Ntziachristos, V.: "Imaging scattering media from a distance: Theory and applications of noncontact optical tomography." *Mod. Phys. Lett. B*, Vol 18, No 28–29, 2004, pp. 1403–1431.

[27] Yu, G. Q., et al.: "Real-time in situ monitoring of human prostate photodynamic therapy with diffuse light." Vol 82, No 5, 2006, pp. 1279–1284.

[28] Li, J., and Zhu, T.: "Real-time treatment planning system for prostate photodynamic therapy." *Med. Phys.*, Vol 33, No 6, 2006, pp. 2133–2133.

[29] Dimofte, A., Finlay, J. C., and Zhu, T. C.: "A method for determination of the absorption and scattering properties interstitially in turbid media." *Phys. Med. Biol.*, Vol 50, No 10, 2005, pp. 2291–2311.

[30] Zhu, T. C., et al.: "Optical properties of human prostate at 732 nm measured during motexafin lutetium-mediated photodynamic therapy." *Photochem. Photobiol.*, Vol 81, No 1, 2005, pp. 96–105.

[31] Pomerleau-Dalcourt, N., and Lilge, L.: "Development and characterization of multi-sensory fluence rate probes." *Phys. Med. Biol.*, Vol 51, No 7, 2006, pp. 1929–1940.

[32] Weersink, R. A., et al.: "Techniques for delivery and monitoring of TOOKAD (WST09)-mediated photodynamic therapy of the prostate: Clinical experience and practicalities." *J. Photochem. Photobiol. B-Biol.*, Vol 79, No 3, 2005, pp. 211–222.

[33] Chin, L. C. L., Whelan, W. M., and Vitkin, I. A.: "Information content of point radiance measurements in turbid media: implications for interstitial optical property quantification." *Appl. Optics*, Vol 45, No 9, 2006, pp. 2101–2114.

[34] Xu, H. P., and Patterson, M. S.: "Determination of the optical properties of tissue-simulating phantoms from interstitial frequency domain measurements of relative fluence and phase difference." *Opt. Express*, Vol 14, No 14, 2006, pp. 6485–6501.

[35] Svensson, T., et al.: "In vivo optical characterization of human prostate tissue using near-infrared time-resolved spectroscopy." Vol 12, No 1, 2007.

[36] Johansson, A., et al.: "Realtime light dosimetry software tools for interstitial photodynamic therapy of the human prostate." *Med. Phys.*, Vol 34, No 11, 2007, pp. 4309–4321.

[37] Lilge, L., et al.: "Sensitivity of normal brain and intracranially implanted VX2 tumour to interstitial photodynamic therapy (vol 73, pg 332, 1996)." *Br. J. Cancer*, Vol 74, No 10, 1996, pp. 1691–1691.

[38] Zeitouni, N. C., Oseroff, A. R., and Shieh, S.: "Photodynamic therapy for nonmelanoma skin cancers—Current review and update." *Mol. Immunol.*, Vol 39, No 17–18, 2003, pp. 1133–1136.

[39] Lehmann, P.: "Methyl aminolaevulinate-photodynamic therapy: a review of clinical trials in the treatment of actinic keratoses and nonmelanoma skin cancer." *Br. J. Dermatol.*, Vol 156, No 5, 2007, pp. 793–801.

[40] Schmidt-Erfurth, U., et al.: "Photodynamic therapy with verteporfin for choroidal neovascularization caused by age-related macular degeneration—Results of retreatments in a phase 1 and 2 study." *Arch. Ophthalmol.*, Vol 117, No 9, 1999, pp. 1177–1187.

[41] Overholt, B. F., et al.: "Five-year efficacy and safety of photodynamic therapy with Photofrin in Barrett's high-grade dysplasia." *Gastrointest. Endosc.*, Vol 66, No 3, 2007, pp. 460–468.

[42] Wainwright, M.: "Local treatment of viral disease using photodynamic therapy." *Int. J. Antimicrob. Agents*, Vol 21, No 6, 2003, pp. 510–520.

[43]   Meijnders, P. J. N., et al.: "Clinical results of photodynamic therapy for superficial skin malignancies or actinic keratosis using topical 5-aminolaevulinic acid." *Lasers Med. Sci.*, Vol 11, No 2, 1996, pp. 123–131.

[44]   Grant, W. E., et al.: "Photodynamic Therapy of Malignant and Premalignant Lesions in Patients with Field Cancerization of the Oral Cavity." *J. Laryngol. Otol.*, Vol 107, No 12, 1993, pp. 1140–1145.

[45]   Baas, P., et al.: "Photodynamic therapy with meta-tetrahydroxyphenylchlorin for basal cell carcinoma: a phase I/II study." Vol 145, No 1, 2001, pp. 75–78.

[46]   Morton, C. A., et al.: "Guidelines for topical photodynamic therapy: report of a workshop of the British Photodermatology Group." Vol 146, No 4, 2002, pp. 552–567.

[47]   Vanstaveren, H. J., et al.: "Integrating Sphere Effect in Whole Bladder Wall Photodynamic Therapy .1. 532 Nm Versus 630 Nm Optical Irradiation." *Phys. Med. Biol.*, Vol 39, No 6, 1994, pp. 947–959.

[48]   vanStaveren, H. J., et al.: "Integrating sphere effect in whole-bladder-wall photodynamic therapy .3. Fluence multiplication, optical penetration and light distribution with an eccentric source for human bladder optical properties." *Phys. Med. Biol.*, Vol 41, No 4, 1996, pp. 579–590.

[49]   Star, W. M.: "The Relationship between Integrating Sphere and Diffusion-Theory Calculations of Fluence Rate at the Wall of a Spherical Cavity." *Phys. Med. Biol.*, Vol 40, No 1, 1995, pp. 1–8.

[50]   van Veen, R. L. P., et al.: "In situ light dosimetry during photodynamic therapy of Barrett's esophagus with 5-aminolevulinic acid." *Lasers Surg. Med.*, Vol 31, No 5, 2002, pp. 299–304.

[51]   Panjehpour, M., et al.: "Results of photodynamic therapy for ablation of dysplasia and early cancer in Barrett's esophagus and effect of oral steroids on stricture formation." Vol 95, No 9, 2000, pp. 2177–2184.

[52]   Grosjean, P., et al.: "Clinical photodynamic therapy for superficial cancer in the oesophagus and the bronchi: 514 nm compared with 630 nm light irradiation after sensitization with Photofrin II." Vol 77, No 11, 1998, pp. 1989–1995.

[53]   Bedwell, J., et al.: "Fluorescence Distribution and Photodynamic Effect of Ala-Induced Pp-Ix in the Dmh Rat Colonic Tumor-Model." Vol 65, No 6, 1992, pp. 818–824.

[54]   Baghdassarian, R., et al.: "The Use of Lipid Emulsion as an Intravesical Medium to Disperse Light in the Potential Treatment of Bladder-Tumors." *J. Urol.*, Vol 133, No 1, 1985, pp. 126–130.

[55]   Poepping, T. L., et al.: "Long exposure growth of in-vivo interstitial laser photocoagulation lesions." *Lasers Med. Sci.*, Vol 14, No 4, 1999, pp. 297–306.

[56]   Thompson, M. S., et al.: "Clinical system for interstitial photodynamic therapy with combined on-line dosimetry measurements." *Appl. Optics*, Vol 44, No 19, 2005, pp. 4023–4031.

[57]   Stepp, H., et al.: "ALA and malignant glioma: Fluorescence-guided resection and photodynamic treatment." *J. Environ. Pathol. Toxicol. Oncol.*, Vol 26, No 2, 2007, pp. 157–164.

[58]   Beck, T. J., et al.: "Interstitial photodynamic therapy of nonresectable malignant glioma recurrences using 5-aminolevulinic acid induced protoporphyrin IX." *Lasers Surg. Med.*, Vol 39, No 5, 2007, pp. 386–393.

[59]   Altschuler, M. D., et al.: "Optimized interstitial PDT prostate treatment planning with the Cimmino feasibility algorithm." *Med. Phys.*, Vol 32, No 12, 2005, pp. 3524–3536.

[60]   Dickey, D. J., et al.: "Light dosimetry for multiple cylindrical diffusing sources for use in photodynamic therapy." *Phys. Med. Biol.*, Vol 49, No 14, 2004, pp. 3197–3208.

[61]   Star, W., M. (1995). "Diffusion Theory of Light Transport." *Optical-Thermal Response of Laser-Irradiated Tissue*, A. J. Welsh and M. J. C. van Gemeert, eds., Plenum, New York, 131–205.

[62] Jacques, S. L.: "Light distributions from point, line and plane sources for photochemical reactions and fluorescence in turbid biological tissues." *Photochem. Photobiol.*, Vol 67, No 1, 1998, pp. 23–32.

[63] Murrer, L. H., Marijnissen, H. P., and Star, W. M.: "Monte Carlo simulations for endobronchial photodynamic therapy: The influence of variations in optical and geometrical properties and of realistic and eccentric light sources." *Lasers Surg. Med.*, Vol 22, No 4, 1998, pp. 193–206.

[64] Wilson, B. C., et al.: "Treatment planning platform for photodynamic therapy: architecture, function, and validation." *SPIE*, Vol 4612, No 2002, pp. 85–92.

[65] Haider, M. A., et al.: "Prostate gland: MR imaging appearance after vascular targeted photodynamic therapy with palladium-bacteriopheophorbide." *Radiology*, Vol 244, No 1, 2007, pp. 196–204.

[66] Trachtenberg, J., et al.: "Vascular targeted photodynamic therapy with palladium-bacteriopheophorbide photosensitizer for recurrent prostate cancer following definitive radiation therapy: Assessment of safety and treatment response." Vol 178, No 5, 2007, pp. 1974–1979.

[67] Jankun, J., et al.: "Diverse optical characteristic of the prostate and light delivery system: implications for computer modelling of prostatic photodynamic therapy." *BJU Int.*, Vol 95, No 9, 2005, pp. 1237–1244.

[68] Rendon, C. A.: "Biological and physical strategies to improve the therapeutic index of Photodynamic therapy," University of Toronto, Toronto,2007.

[69] de Jode, M. L.: "Monte Carlo simulations of the use of isotropic light dosimetry probes to monitor energy fluence in biological tissues." Vol 44, No 12, 1999, pp. 3027–3037.

[70] VanStaveren, H. J.: "Construction, quality assurance and calibration of spherical isotropic fibre optic light diffusers." Vol 10, No 2, 1995, pp. 137–147.

[71] Lilge, L., Haw, T., and Wilson, B. C.: "Miniature Isotropic Optical Fiber Probes for Quantitative Light Dosimetry in Tissue." Vol 38, No 2, 1993, pp. 215–230.

[72] Bays, R.: "Light dosimetry for photodynamic therapy in the esophagus." *Lasers Surg. Med.*, Vol 20, No 3, 1997, pp. 290–303.

[73] Brancaleon, L., and Moseley, H.: "Laser and non-laser light sources for photodynamic therapy." *Lasers Med. Sci.*, Vol 17, No 3, 2002, pp. 173–186.

[74] Lee, L. K., et al.: "An interstitial light assembly for photodynamic therapy in prostatic carcinoma." *BJU Int.*, Vol 84, No 7, 1999, pp. 821–826.

[75] Bellnier, D. A., et al.: "Design and construction of a light-delivery system for photodynamic therapy." *Med. Phys.*, Vol 26, No 8, 1999, pp. 1552–1558.

[76] Ochsner, M.: "Photophysical and photobiological processes in the photodynamic therapy of tumours." *J. Photochem. Photobiol. B-Biol.*, Vol 39, No 1, 1997, pp. 1–18.

[77] Fijan, S., Honigsmann, H., and Ortel, B.: "Photodynamic Therapy of Epithelial Skin Tumors Using Delta-Aminolevulinic-Acid and Desferrioxamine." Vol 133, No 2, 1995, pp. 282–288.

[78] Moseley, H.: "Light distribution and calibration of commercial PDT LED arrays." *Photochem. Photobiol. Sci.*, Vol 4, No 11, 2005, pp. 911–914.

[79] Luksiene, Z., Astrauskas, J., and Kabbara, I.: "LED-based light source for photodynamic inactivation of leukemia cells in vitro." *SPIE*, Vol 5610, No 2004.

[80] Wilson, B. C., et al.: "Metronomic photodynamic therapy (mPDT): concepts and technical feasibility in brain tumor." *SPIE*, Vol 4952, No 2003, pp. 23–31.

[81] Lowe, N. J., and Lowe, P.: "Pilot study to determine the efficacy of ALA-PDT photo-rejuvenation for the treatment of facial ageing." *J Cosmet Laser Ther*, Vol 7, No 3–4, 2005, pp. 159–62.

[82] Babilas, P., et al.: "In vitro and in vivo comparison of two different light sources for topical photodynamic therapy." *Br. J. Dermatol.*, Vol 154, No 4, 2006, pp. 712–718.

[83] Schmidt, M. H., et al.: "Light-emitting diodes as a light source for intraoperative photodynamic therapy." *Neurosurgery*, Vol 38, No 3, 1996, pp. 552–556.

[84] DeJode, M. L., et al.: "A comparison of novel light sources for photodynamic therapy." *Lasers Med. Sci.*, Vol 12, No 3, 1997, pp. 260–268.

[85] Organic light-emitting devices : a survey, 2004, Springer, New York.

[86] Friend, R. H., et al.: "Electroluminescence in conjugated polymers." Vol 397, No 6715, 1999, pp. 121–128.

[87] Samuel, I. D. W., and Ferguson, J. (2005). "Therapeutic light-emitting device." Great Britain.

[88] Whitehurst, C., et al.: "Optimization of Multifiber Light Delivery for the Photodynamic Therapy of Localized Prostate-Cancer." *Photochem. Photobiol.*, Vol 58, No 4, 1993, pp. 589–593.

[89] VanStaveren, H. J., et al.: "Construction, quality assurance and calibration of spherical isotropic fibre optic light diffusers." *Lasers Med. Sci.*, Vol 10, No 2, 1995, pp. 137–147.

[90] vanStaveren, H. J., Bertrams, R. H. P., and Star, W. M.: "Bladder PDT with intravesical clear and light scattering media: Effect of an eccentric isotropic light source on the light distribution." *Lasers Surg. Med.*, Vol 20, No 3, 1997, pp. 248–253.

[91] Hudson, E. J., et al.: "The development of radio-opaque, isotropic, fiberoptic probes for light dosimetry." *Phys. Med. Biol.*, Vol 38, No 10, 1993, pp. 1529–1536.

[92] Marijnissen, J. P. A., and Star, W. M.: "Performance of isotropic light dosimetry probes based on scattering bulbs in turbid media." *Phys. Med. Biol.*, Vol 47, No 12, 2002, pp. 2049–2058.

[93] Star, W. M., and Marijnissen, J. P. A.: "Calculating the Response of Isotropic Light Dosimetry Probes as a Function of the Tissue Refractive-Index So Applied Optics Sn 0740-3224." *Appl. Optics*, Vol 28, No 12, 1989, pp. 2288–2291.

[94] Mizeret, J. C., and vandenBergh, H. E.: "Cylindrical fiberoptic light diffuser for medical applications." *Lasers Surg. Med.*, Vol 19, No 2, 1996, pp. 159–167.

[95] Murrer, L. H. P., Marijnissen, J. P. A., and Star, W. M.: "Improvements in the design of linear diffusers for photodynamic therapy." *Phys. Med. Biol.*, Vol 42, No 7, 1997, pp. 1461–1464.

[96] Lilge, L., Vesselov, L., and Whittington, W.: "Thin cylindrical diffusers in multimode Ge-doped silica fibers." *Lasers Surg. Med.*, Vol 36, No 3, 2005, pp. 245–251.

[97] Ripley, P. M., Mills, T. N., and Brookes, J. A. S.: "Measurement of the emission profiles of cylindrical light diffusers using a video technique." *Lasers Med. Sci.*, Vol 14, No 1, 1999, pp. 67–72.

[98] Rockson, S. G., et al.: "Photoangioplasty—An emerging clinical cardiovascular role for photodynamic therapy." *Circulation*, Vol 102, No 5, 2000, pp. 591–596.

[99] Vesselov, L. M., Whittington, W., and Lilge, L.: "Performance evaluation of cylindrical fiber optic light diffusers for biomedical applications." *Lasers Surg. Med.*, Vol 34, No 4, 2004, pp. 348–351.

[100] Rendon, A., Weersink, R., and Lilge, L.: "Towards conformal light delivery using tailored cylindrical diffusers: attainable light dose distributions." *Phys. Med. Biol.*, Vol 51, No 23, 2006, pp. 5967–5975.

[101] van Veen, R. L. P., et al.: "In vivo fluence rate measurements during Foscan (R)—mediated photodynamic therapy of persistent and recurrent nasopharyngeal carcinomas using a dedicated light applicator." *J. Biomed. Opt.*, Vol 11, No 4, 2006.

[102] Tadir, Y., et al.: "Intrauterine light probe for photodynamic ablation therapy." *Obstet. Gynecol.*, Vol 93, No 2, 1999, pp. 299–303.

[103] Muller, P. J., Wilson, B. C., and Yanche, J. C.: "Intracavitary Photo-Dynamic Therapy (Pdt) of Malignant Primary Brain-Tumors Using a Laser Coupled Inflatable Balloon So Journal of Neuro-Oncology Sn 0167-594x." *J. Neuro-Oncol.*, Vol 4, No 1, 1986, pp. 113–113.

[104]   Selm, B., et al.: "Novel flexible light diffuser and irradiation properties for photodynamic therapy." *J. Biomed. Opt.*, Vol 12, No 3, 2007.

[105]   Kang, J. H., and Shankaran, S.: "Double phototherapy with high irradiance compared with single phototherapy in neonates with hyperbilirubinemia." *Am. J. Perinatol.*, Vol 12, No 3, 1995, pp. 178–180.

[106]   Jackson, S. D., and Lauto, A.: "Diode-pumped fiber lasers: A new clinical tool?" *Lasers Surg. Med.*, Vol 30, No 2, 2002, pp. 184–190.

[107]   Stone, J., and C. A. Burrus, "Neodynium-doped silica lasers in end-pumped fiber geometry," *Appl. Phys. Letter.*, Vol. 23, No. 7, pp. 388–389, 1973.

[108]   Kawauchi, S., et al.: "Influence of light intensity and repetition rate of nanosecond laser pulses on photodynamic therapy with PAD-S31 in mouse renal carcinoma cell line in vitro: study for oxygen consumption and photobleaching AU Kawauchi, S." *SPIE*, Vol 4284, No 2001, pp. 138–143.

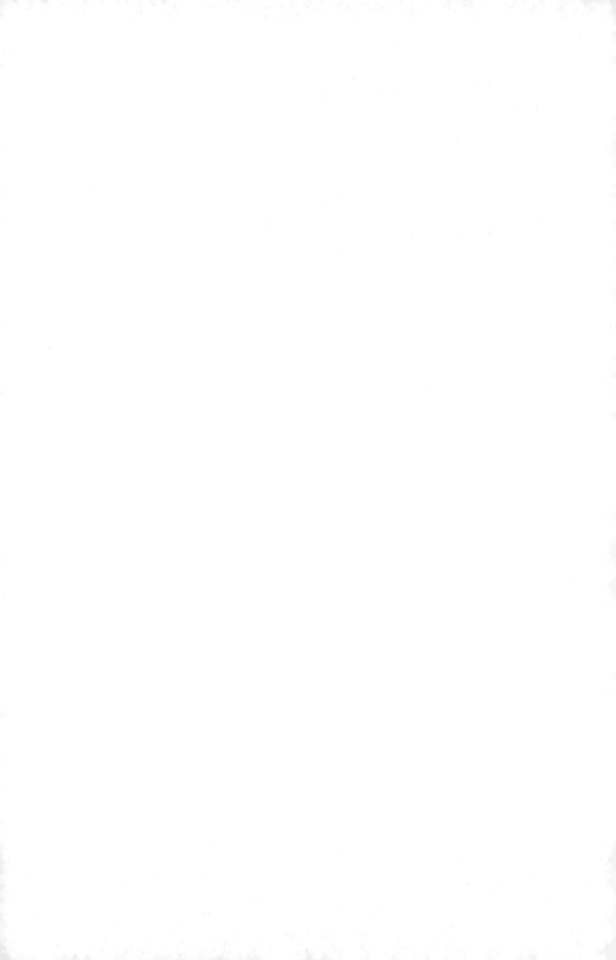

CHAPTER 6

Cell Killing by Photodynamic Therapy

Nancy L. Oleinick, Anna-Liisa Nieminen, and Song-mao Chiu

6.1 Introduction: Direct and Indirect Modes of Cell Death After PDT

Exposure of tumors or other tissues in vivo to PDT leads to the death of cells through multiple pathways. Cell death can result from direct damage to tumor cells and from indirect damage because of PDT-induced vascular collapse or other vessel damage that leads to hypoxia and nutrient deficiency and/or to the release of cytokines and other inflammatory mediators. The indirect mechanisms are considered in other chapters in this book. This chapter will focus on (1) pathways of cell death resulting from direct photodynamic damage to the targeted cells, and (2) the organelle and molecular targets that trigger the direct induction of death pathways.

The literature on cell killing mechanisms by PDT has been summarized and discussed a number of times in the past few years [1–6], including by us [1], and most recently in a very comprehensive and thoughtful review by the Agostinis laboratory [7]. Given the shorter format of the present chapter, for more in-depth coverage the reader is referred to previous reviews for more detailed discussion and more complete references.

6.2 How Cells Die After Direct Exposure to PDT

The earliest studies of cells dying after PDT described cell swelling and lysis, a necrotic process. It is now recognized that cells respond to certain types and amounts of injury by turning on specific genetically programmed enzymatic pathways of cell suicide. These have features associated with genetically encoded pathways for removal of cells during development, termed programmed cell death (PCD). Type I PCD proceeds through cell shrinkage and chromatin condensation (apoptosis), type II PCD occurs through digestion of damaged cellular components by lysosomal enzymes (autophagic death), and type III PCD involves loss of plasma membrane integrity and cell swelling (necrosis). During normal development, these pathways allow for the elimination of abnormal, unnecessary, or damaged cells, and a variety of diseases, including cancer, can be associated with defects in PCD.

6.2.1 Apoptosis

Apoptosis has been demonstrated to occur in many different types of cells and after PDT with many different photosensitizers [1]. The literature on this topic has grown markedly since the first report of the induction of apoptosis by a photosensitizer and light [8]. PDT is an efficient inducer of apoptosis [1, 8] both in cultured cells and in vivo. As with other toxic agents (e.g., hyperthermia), PDT causes necrosis at higher doses than those inducing apoptosis, indicating that one factor in determining the pathway for the final demise of the cell is the overall amount of damage [9–14]. Another factor that can affect the final cell death mechanism is the site(s) of localization of the photosensitizer, as this factor determines the immediate damaged cellular molecules. For some, variable incubation times can result in different localization patterns and culminate in different modes of cell death [15]. Moreover, the initial binding site of some photosensitizers may be different from its preferred damage site in PDT [16]. In addition, different reactive species produced at the same sites can have markedly different cellular effects [17, 18]. Differential sensitivity to PDT occurs among different cell types [19, 20], with lymphoid cells being more sensitive than cells of epithelial or mesenchymal origin. Some of the differential sensitivity is likely due to the activation of diverse signaling pathways that promote or block cell death pathways [1, 4, 21]. In contrast to many other toxic agents, PDT-induced cell death, especially via apoptosis, can occur in any stage of the cell cycle [22, 23] and even despite cell cycle arrest [24].

The mitochondrion is the central processing organelle for the intrinsic pathway to apoptosis (i.e., apoptosis resulting from internal triggers) (Figure 6.1). In this pathway, signals such as Ca^{++} ion released from the ER or the proapoptotic proteins Bax or Bak lead to loss of mitochondrial inner membrane potential ($\Delta\Psi$m), opening of the permeability transition pore complex on the outer membrane, and release of a set of proteins from the intermembrane space into the cytoplasm. These proteins, including cytochrome c, second mitochondrial activator of caspases (SMAC), and apoptosis-inducing factor (AIF), promote the next steps in apoptosis. Cytochrome c combines with cytoplasmic proteins, procaspases-9 and -3, to form the apoptosome, in which the caspases are cleaved and activated. Caspase-3 is the most prominent executioner caspase that cleaves many cellular proteins to ensure the final stages of apoptosis, resulting in nuclear chromatin condensation and DNA fragmentation. In contrast, apoptosis can also be triggered by engagement of death receptors on the cell surface (e.g., TNF-α receptor) that recruit additional cytoplasmic proteins to form a death-inducing signaling complex (DISC) and activate caspases-8 or -10, which can directly activate caspase-3. This pathway can work independently of the mitochondria or can activate the mitochondrial steps through caspase cleavage of the proapoptotic protein Bid that enters mitochondria to promote the intrinsic pathway.

In the context of PDT, a major route to apoptosis involves selective photodamage to cellular components that can trigger the process [1]. The aspects of apoptosis that are unique to PDT are the molecular targets, the types of initial cellular damage, and the immediate consequences of that damage. Many photosensitizers target mitochondria, resulting in changes in the permeability transition pore complex, the apoptotic proteins Bcl-2 and Bcl-xL, and/or phospholipids, especially cardiolipin. Some photosensitizers also target the endoplasmic reticulum, damaging calcium pumps and resulting in the efflux of stored calcium into the cytosol and subsequently mitochondria. With photosensitizers that localize in lysosomes, photoactivation damages the lysosomal membrane, causing release of

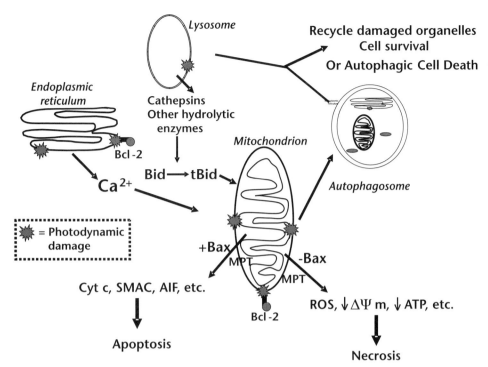

Figure 6.1 A model for the induction of apoptosis and autophagy by photodynamic therapy with photosensitizers localized in various subcellular compartments. Depending upon the photosensitizer, the relative level of damage to these organelles will vary. Photodamage to mitochondria, including to Bcl-2, leads to permeability of the outer membrane and the release of proapoptotic factors from the intermembrane space in a Bax-dependent manner. Damage to the ER leads to the release of Ca^{2+}, which can enter mitochondria. Damage to lysosomes results in the release of various hydrolytic proteins, including cathepsins, which can cleave the proapoptotic protein Bid, allowing tBid to enter mitochondria and promote apoptosis. Damaged organelles can be recycled by autophagy. Autophagosomes merge with lysosomes to hydrolyze damaged cell constituents, allowing cell survival if the damage is not great. In the presence of extensive damage, cell death occurs in spite of or augmented by autophagy. Autophagy or necrosis are dominant modes of cell death when apoptosis is defective.

cathepsins and other hydrolases that can activate apoptosis mediators such as Bid that in turn promote mitochondrial apoptosis. Although the plasma membrane is not commonly a direct target of most photosensitizers, it can be secondarily affected by the release of ligands for membrane receptors, such as Fas ligand. Evidence supporting the roles of each of the organelles in PDT-induced apoptosis is briefly reviewed, and a model is proposed in which mitochondrial damage by PDT directly activates apoptosis, and damage to the endoplasmic reticulum and/or the lysosome promotes the central mitochondrial pathway of apoptosis.

6.2.2 Autophagy

Autophagy is recognized as a cellular program for recycling cell components during starvation or for removing damaged organelles to promote cell survival [7]. When damage becomes extensive, autophagy provides another pathway for cell death. Autophagy is commonly characterized by the formation of double-membrane-enclosed vacuoles (autophagosomes) that can be observed in electron micrographs and by the conversion of the microtubule-associated protein LC3-I to a modified LC3-II form (linked to phosphatidyl ethanolamine and associated with autophagosomes) that can be distinguished by its faster migration on western blots. At low doses of PDT, as with other toxic agents, autophagy can promote cell survival, but upon extensive damage, autophagy contributes to cell death [25].

The induction of autophagy by PDT has been demonstrated in mouse leukemia L1210 cells and in human prostate cancer DU145 cells [26], in human breast cancer MCF-7 cells [27], and in Bax/Bak double-knockout murine embryonic fibroblasts that are defective in apoptosis [28]. Induction of autophagy occurs whether or not apoptosis is blocked or impaired and as a general early response following PDT [26, 27]. To understand the roles of apoptosis and autophagy in cell killing following PDT, Kessel's group has compared cell viability following low- and high-dose PDT in L1210 cells either expressing or knocked down for Bax or Atg7 (an essential enzyme in autophagy). Although the knockdown of Bax markedly suppressed apoptosis, it had no effect on overall photosensitivity, as judged by a clonogenic assay, an observation similar to previous reports in MCF-7 cells lacking caspase-3 [29] and in Bax-deficient DU145 and HCT 116 cells [30, 31]. Atg7-deficient L1210 cells were as sensitive as the wild-type cells from which they were derived to high-dose PDT, but they were more sensitive than wild type cells to low-dose PDT. The data indicate that induction of autophagy by low-dose PDT can enhance cell survival [32]. Moreover, while overexpression of Bcl-2 protects cells from PDT-induced apoptosis, it did not protect cells from nonapoptotic cell death following PDT [27]. This observation is consistent with the notion that the role of Bcl-2 is limited to regulation of the permeabilization of the mitochondrial outer membrane and the release of cytochrome c [33, 34]. Current data appear to suggest that there is crosstalk between autophagy and apoptosis [35]. For example, Atg5, an autophagy-specific protein involved in autophagosome precursor expansion and complexation through a ubiquitin-like conjugation system, can be cleaved following death stimuli and the cleavage product appears to promote apoptosis. In addition, the antiapoptotic protein Bcl-2 can also inhibit autophagy by binding to the autophagic gene product Beclin-1.

6.2.3 Necrosis

This process results either from PDT doses sufficiently high to damage components of the other pathways or from direct photodamage to the plasma membrane, which is described below.

6.3 Subcellular Photosensitizer Localization and Biomolecular Targets

It is now clear that sufficient damage to any cell organelle or essential component can kill the cell. However, most interest is in understanding the roles of more modest, clinically achievable doses of PDT. In this section, we consider evidence for the involvement of photodamage to individual organelles in cell death after PDT. It must be kept in mind that none of the photosensitizers currently approved or in study are absolutely specific for any one cellular site. Most photosensitizers are highly hydrophobic molecules that preferentially accumulate in one or more membrane systems; even those that are water-soluble still contain hydrophobic cores and tend to bind to membranes.

6.3.1 Mitochondria

In general, drugs that interfere with mitochondrial function tend to be more effective in killing cancer cells than the ones that do not affect mitochondria. This is also the case with PDT. Photodynamic damage to mitochondria results in generation of reactive oxygen species (ROS), loss of the mitochondrial membrane potential ($\Delta\Psi m$), and release of proapoptotic factors such as Smac/Diablo, AIF, and cytochrome c into the cytosol. Subsequent activation of the caspases in the presence of ATP results in apoptotic death [1, 4].

An example of a mitochondrion-targeted photosensitizer is Pc 4. By confocal microscopy, Pc 4 localizes to cytosolic membranes, primarily but not exclusively to mitochondria [36, 37]. Formation of mitochondrial ROS then occurs within minutes when cells are exposed to light. This is followed by inner membrane permeabilization, mitochondrial depolarization and swelling, cytochrome c release, and apoptotic death [37]. Thus, PDT represents a mode of apoptosis in which the apoptotic stimulus, in this case the combination of photosensitizer and light, directly affects mitochondrial function.

Mitochondrial dysfunction after PDT may occur by a number of different mechanisms. One model suggests that opening of the mitochondrial permeability transition pores is responsible for release of mitochondrial proteins that reside in the mitochondrial intermembrane space. In the mitochondrial permeability transition (MPT) model, opening of nonselective, highly conductive permeability transition (PT) pores causes the inner membrane of the mitochondria to become permeable to molecules of up to 1,500 Da, which leads to mitochondrial depolarization, uncoupling of oxidative phosphorylation, and large-amplitude mitochondrial swelling [38]. Cyclosporin A (CsA) and a variety of its analogs inhibit PT pore opening. The molecular composition of PT pores remains uncertain. In one model, PT pores form from the adenine nucleotide translocator (ANT) in the inner membrane, the voltage-dependent anion channel (VDAC) and peripheral benzodiazepine receptor (PBR) in the outer membrane, and cyclophylin D (CypD), a CsA binding protein, from the matrix (reviewed in [39, 40]). Recent results showing that the MPT still occurs in mitochondria that are deficient in ANT, VDAC, and even CypD challenge the validity of this model [41–43]. In another model, PT pores form from damaged, misfolded membrane proteins that aggregate at hydrophilic surfaces facing the bilayer to create aqueous transmembrane channels [44]. CypD and other molecular chaperones close these nascent PT pores protecting mitochondria from depolarization and swelling. CypD confers sensitivity to Ca^{2+} by which increased matrix Ca^{2+} opens the PT pores, an action antagonized by CsA. When nascent pores formed by misfolded protein aggregates exceed the chaperones available to regulate their conductance, unregulated PT pore opening occurs. Such unregulated PT pores are insensitive to CsA inhibition and no longer require Ca^{2+} for opening. The protein-misfolding model may explain the occurrence of MPT in ANT-deficient mitochondria [41], since misfolding of other mitochondrial membrane proteins can cause PT pore formation in the absence of ANT.

In spite of uncertainty as to the exact composition of the pore, the above-mentioned components have received much attention as potential targets of PDT. One such component is the 18-kDa PBR, which was suggested to be the critical molecular target for protoporphryin IX (PPIX) and related porphyrins [45–47], based on a strong correlation between a porphyrin's binding affinity to the PBR and cellular photocytotoxicity. For instance, the PBR is a target of the PPIX formed metabolically from exogenously supplied 5-aminolevulinic acid (ALA) [48] and pyropheophorbide ethers [49]. In human lymphoblastic leukemia Reh cells, two specific ligands for the PBR, PK11195 and Ro5-4864, prevented PPIX-PDT-induced apoptosis, suggesting that PBR is a major target of PPIX-PDT. Interestingly, mitochondrial depolarization was not prevented by these two ligands [50]. A recent study suggests that low-level light treatment prior to PDT may increase PBR protein expression in tumor cells, thereby enhancing PDT-mediated cell killing when using ALA-derived PPIX as a photosensitizer. The enhanced cell killing was suggested to be related to enhanced mitochondrial PPIX production [51]. The phthalocyanine Pc 4 also binds to the PBR, but only at concentrations much higher than those needed for efficient photosensitization [52]. Furthermore, two positional isomers of PPIX (PPIII and PPXIII) with similar uptake and mitochondrial binding, and the same ability to photosensitize L1210 leukemia cells as PPIX (as assessed by a clonogenic assay), had significantly lower binding affinity to the PBR than PPIX [53]. Thus, the relationship between PBR binding and photosensitizing efficacy may be limited to certain photosensitizers.

In isolated rat liver mitochondria, hematoporphyrin photosensitization strongly inhibited the 30-kDa ANT and induced onset of the mitochondrial permeability transition [54]. Verteporfin-PDT permeabilized ANT-containing proteoliposomes, a response that could be inhibited by the ANT ligands, ADP and ATP [55]. While intriguing, these observations do not directly prove that ANT is the cellular target of PDT with either photosensitizer. Hexokinase, which is also suggested to be a component of the PT pore, was released into the cytosol and its activity inhibited by hypericin-PDT [56]. Unfortunately, inhibitors of the PT pore opening have provided contradictory results. The loss of $\Delta\Psi m$ after hypericin-PDT was not prevented by CsA or bongkrekic acid [57]. CsA produced a partial inhibition of the PT pore opening in human epidermoid carcinoma A431 cells exposed to Pc 4-PDT, but CsA combined with trifluoperazine strongly inhibited PT pore opening and apoptosis, supporting a transient opening of the PT pore by PDT [37]. Mitochondrial depolarization in isolated mitochondria exposed to PDT with Victoria Blue dyes was CsA-insensitive and was proposed to result from direct effects of the dyes on inner membrane permeability to protons rather than on the MPT [58]. An attractive hypothesis, which is still waiting to be proved, is that PDT-induced MPT may be mediated by clusters of misfolded proteins resulting in unregulated CsA-insensitive pore opening [44]. This hypothesis would explain why CsA was ineffective in preventing onset of the MPT in a number of PDT paradigms.

Inhibition of respiration and oxidative phosphorylation are also common early responses with mitochondrion-localized photosensitization [10, 59, 60].

Photofrin-PDT inhibited electron transport components, including succinate dehydrogenase and cytochome c oxidase, and disrupted the mitochondrial membrane potential [61–63]. Strikingly, the inhibition of respiration caused by Pc 4-PDT in L5178Y-R murine lymphoma cells could largely be restored by addition of exogenous cytochrome c to the permeabilized cells [60], supporting the notion that the inhibition of respiration in that situation primarily resulted from cytochrome c release, rather than from damage to the major enzyme complexes of the electron transport chain.

Recent evidence also suggests that a likely target for the initial lethal damage of PDT with some mitochondrion-specific photosensitizers is cardiolipin (CL). CL is a phospholipid uniquely localized in the mitochondrial inner membrane and in the contact sites of the mitochondrial inner and outer membranes [64]. CL is highly sensitive to oxidation and an attractive candidate for initial singlet oxygen attack after PDT. CL is also important to mitochondrial integrity by providing an attachment site for many mitochondrial proteins, such as respiratory complexes, cytochrome c, and the components of the PT pore [65, 66]. Oxidation of CL by PPIX/ALA may induce the initial loosening of cytochrome c anchorage to CL, resulting in Bax-dependent mitochondrial cytochrome c release [67]. Recently, CL deficiency was reported to free cytochrome c from the mitochondrial inner membrane to the intermembrane space, and sensitize cells to mitochondrial cytochrome c release, and apoptosis after TNFα plus cycloheximide in HeLa cells [68].

The fluorescent dye nonyl-acridine orange (NAO) binds specifically to CL and has been utilized to examine the localization of various photosensitizers in the mitochondrial membranes. Confocal microscopy revealed that NAO competitively inhibited the uptake of Photofrin into mitochondria, suggesting that these two agents were competing for the same site on CL [69]. Oleinick's group showed by FRET analysis that Pc 4 binds on or near CL [70]. Similarly, FRET was also observed between NAO and PPIX (Morris et al., unpublished), suggesting that CL is a likely initial target for these two photosensitizers. Taken together, CL oxidation/deficiency could represent an attractive therapeutic approach by PDT.

6.3.2   Endoplasmic Reticulum

Besides mitochondrial membranes, photosensitizers tend to accumulate also on the membranes of the endoplasmic reticulum (ER) [28, 36, 37, 55, 71–74] (see complete list in Table 1 in [7]). Oxidation of ER proteins due to PDT may cause two major changes in ER function: changes in ER Ca^{2+} homeostasis and aggregation of unfolded and misfolded proteins.

The ER is a major intracellular source of Ca^{2+}. The intracellular release of inositol trisphosphate (IP3) from the plasma membrane causes IP3-induced Ca^{2+} release from the ER into the cytosol through the IP3 receptors. Ca^{2+} is returned to the ER lumen via sarco/endoplasmic Ca^{2+} (SERCA) pumps. Coordinated regulation of Ca^{2+} release and uptake mechanisms maintains the ER free-Ca^{2+} pool at ~500 μM in physiological conditions. Any perturbations of the release and uptake mechanisms eventually affect cytosolic Ca^{2+} concentrations. In HeLa cells, PDT photosensitized by Verteporfin released Ca^{2+} from the ER, which was associated with a rapid caspase-independent inhibition of SERCA-2 [75]. In rat liver microsomes, Ca^{2+}

uptake was impaired after photosensitization with hematoporphyrin or protoporphyrin [76]. In rat pancreatic acini, PDT with gadolinium porphyrin-like macrocycle B or AlPcS4 induced cytosolic Ca^{2+} oscillations by triggering ER Ca^{2+} release through IP3 receptors [77, 78]. AlPc-PDT also induced a rapid transient release of Ca^{2+} from the ER in mouse L5178Y cells [79]. The photosensitizer 9-capronyloxytetrakis (methoxyethyl) porphycene (CPO) localizes predominantly in the ER membranes in murine leukemia L1210 cells, resulting in increased cytosolic Ca^{2+} after PDT [72]. The SERCA pump is damaged by Pc 4-PDT (Oleinick, unpublished observation). Although BAPTA-AM prevented Pc 4-PDT (Nieminen, unpublished observation)- and CPO-PDT [72]-induced cytosolic Ca^{2+} increase, it failed to protect cells from dying by apoptosis [72] (Nieminen, unpublished observation). The data so far suggests that PDT-triggered cytosolic Ca^{2+} increase might not be required for cell death after PDT.

Besides serving as a main free-Ca^{2+} storage in the cell, the ER is also responsible for folding, modifying, and sorting of newly synthesized proteins. Any disturbance in these vital cellular functions leads to ER stress, which may ultimately lead to cell death. For instance, photooxidation of the SERCA pump can induce ER stress and accumulation of photodamaged misfolded proteins by depletion of the ER Ca^{2+} [28].

PDT with photosensitizers that target mitochondria and ER causes photodamage to Bcl-2 and Bcl-xL [13, 71, 73, 80, 81]. Photodamage to these antiapoptotic proteins is observed immediately upon light exposure, and occurs because of direct PDT-produced damage to proteins, and not as the result of any proteolytic or other enzymatic reactions. Bcl-2 photodamage was found in a wide variety of malignant cell lines, and it occurs irrespective of estrogen- or androgen-receptor status, p53 status, or other factors that can contribute to cancer cell resistance to various cancer treatments (reviewed in [1]). The ability of PDT to affect Bcl-2 function doubtless plays a role in the broad spectrum of tumors that can be successfully treated.

Since in most cancer cells Bcl-2/Bcl-xL are found on mitochondrial and ER membranes, it is unclear whether damage to mitochondrial Bcl-2/Bcl-xL is more critical than damage to ER in causing cell death. Kessel's group has shown that the bile acid ursodeoxycholic acid (UDCA) greatly potentiated apoptosis after PDT sensitized by the porphyrin CPO that targets the ER and causes Bcl-2 photodamage [82, 83]. UDCA appeared to act via mitochondria by sensitizing mitochondrial membranes to photodamage. The ER-localizing photosensitizer Foscan was recently shown to cause Bcl-2 photodamage, possibly affecting specifically the ER pool of Bcl-2 in MCF-7 cells [84].

6.3.3 Lysosomes

A number of photosensitizers bind preferentially to lysosomes and upon photoactivation can induce apoptosis [85–88]. Photoactivation of NPe6-loaded murine hepatoma 1c1c7 cells caused a delayed apoptotic response, marked by rapid destruction of the lysosomes, Bid cleavage to generate truncated Bid (tBid), cytochrome c release from mitochondria, and activation of caspases-9 and −3 [87].

It has been demonstrated that lysosomal extracts contain proteolytic activity capable of cleaving Bid [87], at a site in the protein near but not identical to the cleavage site for caspase-8 [89, 90]. Although cathepsins are known to reside in lysosomes and to be released upon lysosomal damage, inhibitors of cathepsins B, D, and L were unable to block apoptosis triggered by NPe6-sensitized PDT [87]. The aryl hydrocarbon receptor (AhR)-deficient cell line, Tao, derived from 1c1c7 cells, was shown to be relatively resistant to cell killing by NPe6-PDT, as judged by a colony-forming assay, in spite of a slightly better uptake of the photosensitizer into its lysosomes [88]. When compared at equal levels of cell killing, apoptosis induction in Tao cells was considerably delayed relative to the induction in 1c1c7 cells. When cells with different levels of AhR were compared, sensitivity to NPe6-PDT tracked with AhR level. Thus, cells with higher levels of AhR, such as 1c1c7 cells, had higher levels of lysosomal proteases available for release, more rapid and extensive cleavage of Bid, activation of caspases-9 and -3, and more rapid and extensive development of morphological apoptosis. PDT with other photosensitizers such as mTHPC and ATX-S10 have also been shown to induce apoptosis through the disruption of lysosomes [91, 92].

Lysosomes are crucial mediators of the final stages of autophagy. Autophagosomes, which enclose organelles and other cytoplasmic constituents, do not contain the necessary hydrolytic enzymes for digestion of their cargo; instead, they merge with lysosomes, and the lysosomal enzymes are responsible for breakdown of the autophagosomal contents either for recycling or for excretion. Most studies of PDT-induced autophagy have focused on the earlier stages of the process involved in formation of the autophagosomes. However, the observation that the autophagosomal component, LC3-II, accumulates in cells in response to PDT [26, 27] may indicate that further processing of the autophagosome is inhibited by PDT-induced damage to lysosomes or to factors needed for the lysosomal stage of autophagy [93]. Future work on PDT will need to consider this possibility.

When cells are exposed to ionizing radiation and certain chemotherapeutic drugs, the increase in cellular ceramide has been shown to be due to activation of lysosomal and other sphingomyelinases, enzymes that cleave sphingomyelin to generate ceramide and phosphorylcholine [94]. The role of ceramide and other sphingolipids in PDT-induced cell death is not yet clear. Ceramide levels were found to increase in a variety of different cells with a PDT dose-response similar to that for induction of apoptosis [22, 95]. This observation suggested that elevated ceramide promotes apoptosis, as has been proposed for other cell stresses [94]. When PDT sensitized by Pc 4 as the triggering agent, either no change or a decrease in lysosomal (acid) sphingomyelinase activity was observed. Instead, the enhanced level of ceramide following PDT was demonstrated to result from inhibition of two enzymes that utilize ceramide for the synthesis of complex sphingolipids, sphingomyelin synthase (SPS), and glucosylceramide synthase (GCS) [96]. With another photosensitizer, PPME, and PDT of human colon cancer HCT-116 cells, the increase in ceramide appeared to involve acid sphingomyelinase, although in that case a contribution of SPS and GCS was not investigated [97]. Furthermore, lymphoblasts from Niemann-Pick patients, which are genetically devoid of acid sphingomyelinase, were unable to either synthesize ceramide or undergo apoptosis in response to PDT, suggesting an important role for acid sphingomyelinase in this system [98]. Thus, the role of ceramide in PDT response may vary with the cell and the photosensitizer.

6.3.4 Microtubules

The cytoplasm of eukaryotic cells contains an array of fibrous proteins that form the cytoskeleton. The cytoskeleton includes microfilaments, built of actin subunits, microtubules, built of tubulin, and intermediate filaments, built of rod-shaped protein subunits, including keratin and actinin. The cytoskeleton is important for cell shape, motility, signal transduction, and separation of duplicated chromosomes during mitosis, and it has been the target of cancer therapy [99]. Cytoskeletal organization can be disrupted by photoactivation of several photosensitizers, including TPPS4, AlPcS4, meso-tetra-(4N-methylpyridyl) porphyrin, TMPyP, Photofrin, and BPD-MA (reviewed by Berg and Moan [100]) in a dose- and time-dependent manner. Whereas a sublethal dose of PDT with Photofrin causes transient microtubule depolymerization, higher doses result in irreversible depolymerization of microtubules and cell death [101]. However, the several components of the cytoskeleton differ in their susceptibility to PDT with different photosensitizers [102]. For example, actin microfilaments and α-actinin are much more severely damaged than keratin filaments by sublethal doses of PDT with ZnPc. Disruption of microtubules by PDT has similar consequences in cells as treatment with inhibitors of microtubules (i.e., disorganization of microtubules and the spindle apparatus resulting in the accumulation of the treated cells in metaphase). Cells late in the cell cycle are more susceptible to PDT-induced mitotic arrest than those at other phases of the cell cycle, probably because they have less time to recover before entering mitosis. Perturbation of microtubules, such as with the microtubule stabilizer Paclitaxel, results in mitotic arrest and the induction of apoptosis, which occurs as a consequence of the activation of the spindle assembly checkpoint leading to accumulation of Bim [103]. Several porphyrins have been shown to bind directly to microtubules and inhibit them from polymerization even in the absence of light. In contrast, raising the intracellular calcium concentration following PDT with Photofrin has been proposed as the cause of the microtubule depolymerization [101].

6.3.5 Plasma Membrane

The most common pathway for apoptosis in response to PDT usually involves the release of cytochrome c followed by activation of caspases-9, and -3; however, other pathways can contribute, especially those through caspase-8, in situations where the dominant pathway is suppressed or when the cells respond by secreting ligands of plasma membrane death receptors (reviewed in [1]). The death receptor complexes can play a role in PDT-induced apoptosis (e.g., expression and secretion of TNFα and FasL [104–108]). Nevertheless, combined effects of death receptor-targeted therapies and PDT remain inconclusive (e.g., whereas treatment with anti-Fas antibody enhanced apoptosis induced by Verteporfin-PDT [109], recombinant human TNFα had no effect on the ability of Pc 4-PDT to induce apoptosis [110]). In a study of murine embryonic fibroblasts from wild-type FADD or FADD knockout mice, the role of these plasma membrane death receptors was further delineated [111]. Both cell lines were equally sensitive to apoptosis after Pc 4-PDT, but the FADD knockout cells were resistant to the induction of apoptosis by TNFα; hence, Pc 4-PDT induced apoptosis does not require functional FADD. Taken together, the role of plasma membrane death receptors in PDT-induced apoptosis appears limited in the case of direct damage to cells in culture. However, in vivo the extrinsic pathway may be more important in responding to changes in cytokine and growth factor levels within the treated tissue.

One possible explanation for the ineffectiveness of death-receptor-therapy in combination with PDT is that PDT may cause a loss or reduction in the levels of these receptors. Indeed, loss of cellular response to epidermal growth factor (EGF) following PDT has been shown to be due to an immediate or delayed reduction in the level of its receptor (EGFR) and other cell surface receptors in both normal and cancer cells [112–114]. Interestingly, the loss of cellular responsiveness to growth factors and cytokines is not limited to PDT with plasma membrane-targeting photosensitizers, such as Photofrin, since the mitochondrion-targeting ALA and Pc 4 also exert the same effect [112, 113]. This observation implies that in addition to photodamage at the plasma membrane, caused by photoactivation of a plasma membrane-targeting photosensitizer, oxidative reactions or signaling mechanisms elicited by PDT at the mitochondria can affect the plasma membrane. Since the recovery of responsiveness to EGF requires 48–72 h after PDT [113], this suggests that in the design of protocols for combined PDT and death-ligand treatments, the timing and sequence of the treatments could be an important factor in determining the efficacy of the interaction.

In studies of Rose Bengal-PDT, photodynamic damage was confined to the plasma membrane of bovine aortic endothelial cells by irradiating the cell monolayer with evanescent wave visible radiation rather than by ordinary transillumination of the cells. In this system, apoptosis was efficiently induced, demonstrating that singlet oxygen produced at the plasma membrane can cause apoptosis [18]. PDT with this photosensitizer also activated Akt/protein kinase B, a component of a prosurvival signaling pathway [114]. However, the activation of Akt by PDT did not involve activation of the plasma membrane-integrated platelet-derived growth factor receptor (PDGFR). In contrast, photoactivation of plasma membrane-targeted Photofrin induced a nonapoptotic cell death in A431 cells [115].

6.3.6 Nuclei

Because of the propensity of the hydrophobic photosensitizers to accumulate in cytoplasmic membranes and membranous organelles and to be excluded from the nucleus (e.g., [36, 37]), there has been relatively little study of DNA damage following PDT. Furthermore, early studies of DNA repair-defective cells by Gomer's group [116, 117] provided strong evidence that whatever DNA damage was produced by PDT was not as important for cell killing as damage to membranes. Despite negligible dye accumulation in the nucleus, damage to nuclear DNA has been reported. Cultured mammalian cells exposed to PDT with porphyrin and porphyrin-like sensitizers produces apparent DNA single-strand breaks and alkali labile sites, nonrepairable DNA-protein cross links, and mutations (reviewed in [118]). However, in other cases, no evidence was found for mutations or for the production of chromosomal aberrations or micronuclei [119, 120]. Most of the apparent DNA strand breaks induced by low-dose PDT are repaired within 24 hours [121]. An important consideration is the assays for detecting effects of PDT on DNA. All of the strand-break studies relied upon assays conducted under alkaline conditions that convert various types of base and sugar alterations to strand breaks. Thus, it is not certain that DNA strand breaks are formed at all in cells by PDT. Furthermore, detection of mutations in cells is very sensitive to the target locus. Thus, a negative result using hypoxanthine-guanine phosphoribosyl transferase (HGPRT) as a target may simply mean that a large deletion of the target included a linked essential gene without which the cell couldn't survive. When the thymidine kinase (TK) locus was studied with Photofrin or Pc 4 as photosensitizer, it was determined that PDT can produce mutations in DNA but the frequency was much lower than for known mutagens, such as ionizing or ultraviolet radiation (reviewed in [122]).

In a novel recent study, estrogen-dependent vascular endothelial cells were loaded with a photosensitizer conjugated to estradiol; photoirradiation of the cells induced DNA damage [123]. It is presumed that binding of the photosensitizer-estradiol conjugate to estrogen receptors on the nuclear membrane directed the photosensitizer to a site allowing DNA damage to occur upon photoactivation of the sensitizer. A combination of low-dose cisplatin and PDT has been shown to greatly enhance DNA damage induction and cytotoxicity [124, 125]. In this combined treatment, electrons are transferred from the excited photosensitizer to cisplatin to produce radicals that damage DNA in a manner independent of oxygen [126]. Such a mechanism could be advantageous for the treatment of hypoxic tumor cells.

6.4 Conclusions

PDT is a highly efficient agent for killing of cells. Photosensitizers that localize to any site within the cell can be photoactivated to damage the sites to which they are bound and secondarily activate or inactivate processes throughout the cell. However, the mechanisms for cell killing can vary with the site of initial damage. PDT can elicit all three forms of PCD. At the lowest doses, autophagy serves as a mechanism to remove damaged cell components and maintain cell viability. As the dose increases, autophagy may be overwhelmed and apoptosis is triggered to remove the damaged cell. At supralethal doses, damage to mediators of autophagy and apoptosis may be too great for those processes, and the cell is destroyed by necrosis.

References

[1] Oleinick, N. L., Morris, R. L., and Belichenko, I., "The role of apoptosis in response to photodynamic therapy: What, where, why, and how," *Photochem. Photobiol. Sci.*, Vol. 1, 2002, pp. 1–21.

[2]   Moan, J., and Peng, Q., "An outline of the hundred-year history of PDT," *Anticancer Res*, Vol. 23, 2003, pp. 3591–3600.

[3]   Almeida, R. D., et al., "Intracellular signaling mechanisms in photodynamic therapy," *Biochim Biophys Acta*, Vol. 1704, 2004, pp. 59–86.

[4]   Granville, D. J., McManus, B. M., and Hunt, D. W., "Photodynamic therapy: Shedding light on the biochemical pathways regulating porphyrin-mediated cell death," *Histol Histopathol*, Vol. 16, 2001, pp. 309–317.

[5]   Girotti, A. W., "Photosensitized oxidation of membrane lipids: Reaction pathways, cytotoxic effects, and cytoprotective mechanisms," *J Photochem Photobiol B*, Vol. 63, 2001, pp. 103–113.

[6]   Ochsner, M., "Photophysical and photobiological processes in the photodynamic therapy of tumours," *Journal of Photochem. Photobiol. (Biology)*, Vol. 39, 1997, pp. 1–18.

[7]   Buytaert, E., Dewaele, M., and Agostinis, P., "Molecular effectors of multiple cell death pathways initiated by photodynamic therapy," *Biochim Biophys Acta*, Vol. 1776, 2007, pp. 86–107.

[8]   Agarwal, M. L., et al., "Photodynamic therapy induces rapid cell death by apoptosis in L5178Y mouse lymphoma cells," *Cancer Res*, Vol. 51, 1991, pp. 5993–5996.

[9]   He, J., and Oleinick, N. L. Cell death mechanisms vary with photodynamic therapy dose and photosensitizer. In: 5th International Photodynamic Association Meeting, Amelia Island, Florida, 1995, pp. 92–96.

[10] Noodt, B. B., et al., "Apoptosis induction by different pathways with methylene blue derivative and light from mitochondrial sites in V79 cells," *Int J Cancer*, Vol. 75, 1998, pp. 941–948.

[11] Noodt, B. B., et al., "Different apoptotic pathways are induced from various intracellular sites by tetraphenylporphyrins and light," *Br J Cancer*, Vol. 79, 1999, pp. 72–81.

[12] Vantieghem, A., et al., "Hypericin-induced photosensitization of HeLa cells leads to apoptosis or necrosis. Involvement of cytochrome c and procaspase-3 activation in the mechanism of apoptosis," *FEBS Lett*, Vol. 440, 1998, pp. 19–24.

[13] Kim, H. R., et al., "Enhanced apoptotic response to photodynamic therapy after bcl-2 transfection," *Cancer Res*, Vol. 59, 1999, pp. 3429–3432.

[14] Lavie, G., et al., "A photodynamic pathway to apoptosis and necrosis induced by dimethyl tetrahydroxyhelianthrone and hypericin in leukaemic cells: possible relevance to photodynamic therapy," *Br J Cancer*, Vol. 79, 1999, pp. 423–432.

[15] Dellinger, M., "Apoptosis or necrosis following Photofrin photosensitization: influence of the incubation protocol," *Photochem Photobiol*, Vol. 64, 1996, pp. 182–187.

[16] Kessel, D., and Poretz, R. D., "Sites of photodamage induced by photodynamic therapy with a chlorin e6 triacetoxymethyl ester (CAME)," *Photochem Photobiol*, Vol. 71, 2000, pp. 94–96.

[17] Kochevar, I. E., et al., "Singlet oxygen, but not oxidizing radicals, induces apoptosis in HL-60 cells," *Photochem Photobiol*, Vol. 72, 2000, pp. 548–553.

[18] Lin, C. P., Lynch, M. C., and Kochevar, I. E., "Reactive oxidizing species produced near the plasma membrane induce apoptosis in bovine aorta endothelial cells," *Exp Cell Res*, Vol. 259, 2000, pp. 351–359.

[19] He, X. Y., et al., "Photodynamic therapy with Photofrin II induces programmed cell death in carcinoma cell lines," *Photochem. Photobiol.*, Vol. 59, 1994, pp. 468–473.

[20] Noodt, B. B., et al., "Apoptosis and necrosis induced with light and 5-aminolaevulinic acid-derived protoporphyrin IX," *Br J Cancer*, Vol. 74, 1996, pp. 22–29.

[21] Allen, C. M., Sharman, W. M., and Van Lier, J. E., "Current status of phthalocyanines in the photodynamic therapy of cancer," *J. Porphyrins Phthalocyanines*, Vol. 5, 2001, pp. 161–169.

[22] Separovic, D., He, J., and Oleinick, N. L., "Ceramide generation in response to photodynamic treatment of L5178Y mouse lymphoma cells," *Cancer Res.*, Vol. 57, 1997, pp. 1717–1721.

[23] Xue, L.-Y., He, J., and Oleinick, N. L., "Rapid tyrosine phosphorylation of HS1 in the response of mouse lymphoma L5178Y-R cells to photodynamic treatment sensitized by the phthalocyanine Pc 4," *Photochem. Photobiol.*, Vol. 66, 1997, pp. 105–113.

[24] Kessel, D., and Luo, Y., "Cells in cryptophycin-induced cell-cycle arrest are susceptible to apoptosis," *Cancer Lett*, Vol. 151, 2000, pp. 25–29.

[25] Eskelinen, E. L., "Doctor Jekyll and Mister Hyde: Autophagy can promote both cell survival and cell death," *Cell Death Differ*, Vol. 12 Suppl 2, 2005, pp. 1468–1472.

[26] Kessel, D., Vicente, M. G., and Reiners, J. J., Jr., "Initiation of apoptosis and autophagy by photodynamic therapy," *Lasers Surg Med*, Vol. 38, 2006, pp. 482–488.

[27] Xue, L. Y., et al., "The death of human cancer cells following photodynamic therapy: apoptosis competence is necessary for Bcl-2 protection but not for induction of autophagy," *Photochem Photobiol*, Vol. 83, 2007, pp. 1016–1023.

[28] Buytaert, E., et al., "Role of endoplasmic reticulum depletion and multidomain proapoptotic BAX and BAK proteins in shaping cell death after hypericin-mediated photodynamic therapy," *ASEB J*, Vol. 20, 2006, pp. 756–758.

[29] Xue, L.-h., Chiu, S.-c., and Oleinick, N. L., "photodynamic therapy-induced death of mcf-7 human breast cancer cells: a role for caspase-3 in the Late Steps of Apoptosis but Not for the Critical Lethal Event," *Exp. Cell Res.*, Vol. 263, 2001, pp. 145–155.

[30] Chiu, S. M., et al., "Bax is essential for mitochondrion-mediated apoptosis but not for cell death caused by photodynamic therapy," *Br J Cancer*, Vol. 89, 2003, pp. 1590–1597.

[31] Chiu, S. M., et al., "Photodynamic therapy-induced death of HCT 116 cells: Apoptosis with or without Bax expression," *Apoptosis*, Vol. 10, 2005, pp. 1357–1368.

[32] Kessel, D., and Reiners, J. J., Jr., "Apoptosis and autophagy after mitochondrial or endoplasmic reticulum photodamage," *Photochem Photobiol*, Vol. 83, 2007, pp. 1024–1028.

[33] Yang, J., et al., "Prevention of apoptosis by Bcl-2: Release of cytochrome c from mitochondria blocked," *Science*, Vol. 275, 1997, pp. 1129–1132.

[34] Kluck, R. M., et al., "The release of cytochrome c from mitochondria: A primary site of Bcl-2 regulation of apoptosis," *Science*, Vol. 275, 1997, pp. 1132–1136.

[35] Luo, S., and Rubinsztein, D. C., "Atg5 and Bcl-2 provide novel insights into the interplay between apoptosis and autophagy," *Cell Death Differ*, Vol. 14, 2007, pp. 1247–1250.

[36] Trivedi, N. S., et al., "Quantitative analysis of Pc 4 localization in mouse lymphoma (LY-R) cells via double-label confocal fluorescence microscopy," *Photochem Photobiol*, Vol. 71, 2000, pp. 634–639.

[37] Lam, M., Oleinick, N. L., and Nieminen, A. L., "Photodynamic therapy-induced apoptosis in epidermoid carcinoma cells. Reactive oxygen species and mitochondrial inner membrane permeabilization," *J Biol Chem*, Vol. 276, 2001, pp. 47379–47386.

[38] Hunter, D. R., Haworth, R. A., and Southard, J. H., "Relationship between configuration, function, and permeability in calcium-treated mitochondria," *J Biol Chem*, Vol. 251, 1976, pp. 5069–5077.

[39] Halestrap, A. P., et al., "Mitochondria and cell death," *Biochem Soc Trans*, Vol. 28, 2000, pp. 170–177.

[40] Crompton, M., "Mitochondrial intermembrane junctional complexes and their role in cell death," *J Physiol*, Vol. 529 Pt 1, 2000, pp. 11–21.

[41] Kokoszka, J. E., et al., "The ADP/ATP translocator is not essential for the mitochondrial permeability transition pore," *Nature*, Vol. 427, 2004, pp. 461–465.

[42] Basso, E., et al., "Properties of the permeability transition pore in mitochondria devoid of Cyclophilin D," *J Biol Chem*, Vol. 280, 2005, pp. 18558–18561.

[43] Baines, C. P., et al., "Voltage-dependent anion channels are dispensable for mitochondrial-dependent cell death," *Nat Cell Biol*, Vol. 9, 2007, pp. 550–555.

[44] He, L., and Lemasters, J. J., "Regulated and unregulated mitochondrial permeability transition pores: a new paradigm of pore structure and function?," *FEBS Lett*, Vol. 512, 2002, pp. 1–7.

[45] Verma, A., Nye, J., and Snyder, S. H., "Porphyrins are endogenous ligands for the mitochondrial (periphera-type) benzodiazepine receptor.," *Mol. Pharmacol.*, Vol. 84, 1987, pp. 2256–2260.

[46] Verma, A., and Snyder, S. H., "Characterization of porphyrin interactions with peripheral type benzodiazepine receptors," *Mol. Pharmacol.*, Vol. 34, 1988, pp. 800–805.

[47] Verma, A., et al., "Photodynamic tumor therapy: Mitochondrial benzodiazepine receptors as a therapeutic target," *Mol. Med.*, Vol. 4, 1998, pp. 40–49.

[48] Ratcliffe, S. L., and Matthews, E. K., "Modification of the photodynamic action of d-aminolaevulinic acid (ALA) on rat pancreatoma cells by mitochondrial benzodiazepine receptor ligads.," *Br. J. Cancer*, Vol. 71, 1995, pp. 300–305.

[49] Dougherty, T. J., et al., "The role of the peripheral benzodiazepine receptor in photodynamic activity of certain pyropheophorbide ether photosensitizers: Albumin site II as a surrogate marker for activity," *Photochem Photobiol*, Vol. 76, 2002, pp. 91–97.

[50] Furre, I. E., et al., "Targeting PBR by hexaminolevulinate-mediated photodynamic therapy induces apoptosis through translocation of apoptosis-inducing factor in human leukemia cells," *Cancer Res*, Vol. 65, 2005, pp. 11051–11060.

[51] Bisland, S. K., et al., "Increased expression of mitochondrial benzodiazepine receptors following low-level light treatment facilitates enhanced protoporphyrin IX production in glioma-derived cells in vitro," *Lasers Surg Med*, Vol. 39, 2007, pp. 678–684.

[52] Morris, R. L., et al., "The peripheral benzodiazepine receptor in photodynamic therapy with the phthalocyanine photosensitizer Pc 4," *Photochem Photobiol*, Vol. 75, 2002, pp. 652–661.

[53] Kessel, D., Antolovich, M., and Smith, K. M., "The role of the peripheral benzodiazepine receptor in the apoptotic response to photodynamic therapy," *Photochem. Photobiol.*, Vol. 74, 2001, pp. 346–349.

[54] Salet, C., et al., "Singlet oxygen produced by photodynamic action causes inactivation of the mitochondrial permeability transition pore," *J. Biol. Chem.*, Vol. 272, 1997, pp. 21938–21943.

[55] Belzacq, A. S., et al., "Apoptosis induction by the photosensitizer verteporfin: identification of mitochondrial adenine nucleotide translocator as a critical target," *Cancer Res*, Vol. 61, 2001, pp. 1260–1264.

[56] Miccoli, L., et al., "Light-induced photoactivation of hypericin affects the energy metabolism of human glioma cells by inhibiting hexokinase bound to mitochondria," *Cancer Res*, Vol. 58, 1998, pp. 5777–5786.

[57] Chaloupka, R., et al., "Over-expression of Bcl-2 does not protect cells from hypericin photo-induced mitochondrial membrane depolarization, but delays subsequent events in the apoptotic pathway," *FEBS Lett*, Vol. 462, 1999, pp. 295–301.

[58] Kowaltowski, A. J., et al., "Mitochondrial effects of triarylmethane dyes," *J Bioenerg Biomembr*, Vol. 31, 1999, pp. 581–590.

[59] Moreno, G., et al., "Photosensitivity of DNA replication and respiration to haematoporphyrin derivative (photofrin II) in mammalian CV-1 cells," *Int J Radiat Biol Relat Stud Phys Chem Med*, Vol. 52, 1987, pp. 213–222.

[60] Varnes, M. E., et al., "Photodynamic therapy-induced apoptosis in lymphoma cells: Translocation of cytochrome c causes inhibition of respiration as well as caspase activation," *Biochem. Biophys. Res. Commun.*, Vol. 255, 1999, pp. 673–679.

[61] Gibson, S. L., and Hilf, R., "Interdependence of fluence, drug dose and oxygen on hematoporphyrin derivative induced photosensitization of tumor mitochondria," *Photochem. Photobiol.*, Vol. 42, 1985, pp. 367–373.

[62] Atlante, A., et al., "Hematoporphyrin derivative (PF II) photosensitization of isolated mito-
      chondria: Impariment of anion translocation," *Biochem. Biophys. Res. Commun.*, Vol.
      141, 1986, pp. 584–590.

[63] Singh, G., et al., "Mitochondrial photosensitization by Photofrin II," *Photochem.
      Photobiol.*, Vol. 46, 1987, pp. 645–649.

[64] Ardail, D., et al., "Mitochondrial contact sites. Lipid composition and dynamics," *J Biol
      Chem*, Vol. 265, 1990, pp. 18797–18802.

[65] Schlame, M., Rua, D., and Greenberg, M. L., "The biosynthesis and functional role of
      cardiolipin," *Prog Lipid Res*, Vol. 39, 2000, pp. 257–288.

[66] McMillin, J. B., and Dowhan, W., "Cardiolipin and apoptosis," *Biochim Biophys Acta*,
      Vol. 1585, 2002, pp. 97–107.

[67] Kriska, T., Korytowski, W., and Girotti, A. W., "Role of mitochondrial cardiolipin
      peroxidation in apoptotic photokilling of 5-aminolevulinate-treated tumor cells," *Arch
      Biochem Biophys*, Vol. 433, 2005, pp. 435–446.

[68] Choi, S. Y., et al., "Cardiolipin deficiency releases cytochrome c from the inner mitochon-
      drial membrane and accelerates stimuli-elicited apoptosis," *Cell Death Differ*, Vol. 14,
      2007, pp. 597–606.

[69] Wilson, B. C., Olivo, M., and Singh, G., "Subcellular localization of Photofrin and
      aminolevulinic acid and photodynamic cross-resistance in vitro in radiation-induced
      fibrosarcoma cells sensitive or resistant to photofrin-mediated photodynamic therapy,"
      Photochem. Photobiol., Vol. 65, 1997, pp. 166–176.

[70] Morris, R. L., et al., "Fluorescence resonance energy transfer reveals a binding site of a
      photosensitizer for photodynamic therapy," *Cancer Res*, Vol. 63, 2003, pp. 5194–5197.

[71] Kessel, D., and Castelli, M., "Evidence that Bcl-2 is the target of three photosensitizers that
      induce a rapid apoptotic response," *Photochem Photobiol*, Vol. 74, 2001, pp. 318–322.

[72] Kessel, D., Castelli, M., and Reiners, J. J., "Ruthenium red-mediated suppression of Bcl-2
      loss and Ca(2+) release initiated by photodamage to the endoplasmic reticulum: scavenging
      of reactive oxygen species," *Cell Death Differ*, Vol. 12, 2005, pp. 502–511.

[73] Xue, L. Y., Chiu, S. M., and Oleinick, N. L., "Photochemical destruction of the Bcl-2
      oncoprotein during photodynamic therapy with the phthalocyanine photosensitizer Pc 4,"
      Oncogene, Vol. 20, 2001, pp. 3420–3427.

[74] Matroule, J.-Y., et al., "Mechanism of colon cancer apoptosis mediated by
      pyropheophorbide-a methylester photosensitization," *Oncogene*, Vol. 20, 2001, pp.
      4070–4084.

[75] Granville, D. J., et al., "Bcl-2 increases emptying of endoplasmic reticulum Ca2+ stores
      during photodynamic therapy-induced apoptosis," *Cell Calcium*, Vol. 30, 2001, pp.
      343–350.

[76] Ricchelli, F., et al., "Photodynamic action of porphyrin on Ca2+ influx in endoplasmic
      reticulum: a comparison with mitochondria," *Biochem J*, Vol. 338 (Pt 1), 1999, pp.
      221–227.

[77] Cui, Z. J., and Kanno, T., "Photodynamic triggering of calcium oscillation in the isolated
      rat pancreatic acini," *J Physiol*, Vol. 504 (Pt 1), 1997, pp. 47–55.

[78] Cui, Z. J., et al., "A novel aspect of photodynamic action: induction of recurrent spikes in
      cytosolic calcium concentration," *Photochem Photobiol*, Vol. 65, 1997, pp. 382–386.

[79] Agarwal, M. L., et al., "Phospholipase activation triggers apoptosis in photosensitized
      mouse lymphoma cells," *Cancer Res.*, Vol. 53, 1993, pp. 5897–5902.

[80] Xue, L. Y., et al., "Photodamage to multiple Bcl-xL isoforms by photodynamic therapy
      with the phthalocyanine photosensitizer Pc 4," *Oncogene*, Vol. 22, 2003, pp. 9197–9204.

[81] Usuda, J., et al., "Domain-dependent photodamage to Bcl-2. A membrane anchorage
      region is needed to form the target of phthalocyanine photosensitization," *J Biol Chem*,
      Vol. 278, 2003, pp. 2021–2029.

[82]   Kessel, D., Caruso, J. A., and Reiners, J. J., Jr., "Potentiation of photodynamic therapy by ursodeoxycholic acid," *Cancer Res*, Vol. 60, 2000, pp. 6985–6988.

[83]   Castelli, M., Reiners, J. J., and Kessel, D., "A mechanism for the proapoptotic activity of ursodeoxycholic acid: effects on Bcl-2 conformation," *Cell Death Differ*, Vol. 11, 2004, pp. 906–914.

[84]   Marchal, S., et al., "Relationship between subcellular localisation of Foscan and caspase activation in photosensitised MCF-7 cells," *Br J Cancer*, Vol. 96, 2007, pp. 944–951.

[85]   Kessel, D., et al., "Determinants of the apoptotic response to lysosomal photodamage," *Photochem Photobiol*, Vol. 71, 2000, pp. 196–200.

[86]   Kessel, D., and Luo, Y., "Intracellular Sites of Photodamage as a Factor in Apoptotic Cell Death," *J Porphyrin. Phthalo.*, Vol. 5, 2001, pp. 181–184.

[87]   Reiners, J. J., Jr., et al., "Release of cytochrome c and activation of pro-caspase-9 following lysosomal photodamage involves Bid cleavage," *Cell Death Differ*, Vol. 9, 2002, pp. 934–944.

[88]   Caruso, J. A., et al., "Differential susceptibilities of murine hepatoma 1c1c7 and Tao cells to the lysosomal photosensitizer NPe6: influence of aryl hydrocarbon receptor on lysosomal fragility and protease contents," *Mol Pharmacol*, Vol. 65, 2004, pp. 1016–1028.

[89]   Stoka, V. V., et al., "Lysosomal protease pathways to apoptosis: cleavage of bid, not Pro-caspases, is the most likely route," *J Biol Chem*, Vol. 276, 2001, pp. 3149–3157.

[90]   Cirman, T., et al., "Selective disruption of lysosomes in HeLa cells triggers apoptosis mediated by cleavage of Bid by multiple papain-like lysosomal cathepsins," *J Biol Chem*, Vol. 279, 2004, pp. 3578–3587.

[91]   Leung, W. N., et al., "Photodynamic effects of mTHPC on human colon adenocarcinoma cells: photocytotoxicity, subcellular localization and apoptosis," *Photochem Photobiol*, Vol. 75, 2002, pp. 406–411.

[92]   Ichinose, S., et al., "Lysosomal cathepsin initiates apoptosis, which is regulated by photodamage to Bcl-2 at mitochondria in photodynamic therapy using a novel photosensitizer, ATX-s10 (Na)," *Int J Oncol*, Vol. 29, 2006, pp. 349–355.

[93]   Tanida, I., et al., "Lysosomal turnover, but not a cellular level, of endogenous LC3 is a marker for autophagy," *Autophagy*, Vol. 1, 2005, pp. 84–91.

[94]   Haimovitz-Friedman, A., et al., "Ionizing radiation acts on cellular membranes to generate ceramide and initiate apoptosis," *J. Exp. Med.*, Vol. 180, 1994, pp. 525–535.

[95]   Separovic, D., Mann, K. J., and Oleinick, N. L., "Association of ceramide accumulation with photodynamic treatment-induced cell death," *Photochem. Photobiol*, Vol. 68, 1998, pp. 101–109.

[96]   Dolgachev, V., et al., "De novo ceramide accumulation due to inhibition of its conversion to complex sphingolipids in apoptotic photosensitized cells," *J Biol Chem*, Vol. 279, 2004, pp. 23238–23249.

[97]   Matroule, J. Y., et al., "Pyropheophorbide-a methyl ester-mediated photosensitization activates transcription factor NF-kappaB through the interleukin-1 receptor-dependent signaling pathway," *J Biol Chem*, Vol. 274, 1999, pp. 2988–3000.

[98]   Separovic, D., et al., "Niemann-Pick human lymphoblasts are resistant to phthalocyanine 4-photodynamic therapy-induced apoptosis," *Biochem Biophys Res Commun*, Vol. 258, 1999, pp. 506–512.

[99]   Jordan, M. A., and Wilson, L., "Microtubules as a target for anticancer drugs," *Nat Rev Cancer*, Vol. 4, 2004, pp. 253–265.

[100] Berg, K., and Moan, J., "Lysosomes and microtubules as targets for photochemotherapy of cancer," *Photochem. Photobiol.*, Vol. 65, 1997, pp. 403–409.

[101] Sporn, L. A., and Foster, T. H., "Photofrin and light induces microtubule depolymerization in cultured human endothelial cells," *Cancer Res.*, Vol. 52, 1992, pp. 3443–3445.

[102] Juarranz, A., et al., "Photodamage induced by Zinc(II)-phthalocyanine to microtubules, actin, alpha-actinin and keratin of HeLa cells," *Photochem Photobiol*, Vol. 73, 2001, pp. 283–289.

[103] Tan, T. T., et al., "Key roles of BIM-driven apoptosis in epithelial tumors and rational chemotherapy," *Cancer Cell*, Vol. 7, 2005, pp. 227–238.

[104] Evans, S., et al., "Effects of photodynamic therapy on tumor necrosis factor production by murine macrophages," *J. Natl. Cancer. Inst*, Vol. 82, 1990, pp. 34–39.

[105] Kick, G., et al., "Strong and prolonged induction of c-jun and c-fos proto-oncogenes by photodynamic therapy," *Br. J. Cancer*, Vol. 74, 1996, pp. 30–36.

[106] Ahmad, N., et al., "Involvement of Fas (APO-1/CD-95) during photodynamic-therapy-mediated apoptosis in human epidermoid carcinoma A431 cells," *J Invest Dermatol*, Vol. 115, 2000, pp. 1041–1046.

[107] Yslas, I., et al., "Expression of Fas antigen and apoptosis caused by 5,10,15, 20-tetra(4-methoxyphenyl)porphyrin (TMP) on carcinoma cells: implication for photodynamic therapy," *Toxicology*, Vol. 149, 2000, pp. 69–74.

[108] Ali, S. M., et al., "Hypericin induced death receptor-mediated apoptosis in photoactivated tumor cells," *Int J Mol Med*, Vol. 9, 2002, pp. 601–616

[109] Jiang, H., et al., "Selective depletion of a thymocyte subset in vitro with an immunomodulatory photosensitizer," *Clin Immunol*, Vol. 91, 1999, pp. 178–187.

[110] Azizuddin, K., et al., "Recombinant human tumor necrosis factor alpha does not potentiate cell killing after photodynamic therapy with a silicon phthalocyanine in A431 human epidermoid carcinoma cells," *Int J Oncol*, Vol. 18, 2001, pp. 411–415.

[111] Nagy, B., et al., "FADD null mouse embryonic fibroblasts undergo apoptosis after photosensitization with the silicon phthalocyanine Pc 4," *Arch Biochem Biophy*, Vol. 385, 2001, pp. 194–202.

[112] Ahmad, N., Kalka, K., and Mukhtar, H., "In vitro and in vivo inhibition of epidermal growth factor receptor-tyrosine kinase pathway by photodynamic therapy," *Oncogene*, Vol. 20, 2001, pp. 2314–2317.

[113] Wong, T. W., et al., "Photodynamic therapy mediates immediate loss of cellular responsiveness to cytokines and growth factors," *Cancer Res*, Vol. 63, 2003, pp. 3812–3818.

[114] Zhuang, S., Ouedraogo, G. D., and Kochevar, I. E., "Downregulation of epidermal growth factor receptor signaling by singlet oxygen through activation of caspase-3 and protein phosphatases," *Oncogene*, Vol. 22, 2003, pp. 4413–4424.

[115] Hsieh, Y. J., et al., "Subcellular localization of Photofrin determines the death phenotype of human epidermoid carcinoma A431 cells triggered by photodynamic therapy: when plasma membranes are the main targets," *J Cell Physiol*, Vol. 194, 2003, pp. 363–375.

[116] Gomer, C. J., et al., "Comparison of mutagenicity and induction of sister chromatid exchange in Chinese hamster cells exposed to hematoporphyrin derivative photoradiation, ionizing radiation, or ultraviolet radiation.," *Cancer Res.*, Vol. 43, 1983, pp. 2622–2627.

[117] Gomer, C. J., Rucker, N., and Murphree, A. L., "Transformation and mutagenic potential of porphyrin photodynamic therapy in mammalian cells," *Int. J. Radiat. Biol.*, Vol. 53, 1988, pp. 651–659.

[118] Oleinick, N. L., et al. Effects of photodynamic treatment on DNA. In: S. Jacques (ed.), Laser-Tissue Interactions II, Vol. 1427, pp. 90–100. *SPIE*, 1991.

[119] Halkiotis, K., Yova, D., and Pantelias, G., "In vitro evaluation of the genotoxic and clastogenic potential of photodynamic therapy," *Mutagenesis*, Vol. 14, 1999, pp. 193–198.

[120] Zenzen, V., and Zankl, H., "In vitro evaluation of the cytotoxic and mutagenic potential of the 5-aminolevulinic acid hexylester-mediated photodynamic therapy," *Mutat Res*, Vol. 561, 2004, pp. 91–100.

[121] Haylett, A. K., Ward, T. H., and Moore, J. V., "DNA damage and repair in Gorlin syndrome and normal fibroblasts after aminolevulinic acid photodynamic therapy: a comet assay study," *Photochem Photobiol*, Vol. 78, 2003, pp. 337–341.

[122] Oleinick, N. L., and Evans, H. H., "The photobiology of photodynamic therapy: Cellular targets and mechanisms," *Radiat. Res.*, Vol. 150, 1998, pp. S146–S156.

[123] El-Akra, N., et al., "Synthesis of estradiol-pheophorbide a conjugates: evidence of nuclear targeting, DNA damage and improved photodynamic activity in human breast cancer and vascular endothelial cells," *Photochem Photobiol Sci*, Vol. 5, 2006, pp. 996–999.

[124] Nonaka, M., Ikeda, H., and Inokuchi, T., "Effect of combined photodynamic and chemotherapeutic treatment on lymphoma cells in vitro," *Cancer Lett*, Vol. 184, 2002, pp. 171–178.

[125] Crescenzi, E., et al., "Photodynamic therapy with indocyanine green complements and enhances low-dose cisplatin cytotoxicity in MCF-7 breast cancer cells," *Mol Cancer Ther*, Vol. 3, 2004, pp. 537–544.

[126] Lu, Q. B., "Molecular reaction mechanisms of combination treatments of low-dose cisplatin with radiotherapy and photodynamic therapy," *J Med Chem*, Vol. 50, 2007, pp. 2601–2604.

CHAPTER 7

The Role of Oxygen in Photodynamic Therapy

Johan Moan and Asta Juzeniene

7.1 Introduction

With few exceptions, solid tumors have regions with little or no oxygen [1–3]. This is due to poor vascularization and is called hypoxia (low oxygen tension) or anoxia (no oxygen). The low oxygen status is a main problem in radiation therapy of cancer, since tissues with low oxygen tension are two to three times less radiation sensitive than the well-oxygenated tissues [3–6]. The oxygen effect in radiation therapy is well documented but not completely understood, since oxygen protects rather than sensitizes biomolecules in solution [7–9]. It is believed that oxygen reacts with radiation products in cells and "fixes" them or contributes to prevent repair [3, 10–15]. For decades, so-called anoxic radiosensitizers, among which misonidazoles are best known, have been sought, since such drugs would help to reduce the oxygen effect and thus make tumors more radiation sensitive [4, 16–19]. Treatment under hyperbaric oxygen tension has also been tried [20–22].

When PDT came on the scene as an anticancer treatment, it was hoped that this treatment would not suffer from any oxygen effect, or at least would be efficient at very low oxygen tensions. There is no a priori reason why the onset of the effect should occur at the same oxygen tension for both treatments, although it was early known that PDT acted mainly via the singlet oxygen mechanism [23, 24]. Still, another photosensitizing pathway may be active, namely type I, or the "radical" mechanism [24–27]. In this case oxygen may or may not, be involved in PDT, since the generated free radicals can be produced and act without any participation of oxygen [24, 28]. Therefore, a great deal of work was done by us [29, 30] and others [31–36] in the early days of PDT to elucidate the oxygen effect. It turned out that the singlet oxygen mechanism (also called type II mechanism or photodynamic action) was the main one and that PDT was inefficient in anoxia [30, 33–35]. However, this is only one of the routes by which oxygen influence the outcome of PDT, and there are several other routes of influence, as will be discussed in this chapter.

7.2 The Primary Effect: Singlet Oxygen Generation

Formation of singlet oxygen is dependent on collision of an excited sensitizer molecule, usually one in the triplet state, and an oxygen molecule in the ground state.

Thus, the ultimate quantum yield is dependent upon three factors: (1) the quantum yield of triplet state formation of sensitizer (usually 0.2–0.9) [37], (2) the influence of quenchers that can react with the triplet state molecules before they collide with molecular oxygen, and (3) the yield of singlet oxygen per collision. The latter two factors are difficult to measure, but they obviously do not play any major role, since the yield of singlet oxygen is not much smaller than that of excited triplet state of a photosensitizer and is about 0.2 to 0.7 [38–42].

Once formed in cells or in extracellular fluids, singlet oxygen can react with quenchers before it reaches a vulnerable biological target. The lifetime of singlet oxygen in cells and its diffusion length are critical parameters [43]. We determined by fluorescence quenching experiments in cells these parameters to be 10 to 40 ns and 10 to 20 nm, respectively [44]. These early determinations have been challenged by later direct measurements of the singlet oxygen fluorescence at 1,270 nm [45, 46]. The later measurements gave much larger lifetimes (<320 ns) [45–48] than we found, but more recent experiments showed lower values (48 ns) [49], almost as low as our values. The problem with these measurements is that they do not distinguish between singlet oxygen formed inside cells and singlet oxygen formed in aqueous phase surrounding them, where the concentration of quenchers is lower, and therefore the lifetime is longer. In any case, it seems clear that the singlet oxygen diffusion length, as well as the triplet molecule diffusion length, are so short that practically all PDT-induced cell and tissue damage occurs in the place where the sensitizer concentration is highest [50–52]. This is extremely important, since it indicates that fluorescence microscopy can be used to identify these targets. In this way the following targets have been identified: all membranes, mitochondria, lysosomes, endoplasmic Reticulum, and Golgi complex [50, 53, 54]. Furthermore, since practically no PDT sensitizers localize in the nucleus (being negatively charged at pH~7), PDT causes little DNA damage and few chromosome changes, indicating a low carcinogenic potential. Experiments have proved this to be true [54–65].

Since the lifetime of the sensitizer molecule in the triplet state in tissues is above 10 μs [48, 66], it is long enough for the triplet excited state to react with oxygen to form singlet oxygen, therefore is dependent on the oxygen concentration. It was, therefore, early realized that the oxygen dependency of PDT in cells was a crucial factor. Lee See et al. [36] measured this using sodium dithionite to reduce the oxygen concentration, while we did it at about the same time by flushing the cell culture with oxygen concentration [30]. The singlet oxygen yield is constant from 100% to 5% oxygen but is halved at 1% oxygen [30]. Similar results were later found in vivo by Henderson et al. [35]. Disappointingly, this oxygen dependency is very similar to that found for ionizing radiation, and PDT cannot kill cells in hypoxic tumor regions. More than that, pressure against a superficial tumor can reduce the blood perfusion and the oxygen concentration to such a degree that PDT does not work [31, 67]. As a curiosity one might mention that UVA solaria, which work partly by photodynamic effects, cause neither erythema nor pigmentation on body parts that press against the transparent floor of the bed.

7.3   Concentrations of Oxygen in Tumors and Other Tissues

Most normal tissues contain about 5% oxygen, which is supplied by blood circulation. The reason why they contain less than 20% (as in the air) is simply respiration. At low vascularization (subnecrotic tumor areas) or at high respiration rates (intense muscular work), oxygen concentrations can be much lower than this [68, 69].

The epidermis is nonvascularized and gets oxygen from direct contact with air and by diffusion from the dermis [70, 71]. Thus, the oxygen concentration in skin changes with distance from the stratum corneum, being at minimum at about 100 μm below the surface and then increasing to 1,700 μm in the vascularized part of the dermis [71]. Therefore, hyperbaric oxygen might increase the oxygen tension in superficial, poorly vascularized tumors [71].

Basal cell carcinomas are often inflamed, well-vascularized, and have slightly higher temperatures than normal surrounding skin [72–76]. This is one of the reasons for the selectivity of PDT for these tumors [77–80].

7.4   Methods to Increase Tumor Oxygenation

Since most normal tissues contain about 5% oxygen, they will not become more sensitive to PDT by increasing the oxygen tension [30]. Hypoxic parts of tumors, however, can be made more vulnerable. Several methods have been proposed to overcome tumor hypoxia: (1) breathing hyperbaric oxygen (HBO), (2) using oxygen-carrying fluorocarbons combined with carbogen (95% oxygen) breathing, (3) using nicotinamide injection and carbogen breathing, (4) using oxygen releasing substances, (5) modulating the oxygen binding capacity of hemoglobin, (6) decreasing the respiration rate, (8) increasing the oxygen solubility, (8) using blood flow modifiers, and (9) destroying hypoxic cells with bioreductive drugs or hypothermia [21]. Several of these methods have been exploited for PDT purposes with promising results in experimental [81–95] and clinical work [96–102].

Tumor hypothermia during PDT can be advantageous for several reasons: the oxygen binding by hemoglobin will increase (the Bohr effect), the metabolic activity will decrease, and repair of sublethal damage will be reduced [103–106]. We tried this and found that the PDT effect was enhanced by cooling the mice tumors to 5°C [107].

7.5   Photosensitization under Anoxia

Type I mechanisms, radical mechanisms, may, in principle, work in the absence of oxygen. PUVA treatment, for instance, is to some extent based on oxygen-independent photosensitized cross-linking of DNA [108, 109]. Also photobleaching of standard sensitizers like Photofrin takes place in the absence of oxygen [49, 110]. However, this does not lead to cell photoinactivation [30, 33, 49], and one may have to wait for efficient anoxic photosensitizers to be found.

7.6   Reduction of the Oxygen Concentration by PDT Itself

7.6.1   Primary Reduction

PDT results in a photooxidation process; one oxygen molecule is consumed for each singlet oxygen that reacts with and oxidizes another molecule. Thus, one can easily compute the rate of oxygen consumption the following parameters are known [111]:

1. The fluence rate of the light exposure, F.
2. The extinction coefficient of the sensitizer, ε, at the relevant wavelength. In case a broadband source is used, convolution integrals have to be determined (i.e., the product, wavelength by wavelength, of the absorption spectrum of the sensitizer, and the emission spectrum of the light source).
3. The concentration of sensitizer, c, in the investigated volume. This concentration varies from point to point, so average values of larger volume elements have to be used.
4. The quantum yield of photooxygenation, Φ. This is usually the same as the quantum yield of singlet oxygen(i.e., in the range 0.2–0.7) [37,112]. The lifetime of singlet oxygen in tissues is much shorter than that in water, indicating that most of the singlet oxygen is reacting. Some quenching without photooxidation may occur, but probably not to any large scale.

It has been shown under clinical conditions that PDT with Photofrin at fluence rates larger than 100 mW/cm^2 leads to oxygen depletion [113–115].

7.6.2   Secondary Reactions

Secondary reactions during PDT take place on a longer time scale than primary reactions of oxygen, and are due to vascular damage [116–124]. Under clinical conditions, with Photofrin and fluence rates of 75 mW/cm^2, such damage is manifested within the first minutes of light exposure [125]. However, the time for vessel damage to be manifested is dependent on tissue, on sensitizer hydrophilicity (hydrophilic sensitizers tend to give more vascular damage than more lipophilic ones), and on time between sensitizer application and light exposure (short time leads to prominent vascular damage because of larger sensitizer concentrations in the blood) [126–129].

7.7   Reoxygenation After PDT

Under certain conditions a mild erythema, an indicator of invasion of inflammatory cells or release of vasoactive substances, occurs after PDT [116, 118, 130–133]. This leads to an increase in blood flow and temperature [73, 134–136]. The increased blood flow leads to higher oxygen concentrations in the treated tissue [114, 134].

7.8   Fluence Rate Effects

The processes mentioned above will play different roles depending on the fluence rate: At high fluence rates, primary oxygen depletion will occur rapidly and lead to over all low PDT efficiency [113–115, 137]. At low fluence rates, long exposure times are required and vessel damage (vasoconstriction and thrombosis) may occur and this will reduce the effect [114, 137, 138]. Therefore, intermediate fluence rates (30 mW/cm^2) may give the best results, since they may offer the possibility to avoid primary oxygen depletion and still give complete tumor destruction before vascular effects are introduced [114, 139–141]. However, after light exposure, vascular effects will contribute substantially to tumor destruction, as first shown by Henderson et al. [121] (Figure 7.1b).

7.9   Fractionated Light Exposure

Fractionated light exposure during PDT may be advantageous for following reasons:

1. Primary oxygen depletion can be avoided and reoxygenation may occur before the next light fraction is given [142–144]. However, the overall timing should not be such that vascular damage starts to play a role during the treatment.
2. Practically all sensitizers are photolabile [145, 146]. Diffusion of fresh sensitizer can occur into the treated volume from the blood, or, in the case of ALA-PDT, be resynthesized in this volume [147–150].
3. Redistribution of photosensitizer to less sensitive locations can occur during light exposure. We have shown that this, indeed, takes place as evidenced by rapid changes in fluorescence quantum yields [151, 152]. Fractionation, on a time scale of minutes, allows the sensitizer to diffuse back to the sensitive targets and give efficient tumor destruction when the next light fraction arrives [151, 152].
4. If the time is long enough between exposures, vasodilatation may occur and thus increase concentration in the treated volume [153, 154].

7.10   Changes of Quantum Yield Related to Sensitizer Relocalization

We have shown by fluorescence measurements that porphyrin sensitizers are relocalized during PDT [155, 156]. This leads to changes in fluorescence yields, and therefore also to changes in photodestruction of tissues [157–159]. In some cases fluorescence microscopy clearly shows relocalization [155, 156, 158, 159]. Good examples are water-soluble phthalocyanines and porphyrins, which are primarily localized outside nuclei, but diffuse into these during light exposure [155, 158, 159]. Little is known about oxygen effects in this context.

7.11   Oxygen Effects on Sensitizer Photobleaching

Photobleaching of sensitizer almost always occurs during PDT [145, 146]. The oxygen dependency of photobleaching is different from that of photokilling of cells [49]. It seems that photobleaching can occur almost under anoxic conditions [49]. Large fluence rates will then lead to destruction of the sensitizer without destruction of the tumor.

7.12   Changes of Optical Penetration Caused by Changes in Oxygen Concentration

Changes in oxygen concentration are extremely important whenever a deep effect of PDT is wanted. The reason for changes in optical penetration is simply that the absorption spectra of hemoglobin (Hb) and oxyhemoglobin (HbO$_2$) are different, as shown in Figure 7.1 [160]. We have shown that as oxygen depletion starts to manifest itself and Hb/HbO$_2$ ratio increases, the optical penetration will increase at 390 to 422, 455 to 500, 530 to 545, and 570 to 585 nm and decrease at 422 to 455, 500 to 530, 545 to570, and 585 to805 nm [161, 162]. Carbogen breathing and other modalities leading to increase in tissue oxygenation may enhance the penetration of red light into the tissue [163].

7.13   Conclusions

The growing realization that the efficacy of PDT in many cases is determined by the tissue availability of oxygen will have an impact both on how the treatment is deliv-

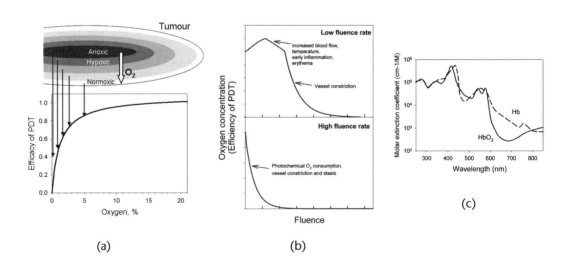

Figure 7.1   (a) Oxygen concentration in tumors; (b) fluence rate effects on PDT efficacy; and (c) Absorption spectra of the oxyhemoglobin (HbO2) and hemoglobin (Hb) [160].

ered, whether tissue oxygen levels should be monitored, and whether tissue oxygen levels can be raised by combination treatments. Although delivery of light at low fluence rates and the adoption of fractionated schedules at traditional fluence rates of 100 mW/cm^2, these procedures may be worth considering to gain the maximum effect on tissue destruction.

Acknowledgments

We appreciate financial support of the Norwegian Cancer Society (Kreftforeningen).

References

[1]   Brown, J. M. and Wilson, W. R., "Exploiting tumour hypoxia in cancer treatment," *Nat. Rev. Cancer*, Vol. 4, No. 6, 2004, pp. 437–447.

[2]   Weinmann, M., Belka, C., and Plasswilm, L., "Tumour hypoxia: impact on biology, prognosis and treatment of solid malignant tumours," *Onkologie*, Vol. 27, No. 1, 2004, pp. 83–90.

[3]   Hoogsteen, I. J., et al., "The Hypoxic Tumour Microenvironment, Patient Selection and Hypoxia-modifying Treatments," *Clin. Oncol. (R. Coll. Radiol.)*, Vol. 19, No. 6, 2007, pp. 385–396.

[4]   Koukourakis, M. I., "Tumour angiogenesis and response to radiotherapy," *Anticancer Res.*, Vol. 21, No. 6B, 2001, pp. 4285–4300.

[5]   Vaupel, P., "Tumor microenvironmental physiology and its implications for radiation oncology," *Semin. Radiat. Oncol.*, Vol. 14, No. 3, 2004, pp. 198–206.

[6]   Gray, L. H., et al., "The concentration of oxygen dissolved in tissues at the time of irradiation as a factor in radiotherapy," *Br. J. Radiol.*, Vol. 26, No. 312, 1953, pp. 638–648.

[7]   Blok, J. and Loman, H., "The effects of gamma-radiation in DNA," *Curr. Top. Radiat. Res. Q.*, Vol. 9, No. 2, 1973, pp. 165–245.

[8]   Quintiliani, M., "The oxygen effect in radiation inactivation of DNA and enzymes," *Int. J. Radiat. Biol. Relat. Stud. Phys. Chem. Med.*, Vol. 50, No. 4, 1986, pp. 573–594.

[9]   Barilla, J. and Lokajicek, M., "The role of oxygen in DNA damage by ionizing particles," *J. Theor. Biol.*, Vol. 207, No. 3, 2000, pp. 405–414.

[10] van Hemmen, J. J., et al., "Letter: On the mechanism of sensitization of living cells towards ionizing radiation by oxygen and other sensitizers," *Int. J. Radiat. Biol. Relat. Stud. Phys. Chem. Med.*, Vol. 25, No. 4, 1974, pp. 399–402.

[11] van Hemmen, J. J., Meuling, W. J., and Bleichrodt, J. F., "Effect of oxygen on inactivation of biologically active DNA by gamma rays in vitro: influence of metalloporphyrins and enzymatic DNA repair," *Radiat. Res.*, Vol. 75, No. 2, 1978, pp. 410–423.

[12] van Hemmen, J. J. and Meuling, W. J., "Inactivation of Escherichia coli by superoxide radicals and their dismutation products," *Arch. Biochem. Biophys.*, Vol. 182, No. 2, 1977, pp. 743–748.

[13] Ewing, D., Koval, T. M., and Walton, H. L., "Radiation sensitization by oxygen of in vitro mammalian cells: is O-2 involved?" *Radiat. Res.*, Vol. 106, No. 3, 1986, pp. 356–365.

[14] Oberley, L. W., et al., "Superoxide Ion as the cause of the oxygen effect," *Radiat. Res.*, Vol. 68, No. 2, 1976, pp. 320–328.

[15] Petkau, A. and Chelack, W. S., "Protection of Acholeplasma laidlawii B by superoxide dismutase," *Int. J. Radiat. Biol. Relat. Stud. Phys. Chem. Med.*, Vol. 26, No. 5, 1974, pp. 421–426.

[16] Palcic, B., "In vivo and in vitro mechanisms of radiation sensitization, drug synthesis and screening: can we learn it all from the high dose data?" *Int. J.Radiat. Oncol. Biol.Phys.*, Vol. 10, No. 8, 1984, pp. 1185–1193.

[17] Brown, J. M., "Sensitizers and protectors in radiotherapy," *Cancer*, Vol. 55, No. 9 Suppl., 1985, pp. 2222–2228.

[18] Coleman, C. N., "Hypoxic cell radiosensitizers: expectations and progress in drug development," *Int. J. Radiat. Oncol. Biol. Phys.*, Vol. 11, No. 2, 1985, pp. 323–329.

[19] Urtasun, R. C., and J. M. Brown, "Chemical Modifiers of Radiation." In *Textbook of Radiation Oncology,* pp. 45–60, S. A. Leibel and T. L. Phillips (eds.), Philadelphia: Saunders, 2004.

[20] Fischer, J. J., Rockwell, S., and Martin, D. F., "Perfluorochemicals and hyperbaric oxygen in radiation therapy," *Int. J. Radiat. Oncol. Biol. Phys.*, Vol. 12, No. 1, 1986, pp. 95–102.

[21] Al-Waili, N. S., et al., "Hyperbaric oxygen and malignancies: a potential role in radiotherapy, chemotherapy, tumor surgery and phototherapy," *Med. Sci. Monit.*, Vol. 11, No. 9, 2005, pp. RA279–RA289.

[22] Bennett, M., et al., "Hyperbaric oxygenation for tumour sensitisation to radiotherapy," *Cochrane Database Syst. Rev.*, No. 4, 2005, pp. CD005007.

[23] Weishaupt, K. R., Gomer, C. J., and Dougherty, T. J., "Identification of singlet oxygen as the cytotoxic agent in photoinactivation of a murine tumor," *Cancer Res.*, Vol. 36, No. 7 PT 1, 1976, pp. 2326–2329.

[24] Ochsner, M., "Photophysical and photobiological processes in the photodynamic therapy of tumours," *J. Photochem. Photobiol. B*, Vol. 39, No. 1, 1997, pp. 1–18.

[25] Foote, C. S., "Mechanisms of Photosensitized Oxidation," *Science*, Vol. 29, 1968, pp. 963–970.

[26] Hariharan, P. V., Courtney, J., and Eleczko, S., "Production of hydroxyl radicals in cell systems exposed to haematoporphyrin and red light," *Int. J. Radiat. Biol. Relat Stud. Phys. Chem. Med.*, Vol. 37, No. 6, 1980, pp. 691–694.

[27] Buettner, G. R. and Oberley, L. W., "The apparent production of superoxide and hydroxyl radicals by hematoporphyrin and light as seen by spin-trapping," *FEBS Lett.*, Vol. 121, No. 1, 1980, pp. 161–164.

[28] Gollnick, K., "Type II photooxygenation reactions in solution," *Adv. Photochem.*, Vol. 6, 1968, pp. 1–122.

[29] Kvello Stenstrom, A. G., et al., "Photodynamic inactivation of yeast cells sensitized by hematoporphyrin," *Photochem. Photobiol.*, Vol. 32, No. 3, 1980, pp. 349–352.

[30] Moan, J. and Sommer, S., "Oxygen dependence of the photosensitizing effect of hematoporphyrin derivative in NHIK 3025 cells," *Cancer Res.*, Vol. 45, No. 4, 1985, pp. 1608–1610.

[31] Gomer, C. J. and Razum, N. J., "Acute skin response in albino mice following porphyrin photosensitization under oxic and anoxic conditions," *Photochem. Photobiol.*, Vol. 40, No. 4, 1984, pp. 435–439.

[32] Holland, R. and Elek, G., "Study on the "toxic oxygen effect" of Janus green B in mouse ascites tumour cells," *Strahlentherapie*, Vol. 154, No. 2, 1978, pp. 127–133.

[33] Mitchell, J. B., et al., "Oxygen dependence of hematoporphyrin derivative-induced photoinactivation of Chinese hamster cells," *Cancer Res.*, Vol. 45, No. 5, 1985, pp. 2008–2011.

[34] Freitas, I., "Role of hypoxia in photodynamic therapy of tumors," *Tumori*, Vol. 71, No. 3, 1985, pp. 251–259.

[35] Henderson, B. W. and Fingar, V. H., "Relationship of tumor hypoxia and response to photodynamic treatment in an experimental mouse tumor," *Cancer Res.*, Vol. 47, No. 12, 1987, pp. 3110–3114.

[36] Lee See K., Forbes, I. J., and Betts, W. H., "Oxygen dependency of photocytotoxicity with haematoporphyrin derivative," *Photochem. Photobiol.*, Vol. 39, No. 5, 1984, pp. 631–634.

[37] Bonnett, R., "Photosensitizers of the Porphyrin and Phthalocyanine Series for Photodynamic Therapy," *Chem. Soc. Rev.*, Vol. 24, 1995, pp. 19–33.

[38] Roeder, B., et al., "Photophysical properties and photodynamic activity in vivo of some tetrapyrroles," *Biophys. Chem.*, Vol. 35, No. 2–3, 1990, pp. 303–312.

[39] Wilkinson, F., Helman, W. P., and Ross, A. B., "Quantum Yields for the Photosensitized Formation of the Lowest Electronically Excited Singlet State of Molecular Oxygen in Solution," *J. Phys. Chem. Ref. Data*, Vol. 22, 1993, pp. 113–262.

[40] DeRosa, M. C. and Crutchley, R. J., "Photosensitized singlet oxygen and its applications," *Coord. Chem. Rev.*, Vol. 233/234, 2002, pp. 351–371.

[41] Lang, K., Mosinger, J., and Wagnerova, D. M., "Photophysical properties of porphyrinoid sensitizers non-covalently bound to host molecules; models for photodynamic therapy," *Coord. Chem. Rev.*, Vol. 248, 2004, pp. 321–350.

[42] Redmond, R. W. and Gamlin, J. N., "A compilation of singlet oxygen yields from biologically relevant molecules," *Photochem. Photobiol.*, Vol. 70, No. 4, 1999, pp. 391–475.

[43] Moan, J., "On the diffusion length of singlet oxygen in cells and tissues," *J. Photochem. Photobiol.B*, Vol. 6, No. 3, 1990, pp. 343–344.

[44] Moan, J. and Berg, K., "The photodegradation of porphyrins in cells can be used to estimate the lifetime of singlet oxygen," *Photochem. Photobiol.*, Vol. 53, No. 4, 1991, pp. 549–553.

[45] Kanofsky, J. R., "Quenching of singlet oxygen by human red cell ghosts," *Photochem. Photobiol.*, Vol. 53, No. 1, 1991, pp. 93–99.

[46] Baker, A. and Kanofsky, J. R., "Quenching of singlet oxygen by biomolecules from L1210 leukemia cells," *Photochem. Photobiol.*, Vol. 55, No. 4, 1992, pp. 523–528.

[47] Dysart, J. S., Singh, G., and Patterson, M. S., "Calculation of singlet oxygen dose from photosensitizer fluorescence and photobleaching during mTHPC photodynamic therapy of MLL cells," *Photochem. Photobiol.*, Vol. 81, No. 1, 2005, pp. 196–205.

[48] Niedre, M., Patterson, M. S., and Wilson, B. C., "Direct near-infrared luminescence detection of singlet oxygen generated by photodynamic therapy in cells in vitro and tissues in vivo," *Photochem. Photobiol.*, Vol. 75, No. 4, 2002, pp. 382–391.

[49] Dysart, J. S. and Patterson, M. S., "Characterization of Photofrin photobleaching for singlet oxygen dose estimation during photodynamic therapy of MLL cells in vitro," *Phys. Med. Biol.*, Vol. 50, No. 11, 2005, pp. 2597–2616.

[50] Peng, Q., Moan, J., and Nesland, J. M., "Correlation of subcellular and intratumoral photosensitizer localization with ultrastructural features after photodynamic therapy," *Ultrastruct. Pathol.*, Vol. 20, No. 2, 1996, pp. 109–129.

[51] Redmond, R. W. and Kochevar, I. E., "Spatially resolved cellular responses to singlet oxygen," *Photochem. Photobiol.*, Vol. 82, No. 5, 2006, pp. 1178–1186.

[52] Juzeniene, A. and Moan, J., "The history of PDT in Norway: Part one: Identification of basic mechanisms of general PDT," *Photodiagn. Photodyn. Ther.*, Vol. 4, No. 1, 2007, pp. 3–11.

[53] Moan, J., et al., "Intracellular localization of photosensitizers," *Ciba Found. Symp.*, Vol. 146, 1989, pp. 95–107.

[54] Oleinick, N. L. and Evans, H. H., "The photobiology of photodynamic therapy: cellular targets and mechanisms," *Radiat. Res.*, Vol. 150, No. 5 Suppl, 1998, pp. S146–S156.

[55] Fiel, R. J., et al., "Induction of DNA damage by porphyrin photosensitizers," *Cancer Res.*, Vol. 41, No. 9 Pt. 1, 1981, pp. 3543–3545.

[56] Boye, E. and Moan, J., "The photodynamic effect of hematoporphyrin on DNA," *Photochem. Photobiol.*, Vol. 31, 1980, pp. 223–228.

[57] Moan, J., Waksvik, H., and Christensen, T., "DNA single-strand breaks and sister chromatid exchanges induced by treatment with hematoporphyrin and light or by x-rays in human NHIK 3025 cells," *Cancer Res.*, Vol. 40, No. 8 Pt 1, 1980, pp. 2915–2918.

[58] Moan, J. and Christensen, T., "Photodynamic effects on human cells exposed to light in the presence of hematoporphyrin. Localization of the active dye," *Cancer Lett.*, Vol. 11, No. 3, 1981, pp. 209–214.

[59] Moan, J. and Boye, E., "Photodynamic effect on DNA and cell survival of human cells sensitized by hematoporphyrin," *Photobiochem. Photobiophys.*, Vol. 2, 1981, pp. 301–307.

[60] Lafleur, M. V. and Loman, H., "Influence of anoxic sensitizers on the radiation damage in biologically active DNA in aqueous solution," *Int. J. Radiat. Biol. Relat. Stud. Phys. Chem. Med.*, Vol. 41, No. 3, 1982, pp. 295–302.

[61] Kvam, E. and Moan, J., "A comparison of three photosensitizers with respect to efficiency of cell inactivation, fluorescence quantum yield and DNA strand breaks," *Photochem. Photobiol.*, Vol. 52, No. 4, 1990, pp. 769–773.

[62] Kvam, E., Stokke, T., and Moan, J., "The lengths of DNA fragments light-induced in the presence of a photosensitizer localized at the nuclear membrane of human cells," *Biochim. Biophys. Acta*, Vol. 1049, No. 1, 1990, pp. 33–37.

[63] Moan, J., K. Berg, and E. Kvam, "Effects of photodynamic treatment on DNA and DNA-related cell functions." In *Photodynamic Therapy of Neoplastic Disease*, pp. 197–209, D. Kessel (ed.), Boca Raton, Ann Arbor, Boston: CRC Press, 1990.

[64] Moan, J., et al., "Effects of PDT on DNA and Chromosomes." In *Photobiology*, pp. 821–829, Riklis E. (ed.), New York: Plenum Press, 1991.

[65] Kvam, E., et al., "Plateau distributions of DNA fragment lengths produced by extended light exposure of extranuclear photosensitizers in human cells," *Nucleic Acids Res.*, Vol. 20, No. 24, 1992, pp. 6687–6693.

[66] Barr, H., et al., "Comparison of Lasers for Photodynamic Therapy with a Phthalocyanine Photosensitizer," *Lasers Med. Sci.*, Vol. 4, No. 1, 1989, pp. 7–12.

[67] Anholt, H., Peng, Q., and Moan, J., "Pressure against the tumor can reduce the efficiency of photochemotherapy," *Cancer Lett.*, Vol. 82, No. 1, 1994, pp. 73–80.

[68] Whipp, B. J. and Ward, S. A., "Pulmonary gas exchange dynamics and the tolerance to muscular exercise: effects of fitness and training," *Ann. Physiol. Anthropol.*, Vol. 11, No. 3, 1992, pp. 207–214.

[69] Zhou, J., et al., "Tumor hypoxia and cancer progression," *Cancer Lett.*, Vol. 237, No. 1, 2006, pp. 10–21.

[70] van der Veen, N., De Bruijn, H. S., and Star, W. M., "Photobleaching during and re-appearance after photodynamic therapy of topical ALA-induced fluorescence in UVB-treated mouse skin," *Int. J. Cancer*, Vol. 72, No. 1, 1997, pp. 110–118.

[71] Fuchs, J. and Thiele, J., "The role of oxygen in cutaneous photodynamic therapy," *Free Radic. Biol. Med*, Vol. 24, No. 5, 1998, pp. 835–847.

[72] Bedlow, A. J., et al., "Basal cell carcinoma—an in-vivo model of human tumour microcirculation?," *Exp. Dermatol.*, Vol. 8, No. 3, 1999, pp. 222–226.

[73] Palsson, S., et al., "Kinetics of the superficial perfusion and temperature in connection with photodynamic therapy of basal cell carcinomas using esterified and non-esterified 5-aminolaevulinic acid," *Br. J. Dermatol.*, Vol. 148, No. 6, 2003, pp. 1179–1188.

[74] Newell, B., et al., "Comparison of the microvasculature of basal cell carcinoma and actinic keratosis using intravital microscopy and immunohistochemistry," *Br. J. Dermatol.*, Vol. 149, No. 1, 2003, pp. 105–110.

[75] Wennberg, A. M., et al., "Delta-aminolevulinic acid in superficial basal cell carcinomas and normal skin-a microdialysis and perfusion study," *Clin. Exp. Dermatol.*, Vol. 25, No. 4, 2000, pp. 317–322.

[76] Stanton, A. W., et al., "Expansion of microvascular bed and increased solute flux in human Basal cell carcinoma in vivo, measured by fluorescein video angiography," *Cancer Res.*, Vol. 63, No. 14, 2003, pp. 3969–3979.

[77] Jori, G., "Tumour photosensitizers: approaches to enhance the selectivity and efficiency of photodynamic therapy," *J. Photochem. Photobiol. B*, Vol. 36, No. 2, 1996, pp. 87–93.

[78] Moan, J., et al., "On the basis for tumor selectivity in the 5-aminolevulinic acid-induced synthesis of protoporphyrin IX," *J. Porphyrins Phthalocyanines*, Vol. 5, 2001, pp. 170–176.

[79] Moan, J., et al., "Tumour selectivity of Photodynamic Therapy." In *Targeted Cancer Therapies. An Odyssey*, pp. 208–211, Ø. S. Bruland and T. Flægstad (eds.), Tromsø: Ravnetrykk, 2003.

[80] Collaud, S., et al., "On the selectivity of 5-aminolevulinic acid-induced protoporphyrin IX formation," *Curr. Med. Chem. Anti-Canc. Agents*, Vol. 4, No. 3, 2004, pp. 301–316.

[81] Pallikaris, I. G., et al., "Histological evaluation of phthalocyanine mediated photodynamic occlusion of corneal neovascularization enhanced by hyperbaric oxygenation," *J. Refract. Surg.*, Vol. 12, No. 2, 1996, pp. S313–S316.

[82] Chen, Q., et al., "Improvement of tumor response by manipulation of tumor oxygenation during photodynamic therapy," *Photochem. Photobiol.*, Vol. 76, No. 2, 2002, pp. 197–203.

[83] Huang, Z., et al., "Hyperoxygenation enhances the tumor cell killing of photofrin-mediated photodynamic therapy," *Photochem. Photobiol.*, Vol. 78, No. 5, 2003, pp. 496–502.

[84] Fingar, V. H., Mang, T. S., and Henderson, B. W., "Modification of photodynamic therapy-induced hypoxia by fluosol-DA (20%) and carbogen breathing in mice," *Cancer Res.*, Vol. 48, No. 12, 1988, pp. 3350–3354.

[85] Schouwink, H., et al., "Photodynamic therapy for malignant mesothelioma: preclinical studies for optimization of treatment protocols," *Photochem. Photobiol.*, Vol. 73, No. 4, 2001, pp. 410–417.

[86] Bremner, J. C., et al., "Increasing the effect of photodynamic therapy on the RIF-1 murine sarcoma, using the bioreductive drugs RSU1069 and RB6145," *Br. J. Cancer*, Vol. 66, No. 6, 1992, pp. 1070–1076.

[87] Baas, P., et al., "Enhancement of interstitial photodynamic therapy by mitomycin C and EO9 in a mouse tumour model," *Int. J. Cancer*, Vol. 56, No. 6, 1994, pp. 880–885.

[88] Bremner, J. C., et al., "Comparing the anti-tumor effect of several bioreductive drugs when used in combination with photodynamic therapy (PDT)," *Int. J. Radiat. Oncol. Biol. Phys.*, Vol. 29, No. 2, 1994, pp. 329–332.

[89] Ma, L. W., et al., "Potentiation of photodynamic therapy by mitomycin C in cultured human colon adenocarcinoma cells," *Radiat. Res.*, Vol. 134, No. 1, 1993, pp. 22–28.

[90] Ma, L. W., et al., "Anti-tumour activity of photodynamic therapy in combination with mitomycin C in nude mice with human colon adenocarcinoma," *Br. J. Cancer*, Vol. 71, No. 5, 1995, pp. 950–956.

[91] Gonzalez, S., et al., "Treatment of Dunning R3327-AT rat prostate tumors with photodynamic therapy in combination with misonidazole," *Cancer Res.*, Vol. 46, No. 6, 1986, pp. 2858–2862.

[92] Henry, J. M. and Isaacs, J. T., "Synergistic enhancement of the efficacy of the bioreductively activated alkylating agent RSU-1164 in the treatment of prostatic cancer by photodynamic therapy," *J. Urol.*, Vol. 142, No. 1, 1989, pp. 165–170.

[93] Evensen, J. F. and Moan, J., "Photodynamic therapy of C3H Tumours in mice: Effect of drug/light dose fractionation and misonidazole," *Lasers Med. Sci.*, Vol. 3, No. 1, 1988, pp. 6.

[94] Jones, G. C., et al., "The effect of cooling on the photodynamic action of hematoporphyrin derivative during interstitial phototherapy of solid tumors. 1983 Second-Place Resident Research Award: basic category," *Otolaryngol. Head Neck Surg.*, Vol. 92, No. 5, 1984, pp. 532–536.

[95]   Griffin, R. J., et al., "Assessing pH and oxygenation in cryotherapy-induced cytotoxicity and tissue response to freezing," *Technol. Cancer Res. Treat.*, Vol. 3, No. 3, 2004, pp. 245–251.

[96]   Maier, A., et al., "Combined photodynamic therapy and hyperbaric oxygenation in carcinoma of the esophagus and the esophago-gastric junction," *Eur. J. Cardiothorac. Surg.*, Vol. 18, No. 6, 2000, pp. 649–654.

[97]   Maier, A., et al., "Hyperbaric oxygen and photodynamic therapy in the treatment of advanced carcinoma of the cardia and the esophagus," *Lasers Surg. Med.*, Vol. 26, No. 3, 2000, pp. 308–315.

[98]   Tomaselli, F., et al., "Acute effects of combined photodynamic therapy and hyperbaric oxygenation in lung cancer—a clinical pilot study," *Lasers Surg. Med*, Vol. 28, No. 5, 2001, pp. 399–403.

[99]   Tomaselli, F., et al., "Photodynamic therapy enhanced by hyperbaric oxygen in acute endoluminal palliation of malignant bronchial stenosis (clinical pilot study in 40 patients)," *Eur. J. Cardiothorac. Surg.*, Vol. 19, No. 5, 2001, pp. 549–554.

[100] Maier, A., et al., "Does new photosensitizer improve photodynamic therapy in advanced esophageal carcinoma?," *Lasers Surg. Med.*, Vol. 29, No. 4, 2001, pp. 323–327.

[101] Maier, A., et al., "Comparison of 5-aminolaevulinic acid and porphyrin photosensitization for photodynamic therapy of malignant bronchial stenosis: a clinical pilot study," *Lasers Surg. Med.*, Vol. 30, No. 1, 2002, pp. 12–17.

[102] Skyrme, R. J., et al., "A phase-1 study of sequential mitomycin C and 5-aminolaevulinic acid-mediated photodynamic therapy in recurrent superficial bladder carcinoma," *BJU Int.*, Vol. 95, No. 9, 2005, pp. 1206–1210.

[103] Moan, J. and Christensen, T., "Photodynamic inactivation of cancer cells in vitro. Effect of irradiation temperature and dose fractionation," *Cancer Lett.*, Vol. 6, No. 6, 1979, pp. 331–335.

[104] Qiu, K. and Sieber, F., "Merocyanine 540-sensitized photoinactivation of leukemia cells: effects of dose fractionation," *Photochem. Photobiol.*, Vol. 56, No. 4, 1992, pp. 489–493.

[105] Gomer, C. J., et al., "Expression of potentially lethal damage in Chinese hamster cells exposed to hematoporphyrin derivative photodynamic therapy," *Cancer Res.*, Vol. 46, No. 7, 1986, pp. 3348–3352.

[106] Dereski, M. O., Madigan, L., and Chopp, M., "The effect of hypothermia and hyperthermia on photodynamic therapy of normal brain," *Neurosurgery*, Vol. 36, No. 1, 1995, pp. 141–145.

[107] Moan, J., Ma, L. W., and Bjorklund, E., "The effect of glucose and temperature on the in vivo efficiency of photochemotherapy with meso-tetra-hydroxyphenyl-chlorin," *J. Photochem. Photobiol. B*, Vol. 50, No. 2–3, 1999, pp. 94–98.

[108] Song, P. S. and Tapley, K. J., Jr., "Photochemistry and photobiology of psoralens," *Photochem. Photobiol.*, Vol. 29, No. 6, 1979, pp. 1177–1197.

[109] Averbeck, D., "Recent advances in psoralen phototoxicity mechanism," *Photochem. Photobiol.*, Vol. 50, No. 6, 1989, pp. 859–882.

[110] Spikes, J. D., "Quantum yields and kinetics of the photobleaching of hematoporphyrin, Photofrin II, tetra(4-sulfonatophenyl)-porphine and uroporphyrin," *Photochem. Photobiol.*, Vol. 55, No. 6, 1992, pp. 797–808.

[111] Foster, T. H., et al., "Oxygen consumption and diffusion effects in photodynamic therapy," *Radiat. Res.*, Vol. 126, No. 3, 1991, pp. 296–303.

[112] Kogan, B. Y., "Nonlinear photodynamic therapy. Saturation of a photochemical dose by photosensitizer bleaching," *Photochem. Photobiol. Sci.*, Vol. 2, No. 6, 2003, pp. 673–676.

[113] Veenhuizen, R. B. and Stewart, F. A., "The importance of fluence rate in photodynamic therapy: is there a parallel with ionizing radiation dose-rate effects?" *Radiother. Oncol.*, Vol. 37, No. 2, 1995, pp. 131–135.

[114] Henderson, B. W., et al., "Photofrin photodynamic therapy can significantly deplete or preserve oxygenation in human basal cell carcinomas during treatment, depending on fluence rate," *Cancer Res.*, Vol. 60, No. 3, 2000, pp. 525–529.

[115] Henderson, B. W., Busch, T. M., and Snyder, J. W., "Fluence rate as a modulator of PDT mechanisms," *Lasers Surg. Med.*, Vol. 38, No. 5, 2006, pp. 489–493.

[116] Fingar, V. H., "Vascular effects of photodynamic therapy," *J. Clin. Laser Med. Surg.*, Vol. 14, No. 5, 1996, pp. 323–328.

[117] Fingar, V. H., et al., "Vascular damage after photodynamic therapy of solid tumors: a view and comparison of effect in pre-clinical and clinical models at the University of Louisville," *In Vivo*, Vol. 14, No. 1, 2000, pp. 93–100.

[118] Krammer, B., "Vascular effects of photodynamic therapy," *Anticancer Res.*, Vol. 21, No. 6B, 2001, pp. 4271–4277.

[119] Abels, C., "Targeting of the vascular system of solid tumours by photodynamic therapy (PDT)," *Photochem. Photobiol. Sci.*, Vol. 3, No. 8, 2004, pp. 765–771.

[120] Chen, B., et al., "Vascular and cellular targeting for photodynamic therapy," *Crit. Rev. Eukaryot. Gene Expr.*, Vol. 16, No. 4, 2006, pp. 279–305.

[121] Henderson, B. W. and Fingar, V. H., "Oxygen limitation of direct tumor cell kill during photodynamic treatment of a murine tumor model," *Photochem. Photobiol.*, Vol. 49, No. 3, 1989, pp. 299–304.

[122] Engbrecht, B. W., et al., "Photofrin-mediated photodynamic therapy induces vascular occlusion and apoptosis in a human sarcoma xenograft model," *Cancer Res.*, Vol. 59, No. 17, 1999, pp. 4334–4342.

[123] Ferrario, A., et al., "Antiangiogenic treatment enhances photodynamic therapy responsiveness in a mouse mammary carcinoma," *Cancer Res.*, Vol. 60, No. 15, 2000, pp. 4066–4069.

[124] Yu, G., et al., "Noninvasive monitoring of murine tumor blood flow during and after photodynamic therapy provides early assessment of therapeutic efficacy," *Clin. Cancer Res.*, Vol. 11, No. 9, 2005, pp. 3543–3552.

[125] Fingar, V. H., et al., "The role of microvascular damage in photodynamic therapy: the effect of treatment on vessel constriction, permeability, and leukocyte adhesion," *Cancer Res.*, Vol. 52, No. 18, 1992, pp. 4914–4921.

[126] Kunzi-Rapp, K., et al., "In vivo uptake and biodistribution of lipophilic and hydrophilic photosensitizers," *Proc. SPIE*, Vol. 2924, 1996, pp. 176–180.

[127] Peng, Q., et al., "Localization of potent photosensitizers in human tumor LOX by means of laser scanning microscopy," *Cancer Lett.*, Vol. 53, No. 2–3, 1990, pp. 129–139.

[128] Peng, Q., et al., "Aluminum phthalocyanines with asymmetrical lower sulfonation and with symmetrical higher sulfonation: a comparison of localizing and photosensitizing mechanism in human tumor LOX xenografts," *Int. J. Cancer*, Vol. 46, No. 4, 1990, pp. 719–726.

[129] Peng, Q. and Nesland, J. M., "Effects of photodynamic therapy on tumor stroma," *Ultrastruct. Pathol.*, Vol. 28, No. 5–6, 2004, pp. 333–340.

[130] Brooke, R. C., et al., "Histamine is released following aminolevulinic acid-photodynamic therapy of human skin and mediates an aminolevulinic acid dose-related immediate inflammatory response," *J. Invest. Dermatol.*, Vol. 126, No. 10, 2006, pp. 2296–2301.

[131] Ormrod, D. and Jarvis, B., "Topical aminolevulinic acid HCl photodynamic therapy," *Am. J. Clin. Dermatol.*, Vol. 1, No. 2, 2000, pp. 133–139.

[132] Lober, B. A. and Fenske, N. A., "Optimum treatment strategies for actinic keratosis (intraepidermal squamous cell carcinoma)," *Am. J. Clin. Dermatol.*, Vol. 5, No. 6, 2004, pp. 395–401.

[133] Alexiades-Armenakas, M., "Laser-mediated photodynamic therapy," *Clin. Dermatol.*, Vol. 24, No. 1, 2006, pp. 16–25.

[134] Pogue, B. W., et al., "Tumor PO(2) changes during photodynamic therapy depend upon photosensitizer type and time after injection," *Comp. Biochem. Physiol. A Mol. Integr. Physiol.*, Vol. 132, No. 1, 2002, pp. 177–184.

[135] Mattiello, J., Hetzel, F., and Vandenheede, L., "Intratumor temperature measurements during photodynamic therapy," *Photochem. Photobiol.*, Vol. 46, No. 5, 1987, pp. 873–879.

[136] Orenstein, A., et al., "Temperature monitoring during photodynamic therapy of skin tumors with topical 5-aminolevulinic acid application," *Cancer Lett.*, Vol. 93, No. 2, 1995, pp. 227–232.

[137] Tsutsui, H., et al., "Optimisation of illumination for photodynamic therapy with mTHPC on normal colon and a transplantable tumour in rats," *Lasers Med. Sci.*, Vol. 17, No. 2, 2002, pp. 101–109.

[138] Xu, T., Li, Y., and Wu, X., "Application of lower fluence rate for less microvasculature damage and greater cell-killing during photodynamic therapy," *Lasers Med. Sci.*, Vol. 19, No. 4, 2005, pp. 257–261.

[139] Coutier, S., et al., "Effect of irradiation fluence rate on the efficacy of photodynamic therapy and tumor oxygenation in meta-tetra (hydroxyphenyl) chlorin (mTHPC)-sensitized HT29 xenografts in nude mice," *Radiat. Res.*, Vol. 158, No. 3, 2002, pp. 339–345.

[140] Ericson, M. B., et al., "Photodynamic therapy of actinic keratosis at varying fluence rates: assessment of photobleaching, pain and primary clinical outcome," *Br. J. Dermatol.*, Vol. 151, No. 6, 2004, pp. 1204–1212.

[141] Sitnik, T. M., Hampton, J. A., and Henderson, B. W., "Reduction of tumour oxygenation during and after photodynamic therapy in vivo: effects of fluence rate," *Br. J. Cancer*, Vol. 77, No. 9, 1998, pp. 1386–1394.

[142] Zilberstein, J., et al., "Light-dependent oxygen consumption in bacteriochlorophyll-serine-treated melanoma tumors: on-line determination using a tissue-inserted oxygen microsensor," *Photochem. Photobiol.*, Vol. 65, No. 6, 1997, pp. 1012–1019.

[143] Oberdanner, C. B., et al., "Photodynamic treatment with fractionated light decreases production of reactive oxygen species and cytotoxicity in vitro via regeneration of glutathione," *Photochem. Photobiol.*, Vol. 81, No. 3, 2005, pp. 609–613.

[144] Togashi, H., et al., "Fractionated photodynamic therapy for a human oral squamous cell carcinoma xenograft," *Oral Oncol.*, Vol. 42, No. 5, 2006, pp. 526–532.

[145] Bonnett, R. and Martinez, G., "Photobleaching of sensitisers used in photodynamic therapy," *Tetrahedron*, Vol. 57, No. 47, 2001, pp. 9513–9547.

[146] Moan, J., P. Juzenas, and S. Bagdonas, "Degradation and transformation of photosensitisers during light exposure." In *Recent Research Developments in Photochemistry and Photobiology*, pp. 121–132, S. G. Pandalai (ed.), Trivandrum: Transworld Research Network, 2000.

[147] Diagaradjane, P., et al., "In vivo pharmacokinetics of d-aminolevulinic acid-induced protoporphyrin IX during pre- and post-photodynamic therapy in 7,12-dimethylbenz(a)nthracene-treated skin carcinogenesis in Swiss mice: a comparison by three-compartment model," *Photochem. Photobiol.*, Vol. 76, No. 1, 2002, pp. 81–90.

[148] De Bruijn, H. S., et al., "Increase in protoporphyrin IX after 5-aminolevulinic acid based photodynamic therapy is due to local re-synthesis," *Photochem. Photobiol. Sci.*, Vol. 6, No. 8, 2007, pp. 857–864.

[149] van den Boogert, J., et al., "Fractionated illumination in oesophageal ALA-PDT: effect on ferrochelatase activity," *J. Photochem. Photobiol. B*, Vol. 56, No. 1, 2000, pp. 53–60.

[150] van den Boogert, J., et al., "Fractionated illumination for oesophageal ALA-PDT: effect on blood flow and PpIX formation," *Lasers Med. Sci.*, Vol. 16, No. 1, 2001, pp. 16–25.

[151] Moan, J., Anholt, H., and Peng, Q., "A transient reduction of the fluorescence of aluminium phthalocyanine tetrasulphonate in tumours during photodynamic therapy," *J. Photochem. Photobiol. B*, Vol. 5, No. 1, 1990, pp. 115–119.

[152] Moan, J. and Anholt, H., "Phthalocyanine fluorescence in tumors during PDT," *Photochem. Photobiol.*, Vol. 51, No. 3, 1990, pp. 379–381.

[153] Stern, S. J., et al., "Photodynamic therapy with chloroaluminum-sulfonated phthalocyanine," *Arch. Otolaryngol. Head Neck Surg.*, Vol. 116, No. 11, 1990, pp. 1259–1266.

[154] Curnow, A., Haller, J. C., and Bown, S. G., "Oxygen monitoring during 5-aminolaevulinic acid induced photodynamic therapy in normal rat colon. Comparison of continuous and fractionated light regimes," *J. Photochem. Photobiol. B*, Vol. 58, No. 2–3, 2000, pp. 149–155.

[155] Peng, Q., et al., "Subcellular localization, redistribution and photobleaching of sulfonated aluminum phthalocyanines in a human melanoma cell line," *Int. J. Cancer*, Vol. 49, No. 2, 1991, pp. 290–295.

[156] Berg, K., et al., "Light induced relocalization of sulfonated meso-tetraphenylporphines in NHIK 3025 cells and effects of dose fractionation," *Photochem. Photobiol.*, Vol. 53, No. 2, 1991, pp. 203–210.

[157] Moan, J., "A change in the quantum yield of photoinactivation of cells observed during photodynamic treatment," *Lasers Med. Sci.*, Vol. 3, 1988, pp. 93–97.

[158] Wood, S. R., Holroyd, J. A., and Brown, S. B., "The subcellular localization of Zn(II) phthalocyanines and their redistribution on exposure to light," *Photochem. Photobiol.*, Vol. 65, No. 3, 1997, pp. 397–402.

[159] Kessel, D., "Relocalization of cationic porphyrins during photodynamic therapy," *Photochem. Photobiol. Sci.*, Vol. 1, No. 11, 2002, pp. 837–840.

[160] Prahl, S., "Tabulated Molar Extinction Coefficient for Hemoglobin in Water," http://omlc.ogi.edu/spectra/hemoglobin/summary.html, 1998.

[161] Nielsen, K. P., et al., "Choice of optimal wavelength for PDT: the significance of oxygen depletion," *Photochem. Photobiol.*, Vol. 81, No. 5, 2005, pp. 1190–1194.

[162] Juzeniene, A., Nielsen, K. P., and Moan, J., "Biophysical aspects of photodynamic therapy," *J. Environ. Pathol. Toxicol. Oncol.*, Vol. 25, No. 1–2, 2006, pp. 7–28.

[163] Mitra, S. and Foster, T. H., "Carbogen breathing significantly enhances the penetration of red light in murine tumours in vivo," *Phys. Med. Biol.*, Vol. 49, No. 10, 2004, pp. 1891–1904.

CHAPTER 8

Photodynamic Therapy and Oxidative Stress

Dominika Nowis and Jakub Golab

8.1 Introduction

As a consequence of aerobic metabolism, cells generate partially reduced forms of O_2, collectively referred to as reactive oxygen species (ROS). This term includes free radicals that contain molecules harboring one or more unpaired electrons on their outermost orbital such as superoxide anion ($O_2^{\cdot-}$), hydroxyl radical ($^{\cdot}OH$), as well as nonradical species such as hydrogen peroxide (H_2O_2) and singlet oxygen ($^1O_2$). A subset of reactive molecules generated in cells that include gaseous nitric oxide (NO) and its derivatives (peroxynitrite, nitrogen dioxide) is termed reactive nitrogen species (RNS). All these molecules produced under normal conditions regulate a number of physiologic processes that include signal transduction, gene expression, or defense against infectious microorganisms. Excessive production or insufficient elimination of ROS leads to a condition collectively referred to as oxidative stress.

Numerous drugs, natural food products, toxins, xenobiotics, and environmental factors (such as solar UV or ionizing radiation, cigarette smoke, etc.) elevate ROS generation. ROS can either directly or indirectly affect the structure and thereby a function of virtually all cellular biomolecules. Abnormal biomolecules accumulate and impair cellular functions leading to their senescence or even cell death. As a consequence ROS contribute to aging, carcinogenesis, or progression of various pathologies that include cardiovascular disorders, neurodegenerative diseases, cancer, or chronic inflammatory illnesses.

8.2 Biochemistry of Reactive Oxygen Species

8.2.1 Superoxide Anion ($O_2^{\cdot-}$)

Superoxide anion is relatively uncreative and is unable to penetrate lipid membranes [1]. It is produced within mitochondrial electron transport chain during an inadvertent leakage of electrons [2]. It has been estimated that approximately 1% to 2% of total oxygen consumed during aerobic metabolism is converted into $O_2^{\cdot-}$ [3], although recent studies indicate that this value is overestimated and does not exceed 0.1% to 0.5% [4]. Superoxide anion is also actively produced in phagocytic cells during innate immune response and in a number of cells by the NOX family of NADPH oxidases [5]. The latter are activated by a variety of growth factors and cytokines such as PDGF, EGF, insulin, angiotensin, and TNF. Additional sources of $O_2^{\cdot-}$ include $5'$-lipoxygenases and xanthine oxidases (XO) [6]. Superoxide anions are frequently referred to as "primary" ROS, as they can be further converted into "secondary" ROS. These reactions are either enzyme- or metal-catalyzed, or can be spontaneous. For example, conversion of $O_2^{\cdot-}$ into H_2O_2 is catalyzed by cytoplasmic or mitochondrial superoxide dismutases (SOD) or can occur through slow disproportionation reaction.

Superoxide-mediated toxicity results primarily from direct oxidation and inactivation of proteins containing iron-sulphur (4Fe-4S) cluster, such as mitochondrial aconitase, complex I NADH dehydrogenase, and to a lesser degree succinate dehydrogenase [7–9]. The reaction produces inactive $[3Fe-4S]^+$ cluster together with free iron ions (Fe^{2+}) and H_2O_2. Free iron and H_2O_2 participate in downstream (Fenton and Haber-Weiss) oxidative reactions (see below) that generate potent hydroxyl radical. $O_2^{\cdot-}$ can also participate in lipid peroxidation (see below) but paradoxically this radical can also terminate lipid peroxidation chain [10].

8.2.2 Hydrogen Peroxide (H_2O_2)

H_2O_2 is usually produced by the catalytic activity of SODs but it can also form spontaneously from molecular oxygen in peroxisomes [11]. Moreover, recent studies indicate that as much as 30% of the total pool of intracellular H_2O_2 is generated by $p66^{Shc}$, which functions as a redox enzyme [12]. Although H_2O_2 is poorly reactive, as compared to other ROS, its significance in oxidative stress is important due to its long half-life and capability to diffuse across cell membranes. H_2O_2 also participates in numerous signal transduction pathways. It can oxidize and thereby alter the activities of many proteins containing deprotonated cysteine residues such as transcriptional regulators, kinases, phosphatases, several metabolic enzymes, and SUMO ligases [13]. Mitochondrial H_2O_2 is becoming a central mediator of cellular aging [2].

8.2.3 Hydroxyl Radical (OH)

Hydroxyl radical has a very unstable electron structure and is therefore short-lived and extremely reactive (Figure 8.1).

The majority of $\cdot$ OH is produced from H_2O_2 and $O_2^{\cdot-}$ in a Haber-Weiss reaction:

$$H_2O_2 + O_2^- \rightarrow O_2 + OH + OH^-$$

or in a transition metal-catalyzed Fenton reaction:

$$Fe^{2+} + H_2O_2 \rightarrow Fe^{3+} + OH + OH^-$$

Barely picogram concentrations of Fe^{2+} are sufficient for this reaction. Other metals that favor $\cdot$ OH generation are Cu^+ and Co^{2+}, but "free pools" of copper are less than a single atom per cell, making the reaction unlikely [14]. Extremely short half-life of $\cdot$ OH (perhaps the shortest among all cellular ROS) limits its reactivity to instant vicinity.

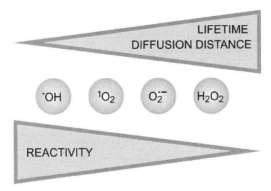

Figure 8.1 Comparison of lifetime, diffusion distance, and reactivity of ROS.

8.2.4   Singlet Oxygen ($^1O_2$)

Singlet oxygen is the only (among other ROS) electronically excited state of molecular oxygen. Therefore, many of its features are unique among oxygen metabolites. While superoxide and H_2O_2 are normally produced during many physiologic processes, $^1O_2$ is mainly a product of photochemical reactions and its chemical synthesis in eukaryotic cells is rather insignificant and limited to specific types of cells such as eosinophils and macrophages [15, 16]. Moreover, $O_2^{\cdot-}$, H_2O_2 and $^{\cdot}OH$ are formed in cascade of reactions while $^1O_2$ cannot directly interconvert to other ROS (nonetheless, it can initiate the formation of other ROS indirectly, see below). Finally, $^1O_2$ exists in excited state for only a short time before losing its reactivity by transferring excess energy to other molecules or by returning to ground state. Other ROS lose their reactivity by reactions with biomolecules or are decomposited enzymatically. There are no known antioxidant enzymes for elimination of singlet oxygen and chemical scavengers that intercept this oxygen metabolite must be present at high concentrations to be effective.

The lifetime of $^1O_2$ in water, which is only up to 4 μs, limits the distance it can diffuse in cells and therefore restricts its reactivity to the so-called "spatially resolved" reactions [17]. In fact, the lifetime of singlet oxygen is usually shortened by reactions with encountered cellular molecules. The maximal diffusion range for $^1O_2$ in water is 200 nm, which is rather a small distance in a cellular scale, where a typical cell is up to 30 μm in diameter, the size of mitochondria is about 500 nm, and a biological membrane is some 10-nm thick. The in vivo lifetime and diffusion range are further reduced due to a high reactivity of $^1O_2$ with cellular constituents. For example, the lifetime of $^1O_2$ in plasma membrane is approximately 60 ns [18] and in vivo luminescence measurements revealed $^1O_2$ lifetime of approximately 200 ns [19].

$^1O_2$ readily reacts with DNA, lipids (mainly unsaturated fatty acids but also cholesterol), and proteins [20–24]. The latter are among the most important targets of $^1O_2$. Among amino acid residues the most reactive with $^1O_2$ are histidine, tryptophan, methionine, cysteine, and tyrosine, which form short-lived endo- or hydroxyperoxides (Figure 8.2). In the presence of redox-reactive metal ions these peroxides undergo decomposition with the formation of reactive radicals that can propagate chain reactions and oxidative damage to other biomolecules [25, 26]. $^1O_2$ has also been shown to induce the formation of protein carbonyls [27] and to mod-

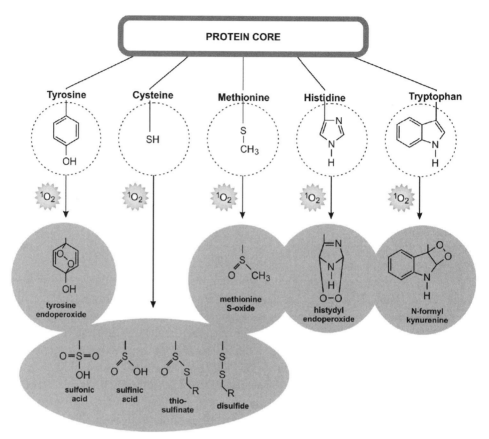

Figure 8.2 Typical changes in aminoacids induced by $^1O_2$-mediated protein oxidation.

ify prosthetic groups within proteins (such as heme in catalase) [28]. Interactions of $^1O_2$ with unsaturated lipids can also trigger downstream reactions. Some longer-lived lipid hydroperoxides can diffuse in cells and initiate chain oxidation reactions at sites remote to initial photodamage. In the presence of Fe^{2+} or Cu^+ lipid peroxides can participate in Fenton-like reactions to produce oxy- (LO) and peroxy- (LOO) radicals capable of inducing DNA damage. An exclusive DNA target of $^1O_2$ is guanine nucleoside and its oxidation product 8-oxo-7,8-dihydroguanine (8-oxoGua) [23].

8.2.5 Reactive Nitrogen Species

Reaction of nitric oxide (NO, or more correctly ˙NO) with $O_2^{˙-}$ yields a short-lived peroxynitrite ($ONOO^-$) anion [29, 30]. This oxidant freely crosses cell membranes and participates in one- and two-electron oxidation reactions with biomolecules. One of the most significant reaction of $ONOO^-$ is with carbon dioxide (CO_2), which leads to the formation of carbonate ($CO_3^{˙-}$) and nitrogen dioxide (˙NO_2) [31]. The latter undergoes radical-radical termination reactions (reactions between two free radicals) with various substrates, resulting in generation of nitrated compounds. Peroxynitrite can also undergo homolytic fission (rupture of a covalent bond in a molecule that yields two products that retain one of the bond electrons) to generate

$\cdot$OH and $\cdot$NO$_2$. This reaction is especially important in hydrophobic environments such as plasma membranes, where it initiates lipid peroxidation [31]. Many biomolecules are targeted by peroxynitrite and its radicals. These include tyrosine residues, DNA (mainly purine nucleotides), unsaturated fatty acids, and thiols [31].

NO can also mobilize redox-active metals from proteins such as heme or 4Fe-4S proteins and bind to and inhibit mitochondrial cytochrome oxidase, thereby increasing ROS formation during electron transport [32].

8.3   Reactive Oxygen Species and Signal Transduction

Robust production of ROS occurs mainly during inflammation. ROS produced in nonimmune cells oxidize only a limited spectrum of molecules, and these more selective reactions possibly serve specific biologic functions. One of these is participation in signal transduction that regulates cell proliferation, differentiation, aging, migration, or cell death. Most aspects of ROS involvement in signaling have been linked with H$_2$O$_2$, perhaps due to its stability and relatively low reactivity.

Activation of receptors for a number of growth factors (such as EGF, PDGF, VEGF, NGF, and insulin) leads to a transient rise in H$_2$O$_2$ concentration [33]. Moreover, neoplastic transformation associated with overexpression of *myc*, BCR/ABL translocation, or Ras mutation leads to enhanced, but to some extent regulated, ROS production [34–36]. These observations explain a long-time observed effect of H$_2$O$_2$ administration to cells in culture [13]. At low concentrations H$_2$O$_2$ promotes cellular proliferation. Among attractive candidates associated with H$_2$O$_2$-mediated signaling are protein tyrosine phosphatases (PTPs) that attenuate signal transduction from activated growth-factor receptors. PTPs inhibited by H$_2$O$_2$ include PTEN, PTP1B, SHP2, CDC25, and many others [2, 13, 33]. PTPs contain reactive cysteine residues within their catalytic domains [37]. These cysteine residues are easily oxidized, leading to phosphatase inactivation. Oxidized cysteinyl thiols can induce formation of disulphide bonds or sulphenic acids, and can undergo glutathionylation [2]. Deglutathionylation seems to participate in the restoration of catalytic activity of some phosphatases, but intriguing observations also indicate that PTP oxidation can be reversed spontaneously [38]. Generation of H$_2$O$_2$ can also activate transcription factors such as HIF-1 and NF-κB [39, 40].

8.4   Generation of Reactive Oxygen Species During Photodynamic Therapy

Singlet oxygen, generated in type II photochemical reactions, is generally considered as the most important mediator of PDT-induced damage [41, 42]. Nonetheless, O$_2$$^{\cdot-}$, H$_2O_2$, $\cdot$OH, NO, and other ROS are also detected in cells and tissues exposed to light and photosensitizers [43]. A number of studies provide evidence for the active role of these metabolites in cytotoxic effects induced by PDT [42, 44]. Unfortunately, we still lack definitive mechanisms explaining how all these ROS are produced during PDT. ROS other than ^{1}O$_2$ might be produced by type I photochemical reactions immediately during illumination, especially when O$_2$ concentration is low

[45]. It is possible however, that they can also be formed secondarily, as a result of $^1O_2$ action [17]. Therefore, even if selective $^1O_2$ scavengers abrogate PDT-induced lesions it is still possible that the damage might have been caused by $^1O_2$-induced secondary ROS.

Altogether, due to their close relatedness and the capacity to interconvert or to generate chain reactions, it is often difficult, if not impossible, to assign a specific biological effect to one or another oxygen species. Experiments with chemical or biologic scavengers are helpful in defining the role of a particular oxygen metabolite, but do not adequately address the potential role of secondary ROS generated in chain reactions. For example, selectivity of the $^1O_2$ scavengers is not absolute. Sodium azide, frequently used as a specific $^1O_2$ quencher, can also, to some extent, react with hydroxyl radicals.

The presence of $O_2^{\cdot-}$, H_2O_2, and $\cdot OH$ during PDT has been demonstrated with flow cytometry (using fluorescence probes) [46, 47], relatively selective quenchers [42] and more directly with electron paramagnetic resonance [48] and spin trapping methods [49]. Fluorescent probes such as $2',7'$-dichlorofluorescein diacetate (H_2DCFDA) and its derivatives were used to show that PDT induces $O_2^{\cdot-}$ and H_2O_2 generation [46, 47, 50]. One caveat with the use of fluorescent probes is that they are not particularly specific. Although H_2DCFDA is insensitive to $^1O_2$ [51], it can react with $^1O_2$-induced peroxyl radicals [51]. Moreover, H_2DCFDA can be oxidized by peroxynitrite [52].

Superoxide generation increases several-fold after Photofrin-mediated PDT [53]. Intracellular production of superoxide ions positively correlates with cell death following 5-ALA and Zn(II) phtalocyanine-mediated PDT [47, 54]. PDT with hematoporphyrin derivative (HPD) induces, in an incompletely understood mechanism, the activity of xanthine oxidase that generates superoxide anions [44]. $^1O_2$ can also directly inactivate primary antioxidant enzymes, thereby decreasing the ROS-scavenging capacity of cells. Photodynamically generated $^1O_2$ was shown to inactivate Cu,Zn-SOD, Mn-SOD, as well as catalase in murine keratinocytes [55]. Contrary to this observation, hypericin-mediated PDT seems to increase enzymatic activity of SOD [56]. Finally, some photosensitizers are effective in inducing PDT-mediated damage despite their inability to generate $^1O_2$ [57].

The involvement of nitric oxide in PDT is even more contentious. NO can act as a potent oxidant, although this activity is usually attributed to its highly active metabolites such as peroxynitrite or nitrogen dioxide. Early studies revealed that NO is produced during PDT and this effect might contribute to cytotoxicity [58]. But PDT also decreases NO generation in endothelial cells, which might explain vessel constriction and blood flow stasis [59]. Tumors generating low levels of NO seem to be more sensitive to Photofrin-PDT than those secreting high amounts of this gas, and selective NOS inhibitors potentiate antitumor effects of PDT [60, 61]. Since NO is a potent vasodilating agent, these latter effects can contribute to potentiated vasoconstriction observed during PDT. NO can also attenuate lipid peroxidation by scavenging lipid-derived radicals, which propagate chain reactions [62]. As a chain-breaking antioxidant NO is 1000-fold more potent than α-tocopherol [63]. These radical-quenching effects contribute to ameliorated cell death during PDT [64, 65]. Moreover, NO can induce delayed cytoprotective responses in tumor cells by inducing expression of heme oxygenase (HO-1) and ferritin, making them resistant to PDT [66].

8.5   ROS-Mediated Damage During Photodynamic Therapy

During photodynamic therapy ROS are usually generated outside of nuclear DNA (photosensitizers poorly localize to the nucleus) in close proximity to cellular membranes. Therefore, ROS generation is usually associated with modification of membrane constituents rather than DNA damage. Although there are articles showing lesions within DNA after PDT, it seems that generally the treatment is not mutagenic and its effectiveness is independent from the activity of p53 (so called "guardian of the genome" responsible for both detection of DNA damage and initiation of its repair) or proteins engaged in the DNA damage repair [67, 68].

8.5.1   Protein Damage

Proteins are major targets (and thereby quenchers) for oxidative reactions as they constitute about 70% of the dry weight of cells, frequently contain endogenous chromophores within their structure, and rapidly react with other excited molecules [22]. Therefore, they can scavenge 50% to 75% of reactive radicals [69]. Radical-induced protein modifications include fragmentation, di- or multimerization, unfolding and structural alterations resulting in functional inactivation or changes in mechanical properties, aggregation, changes in binding of cofactors and metal ions, formation of further reactive species, or accelerated degradation [22].

Protein fragmentation induced by ROS is initiated by abstraction of an α-hydrogen atom from the polypeptide chain. The products of this reaction are H_2O and a carbon-centered radical derivative of the protein that rapidly reacts with O_2, producing a peroxy-radical that is subsequently converted to protein peroxide. Its dismutation leads to formation of alkoxyl derivative that can undergo peptide bond cleavage [70]. The occurrence of oxidative cleavage of proteins has not been thoroughly studied in the setting of PDT. Only a single report is available that shows fragmentation of ion channels after Rose Bengal-mediated PDT [71].

Substantially more studies revealed protein cross-linking after PDT. For example, PDT with mitochondrial photosensitizers leads to effective cross-linking of STAT3, and to a lesser degree STAT1 and STAT4 proteins [72]. Interestingly, these transcription factors are found in the cytosolic and nuclear fractions of cells, in a significant distance from mitochondrial $^1O_2$ production during PDT. Therefore, it seems that other ROS or $^1O_2$-generated radicals participate in these reactions. There are multiple other examples of PDT-induced protein cross-linking: multimerization of proton-translocating ATPase in the inner mitochondrial membrane [73], cross-linking of membrane proteins in human erythrocytes [74], or formation of multimeric complexes of heme-binding proteins [75]. The mechanisms of protein cross-linking following PDT are more difficult to pinpoint because of multiple potential mechanisms. For example, carbonyl groups of oxidized proteins can react with N^ε-amino group of lysine derivative in neighboring protein, oxidation of two cysteins can lead to intramolecular disulfide cross-linked derivatives, or aldehyde groups of malondialdehyde produced during lipid peroxidation can form covalent bonds with separate cysteins on two different proteins [70]. Other mechanisms are also possible.

One of the typical biomarkers for oxidative protein damage is carbonylation. Carbonyl derivatives are formed by a direct metal-catalyzed oxidative modification of proline, arginine, lysine, and threonine [76]. Moreover, secondary reactions with reactive carbonyl groups on lipids and advanced glycation/lipoxidation end products can also lead to formation of carbonyl groups on lysine, threonine, and histidine [77]. Carbonylation is an irreversible process [78] and thus the only way of disposing carbonyls is through enforced degradation [76]. Carbonylation exposes hydrophobic residues that are normally hidden in the interior of soluble proteins. Generation of hydrophobic patches results in protein unfolding, which favors recognition and degradation by proteasomes (Figure 8.3) [79]. It is also possible that carbonylated proteins can be disposed of by autophagy-like mechanisms. Robust carbonylation of proteins results in the formation of large protein aggregates or "aggresomes," which clog proteasomes [80]. A direct evidence of ROS-mediated carbonylation of cellular proteins during PDT was provided by Magi et al. [81]. Specifically, it was shown that Purpurin-18-mediated PDT results in carbonylation of GRP78, HSP60, calreticulin, β-actin and other proteins [81].

PDT-generated $^1O_2$ has been shown to oxidatively modify numerous proteins in various compartments of the cell. Intriguingly, the effects seem to be, at least to some extent, dependent on the type of photosensitizer, which probably results from its subcellular localization. For example, PDT with rhodamine derivatives leads to oxidation of NAD(P)H [82], but this effect is not seen with Photofrin, Verteporfin, AlPcS4, TPPS4, or 5-ALA generated protoporphyrin IX [83], although all of these photosensitizers are presumed to localize in mitochondria. These observations indicate that even within the same organelle different photosensitizers localize in vicinity to different biologic targets and underscore the concept of site-specific or spatially

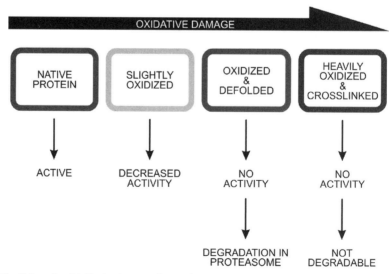

Figure 8.3 Fates of oxidatively-damaged proteins.

resolved effects elicited by $^1O_2$-mediated oxidation. There are multiple other examples of such localized effects in the literature. For example, photosensitization with phthallocyanine 4 (Pc4), which accumulates in mitochondria, leads to crosslinking and functional inactivation of Bcl-2 and Bcl-XL proteins, thereby initiating apoptosis [84]. Interestingly, Bcl-2 truncation mutants that do not localize to mitochondria are not affected by PDT [85]. Moreover, Pc4-mediated photosensitization does not target other mitochondrial membrane proteins such as voltage-dependent anion channel, adenine nucleotide translocator, or a proapoptotic Bax and Bad proteins [84, 85]. Even more selective effects were observed with mitochondria-localizing photosensitizers such as hematoporphyrin IX (HP) and 4,5',8-trimethyl-psoralen (TMP). HP upon illumination leads to site-selective inactivation of discrete functional domains of mitochondrial permeability transition pores resulting from damage to critical histidine residues [86]. In sharp contrast, TMP triggers pore opening [87]. These findings suggest that $^1O_2$ can activate or inactivate a cellular function such as mitochondrial permeability pores depending on the site where it is produced in the mitochondrial membrane.

Hydroxyl radical has been shown, together with $^1O_2$, to participate in HPD-mediated photodestruction of cytochrome P-450 and associated monooxygenases [88]. ˙OH also seems to be responsible for the induction of mitochondrial inner membrane permeabilization and depolarization, two processes that immediately follow induction of apoptosis [50].

Altogether, oxidative protein damage is usually nonrepairable and has deleterious consequences for the cell survival. Therefore, the most important fate of oxidized proteins is their catabolism by proteasomal, lysosomal, or autophagic pathways (see below).

8.5.2 Oxidative Lipid Modifications

The majority of photosensitizers used for PDT are amphiphilic and tend to accumulate in various compartments of the lipid bilayer (lysosomal, endoplasmic reticulum, mitochondrial, or plasma membrane). Therefore, despite lower rate constants of $^1O_2$ reactivity with lipids as compared to proteins, the former become significant targets for PDT-induced oxidative damage. It has been revealed that lipid hydroperoxides (LOOH) are predominant and early products of photosensitization [89]. While ˙OH and other radicals induce lipid peroxidation by hydrogen atom abstraction, $^1O_2$ can react directly with unsaturated fatty acids or cholesterol. The products of these oxidative reactions are different and can be used as molecular fingerprints that prove the existence of respective ROS. For example, $^1O_2$-mediated cholesterol peroxidation generates the following cholesterol hydroperoxides (Ch-OOH): 5α-, 6α-, and 6β-ChOOH [90], while ˙OH typically produces 7α-, and 7β-ChOOH [91].

Although lipid peroxidation is commonly associated with cellular damage, numerous observations indicate that it can also participate in local membrane remodeling, which is associated with endocytosis, exocytosis, receptor-mediated uptake, antigen presentation, and trafficking of intracellular vesicles. Moreover, lipid peroxidation products such as 4-hydroxynonenal (4-HNE) participate in signal transduction.

Phospholipid hydroperoxides (PL-OOH) and fatty acid hydroperoxides (FA-OOH) are dominant lipid peroxidation products that can propagate chain reactions. Fatty acid carbon chains can also undergo spontaneous cleavage, yielding a variety of reactive products such as pentane and ethane radicals, and unsaturated aldehydes. These downstream products exacerbate the effects of primary LOOH, thereby expanding the range of photooxidative damage.

8.6   Intracellular Mechanisms of ROS Scavenging

8.6.1   Superoxide Dismutase (SOD)

Superoxide production in eukaryotic cells is a potentially challenging threat. It has been estimated that a daily superoxide production is about 1×10^{10} radicals per day, so for a 75–kg person it corresponds to 2 kg of superoxide produced per year [92]. No wonder that cells must have developed effective means to deal with this overwhelming exposure.

Superoxide dismutase catalyzes the disproportionation of superoxide radicals to hydrogen peroxide and molecular oxygen [93]:

$$2O_2^- + 2H^+ \xrightarrow{\;\;SOD\;\;} H_2O_2 + O_2$$

There are three different isoforms of SOD: manganese (Mn) located in mitochondrial matrix (also referred to as SOD2), the copper-zinc (Cu,Zn) expressed in cytosol (SOD1), and an extracellular isoform of the enzyme (EC-SOD) [94]. SOD1 is the most abundant isoform in cells, but its levels are relatively constant. The expression of SOD2 is inducible under different stress conditions [95]. EC-SOD is mainly expressed in extracellular fluids such as lymph, synovial fluid and plasma [95].

The protective role of SODs has been shown in a variety of different pathological states known to induce oxidative stress, such as ischemia-reperfusion injury, Parkinson's disease, cancer, AIDS, or chronic obstructive pulmonary disease [94].

8.6.1.1   SOD and PDT

Several studies revealed that PDT induces Mn-SOD expression [96–98]. It seems that SOD activity protects cells from PDT-mediated damage. It has been shown that mice treated with SOD mimetic—β-carotene—had considerably less ear swelling following Photofrin-mediated PDT [99]. Intravenous administration of bacterial SOD decreased the antitumor effects of Photofrin-mediated PDT in three different murine tumor models [61]. Accordingly, sodium diethyldithiocarbamate, a SOD inhibitor, augmented cutaneous photosensitization [99]. Transient transfection with Sod2 gene as well as pretreatment of tumor cells with MnTBAP—a cell-permeable SOD mimetic—rendered tumor cells less susceptible to the cytotoxic effects of PDT [97]. Moreover, another SOD inhibitor and an endogenous estrogen metabolite (2-methoxyestradiol) significantly potentiated antitumor activity of PDT both in vitro and in vivo [97].

8.6.2 Catalase (CAT)

Catalase converts hydrogen peroxide into water and molecular oxygen and together with glutathione peroxidase plays a crucial role in hydrogen peroxide removal [100]:

$$2H_2O_2 \xrightarrow{\;CAT\;} H_2O + O_2$$

Catalase is the main H_2O_2-removing enzyme at high intracellular hydrogen peroxide concentration [100, 101]. Its scavenging activity is one of the highest among known enzymes—every minute it degrades up to 6×10^6 H_2O_2 molecules [102]. Mammalian catalase also has limited peroxidase activity but this is of a relatively slow rate. It seems that at low H_2O_2 concentrations catalase functions as a peroxidase, while the catalatic activity predominates at high H_2O_2 concentrations [101]. Catalase can be found in various cellular organelles (e.g., mitochondria, endoplasmic reticulum) but the majority of the enzyme is expressed in peroxisomes [101].

It has been suggested that catalase might play a cytoprotective role in PDT-treated cells [44, 54, 56, 103]. In the majority of studies the exogenous enzyme was used, but it is unlikely that recombinant enzyme can easily penetrate plasma membrane. Therefore, it is still unresolved whether catalase produced by tumor cells can protect from PDT-mediated damage. Development of genetic engineering techniques and availability of catalase knockout mice may shed some light on this phenomenon in the near future.

8.6.3 Secondary ROS Scavenging Mechanisms

First-line antioxidants such as SOD or CAT do not require glutathione for their function, while secondary antioxidants (glutathione-S-transferases, glutathione peroxidases) rely on its availability [104].

Compounds with thiol (-SH) group regulate the majority of biochemical and pharmacological reactions due to the ease with which they are oxidized and the rapidity of their regeneration.

8.6.3.1 Glutathione

Glutathione is a tripeptide (L-γ-glutamyl-L-cysteinyl-glycine) present in cells at millimolar (~1–10 mM) concentrations [105]. It contains an unusual peptide linkage between the amine group of cysteine and the carboxyl group of the glutamate side chain. Glutathione is abundant in the cytosol, mitochondria, and nuclei and comprises the most important soluble antioxidant in these cellular compartments [102].

Generally, the antioxidant properties of thiol compounds depend on the sulfur ion that can easily accommodate the loss of a single electron. Reduced glutathione reacts with a radical (R$^{\cdot}$) forming a thiyl radical (GS$^{\cdot}$), that further dimerises to form a nonradical product—glutathione disulfide:

$$GSH + R^{\cdot} \rightarrow GS^{\cdot} + RH$$

$$GS^{\cdot} + GS^{\cdot} \rightarrow GSSG$$

where GSH stands for the reduced glutathione, while GSSG stands for glutathione disulfide, often improperly named as "oxidized glutathione."

Subsequently, GSSG is reduced back to GSH in a reaction catalyzed by the enzyme glutathione reductase, which uses NADPH [106]:

$$GSSG + NADPH + H^+ \rightarrow NADP^+ + 2GSH$$

Importantly, a predominant pathway for GSH restoration is de novo synthesis [106]. The ratio of GSH to glutathione disulfide (GSSG) is critical for the maintenance of cellular redox balance. Under physiological conditions, intracellular environment has reducing potential and a GSH/GSSG ratio reaches 100 or more. Thus, the GSH/GSSG system is a major cytosolic redox buffer [105]. Increased amounts of GSSG are usually transient, since GSSG is rapidly reduced to GSH by the glutathione reductase. GSSG can also be exported from the cell in an ATP-dependent mechanism [106]. GSSG can also react with protein sulfhydryls to produce protein-glutathione mixed disulfides in a reaction termed glutathionylation [106]:

$$GSSG + protein - SH \rightarrow protein - SSG + GSH$$

The mixed disulfides have longer half-life than GSSG due to changes in protein folding [106]. This process may contribute to a protection of protein structure and can be reversed by glutaredoxins. Glutaredoxins (GRX) are enzymes that catalyze deglutathionylation of proteins, hence regulate diverse intracellular signaling pathways [107]. No evidence for the role of GRX in PDT-treated cells has been reported yet.

As previously stated, glutathione metabolism is one of the most important antioxidant mechanisms within a cell. Its cytoprotective role is dependent on several unique features of this molecule. Glutathione is a cofactor for several antioxidative enzymes (e.g., glutathione peroxidase, glutathione-S-transferase). Moreover, glutathione itself scavenges hydroxyl radical and singlet oxygen directly and by the action of glutathione peroxidase helps in elimination of hydrogen and lipid peroxides (described below). Glutathione is also able to regenerate vitamin C and E back to their active forms [102].

In the newly proposed "free radical sink" hypothesis, GSH in concert with SOD prevents the oxidative damage [108]. The rationale for this hypothesis can be shown by the following reactions, where $R^{\cdot}$ serves as a carbon-centered radical:

$$R^{\cdot} + GSH \rightarrow RH + GS^{\cdot}$$

$$GS^{\cdot} + GS^- \rightarrow GSSG^{\cdot-}$$

$$GSSG^{\cdot-} + O_2 \rightarrow GSSG + O_2^-$$

$$O_2^- + 2H^+ \xrightarrow{SOD} H_2O_2 + O_2$$

A number of studies have shown the protective effects of sulfhydryl groups against free radicals, especially in radiation-treated cells [109, 110]. Depletion of glutathione with buthionine sulfoximine was shown to potentiate antitumor activity of PDT both in vitro and in vivo. The same effect was observed in the genetically modified cells lacking GSH [111, 112]. Moreover, increase in the intracellular GSH content seems to alleviate the effects of PDT.

8.6.3.2   Thioredoxin (TX)

Thioredoxin (TX) is a small (10–12 kDa) multifunctional disulfide-containing redox protein that contains two redox-active cysteins in its conserved active site (-Trp-Cys-Gly-Pro-Cys-Lys-). TXs, similarly to glutathione, undergo reversible oxidation/reduction cycles of the two cysteine groups. Reduced TX [TX-(SH)$_2$] reduces oxidized proteins and converts into oxidized form [TX-(S-S)]. Oxidized thioredoxin cycles back to its reduced form in an NADPH-dependent reaction catalyzed by thioredoxin reductase (TRX) [113]. TX levels in cells are 100- to 1,000-fold smaller than those of GSH [102].

Thioredoxin serves as antioxidant mainly by being an electron donor for peroxiredoxin (see below). Reduction of thioredoxin peroxidase restores monomeric and active form of this enzyme [114]. Moreover, TX induces thioredoxin peroxidase expression [113].

Thioredoxin reductases (TRXs) are selenoproteins that restore a reduced form of thioredoxin utilizing NADPH produced mainly in the pentose phosphate pathway. TRXs undergo reversible oxidation/reduction cycling. Up to the time of this writing, two TRX isoforms have been cloned in humans, TRX-1 and TRX-2 [113]. Thioredoxin reductases use thioredoxin as a cofactor to reduce other proteins such as insulin or other small molecules such as oxidized ascorbate or hydrogen peroxide [113, 115].

No information on the role of thioredoxin/thioredoxin reductase system in cells treated with PDT has been reported so far.

8.6.3.3   Peroxiredoxins (PRX)

Peroxiredoxins (PRX) are a newly described family of proteins that catalyze the reduction of hydrogen peroxide by the thiol compounds. Sometimes they are also referred to as thioredoxin peroxidases [104]. In their enzymatically active site they have cysteine rather than selenium. The sequence of PRX catalyzed reactions is as follows [106]:

$$H_2O_2 + PRX - S^{\cdot} \rightarrow OH^- + PRX - SOH$$

$$PRX - SOH + GSH \rightarrow PRX - SSG + H_2O$$

$$PRX - SSG + GSH \rightarrow PRX - S^{\cdot} + GSSG$$

Up to the time of this writing, no studies on the role of peroxiredoxins in the effectiveness of PDT have been performed.

8.6.3.4 Glutathione Peroxidase (GPX) and Glutathione-S-Transferase (GST)

Glutathione peroxidase catalyzes decomposition of H_2O_2 with accompanying conversion of reduced glutathione (GSH) to glutathione disulfide (GSSG) [102]:

$$2GSH + H_2O_2 \xrightarrow{GPX} GSSG + 2H_2O$$

Next to catalase, GPX is the most important enzyme engaged in H_2O_2 scavenging. Its affinity to H_2O_2 is several-fold higher than that of catalase [101]. GPX also decomposes organic hydroperoxides (ROOH) to water or alcohol together with oxidizing GSH [102]:

$$2GSH + ROOH \xrightarrow{GPX} GSSG + ROH + H_2O$$

Two different forms of glutathione peroxidase exist. One is selenium-dependent and is referred to as glutathione peroxidase (GPX), and the other is Se-independent and is named glutathione-S-transferase (GST) [102]. Five different isoforms of GPX have been described. GPX1 is cytosolic and mitochondrial and reduces H_2O_2 and fatty acid hydroperoxides. Cytosolic GPX2 and extracellular GPX3 are not well described and poorly expressed. GPX4 reduces phospholipid hydroperoxides, fatty acid hydroperoxides, and cholesterol hydroperoxides, and is located both in cytosol and the membranes fraction. Recently discovered GPX5 is, strikingly, Se-independent and its expression is so far restricted to murine epididymis [116].

Little evidence exists on the role of GPXs in the cellular response to PDT. In HPD-mediated PDT, depletion of selenium significantly increased cytotoxicity [117]. Hypericin-mediated PDT has been shown to decrease enzymatic activity of GPX, accompanied by significant decrease in the intracellular levels of the reduced glutathione [56]. Moreover, GPX4 protected tumor cells from PDT-mediated cytotoxicity, most likely due to reduction of the levels of lipid hydroperoxides within the cells [118, 119].

GST expression has also been described as a factor protecting tumor cells from PDT-induced damage. The mechanism of its cytoprotective function is yet not fully understood. Sequestration of the photosensitizer by GST is one of the possibilities [120].

8.7 Cytoprotective Mechanisms Not Directly Associated with ROS Scavenging

8.7.1 Heme Oxygenase-1 (HO-1)

Heme oxygenase-1 is a rate-limiting enzyme catalyzing oxidative cleavage of heme to biliverdin, carbon monoxide (CO), and Fe^{2+}. Biliverdin is further converted to bilirubin by biliverdin reductase (BVR) (Figure 8.4). Each of these products plays a unique protective role in the human body. Both biliverdin and bilirubin are efficient antioxidants, while carbon monoxide plays a cytoprotective role similar to NO [121]. Free iron upregulates production of ferritin, a protein that sequesters iron ions and makes them inaccessible for Fenton reaction.

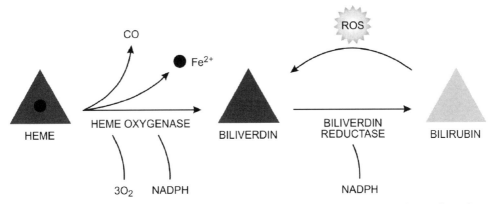

Figure 8.4   A cascade of reactions catalyzed by HO-1 and biliverdin reductase in heme degradation pathway.

Heme oxygenase exists in two different isoforms: an inducible (HO-1) and a constitutively expressed (HO-2) [122]. HO-1 expression is activated by a variety of different stimuli, including oxidative stress, hypoxia, hyperoxia, heat shock, heavy metal salts, ultraviolet A, and tumor promoters and growth factors [123–125].

Major physiological roles of HO-1 include the maintenance of the cellular homeostasis under stressful conditions, reduction of oxidative injury, attenuation of the inflammatory response, tissue-dependent regulation of the cell cycle, and promotion of new blood vessel formation [123]. Several mechanisms seem to account for the protective effects of HO-1. Due to this wide spectrum of functions, HO-1 takes part in the pathogenesis of a vast array of human diseases and pathologies, from sepsis and asthma, via cardiovascular diseases to ischemia-reperfusion injury, transplant graft rejection, neurodegenerative disorders, and finally, cancer [124].

8.7.1.1   Cytoprotective Effects of Heme Degradation Products

For decades, bilirubin was considered just a metabolic waste or even a neurotoxin as observed in neonatal hiperbilirubinemia [126]. The last several years have brought new and attractive evidence that this bile pigment may play an important and protective role as an antioxidative and anti-inflammatory agent.

Bilirubin contains an extended system of conjugated double bonds and a reactive hydrogen atom and thus possesses antioxidant properties [127]. Potent antioxidative effects of bilirubin were confirmed in a vast array of studies. It was found that bilirubin is a potent scavenger of singlet oxygen [128, 129] as well as of superoxide, peroxynitrite, and peroxyl radical [130]. Moreover, bilirubin reacts with superoxide ion, and in the presence of H_2O_2 or organic hydroperoxides, serves as a substrate for peroxidases [130]. At physiological concentrations bilirubin has been shown to prevent fatty acids peroxidation, human LDL, and albumin oxidation and is considered the most effective antioxidant of lipid peroxidation, more potent than α-tocopherol or vitamin C [127, 131]. Additionally, bilirubin prevents formation of protein carbonyls [132]. Inhibition of NADPH oxidase by bilirubin may also decrease superoxide generation [133]. Induction of HO-1 under oxidative stress conditions locally and temporarily increases intracellular bilirubin concentration and may serve as a potent antioxidative mechanism [131].

Carbon monoxide, a low-molecular-weight gaseous product of HO, plays an important role in cytoprotection, exerting antioxidative, anti-inflammatory, antiproliferative, and vasodilatory effects [121]. Degradation of hemoproteins is a major natural source of CO in humans, together with lipid oxidation and xenobiotics metabolism that play a minor role [121]. CO changes conformation of soluble guanylate cyclase (sGC) and thus increases production of cGMP—a potent vasorelaxant and antiaggregation agent [121, 130]. Carbon monoxide also prevents apoptosis by activation of p38 MAPK pathway [134].

By release of free iron from heme, HO-1 potentially contributes to prooxidant state within a cell. However, increased concentration of iron ions stimulates production of ferritin—an iron-sequestering multimeric protein with well-documented cytoprotective function [135]. Interestingly, in some settings ferritin can substitute for HO-1 action, indicating its important role in HO-1-mediated cytoprotection [136]. Moreover, HO-1 induces iron ATPase—an iron-removing pomp, which decreases intracellular iron concentration [137].

8.7.1.2   HO-1 and PDT

PDT increases HO-1 expression, which has been shown in different experimental settings at both mRNA and protein levels [138, 139]. Hemin—a strong inducer of HO-1 expression, decreases sensitivity of tumor cells to Photofrin-mediated PDT [140]. Similarly, transfection with HO-1 gene exerts protective effects in PDT-treated tumor cells in vitro [141]. In vivo, tumors overexpressing HO-1 regrow faster after PDT [141].

HO-1 stimulation by hypericin-mediated PDT is dependent on de novo protein synthesis [142]. Nrf2 seems to be the most important transcription factor involved in this process [142]. As well, p38 and PI3K pathways are necessary for HO-1 induction [142].

Interestingly, the cytoprotective effects of HO-1 in cells undergoing PDT are not dependent on production of antioxidant biliverdin or bilirubin as well as they are on the generation of carbon monoxide [141]. HO-1 protects from PDT-induced cell damage most likely through iron ions-induced expression of ferritin—a potent cytoprotective agent [141]. Moreover, removal of iron ions with desferrioxamine from PDT-treated cells resulted in increased cell death, confirming the crucial role of ferrous ions generation in HO-1-mediated cytoprotection [141]. It has also been shown that nitric oxide protects cells from PDT-mediated damage, mostly due to increased expression of HO-1 and ferritin [66], while spleen apoferritin added to cell culture prevented PDT-induced cell death [143].

8.7.2   ROS-Damaged Proteins Handling: The Role of Molecular Chaperons, Ubiquitin-Proteasome Pathway (UPP), and Autophagy

Singlet oxygen and other ROS generated during photodynamic therapy can damage proteins in various ways. Several amino acid residues can be affected, leading to disrupted enzymatic activities, secondary structure, and spatial organization of a number of vital proteins. Hydrophobic portions are displayed on the surface of protein molecules that triggers protein aggregation [22]. These phenomena can be harmful for cells and can lead to their death. To survive, a cell must activate protective mechanisms that either repair damaged protein structure or eliminate physiologically useless protein waste. Molecular chaperons, ubiquitin-proteasome system of protein degradation, and autophagy are used to repair or to eliminate damaged proteins.

8.7.2.1   Heat Shock Proteins (HSPs)

Molecular chaperons are proteins that help in proteins folding. Usually, they act through repeatable cycles of "client" protein binding and release. It is noteworthy that chaperons do not form any part of the final proteins themselves [144]. Heat shock proteins, a multigene family of proteins from 10 to 150 kDa of weight, were initially described in cellular response to hyperthermia. But HSPs help cells in dealing with a myriad of different stress conditions such as oxidative stress. HSPs, by binding to exposed surfaces, play a role in "fixing" or refolding of oxidatively damaged proteins and protein aggregates.

Photodynamic therapy was found to induce expression of a variety of HSPs including HS1, HSP27, HSP60, HSP70, HSP90, GRP78, and GRP94 [145–149]. For some of these a protective role in PDT-treated cell has been shown. For example, overexpression of HSP27 increased survival of tumor cells exposed to PDT [145]. Cellular levels of HSP60 and HSP70 negatively correlated with tumor cells sensitivity to PDT-induced damage [150, 151].

A combination of PDT with a derivative of the antibiotic geldanamycin resulted in higher apoptosis rate and increased cytotoxicity. Geldanamycin interferes with binding of client proteins by HSP90, among which are phosphorylated survivin (a member of the inhibitors of apoptosis proteins) or phosphorylated Akt and antiapoptotic Bcl-2. Prevention of HSP90-mediated survivin maturation, folding, assembly, and transport seems to significantly augment cytotoxic effects of PDT [152].

The role of HSPs in cellular physiology is far beyond just protein refolding and involves regulation of the cellular signaling mostly due to stabilization or sequestration of various factors. Indeed, some of the "client" proteins for HSPs are involved in survival promoting pathways [153]. Therefore, it is possible that HSPs protect cells not only by enabling a repair of oxidatively damaged proteins but also by less specific inhibition of apoptosis [154].

8.7.2.2   Ubiquitin-Proteasome Pathway (UPP)

Although some oxidatively damaged proteins in PDT-surviving cells can be "repaired" by HSPs, most of them are probably eliminated by intracellular proteolysis. It is likely, that some tumors may have increased capability of proteolysis and cope better with accumulation of the oxidized molecules.

There are two systems of protein degradation in cells. One is dependent on ubiquitylation of useless proteins and their subsequent degradation in the proteasome. The other is referred to as autophagy (that means "self-eating") and is characterized by degradation of dispensable cellular components in lysosome-like structures called autophagosomes.

The ubiquitin-proteasome pathway is responsible for degradation of 80% to 90% of cellular proteins [155]. Proteasomes are multicatalytic complexes present in the majority of living organisms, mostly in the cytoplasm or nucleus of a cell. In eukaryotic cells proteasome consists of a proteolytic core (called 20S subunit) and one or two regulatory subunits placed on its ends called 19S or PA700. Proteolytic core together with regulatory subunit(s) is commonly referred to as 26S proteasome. Barrel-shaped 20S proteasome core is composed of four rings—two inner β rings and two outer α rings. Each ring contains seven distinct subunits. Only three subunits of each β ring possess proteolytic activity: $\beta1$, a post-glutamyl peptide hydrolase-like or caspase-like proteolytic activity, $\beta2$, a trypsin-like proteolytic activity, and $\beta5$, a chymotrypsin-like proteolytic activity. A protein molecule targeted for degradation before getting into proteasome must be flagged with a small polipeptyde called ubiquitin (Ub). The process of Ub attachment is called ubiquitylation and is a multistep energy-consuming procedure engaging a variety of specific Ub-activating, conjugating, and ligating enzymes [156]. Although the majority of proteases cleave peptides into two fragments, 26S proteasome shows progressive fashion of protein degradation and releases just single oligopeptides (Figure 8.5) [157].

Out of 20 amino acids only cysteine and methionine can be reduced to their initial form and thus repaired [158]. The rest of oxidized amino acids cannot be repaired and proteins containing them must be rapidly degraded. If the damage is too heavy degradation is impossible and results in accumulation of aggregates of oxidized proteins known as lipofuscin, and consequently, in cell death [159]. Interestingly, the majority of oxidized proteins accumulate in cytoplasm, while the main cellular localization of proteasomes is the nucleus [160].

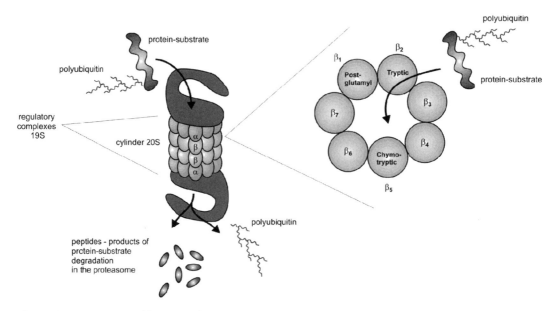

Figure 8.5   Structure and function of proteasome.

In our studies, we observed significant accumulation of ubiquitylated proteins accompanied by decreased proteasome activity in tumor cells subjected to Photofrin-mediated PDT. Moreover, proteasome inhibitors significantly potentiated antitumor activity of PDT both in in vitro and in vivo settings, suggesting crucial protective role of proper functioning proteasome-dependent protein degradation in cells subjected to PDT damage (Makowski et al., submitted).

8.7.2.3   Autophagy

Another potent mechanism of intracellular protein degradation is associated with autophagy. Autophagy was originally described as a survival response in cells subjected to nutrients' deprivation [161]. It is a process in which fragments of cytosol or organelles are engulfed and form vacuoles that fuse with lysosomes and are degraded by lysosomal enzymes. Products of degradation are then released into cytoplasm and reutilized by a cell [161]. It is now well documented that autophagy plays an important role in both cell death induction and cytoprotection [162, 163]. It has been recently shown, that PDT utilizing an ER-localizing photosensitizer induces autophagy [164]. Whether it is a mechanism of cell death induction or a rescue response eliminating oxidatively-damaged molecules remains to be elucidated.

8.8   Summary

Tumor tissue is a heterogeneous and complex structure. The efficacy of PDT directly depends on light, photosensitizer, and oxygen within the tumor mass. Light penetration may not be sufficient to induce phototoxic reaction, especially in the deeper layers of a tumor, resulting in cell death. Thus, cells exposed to sublethal doses of PDT may induce several cytoprotective mechanisms rescuing them from ROS-mediated damage. These surviving cells might be a cause of tumor relapse. The cytoprotective mechanisms are particularly significant in PDT as one of indelible features of this treatment is a highly inhomogeneous light (and therefore its dose) distribution within a tumor. The amount of oxidative stress delivered to a given tumor region depends on multiple factors, including the distance from the light source (many layers of tumor cells absorb the light and decrease the dose delivered to its deepest regions) and vascularization (photosensitizer and oxygen are usually distributed within tumors via blood vessels). These causes explain why some regions of the tumor receive doses of PDT that are below average for the whole lesion. If the cytoprotective mechanisms that preexist or become active in such deep-tumor located cells are sufficient for survival, a relapse of the tumor may occur. Thorough understanding of such mechanisms may allow development of new treatment strategies, possibly including combined therapies, which switch off the cytoprotection and make the below-average dose of PDT capable of killing tumor cells. This, in clinical terms, would decrease the relapse rate and at least partially eliminate one of the limitations of PDT. Not all protective pathways that might play a role in PDT-resistance have been described in this chapter. Several are still to be identified. Hopefully, these efforts, together with further development of different treatment and diagnostic strategies, will allow better control of deadly and devastating neoplastic diseases.

Acknowledgments

The research in the authors' department is supported by grant N401 123 31/2736 from the Ministry of Science and Higher Education. We would like to thank Marek Strauchold for the preparation of figures.

References

[1] Muller, F. L., Liu, Y., and Van Remmen, H., "Complex III releases superoxide to both sides of the inner mitochondrial membrane," *J Biol Chem*, Vol. 279, 2004, pp. 49064–49073.

[2] Giorgio, M., et al., "Hydrogen peroxide: a metabolic by-product or a common mediator of ageing signals?," *Nature Rev Mol Cell Biol*, Vol. 8, 2007, pp. 722–728.

[3] Ott, M., et al., "Mitochondria, oxidative stress and cell death," *Apoptosis*, Vol. 12, 2007, pp. 913–922.

[4] Bayne, A. C., et al., "Enhanced catabolism of mitochondrial superoxide/hydrogen peroxide and aging in transgenic Drosophila," *Biochem J*, Vol. 391, 2005, pp. 277–284.

[5] Lambeth, J. D., "NOX enzymes and the biology of reactive oxygen," *Nat Rev Immunol*, Vol. 4, 2004, pp. 181–189.

[6] Jaeschke, H., "Xanthine oxidase-induced oxidant stress during hepatic ischemia-reperfusion: are we coming full circle after 20 years?" *Hepatology*, Vol. 36, 2002, pp. 761–763.

[7] Fridovich, I., "Superoxide radical and superoxide dismutases," *Annu Rev Biochem*, Vol. 64, 1995, pp. 97–112.

[8] Cadenas, E., and Davies, K. J., "Mitochondrial free radical generation, oxidative stress, and aging," *Free Radic Biol Med*, Vol. 29, 2000, pp. 222–230.

[9] Zhang, Y., et al., "The oxidative inactivation of mitochondrial electron transport chain components and ATPase," *J Biol Chem*, Vol. 265, 1990, pp. 16330–16336.

[10] Nelson, S. K., Bose, S. K., and McCord, J. M., "The toxicity of high-dose superoxide dismutase suggests that superoxide can both initiate and terminate lipid peroxidation in the reperfused heart," *Free Radic Biol Med*, Vol. 16, 1994, pp. 195–200.

[11] Schrader, M., and Fahimi, H. D., "Peroxisomes and oxidative stress," *Biochim Biophys Acta*, Vol. 1763, 2006, pp. 1755–1766.

[12] Giorgio, M., et al., "Electron transfer between cytochrome c and p66Shc generates reactive oxygen species that trigger mitochondrial apoptosis," *Cell*, Vol. 122, 2005, pp. 221–233.

[13] Veal, E. A., Day, A. M., and Morgan, B. A., "Hydrogen peroxide sensing and signaling," *Mol Cell*, Vol. 26, 2007, pp. 1–14.

[14] Rae, T. D., et al., "Undetectable intracellular free copper: the requirement of a copper chaperone for superoxide dismutase," *Science*, Vol. 284, 1999, pp. 805–808.

[15] Kanofsky, J. R., et al., "Singlet oxygen production by human eosinophils," *J Biol Chem*, Vol. 263, 1988, pp. 9692–9696.

[16] Steinbeck, M. J., Khan, A. U., and Karnovsky, M. J., "Extracellular production of singlet oxygen by stimulated macrophages quantified using 9,10-diphenylanthracene and perylene in a polystyrene film," *J Biol Chem*, Vol. 268, 1993, pp. 15649–15654.

[17] Redmond, R. W., and Kochevar, I. E., "Spatially resolved cellular responses to singlet oxygen," *Photochem Photobiol*, Vol. 82, 2006, pp. 1178–1186.

[18] Kanofsky, J. R., "Quenching of singlet oxygen by human red cell ghosts," *Photochem Photobiol*, Vol. 53, 1991, pp. 93–99.

[19] Niedre, M., Patterson, M. S., and Wilson, B. C., "Direct near-infrared luminescence detection of singlet oxygen generated by photodynamic therapy in cells in vitro and tissues in vivo," *Photochem Photobiol*, Vol. 75, 2002, pp. 382–391.

[20] Bachowski, G. J., Pintar, T. J., and Girotti, A. W., "Photosensitized lipid peroxidation and enzyme inactivation by membrane-bound merocyanine 540: reaction mechanisms in the absence and presence of ascorbate," *Photochem Photobiol*, Vol. 53, 1991, pp. 481–491.

[21] Girotti, A. W., "Photosensitized oxidation of cholesterol in biological systems: reaction pathways, cytotoxic effects and defense mechanisms," *J Photochem Photobiol B*, Vol. 13, 1992, pp. 105–118.

[22] Davies, M. J., "Singlet oxygen-mediated damage to proteins and its consequences," *Biochem Biophys Res Commun*, Vol. 305, 2003, pp. 761–770.

[23] Cadet, J., et al., "Singlet oxygen oxidation of isolated and cellular DNA: product formation and mechanistic insights," *Photochem Photobiol*, Vol. 82, 2006, pp. 1219–1225.

[24] Klotz, L. O., Kroncke, K. D., and Sies, H., "Singlet oxygen-induced signaling effects in mammalian cells," *Photochem Photobiol Sci*, Vol. 2, 2003, pp. 88–94.

[25] Wright, A., Hawkins, C. L., and Davies, M. J., "Singlet oxygen-mediated protein oxidation: evidence for the formation of reactive peroxides," *Redox Rep*, Vol. 5, 2000, pp. 159–161.

[26] Wright, A., et al., "Singlet oxygen-mediated protein oxidation: evidence for the formation of reactive side chain peroxides on tyrosine residues," *Photochem Photobiol*, Vol. 76, 2002, pp. 35–46.

[27] Silvester, J. A., Timmins, G. S., and Davies, M. J., "Protein hydroperoxides and carbonyl groups generated by porphyrin-induced photo-oxidation of bovine serum albumin," *Arch Biochem Biophys*, Vol. 350, 1998, pp. 249–258.

[28] Lledias, F., Rangel, P., and Hansberg, W., "Oxidation of catalase by singlet oxygen," *J Biol Chem*, Vol. 273, 1998, pp. 10630–10637.

[29] Gryglewski, R. J., Palmer, R. M., and Moncada, S., "Superoxide anion is involved in the breakdown of endothelium-derived vascular relaxing factor," *Nature*, Vol. 320, 1986, pp. 454–456.

[30] Beckman, J. S., et al., "Apparent hydroxyl radical production by peroxynitrite: implications for endothelial injury from nitric oxide and superoxide," *Proc Natl Acad Sci U S A*, Vol. 87, 1990, pp. 1620–1624.

[31] Szabo, C., Ischiropoulos, H., and Radi, R., "Peroxynitrite: biochemistry, pathophysiology and development of therapeutics," *Nat Rev Drug Discov*, Vol. 6, 2007, pp. 662–680.

[32] Wink, D. A., and Mitchell, J. B., "Chemical biology of nitric oxide: Insights into regulatory, cytotoxic, and cytoprotective mechanisms of nitric oxide," *Free Radic Biol Med*, Vol. 25, 1998, pp. 434–456.

[33] Valko, M., et al., "Free radicals and antioxidants in normal physiological functions and human disease," *Int J Biochem Cell Biol*, Vol. 39, 2007, pp. 44–84.

[34] Irani, K., et al., "Mitogenic signaling mediated by oxidants in Ras-transformed fibroblasts," *Science*, Vol. 275, 1997, pp. 1649–1652.

[35] Nowicki, M. O., et al., "BCR/ABL oncogenic kinase promotes unfaithful repair of the reactive oxygen species-dependent DNA double-strand breaks," *Blood*, Vol. 104, 2004, pp. 3746–3753.

[36] Vafa, O., et al., "c-Myc can induce DNA damage, increase reactive oxygen species, and mitigate p53 function: a mechanism for oncogene-induced genetic instability," *Mol Cell*, Vol. 9, 2002, pp. 1031–1044.

[37] Meng, T. C., Fukada, T., and Tonks, N. K., "Reversible oxidation and inactivation of protein tyrosine phosphatases in vivo," *Mol Cell*, Vol. 9, 2002, pp. 387–399.

[38] Rao, R. K., and Clayton, L. W., "Regulation of protein phosphatase 2A by hydrogen peroxide and glutathionylation," *Biochem Biophys Res Commun*, Vol. 293, 2002, pp. 610–616.

[39] Chandel, N. S., et al., "Reactive oxygen species generated at mitochondrial complex III stabilize hypoxia-inducible factor-1alpha during hypoxia: a mechanism of O2 sensing," *J Biol Chem*, Vol. 275, 2000, pp. 25130–25138.

[40] Schreck, R., Rieber, P., and Baeuerle, P. A., "Reactive oxygen intermediates as apparently widely used messengers in the activation of the NF-kappa B transcription factor and HIV-1," *Embo J*, Vol. 10, 1991, pp. 2247–2258.

[41] Weishaupt, K. R., Gomer, C. J., and Dougherty, T. J., "Identification of singlet oxygen as the cytotoxic agent in photoinactivation of a murine tumor," *Cancer Res*, Vol. 36, 1976, pp. 2326–2329.

[42] Henderson, B. W., and Miller, A. C., "Effects of scavengers of reactive oxygen and radical species on cell survival following photodynamic treatment in vitro: comparison to ionizing radiation," *Radiat Res*, Vol. 108, 1986, pp. 196–205.

[43] Hariharan, P. V., Courtney, J., and Eleczko, S., "Production of hydroxyl radicals in cell systems exposed to haematoporphyrin and red light," *Int J Radiat Biol Relat Stud Phys Chem Med*, Vol. 37, 1980, pp. 691–694.

[44] Chekulayeva, L. V., et al., "Hydrogen peroxide, superoxide, and hydroxyl radicals are involved in the phototoxic action of hematoporphyrin derivative against tumor cells," *J Environ Pathol Toxicol Oncol*, Vol. 25, 2006, pp. 51–77.

[45] Fuchs, J., and Thiele, J., "The role of oxygen in cutaneous photodynamic therapy," *Free Radic Biol Med*, Vol. 24, 1998, pp. 835–847.

[46] Kolarova, H., et al., "Comparison of sensitizers by detecting reactive oxygen species after photodynamic reaction in vitro," *Toxicol In Vitro*, Vol. 21, 2007, pp. 1287–1291.

[47] Gilaberte, Y., et al., "Flow cytometry study of the role of superoxide anion and hydrogen peroxide in cellular photodestruction with 5-aminolevulinic acid-induced protoporphyrin IX," *Photodermatol Photoimmunol Photomed*, Vol. 13, 1997, pp. 43–49.

[48] Viola, A., et al., "ESR studies of a series of phthalocyanines. Mechanism of phototoxicity. Comparative quantitation of O2-. using ESR spin-trapping and cytochrome c reduction techniques," *Free Radic Res*, Vol. 28, 1998, pp. 517–532.

[49] He, Y. Y., An, J. Y., and Jiang, L. J., "EPR and spectrophotometric studies on free radicals (O2.-, Cysa-HB.-) and singlet oxygen (1O2) generated by irradiation of cysteamine substituted hypocrellin B," *Int J Radiat Biol*, Vol. 74, 1998, pp. 647–654.

[50] Lam, M., Oleinick, N. L., and Nieminen, A. L., "Photodynamic therapy-induced apoptosis in epidermoid carcinoma cells. Reactive oxygen species and mitochondrial inner membrane permeabilization," *J Biol Chem*, Vol. 276, 2001, pp. 47379–47386.

[51] Bilski, P., Belanger, A. G., and Chignell, C. F., "Photosensitized oxidation of 2',7'-dichlorofluorescin: singlet oxygen does not contribute to the formation of fluorescent oxidation product 2',7'-dichlorofluorescein," *Free Radic Biol Med*, Vol. 33, 2002, pp. 938–946.

[52] Myhre, O., et al., "Evaluation of the probes 2',7'-dichlorofluorescin diacetate, luminol, and lucigenin as indicators of reactive species formation," *Biochem Pharmacol*, Vol. 65, 2003, pp. 1575–1582.

[53] Salet, C., Moreno, G., and Ricchelli, F., "Effects of Photofrin photodynamic action on mitochondrial respiration and superoxide radical generation," *Free Radic Res*, Vol. 26, 1997, pp. 201–208.

[54] Hadjur, C., et al., "Production of the free radicals O2.- and .OH by irradiation of the photosensitizer zinc(II) phthalocyanine," *J Photochem Photobiol B*, Vol. 38, 1997, pp. 196–202.

[55] Luo, J., et al., "Inactivation of primary antioxidant enzymes in mouse keratinocytes by photodynamically generated singlet oxygen," *Antioxid Redox Signal*, Vol. 8, 2006, pp. 1307–1314.

[56] Hadjur, C., et al., "Photodynamic effects of hypericin on lipid peroxidation and antioxidant status in melanoma cells," *Photochem Photobiol*, Vol. 64, 1996, pp. 375–381.

[57] Skalkos, D., et al., "Iminium salt benzochlorins: structure-activity relationship studies," *Photochem Photobiol*, Vol. 59, 1994, pp. 175–181.

[58] Gupta, S., Ahmad, N., and Mukhtar, H., "Involvement of nitric oxide during phthalocyanine (Pc4) photodynamic therapy-mediated apoptosis," *Cancer Res*, Vol. 58, 1998, pp. 1785–1788.

[59] Gilissen, M. J., et al., "Effect of photodynamic therapy on the endothelium-dependent relaxation of isolated rat aortas," *Cancer Res*, Vol. 53, 1993, pp. 2548–2552.

[60] Henderson, B. W., Sitnik-Busch, T. M., and Vaughan, L. A., "Potentiation of photodynamic therapy antitumor activity in mice by nitric oxide synthase inhibition is fluence rate dependent," *Photochem Photobiol*, Vol. 70, 1999, pp. 64–71.

[61] Korbelik, M., et al., "Nitric oxide production by tumour tissue: impact on the response to photodynamic therapy," *Br J Cancer*, Vol. 82, 2000, pp. 1835–1843.

[62] Korytowski, W., Zareba, M., and Girotti, A. W., "Nitric oxide inhibition of free radical-mediated cholesterol peroxidation in liposomal membranes," *Biochemistry*, Vol. 39, 2000, pp. 6918–6928.

[63] O'Donnell, V. B., et al., "Nitric oxide inhibition of lipid peroxidation: kinetics of reaction with lipid peroxyl radicals and comparison with alpha-tocopherol," *Biochemistry*, Vol. 36, 1997, pp. 15216–15223.

[64] Niziolek, M., Korytowski, W., and Girotti, A. W., "Nitric oxide inhibition of free radical-mediated lipid peroxidation in photodynamically treated membranes and cells," *Free Radic Biol Med*, Vol. 34, 2003, pp. 997–1005.

[65] Niziolek, M., Korytowski, W., and Girotti, A. W., "Chain-breaking antioxidant and cytoprotective action of nitric oxide on photodynamically stressed tumor cells," *Photochem Photobiol*, Vol. 78, 2003, pp. 262–270.

[66] Niziolek, M., Korytowski, W., and Girotti, A. W., "Nitric oxide-induced resistance to lethal photooxidative damage in a breast tumor cell line," *Free Radic Biol Med*, Vol. 40, 2006, pp. 1323–1331.

[67] Fisher, A. M., et al., "Photodynamic therapy sensitivity is not altered in human tumor cells after abrogation of p53 function," *Cancer Res*, Vol. 59, 1999, pp. 331–335.

[68] Schwarz, V. A., et al., "Photodynamic therapy of DNA mismatch repair-deficient and -proficient tumour cells," *Br J Cancer*, Vol. 86, 2002, pp. 1130–1135.

[69] Davies, M. J., et al., "Stable markers of oxidant damage to proteins and their application in the study of human disease," *Free Radic Biol Med*, Vol. 27, 1999, pp. 1151–1163.

[70] Stadtman, E. R., "Protein oxidation and aging," *Free Radic Res*, Vol. 40, 2006, pp. 1250–1258

[71] Kunz, L., et al., "Photodynamic and radiolytic inactivation of ion channels formed by gramicidin A: oxidation and fragmentation," *Biochemistry*, Vol. 34, 1995, pp. 11895–11903.

[72] Liu, W., Oseroff, A. R., and Baumann, H., "Photodynamic therapy causes cross-linking of signal transducer and activator of transcription proteins and attenuation of interleukin-6 cytokine responsiveness in epithelial cells," *Cancer Res*, Vol. 64, 2004, pp. 6579–6587.

[73] Perlin, D. S., et al., "Effects of photosensitization by hematoporphyrin derivative on mitochondrial adenosine triphosphatase-mediated proton transport and membrane integrity of R3230AC mammary adenocarcinoma," *Cancer Res*, Vol. 45, 1985, pp. 653–658.

[74] Girotti, A. W., "Photodynamic action of protoporphyrin IX on human erythrocytes: cross-linking of membrane proteins," *Biochem Biophys Res Commun*, Vol. 72, 1976, pp. 1367–1374.

[75] Vincent, S. H., et al., "Porphyrin-induced photodynamic cross-linking of hepatic heme-binding proteins," *Life Sci*, Vol. 38, 1986, pp. 365–372.

[76] Nystrom, T., "Role of oxidative carbonylation in protein quality control and senescence," *Embo J*, Vol. 24, 2005, pp. 1311–1317.

[77] Dalle-Donne, I., et al., "Protein carbonylation, cellular dysfunction, and disease progression," *J Cell Mol Med*, Vol. 10, 2006, pp. 389–406.

[78] Dalle-Donne, I., et al., "Protein carbonylation in human diseases," *Trends Mol Med*, Vol. 9, 2003, pp. 169–176.

[79] Grune, T., et al., "Selective degradation of oxidatively modified protein substrates by the proteasome," *Biochem Biophys Res Commun*, Vol. 305, 2003, pp. 709–718.

[80] Grune, T., et al., "Decreased proteolysis caused by protein aggregates, inclusion bodies, plaques, lipofuscin, ceroid, and 'aggresomes' during oxidative stress, aging, and disease," *Int J Biochem Cell Biol*, Vol. 36, 2004, pp. 2519–2530.

[81] Magi, B., et al., "Selectivity of protein carbonylation in the apoptotic response to oxidative stress associated with photodynamic therapy: a cell biochemical and proteomic investigation," *Cell Death Differ*, Vol. 11, 2004, pp. 842–852.

[82] Petrat, F., et al., "NAD(P)H, a primary target of 1O2 in mitochondria of intact cells," *J Biol Chem*, Vol. 278, 2003, pp. 3298–3307.

[83] Petrat, F., et al., ""Mitochondrial" photochemical drugs do not release toxic amounts of 1O(2) within the mitochondrial matrix space," *Arch Biochem Biophys*, Vol. 412, 2003, pp. 207–215.

[84] Xue, L. Y., Chiu, S. M., and Oleinick, N. L., "Photochemical destruction of the Bcl-2 oncoprotein during photodynamic therapy with the phthalocyanine photosensitizer Pc 4," *Oncogene*, Vol. 20, 2001, pp. 3420–3427.

[85] Usuda, J., et al., "Domain-dependent photodamage to Bcl-2. A membrane anchorage region is needed to form the target of phthalocyanine photosensitization," *J Biol Chem*, Vol. 278, 2003, pp. 2021–2029.

[86] Salet, C., et al., "Singlet oxygen produced by photodynamic action causes inactivation of the mitochondrial permeability transition pore," *J Biol Chem*, Vol. 272, 1997, pp. 21938–21943.

[87] Moreno, G., et al., "The effects of singlet oxygen produced by photodynamic action on the mitochondrial permeability transition differ in accordance with the localization of the sensitizer," *Arch Biochem Biophys*, Vol. 386, 2001, pp. 243–250.

[88] Das, M., et al., "Role of active oxygen species in the photodestruction of microsomal cytochrome P-450 and associated monooxygenases by hematoporphyrin derivative in rats," *Cancer Res*, Vol. 45, 1985, pp. 608–615.

[89] Girotti, A. W., and Kriska, T., "Role of lipid hydroperoxides in photo-oxidative stress signaling," *Antioxid Redox Signal*, Vol. 6, 2004, pp. 301–310.

[90] Korytowski, W., Wrona, M., and Girotti, A. W., "Radiolabeled cholesterol as a reporter for assessing one-electron turnover of lipid hydroperoxides," *Anal Biochem*, Vol. 270, 1999, pp. 123–132.

[91] Smith, L. L., et al., "Sterol metabolism. 23. Cholesterol oxidation by radiation-induced processes," *J Org Chem*, Vol. 38, 1973, pp. 1763–1765.

[92] Halliwell, B., "Free radicals, antioxidants, and human disease: curiosity, cause, or consequence?," *Lancet*, Vol. 344, 1994, pp. 721–724.

[93] Noor, R., Mittal, S., and Iqbal, J., "Superoxide dismutase?applications and relevance to human diseases," *Med Sci Monit*, Vol. 8, 2002, pp. RA210–215.

[94] Salvemini, D., Riley, D. P., and Cuzzocrea, S., "SOD mimetics are coming of age," *Nat Rev Drug Discov*, Vol. 1, 2002, pp. 367–374.

[95] Fattman, C. L., Schaefer, L. M., and Oury, T. D., "Extracellular superoxide dismutase in biology and medicine," *Free Radic Biol Med*, Vol. 35, 2003, pp. 236–256.

[96] Das, H., et al., "Induction of apoptosis and manganese superoxide dismutase gene by photodynamic therapy in cervical carcinoma cell lines," *Int J Clin Oncol*, Vol., 2000, pp. 97–103.

[97]   Golab, J., et al., "Antitumor effects of photodynamic therapy are potentiated by 2-methoxyestradiol. A superoxide dismutase inhibitor," *J Biol Chem*, Vol. 278, 2003, pp. 407–414.

[98]   Dolgachev, V., et al., "A role for manganese superoxide dismutase in apoptosis after photosensitization," *Biochem Biophys Res Commun*, Vol. 332, 2005, pp. 411–417.

[99]   Athar, M., et al., "In situ evidence for the involvement of superoxide anions in cutaneous porphyrin photosensitization," *Biochem Biophys Res Commun*, Vol. 151, 1988, pp. 1054–1059.

[100] Scibior, D., and Czeczot, H., "Catalase: structure, properties, functions," *Postepy Hig Med Dosw (Online)*, Vol. 60, 2006, pp. 170–180.

[101] Kirkman, H. N., and Gaetani, G. F., "Mammalian catalase: a venerable enzyme with new mysteries," *Trends Biochem Sci*, Vol. 32, 2007, pp. 44–50.

[102] Valko, M., et al., "Free radicals, metals and antioxidants in oxidative stress-induced cancer," *Chem Biol Interact*, Vol. 160, 2006, pp. 1–40.

[103] Curnow, A., and Bown, S. G., "The role of reperfusion injury in photodynamic therapy with 5-aminolaevulinic acid?a study on normal rat colon," *Br J Cancer*, Vol. 86, 2002, pp. 989–992.

[104] Kinnula, V. L., and Crapo, J. D., "Superoxide dismutases in malignant cells and human tumors," *Free Radic Biol Med*, Vol. 36, 2004, pp. 718–744.

[105] Dalle-Donne, I., et al., "S-glutathionylation in protein redox regulation," *Free Radic Biol Med*, Vol. 43, 2007, pp. 883–898.

[106] Dickinson, D. A., and Forman, H. J., "Cellular glutathione and thiols metabolism," *Biochem Pharmacol*, Vol. 64, 2002, pp. 1019–1026.

[107] Gallogly, M. M., and Mieyal, J. J., "Mechanisms of reversible protein glutathionylation in redox signaling and oxidative stress," *Curr Opin Pharmacol*, Vol. 7, 2007, pp. 381–391.

[108] Winterbourn, C. C., "Superoxide as an intracellular radical sink," *Free Radic Biol Med*, Vol. 14, 1993, pp. 85–90.

[109] Deschavanne, P. J., et al., "Radioprotective effect of cysteamine in glutathione synthetase-deficient cells," *Int J Radiat Biol Relat Stud Phys Chem Med*, Vol. 49, 1986, pp. 85–101.

[110] Biaglow, J. E., et al., "The effect of L-buthionine sulfoximine on the aerobic radiation response of A549 human lung carcinoma cells," *Int J Radiat Oncol Biol Phys*, Vol. 12, 1986, pp. 1139–1142.

[111] Granville, D. J., et al., "Nuclear factor-kappaB activation by the photochemotherapeutic agent verteporfin," *Blood*, Vol. 95, 2000, pp. 256–262.

[112] Miller, A. C., and Henderson, B. W., "The influence of cellular glutathione content on cell survival following photodynamic treatment in vitro," *Radiat Res*, Vol. 107, 1986, pp. 83–94.

[113] Biaglow, J. E., and Miller, R. A., "The thioredoxin reductase/thioredoxin system: novel redox targets for cancer therapy," *Cancer Biol Ther*, Vol. 4, 2005, pp. 6–13.

[114] Immenschuh, S., and Baumgart-Vogt, E., "Peroxiredoxins, oxidative stress, and cell proliferation," *Antioxid Redox Signal*, Vol. 7, 2005, pp. 768–777.

[115] Mustacich, D., and Powis, G., "Thioredoxin reductase," *Biochem J*, Vol. 346, Pt 1, 2000, pp. 1–8

[116] Mates, J. M., Perez-Gomez, C., and Nunez de Castro, I., "Antioxidant enzymes and human diseases," *Clin Biochem*, Vol. 32, 1999, pp. 595–603.

[117] Thomas, J. P., and Girotti, A. W., "Role of lipid peroxidation in hematoporphyrin derivative-sensitized photokilling of tumor cells: protective effects of glutathione peroxidase," *Cancer Res*, Vol. 49, 1989, pp. 1682–1686.

[118] Wang, H. P., et al., "Phospholipid hydroperoxide glutathione peroxidase protects against singlet oxygen-induced cell damage of photodynamic therapy," *Free Radic Biol Med*, Vol. 30, 2001, pp. 825–835.

[119] Kriska, T., Korytowski, W., and Girotti, A. W., "Hyperresistance to photosensitized lipid peroxidation and apoptotic killing in 5-aminolevulinate-treated tumor cells overexpressing mitochondrial GPX4," *Free Radic Biol Med*, Vol. 33, 2002, pp. 1389–1402.

[120] Dabrowski, M. J., et al., "Glutathione S-transferase P1-1 expression modulates sensitivity of human kidney 293 cells to photodynamic therapy with hypericin," *Arch Biochem Biophys*, Vol. 449, 2006, pp. 94–103.

[121] Ryter, S. W., Morse, D., and Choi, A. M., "Carbon monoxide and bilirubin: potential therapies for pulmonary/vascular injury and disease," *Am J Respir Cell Mol Biol*, Vol. 36, 2007, pp. 175–182.

[122] Morse, D., and Choi, A. M., "Heme oxygenase-1: from bench to bedside," *Am J Respir Crit Care Med*, Vol. 172, 2005, pp. 660–670.

[123] Was, H., et al., "Overexpression of heme oxygenase-1 in murine melanoma: increased proliferation and viability of tumor cells, decreased survival of mice," *Am J Pathol*, Vol. 169, 2006, pp. 2181–2198.

[124] Alam, J., and Cook, J. L., "How many transcription factors does it take to turn on the heme oxygenase-1 gene?" *Am J Respir Cell Mol Biol*, Vol. 36, 2007, pp. 166–174.

[125] Katavetin, P., et al., "Erythropoietin induces heme oxygenase-1 expression and attenuates oxidative stress," *Biochem Biophys Res Commun*, Vol. 359, 2007, pp. 928–934.

[126] Greenberg, D. A., "The jaundice of the cell," *Proc Natl Acad Sci U S A*, Vol. 99, 2002, pp. 15837–15839.

[127] Stocker, R., et al., "Bilirubin is an antioxidant of possible physiological importance," *Science*, Vol. 235, 1987, pp. 1043–1046.

[128] McDonagh, A. F., "The role of singlet oxygen in bilirubin photo-oxidation," *Biochem Biophys Res Commun*, Vol. 44, 1971, pp. 1306–1311.

[129] McDonagh, A. F., "Evidence for singlet oxygen quenching by biliverdin IX-alpha dimethyl ester and its relevance to bilirubin photo-oxidation," *Biochem Biophys Res Commun*, Vol. 48, 1972, pp. 408–415.

[130] Vitek, L., and Schwertner, H. A., "The heme catabolic pathway and its protective effects on oxidative stress-mediated diseases," *Adv Clin Chem*, Vol. 43, 2007, pp. 1–57.

[131] Tomaro, M. L., and Batlle, A. M., "Bilirubin: its role in cytoprotection against oxidative stress," *Int J Biochem Cell Biol*, Vol. 34, 2002, pp. 216–220.

[132] Neuzil, J., and Stocker, R., "Bilirubin attenuates radical-mediated damage to serum albumin," *FEBS Lett*, Vol. 331, 1993, pp. 281–284.

[133] Kwak, J. Y., et al., "Bilirubin inhibits the activation of superoxide-producing NADPH oxidase in a neutrophil cell-free system," *Biochim Biophys Acta*, Vol. 1076, 1991, pp. 369–373.

[134] Brouard, S., et al., "Carbon monoxide generated by heme oxygenase 1 suppresses endothelial cell apoptosis," *J Exp Med*, Vol. 192, 2000, pp. 1015–1026.

[135] Balla, G., et al., "Ferritin: a cytoprotective antioxidant strategem of endothelium," *J Biol Chem*, Vol. 267, 1992, pp. 18148–18153.

[136] Otterbein, L. E., et al., "Heme oxygenase-1: unleashing the protective properties of heme," *Trends Immunol*, Vol. 24, 2003, pp. 449–455.

[137] Ferris, C. D., et al., "Haem oxygenase-1 prevents cell death by regulating cellular iron," *Nat Cell Biol*, Vol. 1, 1999, pp. 152–157.

[138] Gomer, C. J., et al., "Increased transcription and translation of heme oxygenase in Chinese hamster fibroblasts following photodynamic stress or Photofrin II incubation," *Photochem Photobiol*, Vol. 53, 1991, pp. 275–279.

[139] Bressoud, D., Jomini, V., and Tyrrell, R. M., "Dark induction of haem oxygenase messenger RNA by haematoporphyrin derivative and zinc phthalocyanine; agents for photodynamic therapy," *J Photochem Photobiol B*, Vol. 14, 1992, pp. 311–318.

[140] Lin, F., and Girotti, A. W., "Hyperresistance of leukemia cells to photodynamic inactivation after long-term exposure to hemin," *Cancer Res*, Vol. 56, 1996, pp. 4636–4643.

[141]   Nowis, D., et al., "Heme oxygenase-1 protects tumor cells against photodynamic therapy-mediated cytotoxicity," *Oncogene*, Vol. 25, 2006, pp. 3365–3374.

[142]   Kocanova, S., et al., "Induction of heme-oxygenase 1 requires the p38MAPK and PI3K pathways and suppresses apoptotic cell death following hypericin-mediated photodynamic therapy," *Apoptosis*, Vol. 12, 2007, pp. 731–741.

[143]   Lin, F., and Girotti, A. W., "Hemin-enhanced resistance of human leukemia cells to oxidative killing: antisense determination of ferritin involvement," *Arch Biochem Biophys*, Vol. 352, 1998, pp. 51–58.

[144]   Young, J. C., et al., "Pathways of chaperone-mediated protein folding in the cytosol," *Nat Rev Mol Cell Biol*, Vol. 5, 2004, pp. 781–791.

[145]   Wang, H. P., et al., "Up-regulation of Hsp27 plays a role in the resistance of human colon carcinoma HT29 cells to photooxidative stress," *Photochem Photobiol*, Vol. 76, 2002, pp. 98–104.

[146]   Jalili, A., et al., "Effective photoimmunotherapy of murine colon carcinoma induced by the combination of photodynamic therapy and dendritic cells," *Clin Cancer Res*, Vol. 10, 2004, pp. 4498–4508.

[147]   Xue, L. Y., He, J., and Oleinick, N. L., "Rapid tyrosine phosphorylation of HS1 in the response of mouse lymphoma L5178Y-R cells to photodynamic treatment sensitized by the phthalocyanine Pc 4," *Photochem Photobiol*, Vol. 66, 1997, pp. 105–113.

[148]   Korbelik, M., Sun, J., and Cecic, I., "Photodynamic therapy-induced cell surface expression and release of heat shock proteins: relevance for tumor response," *Cancer Res*, Vol. 65, 2005, pp. 1018–1026.

[149]   Mitra, S., et al., "Activation of heat shock protein 70 promoter with meso-tetrahydroxyphenyl chlorin photodynamic therapy reported by green fluorescent protein in vitro and in vivo," *Photochem Photobiol*, Vol. 78, 2003, pp. 615–622.

[150]   Hanlon, J. G., et al., "Induction of Hsp60 by Photofrin-mediated photodynamic therapy," *J Photochem Photobiol B*, Vol. 64, 2001, pp. 55–61.

[151]   Nonaka, M., Ikeda, H., and Inokuchi, T., "Inhibitory effect of heat shock protein 70 on apoptosis induced by photodynamic therapy in vitro," *Photochem Photobiol*, Vol. 79, 2004, pp. 94–98.

[152]   Ferrario, A., et al., "Survivin, a member of the inhibitor of apoptosis family, is induced by photodynamic therapy and is a target for improving treatment response," *Cancer Res*, Vol. 67, 2007, pp. 4989–4995.

[153]   Brodsky, J. L., and Chiosis, G., "Hsp70 molecular chaperones: emerging roles in human disease and identification of small molecule modulators," *Curr Top Med Chem*, Vol. 6, 2006, pp. 1215–1225.

[154]   Takayama, S., Reed, J. C., and Homma, S., "Heat-shock proteins as regulators of apoptosis," *Oncogene*, Vol. 22, 2003, pp. 9041–9047.

[155]   Glickman, M. H., and Ciechanover, A., "The ubiquitin-proteasome proteolytic pathway: destruction for the sake of construction," *Physiol Rev*, Vol. 82, 2002, pp. 373–428.

[156]   Voorhees, P. M., and Orlowski, R. Z., "The proteasome and proteasome inhibitors in cancer therapy," *Annu Rev Pharmacol Toxicol*, Vol. 46, 2006, pp. 189–213.

[157]   Richardson, P. G., et al., "Proteasome inhibition in the treatment of cancer," *Cell Cycle*, Vol. 4, 2005, pp. 290–296.

[158]   Petropoulos, I., and Friguet, B., "Protein maintenance in aging and replicative senescence: a role for the peptide methionine sulfoxide reductases," *Biochim Biophys Acta*, Vol. 1703, 2005, pp. 261–266.

[159]   Powell, S. R., et al., "Aggregates of oxidized proteins (lipofuscin) induce apoptosis through proteasome inhibition and dysregulation of proapoptotic proteins," *Free Radic Biol Med*, Vol. 38, 2005, pp. 1093–1101.

[160]   Jung, T., Bader, N., and Grune, T., "Oxidized proteins: intracellular distribution and recognition by the proteasome," *Arch Biochem Biophys*, Vol. 462, 2007, pp. 231–237.

[161] Yorimitsu, T., and Klionsky, D. J., "Autophagy: molecular machinery for self-eating," *Cell Death Differ*, Vol. 12 Suppl 2, 2005, pp. 1542–1552.

[162] Gozuacik, D., and Kimchi, A., "Autophagy as a cell death and tumor suppressor mechanism," *Oncogene*, Vol. 23, 2004, pp. 2891–2906.

[163] Eskelinen, E. L., "Doctor Jekyll and Mister Hyde: autophagy can promote both cell survival and cell death," *Cell Death Differ*, Vol. 12 Suppl 2, 2005, pp. 1468–1472.

[164] Kessel, D., Vicente, M. G., and Reiners, J. J., Jr., "Initiation of apoptosis and autophagy by photodynamic therapy," *Lasers Surg Med*, Vol. 38, 2006, pp. 482–488.

CHAPTER 9

Vascular Targeting in Photodynamic Therapy

Bin Chen, Chong He, Peter de Witte, P. Jack Hoopes, Tayyaba Hasan, and Brian W. Pogue

9.1 Introduction

The mechanism of PDT in cancer treatment is complicated and evolves as our understanding of cancer biology and pharmacology progresses. It is now clear that PDT can either directly kill tumor cells or indirectly induce tumor cell death as a result of direct damage to tumor stroma [1]. Adequate and simultaneous deposition of a photosensitizer, light, and oxygen molecules in tumor cells will cause tumor cell death. However, this direct photocytotoxicity is often limited (generally less than 1-log) in tumor cell killing likely due to inadequate supply of photosensitizers, light, and/or oxygen in tumor tissues [2]. Tumor vasculature is an important target of PDT and this indirect tumor targeting mechanism is mainly responsible for the acute decrease of tumor burden after PDT with most photosensitizers [1]. Furthermore, PDT-induced inflammation as well as direct photosensitizing effects on immune cells may activate the body immune system and lead to the generation of tumor-specific immunity, which is important for maintaining long-term tumor control [3].

For most photosensitizers, vascular damage is the predominant PDT effect and primarily responsible for the final treatment outcome [1]. Because of this, vascular-targeting PDT has been developed to further potentiate vascular damage. In this chapter, we will focus on vascular targeting in PDT. This targeting mechanism has led to so far the most successful application of PDT and is showing great promise in cancer treatment as well. We will discuss photodynamic vascular targeting principle, mechanisms, challenges, and strategies to enhance its therapeutic outcome.

9.2 Tumor Vascular Targeting

It is well known that solid tumors cannot grow larger than about 1 mm^3 without developing a vascular network [4]. This is because, similar to normal tissues, tumor tissues require a functional vascular system for the delivery of nutrients and the removal of metabolic waste. To sustain tumor growth, tumor tissues need to depend upon existing host vessels as well as develop new blood vessels for blood supply. Compared to the normal vasculature, tumor blood vessels exhibit significant abnormalities in vessel architecture (e.g., tortuousity, dilatation, irregular branching, and lack of pericyte and basement membrane coverage) and function (e.g., stagnant blood flow, increased vascular permeability) [5]. Although the mechanisms leading to tumor vessel structural and functional abnormalities are not well understood, the imbalance between pro- and antiangiogenic factors and mechanical compression generated by high tumor interstitial pressure and proliferating tumor cells have been suggested to be the major contributing factors [5]. The differences between tumor versus normal vasculature in the vessel molecular signature, structure, and function provide the basis for selective tumor vascular targeting.

Vascular targeting therapy can be divided into antiangiogenic therapy that inhibits the formation of new vessels and vascular disrupting therapy that targets the existing blood vessels [6]. The overall goal of tumor vascular targeting therapy is to selectively disrupt or modulate tumor vascular function for the therapeutic purposes without affecting much normal tissue functions. This modality can be used alone as monotherapy, but more often it is used in combination with other therapies in cancer treatment. Tumor vascular targeting strategy has several apparent advantages over the conventional tumor cellular targeting approach [4, 7]. First, vascular targets are readily accessible to the therapeutic agents delivered intravenously whereas tumor cellular targets are typically difficult to reach due to the existence of various physiological barriers. Second, vascular targeting is highly efficient and potent in tumor cell killing because, unlike tumor cell-targeted therapies, not all the endothelial cells are necessary to be targeted to disrupt tumor vascular function. Instead, damage to a single endothelial cell or a portion of blood vessel may induce catastrophic effect on tumor perfusion, resulting in killing thousands of tumor cells that are dependent upon that vessel for blood supply. Third, because endothelial cells are generally considered to be more genetically stable than tumor cells, the risk of acquiring drug resistance is usually low. These advantages render tumor vascular targeting a promising approach in current cancer therapy.

9.3 Principle of Photodynamic Vascular Targeting

Photodynamic vascular targeting is based on site-directed delivery of photosensitizing agents to the vascular system followed by light irradiation to induce site-specific vascular photosensitizing effects. Since vasculature-directed photosensitizer delivery can be achieved by passive or active means, photodynamic vascular targeting can be further divided into passive or active targeting approach [1]. The passive vasculature-directed photosensitizer delivery is primarily based on the innate photosensitizer pharmacokinetic property that plasma drug level is often high shortly after intravenous administration of a photosensitizer (Color Plate 4). As can be seen, fluorescence image of hypericin (a) and the corresponding H&E staining photograph (b) demonstrate the intravascular localization of hypericin at 30 minutes after i.v. injection of a 5-mg/kg dose of hypericin in the RIF-1 mouse tumor model. Vascular-targeting PDT with hypericin, (i.e., light treatment at 30 minutes after a 5-mg/kg dose of hypericin injection, caused vascular shutdown in central tumor areas). However, some tumor peripheral blood vessels were still functional, as indicated by the presence of Hoechst dye fluorescence (c), which was injected 1 minute before euthanizing the animal. The corresponding H&E staining image (d) confirmed the vessel histology. Vascular-targeting PDT with hypericin (i.e., light treatment at 30 minutes after a 1-mg/kg dose of hypericin injection), significantly inhibited the RIF tumor growth and its antitumor effect was further enhanced by subcutaneous injection of antiangiogenic drug TNP-470 at a dose of 30 mg/kg once every 2 days. Each group included 8 to 10 animals (Figure 9.1).

This time period when photosensitizer is mainly localized inside the vasculature provides a temporal window for the passive vascular targeting. Although the exact location of this temporal window is largely dependent on the plasma kinetics of individual photosensitizer, for most photosensitizers it typically occurs within 60 minutes after injection.

By contrast, active vascular-targeting PDT seeks to achieve vasculature-directed drug delivery by altering photosensitizer pharmacokinetic property through drug structure modification or drug formulation into a targeted delivery system [1]. A targeting moiety that has a high affinity to endothelial cell markers (e.g., integrins, VEGF receptors, tumor endothelial markers) or vessel supporting structures (e.g., fibronectin with ED-B domain) is often used in the photosensitizer modification. The resulting photosensitizer conjugates are expected to be selectively accumulated in the targeted blood vessels, leading to a site-specific photosensitization upon light activation.

9.4   Mechanisms of Photodynamic Vascular Targeting

Photodynamic vascular targeting therapy has been shown to produce reactive oxygen species intravascularly, in particular singlet oxygen, which is believed to be mainly responsible for the subsequent vessel structural and functional alterations [8]. The ultimate goal of vascular-targeting PDT in cancer therapy is to obtain maximal tumor cell killing by inducing tumor vascular shutdown. The mechanism of

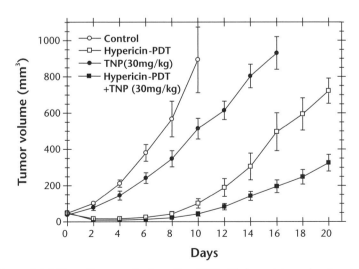

Figure 9.1   Tumor inhibition after vascular-targeting PDT with hypericin and antiangiogenic drug TNP-470.

PDT-induced vascular shutdown is complicated because it likely involves multiple targets in the blood cells and blood vessels, which are interweaved in complex cascades of events. Intravital fluorescence microscopic study demonstrates that microcirculation dysfunction after vascular-targeting PDT is induced by at least two vascular events, vessel occlusion induced by thrombus formation and vessel constriction/collapse caused by mechanic compression and vasoactive substances (Figure 9.2(a) and (b)).

Thrombus formation can be induced by photosensitizing damage to either blood cells or endothelial cells. It has been shown that PDT can cause platelet aggregation and thrombus formation by direct damage to the platelet and red blood cell membranes [9, 10]. Damage to the platelets may further stimulate the release of thromboxane, a vasoactive substance with potent vessel constriction and thrombus formation effects [11]. More often, PDT-induced damage to the blood cells is coupled with damage to the endothelial cells, which might explain why blood cell aggregation is often observed starting from the vessel wall. Since endothelium serves as an interface between blood and underneath tissue, loss of endothelial barrier as a result of vascular photosensitization exposes tissue extracellular matrix to the circulation, which activates platelets and polymorphonuclear leukocytes and induces blood cell adherence to the damaged endothelial cells. Thromboxane release as a result of platelet activation has been shown to contribute significantly to vessel constriction and thrombus formation, which can be inhibited by thromboxane inhibitors aspirin and indomethacin [12] or platelet depletion [11]. Endothelial cells also

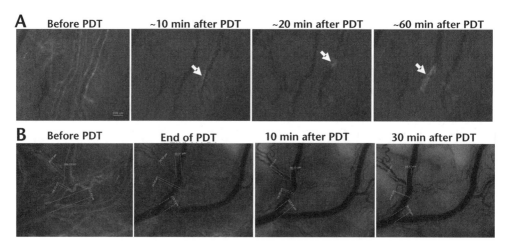

Figure 9.2 (a) Intravital fluorescence microscopic images showing intravascular localization of verteporfin and thrombus formation after vascular-targeting PDT in the orthotopic MatLyLu rat prostate tumor. Rat blood cells were labeled with fluorescent dye DiI and injected (i.v.) into the animals to highlight blood vessels. The MatLyLu tumors were treated with 50-J/cm^2 light (690 nm, at 50 mW/cm^2) at 15 minutes after i.v. injection of 0.25-mg/kg verteporfin to target tumor blood vessels. Blood cell adherence and thrombus formation, indicated by arrows, were clearly visible after vascular-targeting PDT. (b) Intravital fluorescence microscopic imaging of vascular permeability increase and vessel compression after vascular-targeting PDT with verteporfin. Animals were i.v. injected with 10-mg/kg 2,000-kDa FITC-dextran right before irradiation and imaged every 2 minutes for the FITC fluorescence during and after PDT. The images shown are right before PDT, immediately, 10 minutes, and 30 minutes after PDT. Sizes of some blood vessels are labeled on the images.

influence blood clotting balance by releasing von Willebrand factor that facilitates thrombus formation [13] and prostacyclin that inhibits thrombus formation and dilates blood vessels [14]. The net effect likely favors clot formation at least at early stage after vascular photosensitization. Blood clots formed inside vessel lumen cause obstruction to blood flow. However, blood vessels may resume perfusion because not all the clots are stable and some of them can be dissolved and dislodged possibly by body anticoagulants. Only the stable thrombi will finally occlude blood vessels and shut down vascular function. Inhibition of thrombus formation by heparin has been shown to delay PDT-induced blood flow stasis [15]. But it is not able to completely inhibit blood flow decrease, suggesting that thrombus formation is only partially responsible for the vascular damage induced by PDT.

As a spontaneous response to blood vessel damages, vessel constriction is often observed after vascular photosensitization, which also contributes to PDT-induced blood flow stasis (Figure 9.3).

Vessel constriction can be caused by the release of vasoactive substances such as thromboxane and leukotrienes [16]. However, a strong inducer of vessel constriction and even collapse in tumor tissues comes from the increase of interstitial fluid pressure [5]. It is well-established that tumor tissues generally have higher tissue interstitial pressure than the normal tissues because of leaky tumor blood vessels. The mechanic compression generated by high tumor interstitial pressure can collapse tumor blood vessel even without treatment and this is one of the mechanisms involved in acute hypoxia development in tumor tissues [17]. Such vessel compression/collapse effects are aggravated by PDT because PDT is able to cause vascular barrier disruption and therefore further increase tumor interstitial pressure [18, 19].

Since endothelial cells play a critical role in maintaining vascular barrier and perfusion functions, it is important to study how endothelial cells respond to photosensitization at cellular and molecular levels. Studies with different photosensitizers have shown that photosensitization of endothelial cells induces rapid microtubule

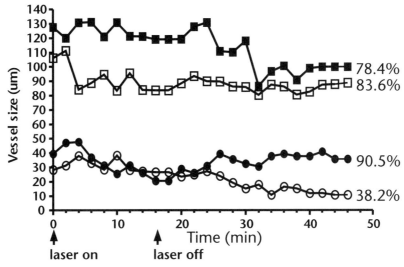

Figure 9.3   The change of blood vessel size during and after vascular-targeting PDT with verteporfin. Sizes of four blood vessels shown in Figure 9.2b were measured and the percentages over pretreatment sizes are shown.

depolymerization followed by stress fiber actin formation and cell rounding [20, 21].

Although it is not clear how microtubule damage results in endothelial cell shape change, microtubule depolymerization is believed to initiate subsequent vessel functional changes because endothelial cell barrier function is dependent on endothelial cell morphology regulated by cell cytoskeleton. Indeed, photosensitization-induced endothelial cell shape change has been shown to be correlated to the permeability increase [21]. Increase in cytosol calcium concentration has been suggested to be the cause of microtubule depolymerization [20]. However, direct photosensitizing damage to the microtubules cannot be ruled out. Vascular permeability increase has been observed in both animal and human studies shortly after PDT [16, 22], suggesting that this is an early event following endothelial cell damage (Figure 9.4).

The disruption of vascular barrier function will trigger the subsequent thrombus formation and vessel compression as described above.

The molecular mechanism involved in endothelial photosensitization is poorly studied. There are reports showing that photosensitization activates nuclear transcriptor NF-κB in endothelial cells through a reactive oxygen species-mediated mechanism [23, 24]. Since NF-κB is major regulator of inflammatory and immune reactions, its activation in endothelial cells plays an important role in vascular photosensitization-induced tumor destruction. Paradoxically, NF-κB activation can cause both tumor inhibition and stimulation [25]. Tumor inhibition is related to its role in enhancing gene expression of cytokines (IL-6, TNF-α), adhesion molecules (intercellular adhesion molecule-1, vascular cell adhesion molecule-1), and possibly heat shock proteins [24, 26]. As a result, vascular photosensitization treatment is able to stimulate blood cells, especially neutrophils adhesion to the endothelial cells, inducing vascular damages. On the other hand, tumor stimulation as a consequence of NF-κB activation is associated with the upregulation of cyclooxygenas-2 (COX-2), matrix metalloproteases (MMPs), and inhibitors of apoptosis [25]. Although there is no report demonstrating the upregulation of COX-2 and

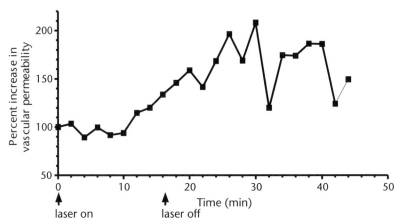

Figure 9.4 The change of vascular permeability during and after vascular-targeting PDT with verteporfin. Vascular permeability change was determined by measuring the 2,000-kDa FITC-dextran fluorescence intensity from the above intravital microscopic images Figure 9.2(b), and normalizing the aftertreatment intensity values to the pretreatment value.

apoptosis inhibitors in endothelial cells, which has been shown in tumor cells, the induction of MMP-9 expression has been confirmed in endothelial cells after PDT, suggesting a role of NF-κB activation in endothelial resistance to photosensitization [25]. Interestingly, pretreatment of endothelial cells with PDT or other oxidative stress inducers has been shown to induce cell adaptation, resulting in the upregulation of heat shock protein and antioxidation enzymes through the p38 MARK pathway. This cellular adaptation to the oxidative stressors indeed renders endothelial cells' resistance to the subsequent treatment [27].

9.5   Therapeutic Challenges of Photodynamic Vascular Targeting

Although vascular-targeting PDT is able to induce extensive tumor vascular shutdown, and consequently, tumor cell death, functional blood vessels are typically detected at tumor peripheral areas following noncurative treatments. The existence of these functional blood vessels can lead to tumor recurrence, which is often observed starting from the peripheral tumor area [28, 29]. Figure 9.5 shows representative tumor fluorescence images after verteporfin-PDT.

In this experiment, we used a lentivirus-transduced MatLyLu prostate tumor cell line that permanently expresses EGFP. The EGFP-MatLyLu tumors were imaged noninvasively for the EGFP fluorescence before and after PDT by using a whole-body fluorescence imaging system. Because dead EGFP-MatLyLu tumor cells were not able to produce EGFP, dead tumor tissues would appear as dark areas and only viable tumor tissues could be visible on tumor EGFP fluorescence images. Control tumors grew rapidly and generally exhibited central necrosis when a tumor reached about 8 to 10 mm in diameter. The 50-J/cm^2 PDT was effective in eradicating tumor tissue and little EGFP fluorescence was detected by 2 days after PDT. However, small EGFP fluorescent spots, indicating the existence of viable tumor cells, were detected at tumor edges several days after treatment. Peripheral viable tumor tissues were found growing rapidly, leading to tumor recurrence.

It is still not clear why tumor peripheral and central blood vessels react differently to the vascular photosensitization. It is hypothesized that such a variation in vascular response is likely related to the differences in tumor interstitial pressure and the structure of blood vessels in tumor central versus peripheral areas. Because

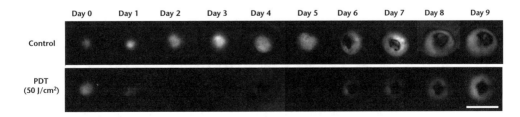

Figure 9.5   Noninvasive fluorescence imaging of tumor response after vascular-targeting PDT with verteporfin. The EGFP-MatLyLu tumors were imaged with a whole-body fluorescence imaging system before and after the vascular-targeting PDT, showing tumor recurrence starting from 3 days after treatment. Images of control tumor receiving no treatment are also shown for comparison. Bar=10 mm.

the tumor central area generally has a higher interstitial pressure than the peripheral area, central blood vessels are more likely to collapse than the peripheral vessels as a result of higher mechanic compression [30, 31]. Moreover, peripheral tumor blood vessels are generally found to be larger and have more vessel supporting structures such as pericytes than the central tumor vessels (Figure 9.6).

Collectively, less tumor interstitial pressure together with more vessel supporting structures might make peripheral tumor vessels more resistant to the vessel compression/collapse imposed by PDT-induced tumor interstitial pressure elevation. Survival of these peripheral blood vessels after vascular photosensitization provides a chance of survival to the tumor cells supported by these vessels.

To maintain tissue integrity and function, biological systems develop sets of well-balanced repairing and adaptive mechanisms to deal with various internal and external damages. Through complicated and often redundant signaling cascades, cells are able to survive nonfatal damages by stimulating cell growth, tissue angiogenesis, and remodeling. Unfortunately, tumor endothelial and tumor cells can hijack these spontaneous responses to obtain their own survival after subcurative treatments, leading to disease recurrence. As mentioned above, photosensitization activates p38 MAPK survival signaling in endothelial cells [27]. The activation of p38 MARK is able to further induce the upregulation of COX-2, which catalyzes the conversion of arachidonic acid to prostaglandins (PGs) [32, 33]. PGs, especially PGE2, have been shown to enhance cell motility, adhesion, and survival, and stimulate tumor angiogenesis by inducing VEGF release. Furthermore, elevated VEGF release can also be obtained via HIF-1-mediated signaling pathway activated by PDT-induced tissue hypoxia [34, 35]. Through the activation of these self-repairing and surviving pathways, tumor endothelial and tumor cells actually create a favorable microenvironment to maintain their survival and growth. It is not unusual to observe that tumor cells after subcurative PDT treatments are actually becoming

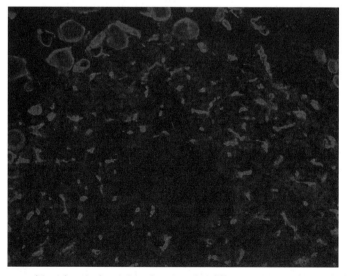

Figure 9.6 Immunohistochemical staining showing the difference in vessel morphology and structure between tumor peripheral and central blood vessels. Blood vessel pericyte marker α-small muscle actin (α-SMA) staining indicates that peripheral vessels are generally bigger and have better pericyte coverage than central vessels. Note the existence of central necrosis.

more aggressive [35, 36]. In the end, noncurative treatments might unintentionally select a small population of cells that are good at manipulating normal physiological pathways to survive therapeutic stressors. Therefore, how to target cell survival signals and adaptation mechanisms represents a major therapeutic challenge for not only photodynamic vascular targeting, but also all other cancer therapies.

9.6   Current Status of Photodynamic Vascular Targeting

Passive vascular-targeting PDT provides an effective way of targeting blood vessels and has been successfully translated into clinical application for diseases characterized by the overproliferation of blood vessels. Based on this mechanism, verteporfin is currently being used for the treatment of age-related macular degeneration (AMD) and more photosensitizers such as tin ethyletiopurpurin (SnET2, Purlytin) and lutetium texaphyrin (Lu-Tex, Optrin) are under clinical trials for AMD. Quite a few photosensitizers have also been evaluated for cancer treatment based on this passive targeting mechanism [1]. Among these photosensitizes, Tookad is at the forefront in the development pipeline. Currently, Tookad is in a phase I/II clinical trial for locally recurrent prostate cancer after radiation therapy [37]. Although limited in the number of studies, active vascular-targeting PDT is being pursued actively for the treatment of cancer and noncancer diseases. Promising results have been obtained from several studies of conjugating photosensitizers to the blood vessel-homing peptides [38–42].

9.7   Strategies to Enhance Photodynamic Vascular Targeting

As combination therapy has been routinely used in cancer treatment, one approach of enhancing photodynamic vascular targeting efficacy is to combine it with other cancer therapies. Combination therapies can be designed based on several different targeting principles. Targeting both tumor vascular and cellular compartments by combining photodynamic vascular targeting therapy with a cancer cell-targeted therapy has been demonstrated to be an effective strategy. For instance, more than additive antitumor effects have been obtained from most early studies exploring the combination of PDT and cancer chemotherapy [43, 44]. Recently, PDT itself has been studied for targeting tumor blood vessels or tumor cells, and enhanced therapeutic effects have been reported from studies with combined PDT regimens that target both tumor compartments. These dual targeting PDT treatments include PDT using a vascular-targeting photosensitizer Photofrin in combination with PDT using a cellular-targeting photosensitizer 5-aminolevulinic acid (5-ALA) [45], PDT regimen based on photosensitizer dose fractionation protocol so that light can be delivered when photosensitizer has been deposited in both vascular and cellular compartments [46], and sequential combination of a cancer cell-targeted PDT followed by a blood vessel-targeted PDT [28].

Although the mechanisms responsible for such enhanced antitumor effects are still not clear, spatial cooperation in tumor cell killing between vascular-targeting PDT and cancer cell-targeted therapies possibly plays a role here. As mentioned above, vascular-targeting PDT is especially effective in inducing central tumor cell death. Cancer cell-targeted therapies however mainly kill peripheral PDT tumor cells because most anticancer agents, including photosensitizers, tend to accumulate more at the tumor periphery presumably because of better perfusion at tumor peripheral areas [47, 48]. Thus, cancer cell-targeted therapies may complement vascular-targeting PDT in reducing some peripheral tumor cells that are otherwise not able to be killed by vascular-targeting PDT. The other mechanism possibly involved in the therapeutic enhancement is that both conventional and vascular-targeting PDT treatments have been shown to improve drug delivery to tumor tissues as a result of PDT-induced vascular permeability increase [21, 49]. Interestingly, we have found that such an enhancement in tumor drug delivery caused by vascular-targeting PDT is actually more pronounced in the tumor peripheral area than in the tumor central area (observation not yet published). The overall increase of the anticancer agent in the tumor tissue, tumor peripheral areas in particular, after vascular-targeting PDT may also account for the improved antitumor effect.

The other important combination strategy is to target the surviving and repairing pathways that tumor endothelial cells as well as tumor cells depend on to maintain their survival after vascular-targeting PDT. An example in this case is the combination of vascular-targeting PDT with antiangiogenic therapy. PDT treatments have been found to stimulate angiogenesis and tumor growth by inducing VEGF upregulation [34, 35]. Depending on the photosensitizer, the type of tumor model, and treatment conditions, the elevation of VEGF can be caused by hypoxia-induced HIF-1 activation [34], COX-2 overexpression [33, 50] and p38 MAPK activation [35]. Thus, combined treatments of PDT with VEGF antibody bevacizumab [51], antiangiogenic drug TNP-470 [52] or COX-2 inhibitor [50] have all been shown to enhance the therapeutic effects. As our understanding regarding tumor/endothelial cell adaptation to therapeutic stressors increases, more such rationale-designed combination regimens will be designed to target crucial cellular and molecular surviving pathways, leading to a synergistic treatment outcome.

9.8 Summary and Conclusions

Vascular damage is the most important mechanism involved in PDT-mediated tumor eradication. Vascular-targeting PDT is designed to further strengthen this vascular photosensitization effect by site-directed delivery of photosensitizing agents to the vascular targets. Being so far the most successful PDT regimen, vascular-targeting PDT has been used clinically in the management of AMD and is showing great promise in cancer treatment as well. However, spatial heterogeneity in the vascular response and tumor/endothelial cell adaptation to the oxidative and hypoxic stressors often result in tumor recurrence. Therefore, a combination therapy with modalities complementary to the vascular-targeting PDT in tumor cell killing or treatments targeting cell surviving and adaptive signaling pathways often shows better results than vascular-targeting PDT alone. These combination regimens should be further evaluated in the clinic. Equally important, we need to further understand the mechanism of vascular-targeting PDT at tissue, cellular, and molecular levels. It is obvious that 100% tumor cure can be achieved in preclinical animal tumor models with photodynamic vascular targeting therapies. The question is whether it is possible to deliver such curative, rather than subcurative, vascular-targeting PDT to the patients, and how.

Acknowledgments

This work was supported by Department of Defense (DOD) Prostate Cancer Research Grant W81XWH-06-1-0148. The authors would like to gratefully acknowledge QLT Inc. for providing verteporfin.

References

[1] Chen, B., et al., "Vascular and cellular targeting for photodynamic therapy," *Crit Rev Eukaryot Gene Expr*, Vol. 16, 2006, pp. 279–305.

[2] Henderson, B. W., and Dougherty, T. J., "How does photodynamic therapy work?" *Photochem Photobiol*, Vol. 55, 1992, pp. 145–157.

[3] Canti, G., De Simone, A., and Korbelik, M., "Photodynamic therapy and the immune system in experimental oncology," *Photochem Photobiol Sci*, Vol. 1, 2002, pp. 79–80.

[4] Siemann, D. W., Chaplin, D. J., and Horsman, M. R., "Vascular-targeting therapies for treatment of malignant disease," *Cancer*, Vol. 100, 2004, pp. 2491–2499.

[5] Fukumura, D., and Jain, R. K., "Tumor microenvironment abnormalities: causes, consequences, and strategies to normalize," *J Cell Biochem*, Vol. 101, 2007, pp. 937–949.

[6] Siemann, D. W., et al., "Differentiation and definition of vascular-targeted therapies," *Clin Cancer Res*, Vol. 11, 2005, pp. 416–420.

[7] Thorpe, P. E., "Vascular targeting agents as cancer therapeutics," *Clin Cancer Res*, Vol. 10, 2004, pp. 415–427.

[8] Gross, S., et al., "Monitoring photodynamic therapy of solid tumors online by BOLD-contrast MRI," *Nat Med*, Vol. 9, 2003, pp. 1327–1331.

[9] Fingar, V. H., Wieman, T. J., and Haydon, P. S., "The effects of thrombocytopenia on vessel stasis and macromolecular leakage after photodynamic therapy using photofrin," *Photochem Photobiol*, Vol. 66, 1997, pp. 513–517.

[10] Ben-Hur, E., et al., "Photodynamic treatment of red blood cell concentrates for virus inactivation enhances red blood cell aggregation: protection with antioxidants," *Photochem Photobiol*, Vol. 66, 1997, pp. 509–512.

[11] Fingar, V. H., Wieman, T. J., and Doak, K. W., "Role of thromboxane and prostacyclin release on photodynamic therapy-induced tumor destruction," *Cancer Res*, Vol. 50, 1990, pp. 2599–2603.

[12] Reed, M. W., et al., "The microvascular effects of photodynamic therapy: evidence for a possible role of cyclooxygenase products," *Photochem Photobiol*, Vol. 50, 1989, pp. 419–423.

[13] Foster, T. H., et al., "Photosensitized release of von Willebrand factor from cultured human endothelial cells," *Cancer Res*, Vol. 51, 1991, pp. 3261–3266.

[14] Henderson, B. W., et al., "Effects of photodynamic treatment of platelets or endothelial cells in vitro on platelet aggregation," *Photochem Photobiol*, Vol. 56, 1992, pp. 513–521.

[15] Dolmans, D. E., et al., "Vascular accumulation of a novel photosensitizer, MV6401, causes selective thrombosis in tumor vessels after photodynamic therapy," *Cancer Res*, Vol. 62, 2002, pp. 2151–2156.

[16] Fingar, V. H., "Vascular effects of photodynamic therapy," *J Clin Laser Med Surg*, Vol. 14, 1996, pp. 323–328.

[17] Vaupel, P., and Mayer, A., "Hypoxia in cancer: significance and impact on clinical out-come," *Cancer Metastasis Rev*, Vol. 26, 2007, pp. 225–239.

[18] Fingar, V. H., Wieman, T. J., and Doak, K. W., "Changes in tumor interstitial pressure induced by photodynamic therapy," *Photochem Photobiol*, Vol. 53, 1991, pp. 763–768.

[19] Leunig, M., et al., "Photodynamic therapy-induced alterations in interstitial fluid pressure, volume and water content of an amelanotic melanoma in the hamster," *Br J Cancer*, Vol. 69, 1994, pp. 101–103.

[20] Sporn, L. A., and Foster, T. H., "Photofrin and light induces microtubule depolymerization in cultured human endothelial cells," *Cancer Res*, Vol. 52, 1992, pp. 3443–3448.

[21] Chen, B., et al., "Tumor vascular permeabilization by vascular-targeting photosensitiza-tion: effects, mechanism, and therapeutic implications," *Clin Cancer Res*, Vol. 12, 2006, pp. 917–923.

[22] Schmidt-Erfurth, U., et al., "Time course and morphology of vascular effects associated with photodynamic therapy," *Ophthalmology*, Vol. 112, 2005, pp. 2061–2069.

[23] Volanti, C., Matroule, J. Y., and Piette, J., "Involvement of oxidative stress in NF-kappaB activation in endothelial cells treated by photodynamic therapy," *Photochem Photobiol*, Vol. 75, 2002, pp. 36–45.

[24] Volanti, C., et al., "Downregulation of ICAM-1 and VCAM-1 expression in endothelial cells treated by photodynamic therapy," *Oncogene*, Vol. 23, 2004, pp. 8649–8658.

[25] Matroule, J. Y., Volanti, C., and Piette, J., "NF-kappaB in photodynamic therapy: discrep-ancies of a master regulator," *Photochem Photobiol*, Vol. 82, 2006, pp. 1241–1246.

[26] Korbelik, M., Sun, J., and Cecic, I., "Photodynamic therapy-induced cell surface expres-sion and release of heat shock proteins: relevance for tumor response," *Cancer Res*, Vol. 65, 2005, pp. 1018–1026.

[27] Plaks, V., et al., "Homologous adaptation to oxidative stress induced by the photosensi-tized Pd-bacteriochlorophyll derivative (WST11) in cultured endothelial cells," *J Biol Chem*, Vol. 279, 2004, pp. 45713–45720.

[28] Chen, B., et al., "Combining vascular and cellular targeting regimens enhances the efficacy of photodynamic therapy," *Int J Radiat Oncol Biol Phys*, Vol. 61, 2005, pp. 1216–1226.

[29] Chen, B., Roskams, T., and de Witte, P. A., "Antivascular tumor eradication by hypericin-mediated photodynamic therapy," *Photochem Photobiol*, Vol. 76, 2002, pp. 509–513.

[30] Boucher, Y., and Jain, R. K., "Microvascular pressure is the principal driving force for interstitial hypertension in solid tumors: implications for vascular collapse," *Cancer Res*, Vol. 52, 1992, pp. 5110–5114.

[31] Rofstad, E. K., et al., "Pulmonary and lymph node metastasis is associated with primary tumor interstitial fluid pressure in human melanoma xenografts," *Cancer Res*, Vol. 62, 2002, pp. 661–664.

[32] Hendrickx, N., et al., "Up-regulation of cyclooxygenase-2 and apoptosis resistance by p38 MAPK in hypericin-mediated photodynamic therapy of human cancer cells," *J Biol Chem*, Vol. 278, 2003, pp. 52231–52239.

[33] Hendrickx, N., et al., "Targeted inhibition of p38alpha MAPK suppresses tumor-associated endothelial cell migration in response to hypericin-based photodynamic therapy," *Biochem Biophys Res Commun*, Vol. 337, 2005, pp. 928–935.

[34] Ferrario, A., et al., "Antiangiogenic treatment enhances photodynamic therapy responsive-ness in a mouse mammary carcinoma," *Cancer Res*, Vol. 60, 2000, pp. 4066–4069.

[35] Solban, N., et al., "Mechanistic investigation and implications of photodynamic therapy induction of vascular endothelial growth factor in prostate cancer," *Cancer Res*, Vol. 66, 2006, pp. 5633–5640.

[36] Momma, T., et al., "Photodynamic therapy of orthotopic prostate cancer with benzoporphyrin derivative: local control and distant metastasis," *Cancer Res*, Vol. 58, 1998, pp. 5425–5431.

[37]   Pinthus, J. H., et al., "Photodynamic therapy for urological malignancies: past to current approaches," *J Urol*, Vol. 175, 2006, pp. 1201–1207.

[38]   Birchler, M., et al., "Selective targeting and photocoagulation of ocular angiogenesis mediated by a phage-derived human antibody fragment," *Nat Biotechnol*, Vol. 17, 1999, pp. 984–988.

[39]   Tirand, L., et al., "A peptide competing with VEGF165 binding on neuropilin-1 mediates targeting of a chlorin-type photosensitizer and potentiates its photodynamic activity in human endothelial cells," *J Control Release*, Vol. 111, 2006, pp. 153–164.

[40]   Ichikawa, K., et al., "Antiangiogenic photodynamic therapy (PDT) by using long-circulating liposomes modified with peptide specific to angiogenic vessels," *Biochim Biophys Acta*, Vol. 1669, 2005, pp. 69–74.

[41]   Reddy, G. R., et al., "Vascular targeted nanoparticles for imaging and treatment of brain tumors," *Clin Cancer Res*, Vol. 12, 2006, pp. 6677–6686.

[42]   Frochot, C., et al., "Interest of RGD-containing linear or cyclic peptide targeted tetraphenylchlorin as novel photosensitizers for selective photodynamic activity," *Bioorg Chem*, Vol. 35, 2007, pp. 205–220.

[43]   Streckyte, G., et al., "Effects of photodynamic therapy in combination with Adriamycin," *Cancer Lett*, Vol. 146, 1999, pp. 73–86.

[44]   Ma, L. W., et al., "Enhanced antitumour effect of photodynamic therapy by microtubule inhibitors," *Cancer Lett*, Vol. 109, 1996, pp. 129–139.

[45]   Peng, Q., et al., "Antitumor effect of 5-aminolevulinic acid-mediated photodynamic therapy can be enhanced by the use of a low dose of photofrin in human tumor xenografts," *Cancer Res*, Vol. 61, 2001, pp. 5824–5832.

[46]   Dolmans, D. E., et al., "Targeting tumor vasculature and cancer cells in orthotopic breast tumor by fractionated photosensitizer dosing photodynamic therapy," *Cancer Res*, Vol. 62, 2002, pp. 4289–4294.

[47]   Jain, R. K., "Delivery of molecular medicine to solid tumors: lessons from in vivo imaging of gene expression and function," *J Control Release*, Vol. 74, 2001, pp. 7–25.

[48]   Pogue, B. W., et al., "Analysis of sampling volume and tissue heterogeneity on the in vivo detection of fluorescence," *J Biomed Opt*, Vol. 10, 2005, pp. 41206.

[49]   Snyder, J. W., et al., "Photodynamic therapy: a means to enhanced drug delivery to tumors," *Cancer Res*, Vol. 63, 2003, pp. 8126–8131.

[50]   Ferrario, A., et al., "Cyclooxygenase-2 inhibitor treatment enhances photodynamic therapy-mediated tumor response," *Cancer Res*, Vol. 62, 2002, pp. 3956–3961.

[51]   Ferrario, A., and Gomer, C. J., "Avastin enhances photodynamic therapy treatment of Kaposi's sarcoma in a mouse tumor model," *J Environ Pathol Toxicol Oncol*, Vol. 25, 2006, pp. 251–259.

[52]   Kosharskyy, B., et al., "A mechanism-based combination therapy reduces local tumor growth and metastasis in an orthotopic model of prostate cancer," *Cancer Res*, Vol. 66, 2006, pp. 10953–10958.

CHAPTER 10

Covalent Photosensitizer Conjugates, Part 1: Antibodies and Other Proteins for Targeted Photodynamic Therapy

Michael R. Hamblin

10.1 Introduction: Photosensitizer Delivery Strategies

Photodynamic therapy (PDT) has inherent dual selectivity due to control of light delivery and to some extent selective photosensitizer (PS) accumulation in tumors. Since the original observation of tumor localizing ability of HPD, many workers have investigated the mechanism of this tendency of PS to preferentially localize in tumors and other specific organs and tissues. There has been much effort made to determine which factors in the chemical structures of the PS are optimal for maximizing the selectivity for the tumor over normal tissue and organs. This has proved quite complicated because the pharmacokinetics can vary dramatically.

One of the particular properties of tetrapyrrole PSs relevant to their tumor localizing ability, is their tendency to bind strongly to serum proteins and to each other. This means that most PSs when injected into the bloodstream behave as macromolecules either because they are more or less firmly bound to large protein molecules or because they have formed intermolecular aggregates of similar size. Many workers have reported on the distribution of PSs between the various classes of serum proteins when mixed with serum in vitro. These are usually divided into albumin and other heavy proteins, high-density lipoprotein (HDL), low-density lipoprotein (LDL), and very low-density lipoprotein (VLDL). It has been argued that PSs that preferentially bind to LDL are better tumor localizers because cancer cells overexpress the LDL (apolipoprotein B/E) receptors. Upregulation of the expression of LDL receptors is one way that rapidly growing malignant cells gain cholesterol necessary for the biosynthesis of lipids needed for the rapid turnover of cellular membranes.

It is useful to make a distinction between selective accumulation and selective retention. The tumor localizing ability of the PS with the faster pharmacokinetics is probably due to selective accumulation in the tumor, while the localization of PS with slower acting pharmacokinetics is more likely due to selective retention. In the selective accumulation model it is thought that the increased vascular permeability to macromolecules typical of tumor neovasculature is chiefly responsible for the preferential extravasation of the PS. These quick-acting PSs frequently bind to albumin, which is of ideal size and Stokes radius to pass through the "pores" in the endothelium of the tumor microvessels. The selective retention of PSs in tumors has been the subject of much speculation. One is that tumors have poorly developed lymphatic drainage, and that macromolecules, which extravasate from the hyperpermeable tumor neovasculature, are retained in the extravascular space. Another involves the macrophages, which infiltrate solid tumors to varying extents. These tumor-associated macrophages have been shown to accumulate up to 13 times the amount of some PSs compared to cancer cells either due to the phagocytosis of aggregates of PSs or the preferential uptake by macrophages of lipoproteins, which have been altered by the binding of porphyrins. Another theory proposes that the low pH commonly found in tumors has the effect of trapping some of the anionic PSs, which are ionized at normal physiological pH. These PS then become neutrally charged and hence more lipophilic when they encounter the lowered pH in the tumor environment.

After experience with treating tumors with PDT using HPD or PF and even newer second generation PS was accumulated, it was realized that in most cases there was suboptimal tumor selectivity. This lack of selectivity is especially important when the intention is to treat multifocal or disseminated disease in a body cavity such as the urinary bladder or the peritoneal cavity and where the use of light delivery to increase selectivity may not be possible. For these applications it may be necessary to achieve higher tumor selectivity by targeting the PS. This generally involves using a targeting vehicle (frequently a macromolecule) to which the PS is covalently attached, and which is recognized by some molecular determinant that is expressed or overexpressed on the target.

In this chapter and Chapter 11 I will discuss several applications of this approach. In the first part I will cover monoclonal antibodies that recognize tumor-associated antigens, and proteins that bind to receptors on particular tumor types. Protein conjugates that target macrophage scavenger receptors will also be discussed. In the second part I will cover polymer-PS conjugates and PSs that can be cleaved from their macromolecular scaffold by enzymes overexpressed in tumors. Conjugates between PSs and small molecules such as vitamins, steroids, or sugars can also be designed to improve cell type-specific targeting. These examples of the use of rationally designed PS-conjugates illustrate a new approach to optimizing PDT and may allow PDT to be applied in hitherto unexplored diseases.

10.2   Monoclonal Antibody PS Conjugates

One of the earliest attempts to actively target PSs to tumors was to take advantage of the development of a number of monoclonal antibodies (Mabs) that recognize human tumor-associated antigens by covalently joining the PS to the IgG molecule in the expectation that the resulting photoimmunoconjugate (PIC) would preferentially deliver the PS to the tumor. The advantages claimed for this approach include those specific to Mabs (high specificity and affinity for their target antigens) and those specific for PS (nontoxic to normal tissues that do not receive light). Because relatively large quantities of immunoconjugates can accumulate in organs such as liver and kidneys, there can be toxicity to normal organs when the cytotoxic moiety is a radioisotope or a protein toxin, but this is avoided if these organs do not receive light. It was thought that in contrast to immunoconjugates with toxin molecules and cytotoxic drugs, PICs could be active if they bound to the plasma membranes of tumor cells, since the reactive species generated upon illumination could diffuse into the cells and produce fatal damage. However, it is now thought that PICs will kill cells more efficiently if they are internalized. In contrast to Mab-toxin or Mab-radionuclide conjugates, photoimmunotargeting requires conjugates with high PS-to-Mab ratios, which makes the synthesis and purification complicated. The goal of any such synthesis should be to retain features essential for both PS and antibody activities and at the same time allow maximal PS incorporation.

Two basic approaches for the synthesis of PICs have been used (Figure 10.1):

1. PSs are linked chemically to Mabs directly; usually by reaction with primary amino groups present on the Mab;
2. PSs are linked to Mabs via polymers or other macromolecular linkers, often to different regions of the Mab.

10.2.1 Direct Antibody-PS Conjugates

One of the first reports [1] conjugated hematoporphyrin to Mabs that recognized the DBA/2J murine myosarcoma M-1. Administration of anti-M-1-HP conjugates i.v. to M-1 tumor-bearing animals followed by exposure to incandescent light resulted in suppression of M-1 growth. The growth-inhibiting properties of the conjugate were M-1-specific; it had no effect on the growth of a C57BL/6J lymphoma EL4 and conjugates made with a nonspecific monoclonal antibody did not have any specific antitumor effect on M-1 growth. Treatment with equivalent doses of

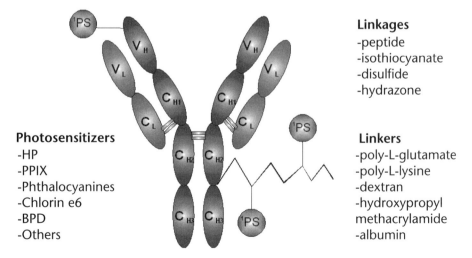

Figure 10.1 Schematic description of the components of the PS-immunoconjugate and examples of antigen targets, linkers, and linkages.

hematoporphyrin or antibody had no significant inhibiting effect on tumor growth. This group of workers then covalently linked Mab (B16G), which recognizes a constant epitope on suppressor T-cells (TsC) to HP, and injected the conjugate i.v. into P815 tumor-bearing mice that were subsequently exposed to light [2]. Tumors underwent permanent regression in 10% to 40% of these mice, while all control animals died within an average of 22 to 24 days after tumor cell injection. It was suggested that tumor regression was facilitated by the elimination of a population of TsC. The B16G-Hp conjugate was capable in vitro of specifically killing cells of a TsC hybridoma, A10. This conjugate had no cytotoxic effect on P815 cells under conditions in which A10 cells were killed.

Donald et al. [3] used the Mab UCD/AB 6.01 conjugated with HpD killed A-431 squamous cell carcinoma cells in vitro, after exposure to light in the 630-nm range. The active tumor cell binding site on the cell surface was found to be on the microvilli, a site at which a 52-kDa protein that is very similar to keratin 8 is found. The clearance of the conjugate from nude mice who have grown an A-431 tumor shows a retention of AB:HPD of approximately 15% and less than 1% in skin and internal organs when measured at 48 hours.

Berki et al. [4] used a-PNAr-I Mab, which binds to the cell surface antigens of gastric cancer cells, conjugated to HP combined with HeNe laser illumination. They could selectively purge a mixed cell population from one component, and in vivo in an animal (nude mice) xenograft tumor model, where human cancer cells were destroyed by the immunotargeting method using monoclonal-antibody-hematoporphyrin (Mab-HP) conjugate and soft laser irradiation. The cell destruction was dependent on the doses of both MAb-HP and He-Ne laser light energy, and occurred only in target cell populations.

A series of papers from van Dongen [5] and coworkers has studied the preparation and in vitro use of PS-antibody conjugates. In the first paper [6], they prepared conjugates between two Mabs and ^{131}I-mTHPC-$(CH_2COOH)_4$ using a labile ester. Insoluble aggregates were not formed when mTHPC-Mab conjugates with a molar ratio of up to 4 were prepared. These conjugates preserved integrity on SDS-PAGE, full stability in serum in vitro, and an optimal immunoreactivity. The head and neck squamous cell carcinoma-selective chimeric Mab U36 gave tumor selectivity in nude mice xenografts. The internalizing murine Mab 425 exhibited more in vitro phototoxicity than the noninternalizing chimeric Mab U36.

The next paper [7] used the model compound TrisMPyP-PhCOH conjugated at a PS:Mab ratio </=3 to the same pair of antibodies and another noninternalizing E48. conjugate. Then they studied aluminum (III) phthalocyanine tetrasulfonate $[AlPc(SO_3H)_4]$ and coupled it to Mabs via the tetra-glycine derivative $AlPc(SO_2Ngly)_4$ [8]. Conjugation was performed to the three Mabs used previously (U36, E48, and 425). Again the internalizing $AlPc(SO_2Ngly)_4$-mMab 425 conjugate performed best and was about 7,500 times more toxic to A431 cells than the free PS. Biodistribution analysis of $AlPc(SO_2Ngly)_4$-^{125}I-U36 conjugates with different PS:Mab ratios in squamous cell carcinoma-bearing nude mice revealed selective accumulation in the tumor, although to a lesser extent than for the unconjugated 125I-U36, whereas tumor:blood ratios were similar. Finally they reported in vitro comparison of mTHPC-Mab and AlPcS(4)-Mab conjugates using five different SCC cell lines as target and three different Mabs (BIWA 4, E48, and 425) [9].

AlPcS($_4$)-BIWA 4 was most consistently effective and mTHPC-Mab conjugates were in general hardly effective.

Our laboratory prepared conjugates between the chimeric antihuman epidermal growth factor receptor monoclonal antibody known as C225 and the fluorescent dye Cy5.5 and also conjugated the PS ce6 to C225 [10]. They were employed for photodiagnosis and PDT of early premalignancy in the hamster cheek pouch carcinogenesis model. Fluorescence levels in the carcinogen-treated tissue correlated with the histological stage of the lesions when the C225-Cy5.5 conjugate was used but did not do so with the irrelevant conjugates. Discrete areas of clinically normal mucosa with high fluorescence (hot spots) were subsequently shown by histology to contain dysplastic areas. The best contrast between normal and carcinogen-treated cheek pouches was found at 4 to 8 days after injection. To test the potential of immunophotodiagnosis as a feedback modality for therapeutic intervention, experiments were conducted with the same Mab conjugated to chlorin(e6) followed by illumination to reduce expression of the EGFR by a photodynamic effect. Subsequent immunophotodiagnosis showed that this treatment led to a significant reduction in fluorescence in the carcinogen-treated cheek pouch compared with nonilluminated areas. This difference between illuminated and dark areas was not seen in the normal cheek pouch.

Savellano and Hasan prepared an improved conjugate with C225 employing the PS, BPD, and with the additional step of modifying the antibody by attachment of polyethylene glycol (PEG) chains [11]. First, a small number of antibody lysines (<3 per antibody) were PEGylated using a 10-kDa branched PEG, which dramatically enhances conjugate solubility and reduces conjugate aggregation. Second, a 50% aqueous DMSO solvent was used to prevent PS aggregation and noncovalent interactions. These measures allowed efficient covalent linkage of BPD to antibody lysines, thorough purification of the resulting photoimmunoconjugates (PICs) (verified by gel electrophoresis), maintenance of PIC antigen-binding activity (verified by cellular binding-uptake assays), and reduction of nonspecific cellular uptake (e.g., macrophage capture) of the PICs. Loading levels were varied controllably in the range < or = 11 BPD/antibody. C225-PICs killed EGFR-overexpressing A-431 cells but did not significantly affect EGFR-negative NR6 cells. Although fluorescence measurements demonstrated that the PICs were quenched by as much as an order of magnitude compared with free BPD, 90% reduction in A-431 cell viability was achieved using 20 J/cm^2 of 690-nm light after a 40-hour incubation with the C225 PICs. In a subsequent report [12], these authors extended the study, giving data on the photophysical and photochemical parameters of the PICS, their cellular uptake of these, subcellular localization, and intracellular degradation. On a per-mole basis, PICs were less phototoxic than free BPD, but PICs were very selective for target cells, whereas free BPD was not.

Savellano and colleagues [13] went on to prepare anti-HER2 photosensitizer PICs from two Mabs, HER50 and HER66, using pyropheophorbide-a (PPA), which required only minor changes to the conjugation procedure. Uptake and phototoxicity experiments using human cancer cells were conducted with the PICs and for comparison, with free PPa. SK-BR-3, and SK-OV-3 cells served as HER2-overexpressing target cells. MDA-MB-468 cells served as HER2-nonexpressing control cells. PICs with PPa/Mab molar ratios up to 10 specifically killed HER2-overexpressing cells but not HER2-negative cells. Multiepitope targeting with a mixture of HER50 and HER66 PICs was significantly more effective than a single anti-HER2 PIC.

Kumova et al. [14] described the synthesis, spectroscopic properties, and intracellular imaging of recombinant antibody single-chain fragment (scFv) anti-HER2 conjugates with pyropheophorbide-a (PPa) and verteporfin (VP) containing on average 10 PS molecules per scFv, with a small contribution (</=20%) from noncovalently bound molecules. Fluorescence microscopy showed cellular uptake of PPa conjugate with the HER2-positive cell line, SKOV-3, but not for the HER2-negative cell line, KB.

Boyle and his coworkers [15] have reported on Mab-PS conjugates mediated via isothiocyanate linkages. Using tris-phenolic and tris-pyridinium porphyrins bearing a single reactive isothiocyanate, they conjugated the PS to Mabs FSP 77 and 17.1A directed against internalizing antigens, and 35A7 that binds to a noninternalizing antigen. With PS-Mab conjugates substituted with 1-3 mol of PS they observed no loss of immunoreactivity. At tumor-to-normal tissue ratios as high as 33.5 were observed using Mab 35A7 conjugates. The internalizing conjugate showed a higher level of phototoxicity as compared to the noninternalizing reagent, using a cell line engineered to express both target antigens. The synthesis of three cationic 5,15-diphenyl porphyrins, bearing an isothiocyanate group for conjugation to proteins was then reported [16].

Staneloudi et al. [17] conjugated isothiocyanato porphyrins to colorectal tumor-specific scFv, derived from an antibody phage display library. The resulting immunoconjugates showed no loss of cell binding and selective photocytotoxic effect on cells. Annexin V and propidium iodide staining of treated cells confirmed that cell death was mediated principally via an apoptotic pathway.

Conlon and Berrios [18] reported a new strategy by which a PS conjugate either with the primary Mab, or with a secondary Mab that recognizes the primary Mab or with streptavidin that recognizes the biotinylated primary antibody, could be used to destroy an enzyme important to the metabolism of cancer cells. Rose bengal, pyropheophorbide, or chlorin (e6) were used to inactivate 8-oxoguanine DNA glycohydrolase (OGG1) via the polyclonal rabbit anti-OGG1 antibody.

A group in Germany has described the actual clinical application of antibody-targeted PDT [19]. Schmidt and coworkers demonstrated selectivity of a conjugate between phthalocyanine and the antiovarian cancer-Mab in photokilling of ovarian cancers cells in vitro [20]. Next they treated three women with advanced ovarian carcinoma (FIGO III) [21]. They showed some evidence of response after PDT by means of an ultramicroscopical analysis demonstrating a selective devitalization of tumor cells.

10.2.2 Antibody-PS Conjugates Via Linkers

In this case the PS is bound to polymeric carriers in the first step, and the carriers are attached to the Mab in a second step. This method allows for a high PS: Mab ratio with only a small number of attachment sites on the Mab itself, and therefore, in principle, minimal losses in the immunoreactivity of the Mab. The first report using the linker conjugation strategy was in 1986. Oseroff et al. [22] coupled chlorin(e6) (ce6) through dextran molecules to an anti-T-cell Mab, anti-Leu-1. Conjugates with Mab/ce6 molar ratios as high as 1:36 retained Mab binding activity, and the absorption spectrum and quantum efficiency for singlet oxygen production of bound chlorin were unchanged from that of the free PS. Phototoxicity, as measured by a clonogenic assay and by uptake of ethidium bromide, was dependent on the doses of both Mab-ce6 and 630- to 670-nm light, was enhanced by deuterium oxide, and was observed only in target populations that bound the Mab. Similarly, free ce6 in solution had no photodynamic effect in amounts 100 times more than that carried by the Mab. For this antibody-targeted system, approximately 10 molecules of singlet oxygen were necessary to kill a cell.

Hasan et al. [23] prepared conjugates between chlorin(e6)-monoethylenediamine monoamide (CMA) as the photosensitizer and an antiovarian carcinoma monoclonal antibody OC125. OC125 is a murine monoclonal antibody, which recognizes the cell surface antigen CA125, a 1,000-kDa glycoprotein expressed by 85% of nonmucinous epithelial ovarian cancers. Phototoxicity after exposure to argon ion-pumped dye laser light at 654 nm was selective for ovarian cancer cells while nonovarian cancer cells were not killed [23]. Dose-response curves revealed reciprocity in photosensitizer concentration and fluence. Next, these workers performed in vivo studies using an ascitic BALB/c nude mouse ovarian cancer model induced by intraperitoneal injection of NIH:OVCAR3 cells [24]. Six weeks after injection, when the animals had developed ascites, biodistribution studies were carried out by injecting the photoimmunoconjugate (PIC) or free PS intraperitoneally and sacrificing the animals and measuring tissue PS by extraction. For both the PIC and free PS, peak tumor concentrations were reached at 24 hours; however, the absolute concentrations for the PIC were always higher. Evaluation of viable tumor cells in ascites following in vivo PDT with a single light exposure demonstrated a dose-dependent relationship with fluence and PIC concentration; however, there was significant treatment-related toxicity at all fluences.

Finally they carried out in vivo PDT of the nude mouse model with the conjugate described [25]. Twenty-four hours after IP injection of 0.5 mg/kg, the intraperitoneal surfaces were illuminated using a cylindrical diffusing tip fiber. The overall treatment was given either once or multiply. No animals died from treatment complications. Twenty-four hours later the percentage of viable tumor cells in the ascites was 34% and 5% of control for one and three treatments, respectively. Mice treated three times and four times had a significant survival advantage compared with controls.

Jiang et al. [26] covalently linked benzoporphyrin derivative monoacid ring A (BPD-MA) to a modified polyvinyl alcohol (PVA) backbone, followed by conjugation to the antibody using heterobifunctional linking technology. PVA was modified with 2-fluoro-1-methyl pyridinium toluene-4-sulfonate and 1,6-hexanediamine to produce side chains containing free amino groups. The free carboxyl group of BPD-MA was utilized to conjugate PS molecules to modified PVA using a standard carbodiimide reaction. Final linkage of the PVA-BPD to a model monoclonal antibody involved further substitution of the carrier with 3-mercaptopropionic acid and carbodiimide to introduce 3-4 sulfhydryl residues per carrier molecule, and introduction of sulfo-m-maleimidobenzoyl-N-hydroxysulfosuccinimide ester residues to the monoclonal antibody (3–4 residues/molecule). They went on [27] to test the conjugate with the Mab 5E8 that recognizes a glycoprotein detected on human squamous cell carcinomas of the lung and showed selective photokilling of the target cell line (A549) over that exhibited by free BPD or a control Mab-PVA-BPD conjugate.

Rakestraw et al. [28] prepared Mab-dextran-tin(IV) chlorin e6 (SnCe6) immunoconjugates by a technique involving the use of reducing, terminal-modified dextran carriers and site-specific modification of the Fc oligosaccharide moiety on the antibodies. The dextran carriers were coupled to the Mab via a single, chain-terminal hydrazide group to prevent aggregation. Conjugates were prepared with antimelanoma Mab 2.1 containing up to 18.9 SnCe6 molecules per Mab. Under neutral conditions, no hydrolysis of the hydrazone bond between the Mab and the dextran carrier could be detected, and the hydrazone was not stabilized by reduction. Analysis of the purified immunoconjugates showed that approximately two dextran carrier chains were attached to a Mab regardless of the number of SnCe6 molecules linked to a dextran carrier. Site-specific covalent attachment of the SnCe6-dextran chains to the Mab was confirmed by SDS-PAGE. HPLC analysis of the conjugates gave a single species eluting in the range of 200 to 240 kDa. As determined by a competitive inhibition radioimmunoassay using viable SK-MEL-2 human malignant melanoma cells, the conjugates showed excellent retention of antigen-binding activity relative to unconjugated Mab. These conjugates (chromophore:antibody molar ratios, 6.8 and 11.2) were used to carry out in vitro photokilling of SK-MEL-2 human melanoma cells that showed both Mab and cell specificity [29]. Phototoxicity, as measured by clonogenic assay, was dependent on the delivered dose of 634-nm light. Finally they studied the photophysical properties of these immunoconjugates with chlorin e6: antibody molar ratios of 18.9:1, 11.2:1, 6.8:1, and 1.7:1. [30] All immunoconjugates retained antigen-binding activity regardless of the chromophore:antibody substitution ratio. In contrast, the ground-state absorption spectra of the immunoconjugates showed features that appeared to be dependent on the chromophore:antibody molar ratio. In addition, the quantum yield of singlet oxygen generated by the conjugated chromophores was observed to be significantly less than that observed with the unbound dye. Time-resolved absorbance spectroscopy of the chromophore excited triplet state indicated that the loss of singlet oxygen quantum yield resulted from diminished chromophore triplet yield.

Shiah et al. [31] prepared conjugates between N-(2-hydroxypropyl)-methacrylamide (HPMA) copolymer-bound doxorubicin (DOX) and mesochlorin e(6) (Mce(6)) targeted with an OV-TL 16 monoclonal antibody (P-DOX-Ab and P-Mce(6)-Ab, respectively). The immunoconjugates were purified by size exclusion chromatography on Superose 6 column and analyzed. The Mce(6) concentration in tissues was determined by a fluorescence assay. P-DOX-Ab and P-Mce(6)-Ab had polymer:drug:protein weight ratios of 32:3:62 and 26:2:72, corresponding to polymer:drug:protein molecular ratios of approximately 4:14:1 and 3:8:1, respectively. The biodistribution results indicated that the percentage of total administered dose of Mce(6) in tumors reached approximately 1% for the nontargeted conjugate at 18 hours after administration, while that of P-Mce(6)-Ab was approximately 13 times higher. Nude mice bearing OVCAR-3 xenografts that received one i.v. dose of

P-DOX-Ab (2.2 mg/kg DOX equivalent) and P-Mce(6)-Ab (1.5 mg/kg Mce(6) equivalent) followed after 18 hours by a light dose of 220 J/cm(2) from a KTP 650-nm dye-laser, led to a cure rate of more than 60%. The incorporation of OV-TL 16 antibody dramatically enhanced the accumulation in tumors with a concomitant increase in the therapeutic efficacy of P-DOX-Ab and P-Mce(6)-Ab in combination therapy, which may probably be attributed to both antibody targeting and enhanced permeability and retention (EPR) effects. Lu et al. [32, 33] described a new polymerizable antibody Fab′ fragment with a PEG spacer (MA-PEG-Fab′) that was prepared from OV-TL 16 antibody, specific against the OA-3 antigen expressed on most human ovarian carcinomas. The MA-PEG-Fab′ possessed a higher reactivity in the copolymerization with N-(2-hydroxypropyl)-methacrylamide (HPMA) than the polymerizable Fab′ fragment MA-Fab′ with a short spacer. The MA-PEG-Fab′ was copolymerized with HPMA and the peptide-linked PS, MA-Gly-Phe-Leu-Gly-Mce(6) producing an Fab′ targeted HPMA copolymer-Mce(6) conjugate. The number and weight average molecular weights of the copolymer were 164,000 and 271,000 Da, respectively. About two MA-PEG-Fab′ fragments per chain were incorporated in the copolymer conjugates. Preliminary in vivo antitumor studies indicated that the Fab′ targeted conjugates showed a higher efficacy of tumor growth inhibition in nude mice than the nontargeted conjugate.

Rancan et al. [34] reported the synthesis of a modular carrier system consisting of a [5:1]-fullerene hexakis adduct with five malonate spacers that can bind two therapeutic units (the PS pyropheophorbide-a) each, for a total of ten, and a longer malonate spacer that serves for the conjugation to the addressing unit, the monoclonal antibody rituximab. Confocal microscopy studies using Epstein-Barr virus-transformed B-lymphocytes and Jurkat cells showed that the antibody conjugate conserves the affinity for its receptor (CD20) and its selectivity toward CD20-positive B-lymphocytes. On the contrary, the antibody-free complex did not show any binding or intracellular uptake.

In our laboratory, we devised a new strategy for linker-mediated attachment of multiple PS to monoclonal antibodies that does not destroy the antibody-recognition sites by binding to the amino-groups of the lysine residues at the antigen recognition sites of the variable region [35]. Since the antigen-binding capabilities of antibodies largely reside in the Fab portion of the antibodies, conjugation at sites removed from these antigen recognition sites are most desirable (termed site-specific). The conjugation strategy involves attaching the PS via a polymeric linker to the partially reduced sulfhydryl groups that bind together the two heavy chains that comprise the IgG molecule. This particular strategy (illustrated in Figure 10.2) is equally applicable to F(ab')2 fragments of Mabs as to whole IgG molecules, in contrast to the oxidized carbohydrate approach that can only be used with entire IgGs as the carbohydrate is lost in F(ab')2 fragments. The linker used is poly-L-lysine (pL) and this allows PICs to be prepared with an overall cationic charge by virtue of the many unreacted epsilon amino groups present on the pL chain. A heterobifunctional (amino-sulfhydryl reactive) reagent is used to attach the preformed pL-ce6 conjugate to a free sulfhydryl group exposed on the Mab. However if the pL-ce6 conjugate is reacted with succinic anhydride after attachment of the heterobifunctional reagent but before binding to the Mab, it can be rendered

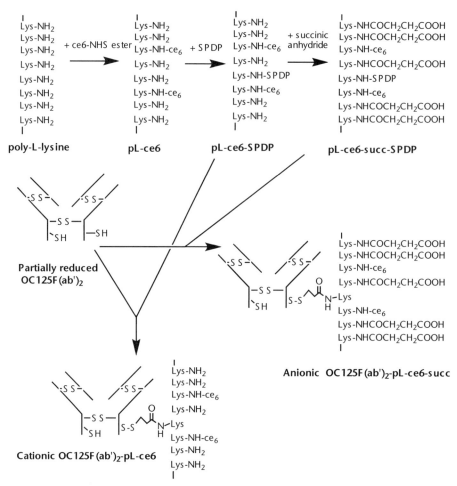

Figure 10.2 Scheme showing preparation of site-specific cationic and anionic photoimmuno-conjugates from OC125F(ab')2 by partial reduction of the interchain disulfide bonds.

polyanionic by virtue of the many free carboxylic acid groups that have replaced the epsilon amino groups in the pL chain. The net result of these manipulations is to be able to compare PICs formed from the same Mab that are identical except for the overall ionic charge. They will have the same number of ce6 molecules attached per Mab and approximately the same molecular weight (succinylated PIC will be slightly heavier).

We first studied PICs between ce6 and the F(ab')2 fragment of the murine antiovarian cancer monoclonal antibody OC125 [36]. PICs were purified by column chromatography and were also radiolabeled with [125]I. PICs with both cationic and anionic charges preserved antigen binding to target cells (OVCAR5) as opposed to nontarget cells (SW1116), as shown by competition studies with native antibody, but the cationic PIC had up to 17 times higher cellular uptake of ce6, probably due to enhanced internalization. The ratio of ce6 to ^{125}I retained by the cells varied with the likelihood of internalization and lysosomal degradation. The phototoxicity of the PICs generally varied with their uptake, but a correlation was found between lysosomal hydrolysis as measured by an increased cellular ratio of ce6: 125I and increased relative phototoxicity. In a subsequent study [37], we compared the effect of the cationic OC125 F(ab′)2-pL-ce6 cationic conjugate on 5 human cancer cell lines (ovarian and breast) and 19 primary cultures from solid and ascites tumor samples obtained from 14 patients with ovarian cancer who were undergoing primary surgery. We tested the hypothesis that PDT could interact synergistically with the cytotoxic drug cisplatin, especially in platinum resistant cells. When all cell types (cisplatin-sensitive and cisplatin-resistant) were considered together, combination treatment yielded cytotoxicity that was, on average, 6.9 times (95% confidence interval = 1.86–11.94) greater than that of cisplatin alone (two-sided $P = 0.023$). Cisplatin-resistant cells showed a synergistic effect of the two treatments (two-sided $P = .044$), while cisplatin-sensitive cells showed an additive effect.

We next investigated the effect of charge modification of these PICs on their biodistribution in a xenograft model of ovarian cancer [38]. Samples were taken from normal organs and tumor at 3 and 24 hours. Tumor to normal ^{125}I ratios showed that the cationic OC125F(ab′)2 PIC had the highest tumor selectivity. Ratios for ce6 were uniformly higher than for ^{125}I, indicating that ce6 became separated from ^{125}I. The amounts of ce6 delivered per gram of tumor were much higher for cationic OC125F(ab′)2 PIC than for other species. The results indicate that cationic charge stimulates the endocytosis and lysosomal degradation of the OC125F(ab′)2-pL- ce6 that has bound to the IP tumor.

We then compared the efficacy of PICs with cationic and anionic molecular charges on IP photoimmunotherapy (PIT) of ovarian cancer xenografts in nude mice [39]. The PIC was injected IP followed after 3 hours by red light delivered through a fiber into the peritoneal cavity. These PIT treatments were repeated three times and the results obtained with the anionic and cationic PICs were compared with those obtained with free ce6 and control. The extent of residual macroscopic disease and death from disease were the evaluable outcomes for tumoricidal and survival studies, respectively: In contrast to other IP PS, mice showed no systemic toxicity or morbidity from the treatment. In this initial study the mean residual tumor weights in all treatment groups were significantly lower compared to untreated controls ($P < 0.0001$) (Figure 10.3(a)), and the response to the cationic conjugate was significantly better than that to the anionic conjugate or free c_{e6} ($P < 0.005$) (Figure 10.3(b)).

We next carried out a series of experiments on an animal model of metastatic tumors in the liver. PICs were prepared between the anticolon cancer monoclonal antibody 17.1A and the ce6 to give cationic or anionic PICs [40]. In in vitro cell culture the cationic PIC delivered four times more ce6 to the cells than the anionic PIC, and both were selective for antigen-positive HT29 cells. Photokilling was much higher for PICs than for free ce6. In the mouse model of colon cancer metastatic to the liver, the PICs were injected i.v. via the tail vein rather than IP [41]. The anionic 17.1A conjugate delivered more than twice as much ce6 to the tumor at 3 hours than other species (five times more than the cationic 17. 1A conjugate) and had a tumor: normal liver ratio of 2.5. Tumor-to-skin ratios were high (>38) for all conjugates but not for free ce6. Cationic species had a high uptake in the lungs compared to anionic species. Mice were treated with interstitial fiber delivery of red light at light at two different fluence rates 3 hours after i.v. injection of the anionic or cationic 17.1A PICs or unconjugated ce6 [42]. There was a significant reduction

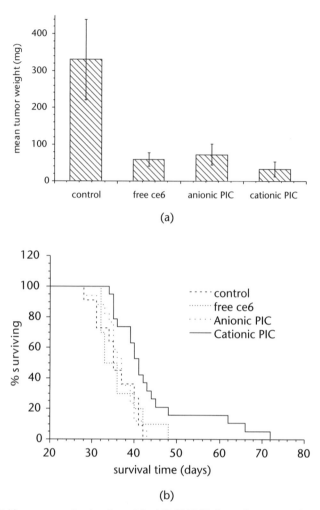

Figure 10.3 PIT (three successive treatments) of IP OVCAR-5 ovarian tumors in nude mice. (a) Mean tumor weights excised from mice sacrificed 26 days after tumor inoculation and 12 days after first PIT treatment with cationic or anionic OC125 PIC or free ce6. (b) Kaplan-Meier curve illustrating survival of mice treated as in (a).

(<20% of controls; $P = 0.0035$) in the weight of the tumors in the mice treated with the anionic PIC (Figure 10.4(a)), and the median survival increased from 62.5 to 102 days ($P = 0.015$) (Figure 10.4(b)). PDT with free ce6 and the cationic PIC produced a smaller decrease in tumor weight and a smaller extension of survival, neither of which were statistically significant. The higher fluence rate prolonged survival significantly more than the lower fluence rate. This may have been because the high fluence rate gave a contribution of laser-induced hyperthermia to the photodamage.

The two sets of experiments described above with two completely different tumor models lead to a very interesting conclusion. The IP ovarian cancer model (OVCAR-5) where the PIC was injected IP showed a much higher tumor localization and tumoricidal effect with the cationic PIC than the anionic PIC. Conversely, the intrahepatic tumor model (HT29), where the PIC was injected i.v. showed the complete opposite effect, with both a higher tumor localization and tumoricidal effect with the anionic PIC compared to the cationic PIC. These results may be

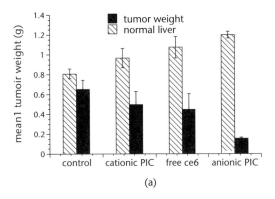

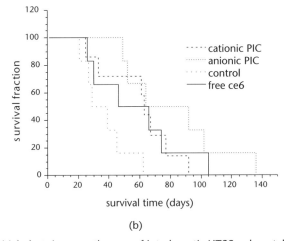

Figure 10.4 Interstitial photoimmunotherapy of intrahepatic HT29 colorectal tumors in nude mice. (a) Mean tumor weights and mean weights of normal liver excised from mice sacrificed 18 days after tumor inoculation and 9 days after PIT treatment with cationic or anionic 17.1A PIC or free ce6. (b) Kaplan-Meier curve illustrating survival of mice treated as in (a).

explained by considering that in the OVCAR-5 model the cationic PIC is injected into the peritoneal cavity where it may directly bind to antigens expressed on the membranes of the tumor cell and leads to increased endocytosis and lysosomal degradation compared to the anionic PIC. In the HT29 model the PIC must be injected i.vi and it is well established that cationic molecules injected i.v. have much higher uptakes in the lungs, and in addition it might be expected that the extravasation of the PIC from the bloodstream into the parenchyma of the liver tumor would be considerably more efficient for molecules with a negative charge than a positive charge.

Another approach to linker-antibody PS conjugates is the use of immuno-liposomes or micelles to encapsulate PS [43]. Poorly soluble meso-tetraphenylporphine (TPP) was solubilized using nontargeted and tumor-targeted polymeric micelles prepared of PEG/phosphatidyl ethanolamine bearing 2C5 Mab. Improved photokilling of murine (LLC, B16) and human (MCF-7, BT20) cancer cells in vitro was achieved. The phototoxic effect depended on the TPP concentration and specific targeting by immunomicelles. This group went on to show that the 2C5-TPP-immunomicelles could be injected into mice bearing Lewis lung carci-

noma [44]. Twenty-four hours after the administration, the tumor sites were illuminated with light (630 nm) for 12 minutes. Microscopic evaluation of tumor response
was conducted in some mice 24 hours after light irradiation, and tumor size was
followed in the remaining animals for another 35 days. The attachment of Mab 2C5
to TPP-loaded immunomicelles provided the maximum level of tumor growth
inhibition as judged by microscopic evaluation of tumor response and following
tumor size. Enhanced tumor accumulation of TPP-loaded Mab 2C5-PEG-PE-
immunomicelles was confirmed by gamma-imaging studies.

10.3   Protein-Photosensitizer Conjugates Recognized by Receptors

Another strategy to enhance the tumor-targeting ability of PS is to form covalent
conjugates between the PS and proteins that are preferentially taken up into cancer
cells. Cells use the process known as receptor-mediated endocytosis to satisfy their
demand for essential nutrients and building blocks that are delivered to normal cells
by well-regulated pathways. Proteins carrying these nutrients are recognized by specific membrane-bound receptors on the cell surface and this recognition triggers
endocytosis into vesicles that are subsequently processed to release the nutrients.
Malignant cells have both faster growth rates and faster metabolic rates than normal
cells, and consequently have a much higher demand for many of these nutrients.
Cancer cells satisfy this increased demand by upregulating the expression of many of
the membrane receptors and this increased expression has been used as the basis for
selectively delivering drugs, radioisotopes, and toxins.

10.3.1   Transferrin Conjugates

One of these approaches to deliver PS to cancer cells in vitro takes advantage of the
transferrin cycle, which is a targeted delivery system designed by nature to supply
iron to cells in proportion to their need. Ferric ions, highly toxic in their free state,
are delivered to cells tightly bound to transferrin. Transferrin binds to specific receptors expressed on the surface of cells and is rapidly endocytosed in coated pits and
enters an acidic endosome compartment having a pH of 5.5. This low pH leads to
release of the iron atoms that are transferred to the cytosol compartment by a process involving reduction to the ferrous state. Most of the apotransferrin is cycled
back to the plasma membrane by the transferrin receptor, exocytosed, and dissoci-
ated into the external medium aided by a fall in receptor affinity on encountering the
elevated pH of the extracellular medium. The transferrin receptor is now primed for
another round of the cycle. The cycle mean transit time is about 17 minutes. Selectivity of transferrin delivery between cells is achieved by the ability of ample cellular
iron stores to downregulate transferrin receptor number by destabilization of receptor mRNA. Rapidly growing cells with large numbers of receptors ($1-3 \times 10^5$) can
acquire iron at the rate of 19,000 molecules/cell/minute for an initial period of 4
hours.

We prepared conjugates of hematoporphyrin (HP) with holotransferrin and
purified them by gel filtration and characterized them by high performance liquid
chromatography, polyacrylamide gel electrophoresis, and spectroscopy [45].

Although the fluorescence was somewhat quenched, the conjugates had similar singlet oxygen quantum yields to free porphyrin. The uptake of HP-transferrin showed evidence of a receptor-mediated component in that it was partially inhibited by native holotransferrin and increased when transferrin receptors were upregulated by pretreatment with an iron chelator. Selective phototoxicity was observed towards cells whose expression of transferrin had been upregulated by iron starvation.

Cavanaugh [46] prepared conjugates between transferring and ce6 using a procedure that involved the preliminary binding of the protein to quaternary amino ethyl-sephadex. The conjugate's singlet oxygen yield was 70% of the efficiency of native ce6. When ce6-transferrin treated human MCF7 and rat MTLn3 mammary adenocarcinoma cells were exposed to toxin-activating visible light, a tumor cell killing effect was achieved in normal (medium plus 10% FBS) culture conditions with an ED50 of approximately 10 to 20 μg/mL.

Transferrin has also been used as a targeting moiety to deliver PSs encapsulated in particulate delivery vehicles to cancer cells expressing the transferrin receptor. Derycke and de Witte prepared sterically stabilized PEG-liposomes containing hypericin and studied the binding to HeLa cells [47]. However, their liposome preparation had problems with hypericin leaking out of the PEG-liposomes, and thus they were unable to demonstrate selective phototoxicity. In a subsequent publication [48], this group studied Tf-conjugated liposomes loaded with aluminum phthalocyanine tetrasulfonate (AlPcS4). HeLa cells that overexpress the transferrin receptor internalized the liposomes by receptor mediated endocytosis. Tf-Lip-AlPcS4 was 10 times more phototoxic than free AlPcS4 whereas Lip-AlPcS4 displayed no phototoxicity at all. Tf-Lip-AlPcS4 gave high uptake by HeLa cells, which could be competed with unmodified transferrin. Next, these workers delivered the targeted and nontargeted liposomes and free PS intravesically to target bladder cancer cells (AY-27) and orthotopic bladder tumors [49]. AY-27 cells incubated with Tf-Lip-AlPcS4 had much higher intracellular AlPcS4 levels than AY-27 cells incubated with Lip-AlPcS4. In rat bladder tumors, intravesical instillation with Tf-Lip-AlPcS4 resulted in higher AlPcS4 fluorescence in tumoral tissue, whereas instillation of free AlPcS4 resulted in nonselective accumulation throughout the whole bladder wall, and Lip-AlPcS4 instillation resulted in no tissue accumulation. PDT of AY-27 cells incubated with Lip-AlPcS4 gave no killing, whileTf-Lip-AlPcS4 or AlPcS4 both gave high kill rates, thus emphasizing the necessity for selectivity in the bladder.

10.3.2   LDL Conjugates

LDL may be a tumor-targeting delivery vehicle for PS and the formation of covalent conjugates between the PS and the apolipoprotein may serve to obviate the possibility of the PS exchanging between LDL and other lipoproteins or cellular membranes. We prepared conjugates between HP and human LDL and they were purified and characterized [50]. HP-LDL was found to be aggregated possibly via interparticle apoB protein cross-linking. Receptor-mediated endocytosis of HP-LDL by NIH 3T3 mouse fibroblast cells was inferred from the increased uptake observed when LDL receptors are upregulated. HP-LDL uptake into HT29 human colorectal cancer cells showed competition from unlabeled LDL, albeit at rather high doses. J774 (a mouse macrophage cell line) avidly accumulated HP-LDL, retaining most of the fluorescence and some of the protein while degrading the remainder. Oxidized LDL species compete in these processes, with the major effect on protein degradation. Chloroquine (a lysosomotropic compound that inhibits intralysosomal degradation by raising pH) had little effect on the fluorescence uptake but inhibited protein degradation (and hence enhanced protein accumulation). We deduced from these results that LDL-HP was recognized by LDL receptors present on 3T3 and HT29 cells, but was also recognized by scavenger-receptors present on macrophages (see next section), and this recognition may lead to higher and faster uptake than that mediated by LDL receptors.

Schmidt-Erfurth et al. [51] prepared covalent conjugates between LDL and ce6 via carbodiimide activation and evaluated them on a fibroblast cell line with defined LDL receptor expression and a retinoblastoma cell line (Y79). Covalent binding to LDL significantly increased the uptake of ce6 measured by spectrofluorimetry for both cell lines by a factor of 4-5. A ce6: LDL binding ratio of 50:1 was optimal. Receptor-mediated uptake was demonstrated by saturability and competitive inhibition by free LDL. Binding also occurred at $2°C$ and was attributed to nonspecific associations. Irradiation with 10 J/cm^2 of 660-nm light after treatment of cells with ce6-LDL conjugate reduced the MTT activity by 80%, while free or LDL-complexed ce6 induced a maximum of 10% reduction in the MTT activity.

10.3.3   Other Protein Conjugates

Tarrago-Trani et al. [52] used Shiga-like toxin B subunit (SLTB) to deliver the photosensitizer, chlorin e6 (Ce6), to Vero cells expressing the Gb3 receptor. Ce6-SLTB after cleanup contained < or =10% noncovalently bound Ce6, and the Ce6-SLTB conjugate was over 10 times more phototoxic to Vero cells than free Ce6. Ce6-SLTB, accumulated in a combination of subcellular sites including mitochondria, Golgi apparatus, ER, and plasma membrane.

10.4   Scavenger Receptor Targeted Photodynamic Therapy

Macrophages are among the most versatile mammalian cells and are found in every tissue in the body. They must perform a number of diverse cellular functions that allow them to kill invading microorganisms, phagocytose particulate matter,and remove senescent cells and altered serum proteins as well as produce growth factors involved in wound healing. They are major players in the functioning of the mammalian immune system, being both professional antigen-presenting cells and the source of many cytokines that upregulate and downregulate many responses of T- and B-lymphocytes. They are one of the most important cellular mediators of inflammation, and are thought to be responsible for many diseases characterized by chronic inflammation. In contrast to previous theories that tumor-associated macrophages (TAMs) were "fighting a valiant but losing battle against the malignant cells," it is now thought that the relationship between the tumor and the TAMs is symbiotic in that both populations help each other to survive and grow in various ways. Mantovani has termed this symbiotic relationship a "ping-pong reciprocal feeding interaction" [53]. Tumors actively recruit macrophages and encourage their growth by expressing chemotactic molecules and growth factors for macrophages/monocytes. In return TAMs can help the tumor to grow and spread in four distinct ways: by secreting tumor growth factors, by secreting proangiogenic factors, by producing matrix metalloproteinases needed for tumor invasion and metastasis, and by helping to suppress the antitumor immune response. For these reasons, TAMs have been called a target for cancer therapy.

Macrophages and monocytes (and to a lesser extent endothelial cells and smooth muscle cells) express several "scavenger" receptors that are membrane proteins that recognize a wide range of ligands, both naturally occurring and synthetic. The ligands are all macromolecules with a pronounced anionic charge, and because of the specificity and high capacity of scavenger receptors many investigators have explored the possibility of preparing covalent conjugates between scavenger receptor ligands and various drugs to produce macrophage targeted therapy

By joining PS to ligands of the scavenger receptor we can specifically target PDT to macrophages, and have the additional advantages that the scavenger receptor of high capacity may lead to efficient degradation of endocytosed molecules in lysosomes, thus releasing the possibly more photoactive free PS [54]. Since the conjugates would be only taken up by macrophage-type cells (that express the scavenger receptor), and the illumination can be confined to the tumor, this should ensure that only macrophages in the tumor or other lesion would be killed. This may be contrasted to other antimacrophage therapies that can also kill circulating monocytes and macrophages in other anatomical locations that may have beneficial antitumor effects such as destroying micrometastases.

10.4.1   LDL-Conjugates

We first observed this specific PS targeting to scavenger receptors with conjugates of hematoporphyrin and lipoproteins. Conjugates between hematoporphyrin (HP) and human low-density lipoprotein (LDL), human high-density lipoprotein (HDL), and bovine HDL were prepared, purified, and characterized (for details see Section 11.3.2).

We went on to test this approach in vitro using maleylated serum albumin, a well-characterized ligand of the Class A scavenger receptor [55]. ce6 was covalently attached to bovine serum albumin (BSA) to give conjugates with molar substitution ratios of 1:1 and 3:1 (dye to protein), and these conjugates could then be further modified by maleylation. All of the purified conjugates were taken up by J774 target macrophage cells and killed them after illumination, while there was only small uptake and no phototoxicity toward nonmacrophage OVCAR-5 cells, as shown in Figure 10.5(a) and (b).

The uptake and phototoxicity by J774 cells were decreased after incubation at 4°C demonstrating internalization, and confocal microscopy with organelle-specific green fluorescent probes showed largely lysosomal localization (Color Plate 5). Uptake and phototoxicity by J774 cells could both be competed by addition of the scavenger receptor ligand, maleylated BSA.

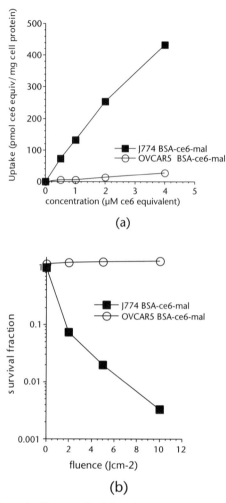

(a)

(b)

Figure 10.5   Demonstration of cell-type selectivity of scavenger-receptor targeted PS conjugates for J774 macrophages compared to OVCAR-5 cancer cells. (a) Cellular uptake of BSA-ce6.-mal incubated at 2 μM concentration for 24 hours by J774 mouse macrophages and OVCAR-5 human ovarian cancer cells. (b) Phototoxicity determined by MTT assay of cells incubated as in Figure 9A and exposed to 660 nm of light.

Next, we explored the effect of macrophage activation state and scavenger receptor class A (SRA) expression on this targeting in two murine macrophage tumor cell lines (RAW264.7 and P388D1) and a control murine mammary sarcoma cell line (EMT-6) [56]. Cells were pretreated with interferon gamma (IFN gamma) and/or lipopolysaccharide (LPS) followed by BSA-ce6-mal addition. The SRA expression, tumor necrosis factor alpha (TNF alpha) release, conjugate uptake, and PDT killing were measured. Both macrophage cell lines expressed SRA and took up conjugate specifically in an SRA-dependent manner, but differences were observed in their response to activation. RAW264.7 expressed increasingly more SRA and took up increasingly more BSA-ce6-mal in response to IFN gamma, LPS, and IFN gamma + LPS, respectively. The PDT killing did not follow the same pattern as the uptake of the photosensitizer. The increase in uptake in the IFN gamma-treated cells did not lead to an increase in PDT killing, while stimulation with LPS or IFN gamma

+ LPS resulted in a significant protection against PDT, despite a significant increase in photosensitizer uptake. P388D1 was not responsive to IFN gamma, LPS, or IFN gamma + LPS with respect to SRA expression, conjugate uptake, and PDT killing.

We next asked whether these conjugates could be used to target PS to macrophage-rich tumors in vivo [57]. We tested the intravenous (i.v.) injection of a conjugate between maleylated albumin and chlorin(e6) to BALB/c mice bearing three tumor types with differing proportions of tumor-associated macrophages. The accumulation of PS within the tumors after i.v. injection and 24 hour-incubation time was disappointing, and we therefore investigated intratumoral (IT) injection. This gave 20 to 50 times greater concentrations of PS within the tumor compared to i.v. injection as determined by tissue extraction. Furthermore, the amounts of PS in each tumor type correlated well with the numbers of macrophages both as determined by extraction from bulk tumor and fluorescence quantification and as determined by tissue dissociation to a single-cell suspension and two-color flow cytometry with macrophage-specific antibodies. IT injection of nonconjugated PS gave lower tumor accumulation that did not correlate with macrophage content.

Brasseur et al. [58] conjugated aluminum tetrasulfophthalocyanine (AlPcS4) to maleylated bovine serum albumin (mal-BSA), at a 9:1 molar ratio via one or two sulfonamide-hexanoic-amide spacer chains, followed by treatment with maleic anhydride to yield the mal-BSA-phthalocyanine conjugates. The latter were tested for singlet oxygen production, receptor-mediated cell uptake, and phototoxicity toward J774 cells of macrophage origin and nonphagocytic EMT-6 cells. Cell uptake of ^{125}I-mal-BSA showed specific binding for J774 cells but not for EMT-6 cells. Competition studies of the conjugates with ^{125}I-mal-BSA showed that coupling of AlPcS4 to BSA resulted in recognition of the conjugate by the scavenger receptor, whereas coupling to mal-BSA further enhanced its binding affinity. This suggests that affinity for the scavenger receptor is related to the overall negative charge of the protein. Phototoxicity of the conjugates toward J774 cells paralleled their relative affinity, with mal-BSA-AlPcS4 coupled via two spacer chains showing the highest activity. The conjugates were less phototoxic toward the EMT-6 cell line. The activities in both cell lines of all conjugated AlPcS4 preparations were, however, lower than that of the free disulfonated AlPcS2.

One of the most important applications of scavenger–receptor-mediated targeting of PS to macrophages is in atherosclerosis where the macrophage is the key pathologic cell type. This approach is covered in detail in Chapter 21.

10.5 Conclusion

The preparation and use of covalent conjugates between PS and protein targeting vehicles has the potential to dramatically improve the selectivity and efficacy of PDT. Conjugates should be rationally designed for their particular application, taking into account the cellular or tissular target, delivery route, pharmacokinetics, photochemical efficiency, and attainable PS and light doses. Although in many cases the process of forming covalent conjugates between PS and macromolecules such as antibodies or proteins can significantly reduce the quantum yield of phototoxic species, this reduction may be compensated by increased selectivity and reduced collateral damage to nontarget tissue. Factors such as the molecular size and charge of the conjugates should be taken into account in deciding the delivery route and the time interval before illumination. The use of PS conjugates as PDT sensitizers means that the actual dye molecule can be chosen on its photochemical, photophysical properties, allowing the targeting to be carried out by the macromolecule. With advances constantly being made in the design of targeting vehicles used for delivering therapies for cancer such as radioisotopes, toxins, and cytotoxic drugs, this will lead to the further diverse applications of similar techniques to target PS more selectively and to a wider array of targets on both the molecular, cellular, and tissular levels.

References

[1]   Mew, D., et al., "Photoimmunotherapy: treatment of animal tumors with tumor-specific monoclonal antibody-hematoporphyrin conjugates," *J Immunol*, Vol. 130, 1983, pp. 1473–1477.

[2]   Steele, J. K., et al., "Suppressor deletion therapy: selective elimination of T suppressor cells in vivo using a hematoporphyrin conjugated monoclonal antibody permits animals to reject syngeneic tumor cells," *Cancer Immunol Immunother*, Vol. 26, 1988, pp. 125–131.

[3]   Donald, P. J., et al., "Monoclonal antibody-porphyrin conjugate for head and neck cancer: the possible magic bullet," *Otolaryngol Head Neck Surg*, Vol. 105, 1991, pp. 781–787.

[4]   Berki, T., and Nemeth, P., "Photo-immunotargeting with haematoporphyrin conjugates activated by a low-power He-Ne laser," *Cancer Immunol Immunother*, Vol. 35, 1992, pp. 69–74.

[5]   van Dongen, G. A., Visser, G. W., and Vrouenraets, M. B., "Photosensitizer-antibody conjugates for detection and therapy of cancer," *Adv Drug Deliv Rev*, Vol. 56, 2004, pp. 31–52.

[6]   Vrouenraets, M. B., et al., "Development of meta-tetrahydroxyphenylchlorin-monoclonal antibody conjugates for photoimmunotherapy," *Cancer Res*, Vol. 59, 1999, pp. 1505–1513.

[7]   Vrouenraets, M. B., et al., "Targeting of a hydrophilic photosensitizer by use of internalizing monoclonal antibodies: A new possibility for use in photodynamic therapy," *Int J Cancer*, Vol. 88, 2000, pp. 108–114.

[8]   Vrouenraets, M. B., et al., "Targeting of aluminum (III) phthalocyanine tetrasulfonate by use of internalizing monoclonal antibodies: improved efficacy in photodynamic therapy," *Cancer Res*, Vol. 61, 2001, pp. 1970–1975.

[9]   Vrouenraets, M. B., et al., "Comparison of aluminium (III) phthalocyanine tetrasulfonate- and meta-tetrahydroxyphenylchlorin-monoclonal antibody conjugates for their efficacy in photodynamic therapy in vitro," *Int J Cancer*, Vol. 98, 2002, pp. 793–798.

[10] Soukos, N. S., et al., "Epidermal growth factor receptor-targeted immunophotodiagnosis and photoimmunotherapy of oral precancer in vivo," *Cancer Res*, Vol. 61, 2001, pp. 4490–4496.

[11] Savellano, M. D., and Hasan, T., "Targeting cells that overexpress the epidermal growth factor receptor with polyethylene glycolated BPD verteporfin photosensitizer immunoconjugates," *Photochemistry and photobiology*, Vol. 77, 2003, pp. 431–439.

[12] Savellano, M. D., and Hasan, T., "Photochemical targeting of epidermal growth factor receptor: a mechanistic study," *Clinical cancer research: an official journal of the American Association for Cancer Research*, Vol. 11, 2005, pp. 1658–1668.

[13] Savellano, M. D., et al., "Multiepitope HER2 targeting enhances photoimmunotherapy of HER2-overexpressing cancer cells with pyropheophorbide-a immunoconjugates," *Cancer Res*, Vol. 65, 2005, pp. 6371–6379.

[14] Kuimova, M. K., et al., "Fluorescence characterisation of multiply-loaded anti-HER2 single chain Fv-photosesitizer conjugates suitable for photodynamic therapy," *Photochem Photobiol Sci*, Vol. 6, 2007, pp. 933–939.

[15] Hudson, R., et al., "The development and characterisation of porphyrin isothiocyanate-monoclonal antibody conjugates for photoimmunotherapy," *Br J Cancer*, Vol. 92, 2005, pp. 1442–1449.

[16] Malatesti, N., et al., "Synthesis and in vitro investigation of cationic 5,15-diphenyl porphyrin-monoclonal antibody conjugates as targeted photodynamic sensitisers," *Int J Oncol*, Vol. 28, 2006, pp. 1561–1569.

[17] Staneloudi, C., et al., "Development and characterization of novel photosensitizer: scFv conjugates for use in photodynamic therapy of cancer," *Immunology*, Vol. 120, 2007, pp. 512–517.

[18] Conlon, K. A., and Berrios, M., "Site-directed photoproteolysis of 8-oxoguanine DNA glycosylase 1 (OGG1) by specific porphyrin-protein probe conjugates: a strategy to improve the effectiveness of photodynamic therapy for cancer," *J Photochem Photobiol B*, Vol. 87, 2007, pp. 9–17.

[19] Schmidt, S., "Antibody-targeted photodynamic therapy," *Hybridoma*, Vol. 12, 1993, pp. 539–541.

[20] Schmidt, S., et al., "Photodynamic laser therapy with antibody-bound dyes. A new procedure in therapy of gynecologic malignancies," *Fortschr Med*, Vol. 110, 1992, pp. 298–301.

[21] Schmidt, S., et al., "Clinical use of photodynamic therapy in gynecologic tumor patients—antibody-targeted photodynamic laser therapy as a new oncologic treatment procedure.," *Zentralbl Gynakol,* Vol. 114, 1992, pp. 307–311.

[22] Oseroff, A. R., et al., "Antibody-targeted photolysis: selective photodestruction of human T-cell leukemia cells using monoclonal antibody-chlorin e6 conjugates," *Proc. Natl. Acad. Sci. U S A*, Vol. 83, 1986, pp. 8744–8748.

[23] Hasan, T., Lin, C. W., and Lin, A., "Laser-induced selective cytotoxicity using monoclonal antibody-chromophore conjugates," *Prog Clin Biol Res*, Vol. 288, 1989, pp. 471–477.

[24] Goff, B. A., et al., "Photoimmunotherapy and biodistribution with an OC125-chlorin immunoconjugate in an in vivo murine ovarian cancer model," *Br J Cancer*, Vol. 70, 1994, pp. 474–480.

[25] Goff, B. A., et al., "Treatment of ovarian cancer with photodynamic therapy and immunoconjugates in a murine ovarian cancer model,"*Br J Cancer*, Vol. 74, 1996, pp. 1194–1198.

[26] Jiang, F. N., et al., "Development of technology for linking photosensitizers to a model monoclonal antibody," *J Immunol Methods*, Vol. 134, 1990, pp. 139–149

[27] Jiang, F. N., et al., "Photodynamic killing of human squamous cell carcinoma cells using a monoclonal antibody-photosensitizer conjugate," *J Natl Cancer Inst*, Vol. 83, 1991, pp. 1218–1225.

[28] Rakestraw, S. L., Tompkins, R. G., and Yarmush, M. L., "Preparation and characterization of immunoconjugates for antibody-targeted photolysis," *Bioconjug Chem*, Vol. 1, 1990, pp. 212–221.

[29] Rakestraw, S. L., Tompkins, R. G., and Yarmush, M. L., "Antibody-targeted photolysis: in vitro studies with Sn(IV) chlorin e6 covalently bound to monoclonal antibodies using a modified dextran carrier," *Proc Natl Acad Sci USA*, Vol. 87, 1990, pp. 4217–4221.

[30] Rakestraw, S., et al., "Antibody-targeted photolysis: in vitro immunological, photophysical, and cytotoxic properties of monoclonal antibody-dextran-Sn(IV) chlorin e6 immunoconjugates," *Biotechnol Prog*, Vol. 8, 1992, pp. 30–39.

[31] Shiah, J. G., et al., "Combination chemotherapy and photodynamic therapy of targetable N-(2-hydroxypropyl)methacrylamide copolymer-doxorubicin/mesochlorin e(6)-OV-TL 16 antibody immunoconjugates," *J Control Release*, Vol. 74, 2001, pp. 249–253.

[32] Lu, Z. R., Kopeckova, P., and Kopecek, J., "Polymerizable Fab' antibody fragments for targeting of anticancer drugs," *Nat Biotechnol*, Vol. 17, 1999, pp. 1101–1104.

[33] Lu, Z. R., et al., "Preparation and biological evaluation of polymerizable antibody Fab' fragment targeted polymeric drug delivery system," *J Control Release*, Vol. 74, 2001, pp. 263–268.

[34] Rancan, F., et al., "Synthesis and in vitro testing of a pyropheophorbide-a-fullerene hexakis adduct immunoconjugate for photodynamic therapy," *Bioconjug Chem*, Vol. 18, 2007, pp. 1078–1086.

[35] Hamblin, M. R., "Covalent photosensitizer conjugates for targeted photodynamic therapy," *Trends Photochem Photobiol*, Vol. 9, 2002, pp. 1–24.

[36] Hamblin, M. R., Miller, J. L., and Hasan, T., "Effect of charge on the interaction of site-specific photoimmunoconjugates with human ovarian cancer cells," *Cancer Res*, Vol. 56, 1996, pp. 5205–5210.

[37] Duska, L. R., et al., "Combination photoimmunotherapy and cisplatin: effects on human ovarian cancer ex vivo.," *J Natl Cancer Inst*, Vol. 91, 1999, pp. 1557–1563.

[38] Duska, L. R., et al., "Biodistribution of charged F(ab')2 photoimmunoconjugates in a xenograft model of ovarian cancer," *Br J Cancer*, Vol. 75, 1997, pp. 837–844.

[39] Molpus, K. L., et al., "Intraperitoneal photoimmunotherapy of ovarian carcinoma xenografts in nude mice using charged photoimmunoconjugates," *Gynecol Oncol*, Vol. 76, 2000, pp. 397–404.

[40] Del Governatore, M., et al., "Targeted photodestruction of human colon cancer cells using charged 17.1A chlorin e6 immunoconjugates," *Br J Cancer*, Vol. 82, 2000, pp. 56–64.

[41] Hamblin, M. R., et al., "Biodistribution of charged 17.1A photoimmunoconjugates in a murine model of hepatic metastasis of colorectal cancer," *Br J Cancer*, Vol. 83, 2000, pp. 1544–1551.

[42] Del Governatore, M., et al., "Experimental photoimmunotherapy of hepatic metastases of colorectal cancer with a 17.1A chlorin(e6) immunoconjugate," *Cancer Res*, Vol. 60, 2000, pp. 4200–4205.

[43] Roby, A., Erdogan, S., and Torchilin, V. P., "Solubilization of poorly soluble PDT agent, meso-tetraphenylporphin, in plain or immunotargeted PEG-PE micelles results in dramatically improved cancer cell killing in vitro," *Eur J Pharm Biopharm*, Vol. 62, 2006, pp. 235–240.

[44] Roby, A., Erdogan, S., and Torchilin, V. P., "Enhanced In Vivo Antitumor Efficacy of Poorly Soluble PDT Agent, Meso-Tetraphenylporphine, in PEG-PE-Based Tumor-Targeted Immunomicelles," *Cancer Biol Ther*, Vol. 6, 2007.

[45] Hamblin, M. R., and Newman, E. L., "Photosensitizer targeting in photodynamic therapy. I. Conjugates of haematoporphyrin with albumin and transferrin," *J Photochem Photobiol B*, Vol. 26, 1994, pp. 45–56.

[46] Cavanaugh, P. G., "Synthesis of chlorin e6-transferrin and demonstration of its light-dependent in vitro breast cancer cell killing ability," *Breast Cancer Res Treat*, Vol. 72, 2002, pp. 117–130.

[47] Derycke, A. S., and De Witte, P. A., "Transferrin-mediated targeting of hypericin embedded in sterically stabilized PEG-liposomes," *Int J Oncol*, Vol. 20, 2002, pp. 181–187.

[48] Gijsens, A., et al., "Targeting of the photocytotoxic compound AlPcS4 to Hela cells by transferrin conjugated PEG-liposomes," *Int J Cancer*, Vol. 101, 2002, pp. 78–85.

[49] Derycke, A. S., et al., "Transferrin-conjugated liposome targeting of photosensitizer AlPcS4 to rat bladder carcinoma cells," *J Natl Cancer Inst*, Vol. 96, 2004, pp. 1620–1630.

[50] Hamblin, M. R., and Newman, E. L., "Photosensitizer targeting in photodynamic therapy. II. Conjugates of haematoporphyrin with serum lipoproteins," *J Photochem Photobiol B*, Vol. 26, 1994, pp. 147–157.

[51] Schmidt-Erfurth, U., et al., "Photodynamic targeting of human retinoblastoma cells using covalent low-density lipoprotein conjugates," *Br J Cancer*, Vol. 75, 1997, pp. 54–61.

[52] Tarrago-Trani, M. T., et al., "Shiga-like toxin subunit B (SLTB)-enhanced delivery of chlorin e6 (Ce6) improves cell killing," *Photochem Photobiol*, Vol. 82, 2006, pp. 527–537.

[53] Bottazzi, B., et al., "A paracrine circuit in the regulation of the proliferation of macrophages infiltrating murine sarcomas," *J Immunol*, Vol. 144, 1990, pp. 2409–12

[54] Demidova, T. N., and Hamblin, M. R., "Macrophage-targeted photodynamic therapy," *Int.J.Immunopathol.Pharmacol.*, Vol. 17, 2004, pp. 117–126.

[55] Hamblin, M. R., Miller, J. L., and Ortel, B., "Scavenger-receptor targeted photodynamic therapy," *Photochem Photobiol*, Vol. 72, 2000, pp. 533–540.

[56] Liu, Q., and Hamblin, M. R., "Macrophage-targeted photodynamic therapy: scavenger receptor expression and activation state," *Int J Immunopathol Pharmacol*, Vol. 18, 2005, pp. 391–402.

[57] Anatelli, F., et al., "Macrophage-targeted photosensitizer conjugate delivered by intratumoral injection," *Mol Pharm*, Vol. 3, 2006, pp. 654–664.

[58] Brasseur, N., et al., "Receptor-mediated targeting of phthalocyanines to macrophages via covalent coupling to native or maleylated bovine serum albumin," *Photochem Photobiol*, Vol. 69, 1999, pp. 345–352.

CHAPTER 11

Covalent Photosensitizer Conjugates, Part 2: Peptides, Polymers, and Small Molecules for Targeted Photodynamic Therapy

Michael R. Hamblin

11.1 Introduction

Chapter 10 discussed conjugates between PS and proteins such as antibodies, transferrin, or scavenger receptor ligands that could target or be accumulated by cells expressing specific cell surface markers or receptors. However, proteins tend to be large molecules and can experience difficulties in exiting blood vessels after IV injection. Antibodies in particular can also have difficulties in moving through the interstitial space of the tumors when they have come out of the blood vessels. The present chapter will look at some other targeting vehicles to which PSs have been covalently attached. Peptides can have the same sequence of amino acids and can therefore be recognized by receptors in the same fashion as some proteins. Growth factors tend to be polypeptides with lower molecular weights than most proteins. Polymer-PS conjugates can be used to take advantage of leaky tumor vasculature and poor lymphatic drainage by the phenomenon known as enhanced permeability and retention. PS that can be cleaved from their macromolecular scaffold by enzymes overexpressed in tumors that recognize specific peptide linkage sequences can add an additional layer of selectivity. Conjugates between PSs and small molecules such as vitamins, steroids, or sugars can also be designed to improve cell type-specific targeting. These examples of the use of rationally designed PS-conjugates illustrate a new approach to optimizing PDT and may allow PDT to be applied in hitherto unexplored diseases.

11.2 Peptide or Growth Factor Conjugates

To overcome the difficulties inherent in using large proteins such as antibodies as targeting vehicles, there have been efforts to use much smaller peptides as targeting vehicles. These peptides recognize fairly specific receptors that in some circumstances may be expressed or overexpressed on tumor cells.

Epidermal growth factor is a 53-aminoacid peptide that is avidly recognized by EGF receptors that can be highly overexpressed on some tumor cells such as squamous cell carcinoma, lung cancer, colon cancer, and many others. Conjugates of EGF to Sn(IV)Ce6 were synthesized [1] through a dextran or polyvinylalcohol (PVA) carrier. EGF targeted conjugates were compared to conjugates of the PS to dextran or to PVA alone. The EGF-Dex-SnCe6 conjugates bound specifically to the EGF receptors of the human squamous carcinoma cell line A431 in contrast to EGF-PVA-SnCe6. However, EGF-PVA-SnCe6 exhibited a higher phototoxicity than EGF-Dex-SnCe6 and SnCe6. PVA-SnCe6 had a similar phototoxicity to EGF-PVA-SnCe6, indicating that PVA, more than EGF, played a determinant role in the uptake of the conjugates by A431 cells. A second report [2] used a related PS, Sn-(IV)Ce6 monoethylenediamine [SnCe6(ED)] attached to EGF via carriers such like human serum albumin (HSA) or dextran, and tested the phototoxicity on the EGF receptor-overexpressing MDA-MB-468 breast adenocarcinoma cell line. The affinity of EGF for its receptor was substantially impaired when conjugated in EGF-Dex-SnCe6(ED), in contrast to EGF-HSA-SnCe6(ED). In corresponding results, EGF-HSA-SnCe6(ED) displayed a high phototoxicity (IC50, 63 nM) on MDA-MB-468 cells at a light dose of 27 kJ/m^2, whereas EGF-Dex-SnCe6(ED) showed very limited phototoxicity. EGF-HSA-SnCe6(ED) was no longer phototoxic in the presence of a competing EGF concentration. The high phototoxicity of EGF-HSA-SnCe6(ED) was shown to be the result of a high intracellular concentration in MDA-MB-468 cells, which could be lowered dramatically by incubating the conjugate with a competing EGF concentration. In contrast, EGF-Dex-SnCe6(ED) accumulated poorly in MDA-MB-468 cells, in agreement with its low EGF receptor affinity and phototoxicity. EGF-HSA-SnCe6(ED) produced much more intracellular reactive oxygen species on light irradiation than EGF-Dex-SnCe6(ED).

Rahimipour et al. [3] conjugated protoporphyrin IX (PpIX) to a gonadotropin-releasing hormone (GnRH) receptor agonist, [d-Lys6]GnRH, or to a GnRH antagonist, [d-pGlu1, d-Phe2, d-Trp3, d-Lys6]GnRH. The condensation of the peptide with PPIX was carried out in a homogeneous solution using benzotriazole-1-yloxytris(pyrrolidinophosphonium) hexafluorophosphate as a coupling reagent. Although these conjugates had lower binding affinity to rat pituitary GnRH receptors than their parent analogues, they fully preserved their agonistic or antagonistic activity in vitro and in vivo. The GnRH agonist conjugate proved to be long-acting in vivo. The conjugates, notably the agonist, were more phototoxic toward pituitary gonadotrope alphaT3-1 cell line than was free PPIX. The phototoxicity of the conjugates (but not PPIX) toward alphaT3-1 cells or to human breast cancer cells (MCF-7 cells that were transfected with human GnRH receptors) was competed by coincubation with the parent peptide. The selectivity of the GnRH antagonist conjugate to gonadotrope cells in a primary pituitary culture was approximately 10 times higher than that of the free PPIX.

A series of papers from Sobolev and colleagues in Russia described conjugates between bovine serum albumin (BSA) and the 51-aminoacid peptide hormone, insulin, as a vehicle to deliver chlorin e6 [4, 5]. Experiments with insulin expressing human hepatoma PLC/PRF/5 cells involving the use of two different tests (colony formation and trypan blue exclusion) demonstrated a significantly higher photosensitizing activity of conjugates after receptor-mediated endocytosis. Further studies on the same system looked at inhibition of endocytosis of the conjugate that abrogated the enhanced photokilling [6]. Endocytosis and subsequent localization around and in the cell nucleus was visualized using both FITC-labeled conjugate and 2′,7′-dichlorofluorescin diacetate, a fluorescent indicator of the production of active oxygen species due to ce6 activation. A subsequent paper went a step further, in which variants of the simian virus SV40 large tumor antigen nuclear localization signal (NLS) were linked to the conjugate in order to deliver the PS to the nucleus, a hypersensitive site for ROS-induced damage [7]. NLSs were either included as peptides cross-linked to the carrier BSA or encoded within the sequence of a beta-galactosidase fusion protein carrier. The presence of NLSs further increased the photokilling of chlorin e6 by a factor of over 2,000-fold. Finally, they reported that attenuated adenoviruses could be used to increase the nuclear delivery of conjugates through their endosomal-membrane-disrupting activity [8]. In the case of the NLS-containing-conjugate, coincubation with adenovirus increased the proportion of cells whose nuclear photosensitizing activity was higher than that in the cytoplasm by 2.5-fold.

Bisland et al. [9] coupled ce6 to a nucleus-directed linear peptide or a branched peptide (loligomer) composed of eight identical arms displaying the same sequence. These constructs incorporated signals guiding their cytoplasmic uptake and nuclear localization. Ce6-peptide and Ce6-loligomer displayed an enhanced photokilling of CHO and RIF-1 cells by 1 or more orders of magnitude compared to free ce6. Constructs were internalized by cells within an hour and by 6 hours, the release of reactive oxygen species could be observed within the nucleus of cells pretreated with Ce6-loligomer.

Frochot et al. conjugated a PS (5-(4-carboxyphenyl)-10,15,20-triphenylchlorin or porphyrin) to the alpha(v)beta(3) integrin specific peptide RGD (H-Arg-Gly-Asp-OH) motif that is able to specifically recognize and bind to alpha(V)beta3 intergrins present on tumor microvascular endothelial cells [10]. Using efficient solid-phase synthesis they prepared conjugates with linear or cyclic[RGDfK] RGD motif and compared in vitro selectivity and PDT activity. The conjugates were characterized by (^{1})H NMR, MALDI, UV-visible spectroscopy, and singlet oxygen formation was performed. Chlorins containing linear and constrained RGD motif were incorporated up to 98- and 80-fold more, respectively, than the unconjugated photosensitizer over a 24-hour exposure in human umbilical vein endothelial cells (HUVEC) overexpressing alpha(v)beta(3) integrin. Peptidic moiety also led to a nonspecific increase in cellular uptake by murine mammary carcinoma cells (EMT-6), lacking RGD binding receptors. Survival measurements demonstrated that HUVEC were greatly sensitive to conjugate-mediated PDT.

In another approach, these workers also targeted tumor neovasculature endothelial cells by conjugating a PS, [5-(4-carboxyphenyl)-10,15,20-triphenylchlorin (TPC)], via a spacer [6-aminohexanoic acid (Ahx)], to a vascular endothelial growth factor receptor-specific heptapeptide [H-Ala-Thr-Trp-Leu-Pro-Pro-Arg-OH (ATWLPPR)] and showed that TPC-Ahx-ATWLPPR binds to neuropilin-1 [11]. Because peptides often display low stability in biological fluids, they examined the in vivo and in vitro stability of this conjugate by high-performance liquid chromatography and matrix-assisted laser desorption ionization/time of flight mass spectrometry. TPC-Ahx-ATWLPPR was stable in vitro in human and mouse plasma for at least 24 hours at 37°C, but following IV injection in glioma-bearing nude mice, was degraded in vivo to various rates, depending on the organ considered.

TPC-Ahx-A was identified as the main metabolic product, and biodistribution studies suggested that its appearance in plasma mainly resulted from the degradation of the peptidic moiety into organs of the reticuloendothelial system. In vitro TPC-Ahx-ATWLPPR mostly localized into lysosomes, and when HUVEC cells were treated with the lysosomal enzyme inhibitor ammonium chloride, this resulted in a significant decrease of the peptide degradation.

In a subsequent report, the same authors demonstrated selectivity of TPC-Ahx-ATWLPPR to neuropilin-1 (NRP-1) recombinant chimeric protein but was found to be devoid of affinity for VEGF receptor type 2 (VEGFR-2, KDR), to which ATWLPPR was initially thought to bind [12]. TPC-Ahx-ATWLPPR was incorporated up to 25-fold more in HUVEC cells than TPC over a 24-hour period, and the addition of 8-mM ATWLPPR induced a significant decrease of this uptake corroborating a receptor-mediated incorporation. Slightly less cytotoxic in the dark, TPC-Ahx-ATWLPPR exhibited enhanced in vitro PDT activity compared to TPC. Pharmacokinetic analysis in nude mice xenografted with U87 human malignant glioma cells revealed relevant tumor levels as soon as 1 hour after IV injection of TPC-Ahx-ATWLPPR, and a rapid elimination from the blood compartment.

Another peptide-conjugation approach was taken by Choi et al. [13] who conjugated a membrane-penetrating arginine-oligopeptide (R7) to 5-[4-carboxyphenyl]-10,15,20-triphenyl-2,3-dihydroxychlorin (TPC). The resulting conjugate (R7-TPC) enhanced intracellular TPC uptake, which increased proportionally with the incubation time of the conjugate. The water solubility of the highly hydrophobic TPC photosensitizer was also improved after conjugation. Increased phototoxicity of R7-TPC to tumor cells after 30 minutes incubation involved apoptosis at lower concentrations of R7-TPC, whereas necrotic cell damage became prevalent at higher concentrations.

11.3   Polymer-PS Conjugates

In recent years, much progress has been made in the use of conjugates between cytotoxic drugs and polymeric carriers to increase the therapeutic ratio of tumor treatment (i.e., to increase tumor selectivity while simultaneously reducing toxicity to normal organs). Similar arguments have been made in favor of the use of polymeric PS conjugates to increase the targeting ability of PS. Many of the synthetic schemes for preparing polymer-PS conjugates have arisen from work on conjugates between Mabs and PSs (see Chapter 10). The preparation of conjugates between tetrapyrrole PS and polymers poses special challenges. They may aggregate to a greater or lesser extent due to the amphiphilic nature of hydrophobic tetrapyrroles joined to hydrophilic polymer chains. Water-soluble PS-polymer conjugates must be relatively hydrophilic, but may bear net cationic, anionic, or neutral charges.

The first example was reported by Davis et al. [14] based on their Mab conjugates [15] described in Chapter 10. They conjugated BPD to modified polyvinyl alcohol; PVA, molecular weight = 10,000 at loading ratios of 1:12, 1:25, 1:50, 1:75, and 1:100. Most of the work was carried out with a conjugate having a 1:25 molar ratio. In vitro photosensitization was tested using A549 (human lung carcinoma), A432 (human epidermoid carcinoma), and P815 (mastocytoma of DBA/2 mice) and

PVA-BPD conjugates were at least as efficient in photosensitization of tumor cells as an equivalent number of free BPD molecules, both in the presence and in the absence of serum. Biodistribution studies were carried out using M1 tumor-bearing DBA/2 mice and either free 3H-BPD or PVA-3H BPD. The conjugate (1:25) reached slightly higher levels in the blood, kidney, lung, and spleen, and lower levels in the liver, brain, skin, and muscle in comparison with free BPD. Photosensitization of M1 (rhabdomyosarcoma of DBA/2 mice) tumors was tested in an in vivo/in vitro assay, in which tumor-bearing mice were injected intravenously with free or conjugated 3H-BPD and 3 hours later light activation of tumor cells was carried out in vitro.

A series of papers from Kopecek's laboratory examined the combination of PDT with N-(2-hydroxypropyl) methacrylamide copolymer conjugated PS and also conjugated cytotoxic anticancer drugs [16]. The first paper [17] compared the efficacy and toxicity of (a) free Adriamycin and N-(2-hydroxypropyl) methacrylamide (HPMA) copolymer-Adriamycin conjugate (P-A), (b) free and HPMA copolymer-meso-chlorin e6 monoethylene diamine disodium salt (Mce6) conjugate (P-C) and PDT, and (c) combinations of the HPMA copolymer conjugates (P-A and P-C) in the destruction of human epithelial ovarian carcinoma heterotransplanted in the nude mouse (OVCAR-3). Nude mice were injected in both flanks with OVCAR-3 solid tumor dispersed in media. Adriamycin (1 mg/kg) and P-A (30-mg/kg. 2.2-mg/kg Adriamycin equivalent) caused less than a 10% weight loss, and treated tumor volumes (days 10–32) were significantly less than those of controls. PDT with free Mce6 or P-C demonstrated significant tumor destruction but not complete ablation. The combinations of P-A plus P-C with light resulted in tumor volumes that were significantly less than control and the tumor volumes of mice receiving either P-A alone or P-C with light alone. Mce6-PDT added to P-A resulted in complete tumor ablation. Free Mce6 demonstrates a narrow margin of safety, which is extended by incorporation into HPMA copolymers.

The next paper reported the effects of the combination therapy in OVCAR3 cells in vitro [18]. The effects of each agent (free drugs and HPMA copolymer bound) alone and in combination were measured simultaneously utilizing two measures of cell viability:MTT assay and tritiated thymidine incorporation assay. Adriamycin (free and bound) was added at time zero, 24 hours later PS (free or bound) was added and 24 hours later light delivered. Assays were performed at 72 and 144 hours. Adriamycin plus Mce6/light acted cooperatively to increase the percentage of cells inhibited. Compared to free drugs, both HPMA copolymer bound adriamycin (P-A) and HPMA copolymer bound Mce6/light (P-C) required a 10-fold increase in drug concentration to show equivalency with free drugs. Dose response curves demonstrated a reduced slope compared to free drugs in the same dose ranges. HPMA-adriamycin added to HPMA-Mce6-PDT improved the efficacy.

Another in vivo study measured concentrations of Mce6 and adriamycin in blood and tissues, after injection in free or HPMA copolymer-bound form [19]. The peak concentration of HPMA copolymer-Mce6 conjugate in tumor was achieved 18 hours after administration. PDT with HPMA copolymer-Mce6 conjugate resulted in significant suppression of the growth of OVCAR-3 tumors. Single PDT plus multiple CHEMO exhibited significantly greater therapeutic efficacy than multiple CHEMO. However, 10 of 12 tumors exhibited complete responses in the group of mice receiving multiple PDTMC plus multiple CHEMO. PDT using HPMA copolymer-Mce6 conjugate with multiple light irradiations was a better therapy than that with single light irradiation. Other reports on this system have looked at subcellular localization of HPMA copolymer-Mce6 conjugates in OVCAR3 cells [20, 21] mechanisms of cell killing after in vitro PDT with free Mce6 or HPMA copolymer-Mce6 conjugates [22], and demonstration that chronic exposure of OVCAR3 cells to free or HPMA copolymer-bound mce6 does not induce P-glycoprotein-mediated multidrug resistance [23].

Our laboratory studied the effect of charge on the cellular uptake, localization, and phototoxicity of conjugates between ce6 and pL (described in Section 10.2 for their reaction with Mabs) [24]. These conjugates (average MW 35-55 kDa) were synthesized to have polycationic, polyanionic, or neutral charges (see Figure 11.1). Two human cell lines (A431 epidermoid carcinoma cells and EA.hy926 hybrid endothelial cells) were studied in vitro and the cellular uptake of ce6 was time- and concentration-dependent and temperature-dependent in the case of neutral and anionic conjugates. Relative uptake at 6 hours for A431 cells was 73:15:4:1 and for EA.hy926 cells was 63:11:3:1 for cationic, anionic, neutral, and free ce6, respectively, but EA.hy926 cells took up 1.5 to 2 times as much ce6 from all the conjugates as A431 cells. Localization as studied by fluorescence microscopy indicated that the cationic conjugate was in aggregates bound to the plasma membrane, while the other forms were internalized in organelles and membranes. In contrast to the

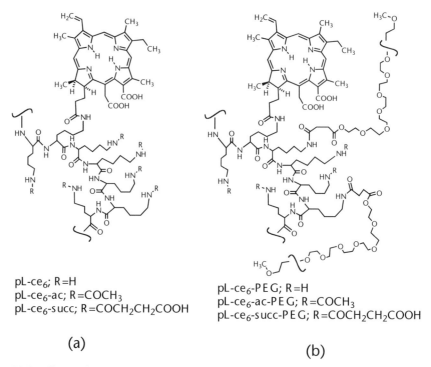

pL-ce6; R=H
pL-ce6-ac; R=COCH3
pL-ce6-succ; R=COCH2CH2COOH

pL-ce6-PEG; R=H
pL-ce6-ac-PEG; R=COCH3
pL-ce6-succ-PEG; R=COCH2CH2COOH

(a)

(b)

Figure 11.1 Chemical structures of conjugates between poly-L-lysine and chlorin (e6). Conjugates are modified from cationic (R=H) pL-ce6 (a), or from the same cationic (R=H) conjugate that has been pegylated, pL-ce6-PEG (b). Modifications produce a neutral form of the conjugate by acetylation (R=COCH3), or produce an anionic form by succinylation (R=COCH2CH2COOH).

uptake, the order of phototoxicity for both cell types per mole of ce6 uptake per cell was neutral >> anionic > cationic > free ce6.

Polymeric drug conjugates are used in cancer therapy, and varying their molecular size and charge, will affect their in vivo transport and extravasation in tumors. Partitioning between tumor vasculature and tumor tissue will be of particular significance in the case of PS conjugates used in PDT, where this partitioning can lead to different therapeutic effects. PL- ce6 conjugates (derived from polymers of average Mr 5000 and 25000, and referred to as small and large, respectively) were prepared both in a cationic state and by poly-succinylation in an anionic state (see Figure 11.2).

A fluorescence-scanning laser microscope was used to follow the pharmacokinetics of these conjugates in vivo in an orthotopic rat prostate cancer model obtained with MatLyLu cells [25]. Fluorescence was excited with the 454- to 528-nm group of lines of an argon laser and a 570-nm long-pass filter used to isolate the emission. Image processing software was used to quantify the fluorescence in various tissue compartments. Examples of images captured from the fluorescence imaging studies are shown in Figure 11.3(a–h). The initial images (Figure 11.3(a), (c), (e), (g)) were usually less fluorescent but in better focus than the intermediate images, while the focus improved towards the end of the imaging (Figure 11.3(b), (d), (f), (h)) when the vasculature became negative with respect to the rest of the tissue. Considerable heterogeneity was observed in the degree to which different types of tumor vasculature extravasated fluorescence. Areas where the blood vessels were convoluted were especially "leaky" (Figure 11.3(a), (b)), while large straight vessels were less leaky and small straight vessels the least. Fluorescence can be seen on the vessel wall in Figure 11.3(e), (g). With some conjugates there was a significant "lag" period after the fluorescence had leaked out into the tissue, and the blood vessels

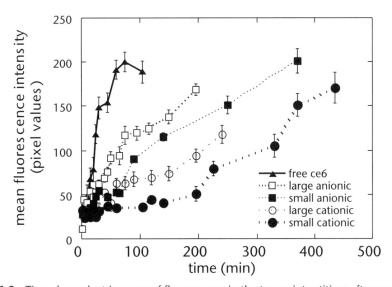

Figure 11.2 Time-dependent increase of fluorescence in the tumor interstitium after prostate tumor bearing rats were injected IV with pl-ce6 conjugates or free ce6. Images were captured at intervals by confocal laser fluorescence microscope and the grayscale levels of at least 100 pixels in the tissue compartment were averaged for each image, values are the means of these mean values for three rats at each time point, and bars are SEM.

had become negative, before the fluorescence intensity in the tissue rose dramatically.

The anionic conjugates produced tissue fluorescence faster than the cationic ones, and surprisingly, the larger Mr conjugates produced tissue fluorescence faster than the smaller ones with the same charge as shown in Figure 11.2. This latter finding was explained by the increased tendency of the small Mr conjugates to aggregate

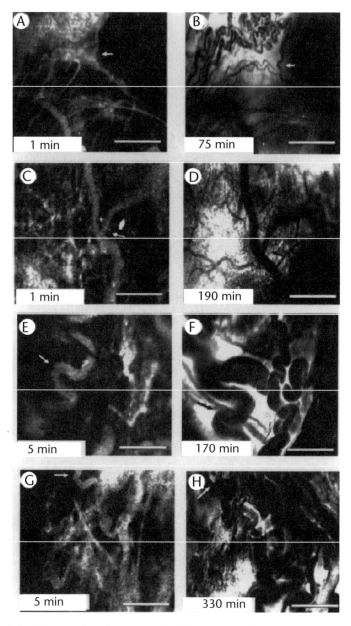

Figure 11.3 Pairs of images from laser scanning fluorescence microscopy, one at an early time point and one at a late time point. Arrows indicate landmarks for orientation in pairs of images. The grayscale values of these images have been optimized for brightness and contrast for printing, and are only proportional to the grayscale values that were used for calculation of pharmaco-kinetics. (a, b) Free ce6; (c, d) small anionic; (e, f) large cationic; and (g, h) small cationic. Scale bar is 500 μm in every case.

in serum and thus to behave as if they were actually larger than the large Mr conjugates.

The conjugation of polyethylene glycol (PEG) to macromolecules that are administered IV has been used to extend serum half-life and reduce the immunogenicity of injected proteins. PEG has also found wide application in the preparation of sterically stabilized (Stealth) liposomes that show reduced uptake by macrophages, and has been shown to increase solubility and reduce aggregation. We reported on an approach to improve tumor targeting by exploiting differences between cell types and by chemical modification of a PS conjugate [26]. Attachment of PEG (pegylation) to a polyacetylated conjugate between pL and ce6 increased the relative phototoxicity in vitro toward an ovarian cancer cell line (OVCAR-5) while reducing it toward a macrophage cell line (J774), compared to the nonpegylated conjugate. Surprisingly, the increased phototoxicity of the pegylated conjugate correlated with reduced oxygen consumption. Pegylation also reduced the tendency of the conjugate to aggregate and reduced the consumption of oxygen when the conjugates were illuminated in solution in serum containing medium, suggesting a switch in photochemical mechanism from type II (singlet oxygen) to type I (radicals or electron transfer). Pegylation led to more mitochondrial localization as shown by confocal fluorescence microscopy in OVCAR-5 cells, and upon illumination produced a switch in cell death mechanism towards apoptosis not seen with J774 cells. Conjugates were injected IP into nude mice bearing IP OVCAR-5 tumors and the pegylated conjugate gave higher amounts of photosensitizer in tumor, higher tumor to normal tissue ratios, and increased the depth to which the ce6 penetrated into the peritoneal wall (Color Plate 6).

A subsequent study from our lab [27] explored the effect of pegylation on corresponding conjugates with either cationic or anionic charges in the same two cell lines. The cationic conjugate after pegylation became less aggregated, consumed less oxygen, and had reduced cellular uptake. However, the phototoxicity corrected for cellular uptake increased three- to five-fold. In contrast, the anionic succinylated conjugate on pegylation became more aggregated, consumed similar amounts of oxygen, and had higher cellular uptake. The anionic conjugate showed the highest relative phototoxicity towards both cell lines (compared to the other three conjugates) and it decreased most towards the macrophages after pegylation. Pegylation reduced the amount of oxygen consumed per ce6 molecule when photosensitized cells were illuminated. These in vitro studies suggest that pegylation alters the phototoxicity of PS conjugates depending on the effect produced on the aggregation state.

A series of studies from our laboratory and from the laboratory of Jori had examined the use of polycationic conjugates of PS with polymers such as pL and polyethyelenimine with the aim of targeting PS to pathogenic microbes such as bacteria and fungi. These studies are covered in Chapter 18.

11.4 Enzyme Cleavable PS Conjugates

Another method of increasing specificity for tumors and many other nonmalignant diseases is to take advantage of the lesion-specific expression of enzymes such as proteases. If the PS conjugate is in a quenched form before injection but the linker between PS and quencher is subject to specific enzyme-mediated cleavage, then the cleavage of the PS from the quencher by the enzyme present at the target lesion will release it in a photoactive form and PDT activity will be selectively enhanced. The principle is graphically illustrated in Figure 11.4.

This technique was first reported in 2004 by Chen et al. [28] who constructed a caspase 3 cleavable construct consisting of GDEVDGSGK as the peptide sequence, for which there is a well-established assay for the caspase-3-specific fluorogenic substrate, and conjugated to pyropheophorbide as the PS and a carotenoid as the quencher moiety, since caretonoids (CAR) are well known both to quench triplet excited states and also to scavenge singlet oxygen. When the CAR moiety is held in close proximity to the PS by the short peptide sequence, it efficiently decreases singlet oxygen generation and lifetime, while addition of caspase-3 increased singlet oxygen production. Cleavage of these constructs by caspase 3 means that the compound can be used as an "apoptosis sensor" giving an increased fluorescent signal when caspase 3 liberates the fluorophore [29]. Caspase 3 is one of the major executioner caspase enzymes whose activity is greatly increased when cells undergo apoptosis These constructs can also contain a targeting moiety such as folate [30] (see Section 11.5.1). PDT-triggered cleavage of the peptide linker by caspase 3 resulted in a detectable increase in fluorescence in folate receptor-overexpressing cancer cells and tumors. The presence of apoptosis was confirmed in vitro by flow cytometry and ex vivo by Apoptag assay, supporting the ability of TaBIAS to specifically induce and image apoptosis in situ. Molecular beacons that use near-infrared fluorescence imaging (NIRF-I) to identify the unique cellular and metabolic markers characteristic of cancer can be combined with PDT [31]. Guided by the beacon's restored fluorescence, the PDT laser could be focused on affected sites, killing the cancer cells using the enhanced photoactivity of the same beacon. Or vice versa—the restored fluorescence from the cleaved beacon could be used as an indication of the beacon's own therapeutic success, imaging the post-PDT apoptotic cells. Another manifestation of this approach was the construction of a matrix metalloproteinase-7 (MMP7)-triggered photodynamic molecular beacon (PMB) [32] and achieving not only MMP7-triggered production of singlet oxygen in solution but also

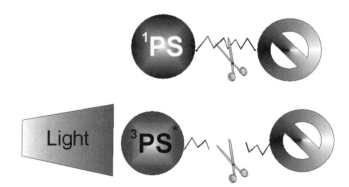

Figure 11.4   Schematic representation of a cleavable-conjugate between a PS and a quencher. The linker typically has an amino-acid sequence that is susceptible to cleavage by an enzyme that is overexpressed in the target tissue.

MMP7-mediated photodynamic cytotoxicity in cancer cells. Preliminary in vivo studies also revealed the MMP7-activated PDT efficacy of this PMB.

Campo et al. prepared polymeric photosensitizer prodrugs (PPPs) in which multiple PS units are covalently coupled to a polymeric backbone via protease-cleavable peptide linkers [33]. These initially quenched PS become fluorescent and phototoxic after enzymatic cleavage of the peptide linkers. PL conjugates to pheophorbide(a), sensitive to trypsin-mediated cleavage, gave rise to a fluorescence increase and to more efficient generation of reactive oxygen species upon light irradiation. In vitro tests using the T-24 bladder carcinoma cell line and ex vivo experiments using mouse intestines illustrated the ability of these PPP to fluoresce and induce phototoxicity upon enzymatic activation.

Gabriel et al. further elaborated this approach [34] with different pheophorbide a-peptide loading ratios and backbone net charges were evaluated with respect to their solubility, "self-quenching" capacity of fluorescence emission, and reactive oxygen species (ROS) generation. In addition, linker sequence impaired selectivity toward enzymatic cleavage was demonstrated either by incubating PPPs with different enzymes having trypsin-like activity or by introducing a single d-arginine mutant in the peptide sequence. In vitro cell culture tests confirmed dose-dependent higher phototoxicity of enzymatically activated PPPs compared to the nonactivated conjugate after irradiation with white light.

Another approach involved designing chlorin e6 (ce6)-containing macromolecules, which are sensitive to tumor-associated proteases [35]. The agents were nontoxic in their native state but became fluorescent and produced singlet oxygen on protease conversion. Coupled with optimized delivery systems, they showed that (a) the agents efficiently accumulated in tumors due to the enhanced permeability and retention effect, (b) the agents were locally activated by proteases, (c) local drug concentrations could be measured by quantitative fluorescence tomography, and (d) light-treated tumors showed reduced growth [36]. A single low dose of PDT (0.125 mg Ce6 equivalent/kg) was sufficient to suppress tumor growth by >50%.

11.5 Small Molecule-PS Conjugates

Several small molecule conjugates with PS have been proposed to increase tumor targeting of PSs or to modify their tissue biodistribution. The examples that will be covered in this section are (1) folic acid, (2) steroid hormones, and (3) sugars (schematically illustrated in Color Plate 7).

11.5.1 Folic Acid Conjugates

Folate is involved in the synthesis, repair, and functioning of DNA and a deficiency of folate may result in damage to DNA that may lead to cancer. Folate is important for cells and tissues that rapidly divide, and therefore rapidly dividing cancer cells tend to overexpress folic acid receptors to ensure that they obtain a sufficient supply. This overexpression combined with the high affinity recognition displayed by the receptor ligand binding has meant that folate receptors have become a popular tumor target by conjugating folic acid to anticancer molecules.

Schneider et al. synthesized two new conjugates of three components, folic acid/hexane-1,6-diamine/4-carboxyphenylporphyrine 1 and folic acid/2,2' -(ethylenedioxy)-bis-ethylamine/4-carboxyphenylporphyrine 2 [37]. The conjugates were characterized by 1H NMR, MALDI, UV-visible spectroscopy, and fluorescence quantum yield. The targeted delivery of these photoactive compounds to KB nasopharyngeal cell line, which is one of the numerous tumor cell types that overexpress folate receptors, was studied. It was found that after 24-hour incubation, conjugates 1 and 2 cellular uptake was on average sevenfold higher than tetraphenylporphyrin (TPP) used as reference and that 1 and 2 cellular uptake kinetics increased steadily over the 24-hour period, suggesting an active transport via receptor-mediated endocytosis. In corresponding results, conjugates 1 and 2 accumulation displayed a reduction of 70% in the presence of a competitive concentration of folic acid. Survival measurements demonstrated that KB cells were significantly more sensitive to conjugated porphyrins-mediated PDT. Under the same experimental conditions and the same photosensitizer concentration, TPP displayed no photocytotoxicity while conjugates 1 and 2 showed photodynamic activity with light dose values yielding 50% growth inhibition of 22.6 and 6.7 J/cm^2, respectively.

Stefflova et al. prepared a construct (pyro-peptide-folate, PPF) consisting of three components: (1) pyropheophorbide(a) as the PS, (2) peptide sequence as a stable linker, and (3) folate as a targeting moiety [38]. They found a higher accumulation of PPF in KB cancer cells (FR+) compared to HT 1080 cancer cells (FR-), resulting in a more effective post-PDT killing of KB cells over HT 1080 or normal CHO cells. The accumulation of PPF in KB cells can be up to 70% inhibited by an excess of free folic acid. The effect of folate on preferential accumulation of PPF in KB tumors (KB versus HT 1080 tumors 2.5:1) was also confirmed in vivo. In contrast, no significant difference between the KB and HT 1080 tumor was observed in the case of the untargeted probe (pyro-peptide, PP). A short peptide sequence considerably improved the delivery efficiency of the probe demonstrated by a 50-fold reduction in PPF accumulation in liver and spleen when compared to a peptide-lacking probe.

11.5.2 Steroid Hormones

Covalent attachment of steroid hormone receptor ligands to molecules can be used to target tumors such as breast, prostate, endometrial, and testicular cancer that tend to overexpress estrogen or androgen receptors. This approach could potentially deliver drugs more selectively to specific target tissues, but they could also be used to target different subcellular locations inside a cell. Even though the targets of these conjugates are believed to be intracellular, conjugates can still enter cells and elicit cellular responses. Increasing evidence suggests that steroid hormones can elicit cellular responses from different locations in the cell such as the plasma membrane and endoplasmic reticulum.

James et al. synthesized a tetraphenylporphyrin-C11-beta-estradiol conjugate and demonstrated by competitive binding assay that conjugate binds specifically to estrogen receptor (ER)-ligand-binding domain with high affinity [39]. Cellular uptake studies with ER-positive MCF-7 and ER-negative HS578t human breast cancer cells revealed that the conjugate was taken up by MCF-7 cells in a dose-dependent manner, which was obliterated by coincubation with a large excess of estradiol [40]. There was very little uptake of the unconjugated porphyrin by MCF-7 and Hs578t cells and HS578t cells also showed insignificant uptake of the conjugate.

These workers then synthesized four conjugates of C17-alpha-alkynylestradiol and ce6-dimethyl ester with varying tether lengths, and showed that all these conjugates specifically bound to recombinant ER alpha [41]. In a cellular uptake assay with ER-positive MCF-7 and ER-negative MDA-MB 231 human breast cancer cell-lines, they observed that one conjugate (E17-POR, XIV) was selectively taken up in a dose-dependent and saturable manner by MCF-7 cells, but not by MDA-MB 231 cells. Furthermore, MCF-7 cells, but not MDA-MB 231 cells, were selectively and efficiently killed by exposure to red light after incubation with E17-POR. Finally, they prepared a tamoxifen (TAM)-pyropheophorbide conjugate that specifically binds to ER alpha, and caused selective cell-kill in MCF-7 breast cancer cells upon light exposure [42]. Another group also prepared estradiol-pheophorbide a conjugates [43]. They showed higher cellular uptake of the conjugate by ER-positive MCF-7 cells compared with ER-negative SKBR3 cells and endothelial cells that correlated with higher phototoxicity. Fluorescence microscopy showed evidence of nuclear localization of the conjugate in ER+ cells not seen with the PS alone.

11.5.3 Saccharides

The rationale for conjugating sugar residues or saccharides to PS is to take advantage of the avid recognition and binding of various sugar residues by lectins. Lectins bind carbohydrate moieties as such free in solution or a carbohydrate moiety that is a part of protein/particulate body. They agglutinate cells and/or precipitate glycoconjugates. There are lectins found on the surface of mammalian liver cells that specifically recognize galactose residues. It is believed that these cell-surface receptors are responsible for the removal of certain glycoproteins from the circulatory system. Another example is the mannose-6-phosphate receptor that recognizes hydrolytic enzymes containing this residue and subsequently targets these proteins for delivery to the lysosomes. Lectins serve many different biological functions from the regulation of cell adhesion to glycoprotein synthesis and the control of protein levels in the blood. Lectins are also known to play important roles in the immune system by recognizing carbohydrates that are found exclusively on pathogens, or that are inaccessible on host cells. Examples are the lectin complement activation pathway and Mannose binding lectin.

Lectins have been reported to be overexpressed in many types of cancer cells including liver, breast, prostate, lung, and bile duct cell types, and have therefore become a popular target for glycoconjugated anticancer molecules. Di Stasio et al. synthesized mono- (1) and di-glucosylated (2) porphyrins, and monoglucosylated chlorin (3) and showed HT29 human adenocarcinoma cells were significantly more sensitive to asymmetric and less hydrophobic glucosylated PS-mediated PDT (1, 3), compared to tetraphenylporphyrin (TPP) [44]. The lowest photosensitivity observed for TPP was consistent with the lowest uptake. Moreover, the most pronounced PDT activity measured for 3 was in relation with the improvement of cellular uptake, the singlet oxygen quantum yield, and the high extinction coefficient value at 650 nm compared to porphyrins. Cellular localization analysis showed that 1 and 3 accumulated mainly inside the endoplasmic reticulum.

Frochot reported the synthesis and the photophysical properties (absorption, fluorescence, singlet oxygen formation) of new glycosylated porphyrins [45]. In vitro photocytotoxic properties were evaluated on the human colon adenocarcinoma cell line HT29. Zheng et al. reported [46] on the synthesis and biological evaluation of beta-galactose-conjugated purpurinimides (a class of chlorins containing a six-membered fused imide ring system) with the aim of these conjugates being recognized by Gal-1 (galectin-1). They synthesized them from purpurin-N-propargylimide via enyne metathesis and obtained a crystal structure of the galectin-1 N-acetyllactose amine conjugate. Molecular modeling analysis utilizing the modeled photosensitizers and the available crystal structures of galectin-carbohydrate complexes indicated that addition of the photosensitizer to the carbohydrate moiety at an appropriate position does not interfere with the galectin-carbohydrate recognition. Compared to the free purpurinimide analogue, the purpurinimides conjugated either with galactose or with lactose (Gal(beta1-4)-Glc) produced a considerable increase in photosensitizing efficacy in vitro.

Chen et al. [47] reported a two-step method to make nonhydrolyzable saccharide-porphyrin conjugates in high yields using a tetra(pentafluorophenyl)-porphyrin and the thio derivative of the sugar. Different malignant cell types take up one type of saccharide-porphyrin conjugate preferentially over others; for example, human breast cancer cells (MDA-MB-231) absorb a tetraglucose-porphyrin conjugate over the corresponding galactose derivative. Dosimetric studies revealed that these saccharide-porphyrin conjugates exhibited varying PDT responses depending on drug concentration and irradiation energy including necrosis, apoptosis, and a reduction in cell migration is observed.

11.6   Conclusion

The preparation and use of covalent conjugates between PSs and targeting vehicles has the potential to dramatically improve the selectivity and efficacy of PDT. Conjugates should be rationally designed for their particular application, taking into account the cellular or tissue targets, delivery route, pharmacokinetics, photochemical efficiency, and attainable PS and light doses. Although in many cases the process of forming covalent conjugates between PS and macromolecules can significantly reduce the quantum yield of phototoxic species, this reduction may be compensated by increased selectivity and reduced collateral damage to nontarget tissue. Factors such as the molecular size and charge of the conjugates should be taken into account in deciding the delivery route and the time interval before illumination. The use of PS conjugates as PDT sensitizers means that the actual dye molecule can be chosen on its photochemical, photophysical properties, allowing the targeting to be carried out by the macromolecule. With advances constantly being made in the design of targeting vehicles used for delivering therapies for cancer such as radioisotopes, toxins, and cytotoxic drugs, this will lead to the further diverse applications of similar techniques to target PSs more selectively and to a wider array of targets on both the molecular, cellular, and tissular levels.

References

[1] Gijsens, A., and De Witte, P., "Photocytotoxic action of EGF-PVA-Sn(IV)chlorin e6 and EGF-dextran-Sn(IV)chlorin e6 internalizable conjugates on A431 cells," *Int J Oncol*, Vol. 13, 1998, pp. 1171–1177.

[2] Gijsens, A., et al., "Epidermal growth factor-mediated targeting of chlorin e6 selectively potentiates its photodynamic activity," *Cancer Res*, Vol. 60, 2000, pp. 2197–2202.

[3] Rahimipour, S., et al., "Receptor-mediated targeting of a photosensitizer by its conjugation to gonadotropin-releasing hormone analogues," *J Med Chem*, Vol. 46, 2003, pp. 3965–3974.

[4] Sobolev, A. S., et al., "Internalizable insulin-BSA-chlorin E6 conjugate is a more effective photosensitizer than chlorin E6 alone," *Biochem Int*, Vol. 26, 1992, pp. 445–450.

[5] Akhlynina, T. V., et al., "The use of internalizable derivatives of chlorin E6 for increasing its photosensitizing activity," *Photochem Photobiol*, Vol. 58, 1993, pp. 45–48.

[6] Akhlynina, T. V., et al., "Insulin-mediated intracellular targeting enhances the photodynamic activity of chlorin e6," *Cancer Res*, Vol. 55, 1995, pp. 1014–1019.

[7] Akhlynina, T. V., et al., "Nuclear targeting of chlorin e6 enhances its photosensitizing activity," *J Biol Chem*, Vol. 272, 1997, pp. 20328–20331.

[8] Akhlynina, T. V., et al., "Adenoviruses synergize with nuclear localization signals to enhance nuclear delivery and photodynamic action of internalizable conjugates containing chlorin e6," *Int J Cancer*, Vol. 81, 1999, pp. 734–740.

[9] Bisland, S. K., Singh, D., and Gariepy, J., "Potentiation of chlorin e6 photodynamic activity in vitro with peptide-based intracellular vehicles," *Bioconjug Chem*, Vol. 10, 1999, pp. 982–992.

[10] Frochot, C., et al., "Interest of RGD-containing linear or cyclic peptide targeted tetraphenylchlorin as novel photosensitizers for selective photodynamic activity," *Bioorg Chem*, Vol. 35, 2007, pp. 205–220.

[11] Tirand, L., et al., "Metabolic profile of a peptide-conjugated chlorin-type photosensitizer targeting neuropilin-1: an in vivo and in vitro study," *Drug Metab Dispos*, Vol. 35, 2007, pp. 806–813.

[12] Tirand, L., et al., "A peptide competing with VEGF165 binding on neuropilin-1 mediates targeting of a chlorin-type photosensitizer and potentiates its photodynamic activity in human endothelial cells," *J Control Release*, Vol. 111, 2006, pp. 153–164.

[13] Choi, Y., et al., "Conjugation of a photosensitizer to an oligoarginine-based cell-penetrating peptide increases the efficacy of photodynamic therapy," *ChemMedChem*, Vol. 1, 2006, pp. 458–463.

[14] Davis, N., et al., "Modified polyvinyl alcohol-benzoporphyrin derivative conjugates as phototoxic agents," *Photochem Photobiol*, Vol. 57, 1993, pp. 641–647.

[15] Jiang, F. N., et al., "Development of technology for linking photosensitizers to a model monoclonal antibody," *J Immunol Methods*, Vol. 134, 1990, pp. 139–149.

[16] Peterson, C. M., et al., "HPMA copolymer delivery of chemotherapy and photodynamic therapy in ovarian cancer," *Adv Exp Med Biol*, Vol. 519, 2003, pp. 101–123.

[17] Peterson, C. M., et al., "Combination chemotherapy and photodynamic therapy with N-(2-hydroxypropyl) methacrylamide copolymer-bound anticancer drugs inhibit human ovarian carcinoma heterotransplanted in nude mice," *Cancer Res*, Vol. 56, 1996, pp. 3980–3985.

[18] Lu, J. M., et al., "Cooperativity between free and N-(2-hydroxypropyl) methacrylamide copolymer bound adriamycin and meso-chlorin e6 monoethylene diamine induced photodynamic therapy in human epithelial ovarian carcinoma in vitro," *Int J Oncol*, Vol. 15, 1999, pp. 5–16.

[19] Shiah, J. G., et al., "Antitumor activity of N-(2-hydroxypropyl) methacrylamide copolymer-Mesochlorine e6 and adriamycin conjugates in combination treatments," *Clin Cancer Res*, Vol. 6, 2000, pp. 1008–1015.

[20] Tijerina, M., Kopeckova, P., and Kopecek, J., "The effects of subcellular localization of N-(2-hydroxypropyl)methacrylamide copolymer-Mce(6) conjugates in a human ovarian carcinoma," *J Control Release*, Vol. 74, 2001, pp. 269–273.

[21] Tijerina, M., Kopeckova, P., and Kopecek, J., "Correlation of subcellular compartmentalization of HPMA copolymer-Mce6 conjugates with chemotherapeutic activity in human ovarian carcinoma cells," *Pharm Res*, Vol. 20, 2003, pp. 728–737.

[22] Tijerina, M., Kopeckova, P., and Kopecek, J., "Mechanisms of cytotoxicity in human ovarian carcinoma cells exposed to free Mce6 or HPMA copolymer-Mce6 conjugates," *Photochem Photobiol*, Vol. 77, 2003, pp. 645–652.

[23] Tijerina, M., et al., "Chronic exposure of human ovarian carcinoma cells to free or HPMA copolymer-bound mesochlorin e6 does not induce P-glycoprotein-mediated multidrug resistance," *Biomaterials*, Vol. 21, 2000, pp. 2203–2210.

[24] Soukos, N. S., Hamblin, M. R., and Hasan, T., "The effect of charge on cellular uptake and phototoxicity of polylysine chlorin(e6) conjugates," *Photochem Photobiol*, Vol. 65, 1997, pp. 723–729.

[25] Hamblin, M. R., et al., "In vivo fluorescence imaging of the transport of charged chlorin e6 conjugates in a rat orthotopic prostate tumour.," *Br J Cancer*, Vol. 81, 1999, pp. 261–268.

[26] Hamblin, M. R., et al., "Pegylation of a chlorin(e6) polymer conjugate increases tumor targeting of photosensitizer," *Cancer Res*, Vol. 61, 2001, pp. 7155–7162.

[27] Hamblin, M. R., et al., "Pegylation of charged polymer-photosensitiser conjugates: effects on photodynamic efficacy," *Br J Cancer*, Vol. 89, 2003, pp. 937–943.

[28] Chen, J., et al., "Protease-triggered photosensitizing beacon based on singlet oxygen quenching and activation," *J Am Chem Soc*, Vol. 126, 2004, pp. 11450–11451.

[29] Stefflova, K., et al., "Photodynamic therapy agent with a built-in apoptosis sensor for evaluating its own therapeutic outcome in situ," *J Med Chem*, Vol. 49, 2006, pp. 3850–3856.

[30] Stefflova, K., et al., "Targeted photodynamic therapy agent with a built-in apoptosis sensor for in vivo near-infrared imaging of tumor apoptosis triggered by its photosensitization in situ," *Mol Imaging*, Vol. 5, 2006, pp. 520–532.

[31] Stefflova, K., Chen, J., and Zheng, G., "Using molecular beacons for cancer imaging and treatment," *Front Biosci*, Vol. 12, 2007, pp. 4709–4721.

[32] Zheng, G., et al., "Photodynamic molecular beacon as an activatable photosensitizer based on protease-controlled singlet oxygen quenching and activation," *Proc Natl Acad Sci USA*, Vol. 104, 2007, pp. 8989–8994.

[33] Campo, M. A., et al., "Polymeric photosensitizer prodrugs for photodynamic therapy," *Photochem Photobiol*, Vol. 83, 2007, pp. 958–965.

[34] Gabriel, D., et al., "Tailoring Protease-Sensitive Photodynamic Agents to Specific Disease-Associated Enzymes," *Bioconjug Chem*, Vol., 2007.

[35] Choi, Y., Weissleder, R., and Tung, C. H., "Protease-mediated phototoxicity of a polylysine-chlorin(E6) conjugate," *ChemMedChem*, Vol. 1, 2006, pp. 698–701.

[36] Choi, Y., Weissleder, R., and Tung, C. H., "Selective antitumor effect of novel protease-mediated photodynamic agent," *Cancer Res*, Vol. 66, 2006, pp. 7225–7229.

[37] Schneider, R., et al., "Design, synthesis, and biological evaluation of folic acid targeted tetraphenylporphyrin as novel photosensitizers for selective photodynamic therapy," *Bioorg Med Chem*, Vol. 13, 2005, pp. 2799–2808.

[38] Stefflova, K., et al., "Peptide-based pharmacomodulation of a cancer-targeted optical imaging and photodynamic therapy agent," *Bioconjug Chem*, Vol. 18, 2007, pp. 379–388.

[39] James, D. A., et al., "Synthesis and estrogen receptor binding affinity of a porphyrin-estradiol conjugate for targeted photodynamic therapy of cancer," *Bioorg Med Chem Lett*, Vol. 9, 1999, pp. 2379–2384.

[40] Swamy, N., et al., "An estradiol-porphyrin conjugate selectively localizes into estrogen receptor-positive breast cancer cells," *Bioorg Med Chem*, Vol. 10, 2002, pp. 3237–3243.

[41] Swamy, N., et al., "Nuclear estrogen receptor targeted photodynamic therapy: selective uptake and killing of MCF-7 breast cancer cells by a C17alpha-alkynylestradiol-porphyrin conjugate," *J Cell Biochem*, Vol. 99, 2006, pp. 966–977.

[42] Fernandez Gacio, A., et al., "Photodynamic cell-kill analysis of breast tumor cells with a tamoxifen-pyropheophorbide conjugate," *J Cell Biochem*, Vol. 99, 2006, pp. 665–670.

[43] El-Akra, N., et al., "Synthesis of estradiol-pheophorbide a conjugates: evidence of nuclear targeting, DNA damage and improved photodynamic activity in human breast cancer and vascular endothelial cells," *Photochem Photobiol Sci*, Vol. 5, 2006, pp. 996–999.

[44] Di Stasio, B., et al., "The 2-aminoglucosamide motif improves cellular uptake and photodynamic activity of tetraphenylporphyrin," *Eur J Med Chem*, Vol. 40, 2005, pp. 1111–1122.

[45] Frochot, C., et al., "New glycosylated porphyrins for PDT applications," *Oftalmologia*, Vol. 56, 2003, pp. 62–66.

[46] Zheng, G., et al., "Synthesis of beta-galactose-conjugated chlorins derived by enyne metathesis as galectin-specific photosensitizers for photodynamic therapy," *J Org Chem*, Vol. 66, 2001, pp. 8709–8716.

[47] Chen, X., et al., "Efficient synthesis and photodynamic activity of porphyrin-saccharide conjugates: targeting and incapacitating cancer cells," *Biochemistry*, Vol. 43, 2004, pp. 10918–10929.

CHAPTER 12

Emerging Strategies in Photodynamic Therapy

Brian C. Wilson

12.1 Introduction

Virtually all photodynamic therapy as currently practiced clinically utilizes essentially the same basic technique, summarized in Table 12.1. Also listed are strategies currently under development that diverge in some fundamental way from these standard conditions (i.e., that represent nonincremental advances). These alternative strategies are the subject of this chapter and each of these will be introduced in turn, together with a critical discussion of the potential advantages and the barriers to the development and/or implementation.

12.2 Photosensitizer-Based Strategies

Several options have been identified that use a different approach from the traditional molecular-dye type of photosensitizer (PS). There are many examples of the

Table 12.1 Standard and Novel PDT Strategies

Focus of Strategy	Standard PDT Technique	Novel PDT Strategies
Photosensitizer (PS)	Organic molecular PS	Nanoparticle (NP)-based photosensitizers: Inorganic NPs as photosensitizers / NP-PS FRET conjugates / NPs as PS delivery vehicles
	Passive (intrinsic) PS targeting	active targeting at the tissue, cell or sub-cellular organelle level
	PS always activatable	PDT molecular beacons
light (γ)	CW or quasi-CW single-photon (1-γ) activation	short-pulsed 2-γ activation: simultaneous (resonant) 2-γ absorption / sequential 2-photon, 2-wavelength (2-γ/2-λ) activation
PS and γ dose rates	acute (high dose-rate) treatment	metronomic PS and γ delivery
photobiological effect	cell kill/tissue destruction as the primary objective	modulation of cell/tissue function/structure

latter, discussed elsewhere in this book. Most of the ongoing development of PDT photosensitizers is focused on the design and synthesis of new organic molecules with improved properties such as high optical extinction (molar absorption coefficient) at long wavelengths (>~700–850 nm) to achieve greater light penetration in tissue, high quantum yield for the primary cytotoxic photoproduct singlet oxygen, water solubility to simplify systemic administration without the use of a delivery vehicle, altered pharmacokinetics (e.g., rapid uptake and clearance to achieve primarily vascular targeting, and low skin photosensitization) or practical considerations such as ease of synthesis and scale-up, purity, and cost. Photodynamic bacterial decontamination [1] poses different challenges from targeting mammalian cells/tissues, particularly penetration and destruction of the thick bacterial cell wall.

12.2.1 Nanoparticles

One novel strategy is the use of nanoparticles (NPs) for PDT, of which there are three main classes (see Figure 12.1): (1) NPs that are themselves photodynamically active, (2) NPs that serve as an "energy transducer" to absorb the light and transfer the energy to a photosensitizer molecule, and (3) NPs that act as carriers for conventional photosensitizers.

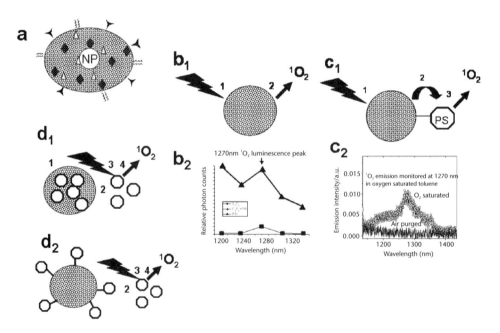

Figure 12.1 Schematic illustrations of the different classes of NP applications in PDT. (a) NPs as a generic platform for drug delivery, with surface targeting and biocompatibility molecules. (b) NPs as photosensitizers with an example (b2) of the singlet oxygen near-infrared luminescence from porous silicon NPs in aqueous suspension (courtesy Dr. B. Li). (c) NP-photosensitizer FRET conjugates showing the light absorption by the NP, followed by resonant energy transfer to the photosensitizer molecule, which then is excited and generates $^1O_2$ through a type-II process. (c2) example of the $^1O_2$ luminescence spectrum from Qdot-phthalocyanine conjugates under oxygenated (upper curve) and anoxic (lower) conditions (adapted from [7], with permission). (d) NPs as photosensitizer carriers for targeted delivery of high PS payload (d1-encapsulated, d2-decorated)

These developments in PDT should be seen in the context of the intense effort over the past few years on developing NPs of many different types for a variety of analytic, diagnostic, and therapeutic applications [2]. One driving force for this is the fact that fundamental changes can take place in the physical properties of materials, including their optical properties, when they are in the form of nanoparticles compared to the bulk-material properties: "nano" is defined here as in the range of 1 to 100 nm, in keeping with the operational definition of the National Institutes of Health (USA) [3].

In the first class (i.e,. NPs as photosensitizers), it has been shown, for example, that porous silicon NPs can generate singlet oxygen ($^1O_2$) or other reactive-oxygen species [4]. This is illustrated in Figure 12.1(b) by the detection in an aqueous medium of the luminescence decay of $^1O_2$ at 1270 nm. This altered property compared with bulk silicon is associated with the large surface-to-volume ratio in the porous silicon nanoparticles, which enables efficient dipole-dipole or direct electron exchange due to coupling between the excitons confined in the nanostructure and molecular oxygen. What has not yet been shown is that this can result in cytotoxicity, either in vitro or in vivo. There are two main issues to make this a reality: the first is how to deliver the NPs to the target tissue and to have them be internalized within cells, and the second is whether the $^1O_2$ generated within the NP porous matrix can "escape" to the biological target(s). Advantage of porous Si NPs should be their low intrinsic (dark) toxicity and low cost of production. However, it is not obvious what would be the real photobiological advantage over molecular dyes, unless, for example, it was possible to achieve very specific subcellular (e.g., nuclear) targeting. In principle, this could be achieved, since the concept of using NPs as the photosensitizer in PDT means that the photophysical properties can be uncoupled from the pharmacokinetic behavior.

A second example of NPs as direct photosensitizers is the use of photosensitizer nanocrystals, which has been recently reported in vitro as a means of delivering the hydrophobic pyropheophorbide sensitizer HPPH without the use of a carrier [5]. In this case the mechanisms of cellular uptake are not fully understood. The in vivo PDT efficacy in a tumor model was comparable to that achieved by administrating the photosensitizer in a delivery formulation (Tween-80). This approach is also being explored for other hydrophobic therapeutic drugs.

A third example of NPs as direct photosensitizers is that of quantum dots (Qdots), that are composed of semiconductor materials (e.g., CdSe, InP, InAs.), usually in the form of a core of one material and a shell of a different material. The surface can then be "passified" in order to stabilize the Qdots and to facilitate coating with ligands (e.g., antibodies or peptide sequences) to target specific cell receptors. This was demonstrated, for example, by Bharali et al. [6], who targeted Qdots to the folate receptor that is expressed on the surface of many cancer cells. There is great interest in Qdots because of their unique optical properties: high fluorescence quantum yield, low photobleaching, broad excitation spectrum, large Stokes shift and narrow emission spectra, which hold the promise of high-order spectral multiplexing for fluorescence imaging and diagnostics. For PDT, the interest is two-fold. First, Qdots have very high 2-photon cross sections, typically >50,000 GM units: as will be discussed in detail below, this makes them potentially useful for (simultaneous) 2-γ activation. Second, they can be used for Föster Resonant Energy Transfer (FRET), which represents the second class of NP-based PDT strategies [7].

In this second class (i.e., NPs as energy transducers), a conjugate is made comprising the Qdot and a (conventional, organic dye-based) photosensitizer molecule. The light is then absorbed by the Qdot. If there is good overlap between the PS absorption and Qdot emission spectra, then resonant energy transfer takes place and the photosensitizer is raised to an excited electronic singlet state, from which it proceeds to generate $^1O_2$ by the normal type-II photophysical process (see below). This has been demonstrated in solu by Samia et al. [7, 8]. The potential advantage of this approach is that it could allow more flexibility in selecting the spectral properties of the PS so that its other properties could be optimized. The penalty is the greater complexity of the conjugate, and, as with the other applications of Qdots, the possibility of dark toxicity due to the heavy-metal content of the semiconductor materials. In vivo delivery of the Qdots is also a major challenge [8]. This FRET approach has also been investigated using dye aggregates as the optical absorber for 2-photon excitation (see below).

In the first two NP strategies above, the critical element is that the NPs have some novel optical property that is not present in the bulk material. In the third class of nanoparticle-based PDT, the approach is to use NPs as delivery vehicles. Generically, this is shown in Figure 12.1(a), which also schematically illustrates the potential of NPs to carry multiple therapeutic drugs or image contrast materials as payloads and to be decorated with targeting and other biocompatible moieties to facilitate in vivo delivery. In the same way, NPs can be used to carry a payload of photosensitizing molecules, including hydrophobic drugs, either encapsulated in the NP or attached to the surface, as in Figure 12.1(d). This approach is not new in PDT: for example, in the commercial formulation of benzoporphyrin used to treat macular degeneration the photosensitizer is encapsulated in liposomes (i.e., in lipid nanoparticles) [9].

There are several reports of other forms of NP used for photosensitizer delivery, either with the NPs encapsulating the photosensitizer molecules or with photosensitizer covalently attached to the NP surface. Various NP materials have been investigated, both inorganic and organic (LDLs), including gold, organically-modified silica, cyclodextrin, low-density lipoproteins, coblock polymer micelles, polylactic acid, and polylactic-coglycolic acid (see for example [10–14]). Increased cell uptake and in vivo tumor targeting in preclinical models has been achieved and improved PDT cytotoxicity has been reported in some cases. NPs such as LDLs and liposomes have the advantage that these are made from biomaterials and so have high biocompatibility and low toxicity; the use of high-density lipoproteins enables low sequestering of the NPs in the reticuloendothelial system in vivo, with resulting high-target tissue (e.g., tumor) uptake [15]. Most work has been aimed at solid tumor treatments and a variety of photosensitizers have been used to demonstrate proof-of-principle. Recently, Gil-Thomás and colleagues [16] reported a toluidine blue O (TBO)-tiopronin-gold NP conjugate that gave a fourfold reduction in the minimum bacterial concentration compared to the unconjugated dye in PDT killing of *Staphylococcus aureus*. In this formulation, there were 11–15 TBO molecules per 2- to 3-nm diameter NP.

The general advantage of nanoparticles as photosensitizer delivery vehicles is that they can provide very high payloads, including hydrophobic agents, and they can be decorated at relatively high density with targeting moieties. This is to be compared with traditional PS targeting, for example antibody-PS conjugates, where a major barrier is that only a few PS molecules can be attached to each antibody without interfering with the ability to bind to the target antigen. In addition, it would be possible to deliver more than one photosensitizer in a single NP or to use multiple NPs with different targets (say, tumor cells and vasculature) with the same or different photosensitizers. It would also be possible to combine PS delivery with simultaneous delivery of a second, mechanistically-complementary (nonphotoactive) cytotoxic agent.

A further advantage of NPs as delivery vehicles is that they can be multifunctional, for example incorporating a contrast agent for magnetic resonance imaging [17, 18] of their localization in vivo. For PDT such capability could be achieved by conjugating the photosensitizer to a nanoparticle, such as iron oxide or magnetite, that has intrinsic image-contrast capability [19]. A further possibility with magnetic NPs is to apply megnetophoretic control (magnetic guidance) to improve targeting [20].

The bimodal concept can also be applied to enhance the efficacy of PDT by using a photosensitizer coupled to an iron oxide nanoparticle that could enhance the localized absorption of EM radiation in order to produce hyperthermia [21], which has been shown many years ago to be synergistic with PDT. Another approach is to use photosensitizer-NP conjugates where the NPs are made of a material that luminesces upon absorption of X-rays, thereby activating the photosensitizer [22]. This could be thought of either as a way to reduce the required dose of ionizing radiation or as a way to achieve X-ray activation of photosensitizers that would overcome the limitations of light penetration in tissue. However, the total energy absorbed per gm of tissue in radiation therapy (e.g., 50 Gy radical treatment $\cong$ 50 mJ per gm) is 1 to 3 orders of magnitude less than in typical PDT (~1–100 J per gm), so that this may be energetically unfavorable.

These multiple and varied potential gains that could, in principle, be achieved through the use of NPs in PDT have to be balanced against the many barriers, both fundamental and practical, to them becoming a reality in clinical use, including their likely cost due to complexity of synthesis, conjugation, and scale-up to production level and in some cases their possible toxicity. Nevertheless, the sheer quantity of research and development in nanotechnologies in general seem certain to lead to NPs penetrating the practice of PDT in some form or another and could potentially revolutionize it.

12.2.2 PS Targeting

The last examples above represent attempts to actively target the PS, exploiting the special properties of nanoparticles. There are an increasing range of other approaches to targeting in PDT. These are both passive and active [23]. The former includes exploiting the rapid uptake and clearance of some photosensitizers, so that, if the light is applied during this period, there is effectively vascular targeting. Examples of this are the well-established use of Visudyne® (QLT, Canada) to treat AMD and palladium bacteriopheophorbide (TOOKAD®, Steba, France), which is in clinical trials for treatment of prostate cancer [24]. Active targeting [23, 25] includes the use of antibody (Ab)-PS conjugates, peptides [26] and hormones [27] targeted to specific receptors that are overexpressed compared to normal tissues/cells. Other strategies have included targeting tumor-associated macrophages [28] and bacteriophage-photosensitizers conjugate to target bacteria [29].

A different approach has been to target PSs to specific subcellular organelles. Most photosensitizers in clinical use tend to accumulate naturally in cell membranes, particularly mitochondria. The efficacy of the hormone (estradiol)-photosensitizer conjugates referred to above [27] appears to be through its nuclear targeting. Active nuclear targeting of the chlorine photosensitizer Cle6 by conjugating it to polymeric peptides (loligomers) was reported by Bisland et al. in 1999 [30], resulting in a tenfold reduction in the concentration of photosensitizer required to achieve the same level of PDT cell kill in vitro compared with untargeted PS. Cle6 was also used by Akhlynina and colleagues [31] conjugated to insulin and linked to SV40 simian viruses and gave a 2,000-fold reduction in the photosensitizer dose required to kill insulin receptor-positive cells in vitro. Recently, S. Kelly and colleagues [32] have reported conjugates of the photosensitizer thiozole orange (TO) with short peptide sequences that have very high preferential localization to specific subcellular organelles, with nuclear and mitochondrial targeting demonstrated to date, as illustrated in Figure 12.2. The improvement in photocytotoxicity compared with untargeted PS has not yet been reported.

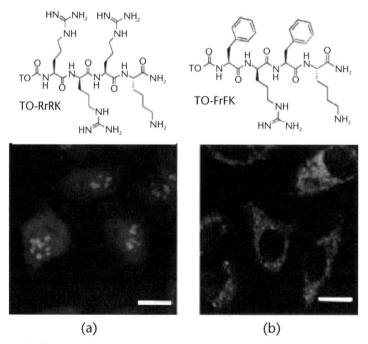

Figure 12.2 Subcellular organelle targeting of peptide-photosensitizer (thiazine orange) conjugates: (a) nuclear localization, and (b) mitochondrial localization shown by fluorescence microscopy. The corresponding peptide structures are also shown (adapted from [32] with permission).

Parenthetically, the absence of nuclear localization and consequent DNA damage has been long considered an advantage of PDT, since it differentiates its mechanism of action from that of ionizing radiation and many antineoplastic drugs, so that PDT and these established therapies are not contraindicated.

Overall, the potential advantages of active photosensitizer targeting are clear and address one of the central limitations of current PDT, namely the disappointingly low intrinsic specificity of most photosensitizers, including many of those in clinical use or trials. Of course, this is compensated in part by the generally low systemic and dark toxicity of most PSs and the additional targeting provided by the application of the light. The limitations of the above strategies will be the same as those encountered with targeting any other cytotoxic or image contrast agent. An additional issue with PS targeting is that it must leave the photophysical properties of the photosensitizer intact.

12.2.3   Photodynamic Molecular Beacons

A radically different approach to increased target specificity is provided by PDT molecular beacons (PMBs), introduced by Zhang and colleagues in 2004 [33], that are analogous to beacons developed for fluorescence diagnostics. The concept is illustrated in Figure 12.3, and as with the Qdot-photosensitizer conjugates discussed above, exploits the FRET effect.

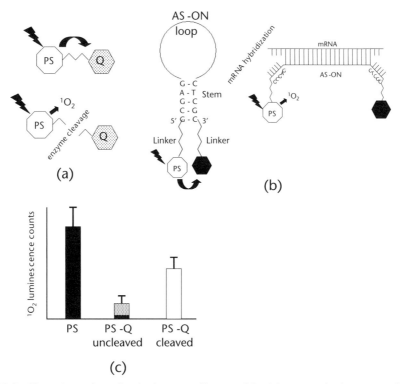

Figure 12.3   Photodynamic molecular beacons, illustrated for (a) enzymatic cleavage and (b) opening of an antisense oligonucleotide loop by hybridization to specific target mRNA, and (c) singlet oxygen photoproduction in solution from pyropheophorbide (PS)-carotenoid (Q) beacon before and after caspase cleavage, compared with that from the photosensitizer alone [33].

A PMB comprises three elements: (1) the photosensitizer, (2) a quenching moiety to which the optical energy absorbed by the PS molecule is transferred when the two are in close proximity ($1/r^6$ dependence on the separation, r), thereby silencing the photoactivation of the PS, and (3) a linker that joins these two elements. The PBM is designed to be in the OFF state when it is administered but the PS becomes active (ON) when it is physically separated from the quencher upon reaching the biological target. This can be accomplished in several ways, for example enzymatic cleavage of a liker consisting of a peptide sequence (Figure 12.3(a)) or opening, by hybridization to complementary mRNA, of a linker in the form of an antisense loop (Figure 12.3(b)). The key point is that the breaking or opening of the linker can be made highly target specific.

This high specificity of the quenching and unquenching of singlet oxygen generation with both forms of PMB has been demonstrated through direct measurements of the $^1O_2$ near-infrared luminescence, as illustrated in Figure 12.3(c). Enzyme-based PMBs have been demonstrated to date in tumors, both in vitro and in vivo, where the peptide linker has been designed to be cleaved by, for example, matrix metalloproteinase MMP7 [34]. Here, in solution, the quenching of the PS (pyropheophorbide) by the so-called black-hole quencher reduced the $^1O_2$ generation 18-fold due to the self-folding of the linker, while addition of MMP7 fully restored the photoactivity. Likewise, high photocytotoxicity was found in vitro in tumor cells expressing MMP7, while MMP7-negative cells showed no measurable PDT response. The former, grown as solid tumor xenografts also showed PDT-induced necrosis when treated in vivo.

To date, mRNA-dependent unquenching has been shown in solution and in tumor cells in vitro [35]. In solution, 15-fold less $^1O_2$ was generated in the quenched beacon than in unconjugated PS and this was then increased by ninefold upon addition of the target mRNA; the PS fluorescence increased 13-fold upon hybridization with the target mRNA but only by threefold when there was a single base-pair mismatch present. Fluorescence microscopy also showed that this PMB was internalized in tumor cells in vitro. Interestingly, and for reasons that are not entirely clear, these PMBs appear to have some degree of intrinsic tumor cell localization. This may help address one of the issues with PMBs, namely how to deliver them to the target in sufficient concentration. Other potential barriers to the development and successful in vivo/clinical use of PMBs are the complex synthesis required, which may be difficult or costly to scale up, and the limited density of receptor targets, which are preferably intracellular in order to target PDT-sensitive organelles. Nevertheless, the potential advantage of triple specificity (beacon delivery, light delivery, and photoactivation) is compelling.

Interesting variants of the PMB concept include (a) coupling of multiple photosensitizer molecules onto a polymeric backbone via enzyme-cleavable amino acid sequences, in which the photosensitizer molecules self-quench due to high local concentration [36], (b) the use of Qdots as the photosensitizer, with gold nanoparticles as the quencher, which has been shown in fluorescence mode [37], and (c) self reporting photosensitizers [38], where the beacon is taken up into cells intact and becomes fluorescent only upon cleavage by caspases that are upregulated as part of the apoptosis signaling pathway following PDT damage (see Color Plate 8).

12.3   Light-Based Strategies

12.3.1   Simultaneous Two-Photon PDT

The Jablonski energy-level diagram for conventional single-photon (1-γ), type-II photosensitization is shown in Figure 12.4(a).

As is well known, the absorption of a photon of appropriate wavelength (energy) excites the PS molecule from the ground state (S_0) to the S_1 state, whereupon it can undergo intersystem crossing to the excited triplet (T_1) state (or de-excite nonradiatively or by fluorescence emission). T_1 is long-lived (~μs) and can exchange energy with triplet ground-state molecular oxygen ($^3O_2$) to generate $^1O_2$. There are two main alternates to this scheme in which two photons are involved. The first (Figure 12.4(b)) requires simultaneous absorption of two photons by S_0. Thereafter, the processes are the same as in 1-γ absorption. The total energy required (S_1-S_0) is also the same, so that if the two photons are of the same wavelength, then each requires about half the energy of the 1-γ case (i.e., have double the wavelength). Whereas 1-γ absorption is a linear process, the probability of 2-γ absorption increases as the square of the local light intensity, I. That is, for equal PS concentrations,

$$1-\gamma: \qquad Probability \propto \varepsilon.I \qquad\qquad (12.1a)$$

$$2-\gamma: \qquad Probability \propto \sigma.I^2 \qquad\qquad (12.1b)$$

where ε is the 1-γ extinction coefficient (cm^{-1}) and σ is the 2-γ absorption cross section, usually expressed in GM units (named after the 1963 Nobel Laureate Maria Goeppert-Mayer, who first proposed this phenomenon; 1GM unit = 10–50 cm^{-4}.s.photon^{-1}). σ is extremely small for most photosensitizers designed for 1-γ activation, so that 2-γ activation is negligible under normal continuous-wave (CW) or

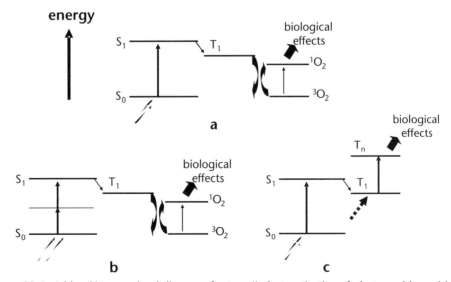

Figure 12.4   Jablonski energy level diagrams for type II photoactivation of photosensitizers: (a) 1-γ PDT, (b) simultaneous 2-γ PDT, and (c) 2-γ/2−λ PDT.

quasi-CW illumination. For example, at the peak of the 2-γ absorption spectra of Photofrin (~800 nm) and benzoporphyrin, BPD, (>~900 nm), Karotki et al. [39] measured σ values of about 10 and 50 GM, respectively (see Color Plate 9a). The only way to get significant 2-γ PDT activation is then to increase and/or I.

Consider first the option of increasing the light intensity to exploit the quadratic dependence. Since the same photophysics, photochemistry, and photobiological effects take place after exciting the S1 state by 2-γ as by 1-γ absorption, the total light energy, E, required is the same in both modes. Hence, the only way to increase I without concomitant increase in E is to use very short pulses of light, of length τ, since the peak pulse power (and I) is proportional to E/τ. The optimum value of τ appears to be around 100 fs (10^{-13}s); longer than this does not produce high enough instantaneous values of I^2, while use of shorter pulses can generate photomechanical damage to cells, through plasma formation and resultant shock-wave generation that is independent of the photosensitizer, thereby losing the potential photobiological advantages of PDT. Using pulsed lasers in the 100-fs range can lead to measurable 1-γ activation even with photosensitizers that are not specially designed for this purpose. For example, in vitro cell killing in vascular endothelial cell cultures has been shown for both Photofrin and BPD [40] and vascular shutdown has been shown also using BPD (Visudyne®) in vivo in the chick chorioallantoic membrane model [41]. The irradiation wavelength used in these studies was 865 nm, which is well beyond the 1-γ absorption peak of these photosensitizers. Note, however, that these measurements have to be done with meticulous attention to the controls, since even a very small residual 1-γ absorption can be misinterpreted as a 2-γ effect. The limitation of these results is that the in vitro cell kill required total energy doses that are orders of magnitude higher than that required for equivalent cell kill with 1-γ activation. This would result in exposure times that are too long to be clinically practical. The option of increasing I was explored, but direct photomechanical damage occurred at the intensities far below those needed to reach comparable treatment times [40]. It, therefore, seems impractical to use conventional 1-γ photosensitizers in 2-γ mode in order to treat a whole area of neovascularization. One option is to target only individual feeder vessels, as done in the CAM model [41], but the efficacy of this is not known for AMD treatment.

Recently, there have been several independent attempts to synthesize photosensitizers that have high σ values. One option [42] is to employ a FRET-like strategy, with a molecular complex that has both high σ photoactivatable components. This has achieved values of σ>~500 GM units. A second example is to use conjugated porphyrin dimers, which have been reported to have σ~5,000 GM units [43]. Recently, successful microvessel closure in vivo by 2-γ PDT has been accomplished with one such photosensitizer (which also has the advantage of being water soluble), delivered systemically in a mouse model, as illustrated in Color Plate 9c, with irradiation parameters that are realistic for potential clinical translation.

There are also nanoparticle-based strategies to achieve high 2-photon efficiency. One option is to use Qdots themselves, since these have σ>~50,000 GM units, as has been investigated for multiphoton fluorescence microscopy [6]. A second is to use NPs to encapsulate fluorophores and photosensitizers such that there is a high concentration of the former to cause self-aggregation, leading to enhanced 2-photon cross-section and FRET activation of the sensitizer [44].

Given the many technical complexities of 2-γ PDT, why would one attempt this strategy? There are two main reasons, both relating to the delivery of the light. Firstly, long wavelength (near infrared) light can be used, unlike 1-γ activation where increasing the wavelength too far into the near infrared means either that there is not enough energy to generate the S_1 state efficiently and/or that the photosensitizer molecules are photolabile and unstable. Hence, one can maximize the penetration of the light in the target tissue, allowing, for example, treatment of deeper or larger tumors [42]. However, one caveat is that I^2 decreases more rapidly than I with increasing depth, which counters the decrease in the optical attenuation by the tissue. In addition, the high scattering of light in tissue means that there is a background of 1-γ events unless the linear extinction coefficient (ε) of the PS is truly negligible at the 2-γ excitation wavelength. Nevertheless, the concept is appealing, considering that depth of the PDT treatment effect can be a significant limitation in some applications.

The second reason is that, if the laser beam is focused to a point in or on the tissue, then the quadratic (I^2) dependence makes the effective activation volume very small (in the femtoliter range). In essence, one obtains exquisite spatial confinement of the treatment. This is analogous to the use of 2-γ confocal fluorescence microscopy that provides submicron spatial resolution. In addition, there is minimal photodynamic effect in the tissues above or below the focal plane, since the intensity is not high enough. (Again, this is analogous to the reduced photobleaching of the sample in 2-γ microscopy.) The application for which most work has been done to exploit these effects is 2-γ PDT for AMD [40, 41, 43], driven by the possibility that this would minimize the collateral damage to normal retinal structures that may, in part, be responsible for the need to re-treat multiple times with 1-γ PDT.

Since 2-γ PDT is a point-by-point treatment, some form of image guidance and control of the laser beam is required, such as the use of a scanning laser ophthalmoscope in the case of AMD. While conceptually compelling, there are several potential limitations, including degradation of the focus by the limited numerical aperture and optical aberrations of the eye (especially in the elderly), pulse dispersion in the beam as it propagates to and within the eye, and the need for high-speed tracking to compensate for eye movement. Other applications can be envisaged where precise spatial confinement of the PDT treatment might be of use, such as in other ocular diseases (diabetic retinopathy, ocular melanoma) and (micro) bonding of tissues (see below).

12.3.2 Two-Photon/2-Wavelength PDT

The other form of 2-γ activation considered here is shown in Figure 12.4(c). In this case the first photon is absorbed by the PS, as in 1-γ activation. A second photon is then absorbed by the triplet (T_1) state, raising it to a higher energy triplet, T_n. This can then react with biomolecules by processes that do not require oxygen, which is the main motivation to explore this strategy. In principle, this process can occur during conventional PDT with a broadband CW light source. For example, Mir et al. [45] have shown that copper tetrasulfophthalocyanine irradiated in solution simultaneously with 514- and 670-nm CW light at modest power densities (183 and 86 mWcm^{-2}, respectively) increased the photoinactivation of the enzyme acetylcholinesterase compared to using only one wavelength at a time. However, relative to 1-photon excitation this has low probability, since the instantaneous ratio of T_1 to S_0 states is low. This group has, nevertheless, shown 2-γ/2-λ PDT killing of cells in vitro using the same photosensitizer but activated with pulsed laser light [46].

The oxygen independence of 2-γ/2-λ PDT was demonstrated in vitro by Smith et al. [47] using rose bengal as the photosensitizer. With 1-γ activation there was good cell killing under oxygenated conditions, which was eliminated under nitrogen purging of the cells; by contrast, cytotoxicity was retained, albeit at a lower level, with 2-γ/2-λ treatment, demonstrating the photocytotoxicity of oxygen-independent pathways from the higher excited triplet state. The potential value of this observation lies in the poor oxygenation of many solid tumors, which may limit the efficacy of 1γ PDT.

Photosensitizers for 2-γ/2-λ need to have suitable photophysical properties, including long wavelength absorption in both the S_0 and T_1 states in order to retain good light penetration in tissue. A second major challenge is to develop practical light sources for this technique. Laser systems that can generate the requisite pulse characteristics (λ_1, λ_2, pulse-pulse time interval, adequate pulse energies, and repetition rates) are large, complex scientific instruments and this technology is a long way from an affordable, compact source in which the user could "dial up" the best parameters to match the specific photosensitizer.

12.4 Photosensitizer and Light Dose-Rate Strategies

12.4.1 Metronomic PDT

As stated earlier, the standard PDT strategy has been to administer the highest possible photosensitizer and light doses in a single, acute treatment in order to achieve maximum target cell or tissue destruction. The administered light fluence rate (power density) is also usually the highest possible, while avoiding tissue heating from the optical energy absorption in the tissue, or photochemical oxygen depletion. Typically, for surface irradiation, hyperthermia occurs at >~100–200 mWcm^{-2}, depending on the wavelength (and, hence, volume distribution of the light) and on the blood perfusion rate of the tissue. Correspondingly, with interstitial fiberoptic point or cylindrically diffusing light delivery, about 100 mW or 100–200 mW.cm^{-1}, respectively, are typically acceptable in terms of avoiding significant heating (i.e., less than a few degrees). Photochemical oxygen consumption can occur, however, at lower power levels. With devices such as interstitial linear light-emitting diode (LED) arrays that do not incorporate active cooling, the power that can be used in more typically in the tens of mW per cm length. In this case, since LEDs have electrical-to-optical conversion efficiencies of only 10% to 15%, it is the self-heating of the source that is the limiting factor rather than the light absorption by the tissue.

There has, for practical reasons, been little motivation to pursue low drug and/or light dose rates or to deliver treatment in multiple small fractions. Indeed, one of the putative advantages of PDT has always been the fact that it can be given as a single-shot treatment, in contrast for example to radiation or chemotherapy where many fractions are administered over days or weeks. However, it may be possible to increase the ratio between, say, tumor destruction and damage to the adjacent normal host tissues, by using so-called metronomic PDT (mPDT) [48], in which the photosensitizer and light are administered at very low rates over an extended period (days). The evidence for this has, to date, come primarily from studies to optimize PDT of malignant brain tumors. In this application, both clinical and preclinical observations have shown that the normal brain is exquisitely sensitive to PDT damage [49], probably because the photosensitizer is localized in the vascular endothelium in brain regions with intact blood-brain barrier. In the case of ALA-PpIX, it was shown that there was high PpIX concentration in tumor compared with normal white matter (in which 80% of adult gliomas occur), and to a lesser extent, with gray matter (cortex) [50]. However, despite this, necrosis could still be induced in the normal tissue at clinically relevant drug and light doses. It is well established that induction of tissue necrosis in PDT is a threshold phenomenon (i.e., for a given photosensitizer and tissue there is a well-defined drug-light product at any point in the tissue below which necrosis does not occur, and that this threshold is very sharp). Since necrotic damage, even to tumor tissue, can cause secondary inflammatory response in the brain, the ALA and light doses still given in a single treatment were reduced below the threshold(s), and it was found possible still to produce apoptotic cell death (which has a stochastic rather than threshold response) in both tumor and normal brain. At low enough dose rates, it was possible to produce tumor cell-selective apoptosis [48, 51], as illustrated in Color Plate 10a. Thus, mPDT seeks to bias the mechanism of cell death towards apoptosis. (Note that this is conceptually different from using low-light fluence rates or ON-OFF light regimes to avoid the well-known phenomenon of photochemical depletion of oxygen of tissues and is also different from fractionating the light so as to allow oxygen or photosensitizer replenishment.)

Several questions arise from these observations:

1. Is it feasible to achieve an adequate level of tumor cell kill in this way (i.e., can one kill tumor cells faster that they proliferate)?
2. Is mPDT applicable to other photosensitizers and/or tissues and pathologies?
3. Would mPDT be of value in situations where inducing tumor necrosis would be acceptable?
4. How could mPDT be administered in practice, both in terms of the drug and the light if both must be delivered over an extended period or days or weeks?

There has been little work to date on addressing questions 2 and 3. The answer to the first question will clearly depend on balancing the rate of induced apoptosis with the rate of tumor cell repopulation, while keeping below the necrosis thresholds of the target and normal tissues. Color Plate 10b shows recent results in an intracranial brain tumor model that demonstrate that this can be done. In this case, ALA was administered orally over a period of up to 5 days at a rate of 100-mg/kg body weight per day and light was delivered by an interstitial optical fiber at a rate of 44 joules per day (~500 μW).

For question 4, there are different challenges around the photosensitizer and the light. One of the key issues is the potential toxicity of photosensitizer delivered over an extended period at a rate that produces adequate uptake in the target. In the case of ALA given orally, a dose of above about 200 mg/kg/day produces detectable neurotoxicity in rats, while 100 mg/kg/day appears to produce adequate tumor cell uptake. Extended drug delivery is common practice in chemotherapy of tumors, using for example an implanted infusion pump. Alternatively, the sensitizer could be given in hyperfractionated fashion, with the time interval between fractions determined by the uptake and clearance rates in the tumor. For applications such as photodynamic decontamination of chronic infected skin wounds, the drug could be applied topically using a continuous-delivery surface device.

In terms of light application, there are various options, depending on whether the target is superficial or deep-seated. For brain tumors, the major challenge is that it will be necessary to place an implant within the brain, most likely at the time of surgical debulking of the tumor. This is feasible, for example using implanted optical fibers that are then connected to an external laser or LED source, as illustrated preclinically in Color Plate 10b. A balloon-type applicator, based on a system for delivering radioactive sources for postoperative brachytherapy of gliomas, has also been reported [52]. One could also envisage distributing the light through the target volume by either multiple laser-couple optical fibers or by using interstitial linear LED arrays [53] that have been used in other tumor sites. For surface treatments, there are several possible technologies. Examples are a fiber-optic mesh, semiconductor LED arrays [54], or as recently reported, an organic LED (OLED) patch [55]. In the case of OLEDs, mPDT is de facto the mode of light delivery, since at present the output power levels are very low.

12.5   Photobiology-Based Strategies

Most PDT has been in applications where cell death is the objective, for example, tumor cells, vascular endothelial cells, or micro-organisms. Here, we will briefly give examples of other potential applications where, rather than cytotoxicity, sublethal modification of cell/tissue function or other effects of photodynamic activation are exploited.

12.5.1   PDT Treatment of Epilepsy

E. Zusman and colleagues have carried out initial studies of PDT to reduce neuronal cell hyperexcitability for treatment of epilepsy [56], based on the observation that enhanced ALA-induced PpIX synthesis is seen in such cells, both in vitro and in (rat) brain tissue in vivo compared with normal quiescent cells. This could be done clinically by local application of light, either during open surgery or by interstitial fiber placement through a burr hole. It may also be possible to use the fluorescence of ALA-induced PpIX as an aid in localization of the epileptic focus, instead of or as an adjuvant to electrical mapping.

12.5.2   PDT to Modulate (Bone) Growth

PDT is under development to treat metastatic and primary cancers in bone [57] and bone infection (osteomyelitis) [58]. A concern arising from this work (as it should for any organ) was whether or not the treatment would have adverse effects on bone integrity, either structural or functional. Biomechanical tests indicated that, surprisingly, the opposite could happen, namely that bone could be strengthened by PDT treatment. This led to studies of the use of PDT more generally to modulate bone growth, either stimulatory or inhibitory. The outcome is not clear at this stage, but it appears that both phenomena are possible. In particular, the inhibition of bone growth appears to be the result of PDT-induced angiogenesis in the growth plate [59], which is a natural signal to close the plate. Potential applications would be to correct asymmetric bone growth, for example in the legs or spine. Clinically, there would be advantages in some cases if growth could be stimulated, and some of the control experiments in the above work [59] suggest that this can happen in the absence of administered photosensitizer (i.e., by light treatment only).

12.5.3 PDT and Low-Level Light Therapy

This last observation opens up the question as to whether, and to what extent, can some of the effects reported in so-called low-level light therapy (also known as photobiomodulation or soft laser therapy) be considered photodynamic in nature. This field is a minefield of confusing information, with rigorous research having been reported in many in vitro studies (in both plant and mammalian cells), a more limited set of reliable data in preclinical animal models in vivo, but a paucity of controlled clinical trials [60]. In spite of, or perhaps because of this, such treatments are used widely for conditions ranging from control of chronic wounds and chronic pain to behavioral modification such as stopping smoking. Since exogenous photosensitizers are not administered, any photodynamic mechanisms would be through excitation of exogenous chromophores. Most of the in vitro studies suggest that the main photobiological effects are mediated by modifications to the cell energy metabolism. Little has been done to look explicitly for synergy or antagonism between such effects and conventional PDT: one example is a recent study showing increased ALA-induced PpIX in glioma cells in vitro following low-level light therapy due to upregulation of the mitochondrial bezodiazapine receptor [61].

12.5.4 Photodynamic Tissue Bonding

The use of PDT to bond or weld tissues is not new. However, there has recently been revived interest. It is based on photochemical cross-linking of proteins, including collagen, which should cause less damage to the tissues than more conventional (photo) thermal bonding [62]. For example, I. Kochevar, R. Redmond, and colleagues in Boston have reported successful bonding of a variety of tissues, including skin, cornea, tendon, and artery and functional repair of sciatic nerve damage in rats in vivo using rose bengal as the photosensitizer [63 and references therein]. Depending on the site, especially the thickness of the tissue to be bonded, challenges in PDT for these surgical applications include delivery of the photosensitizer uniformly and at the optimum concentration across the surfaces to be bonded, and similarly, achieving adequate light irradiation throughout the full thickness. The latter would be facilitated by use of photosensitizers activated at long wavelengths, in the red or near-infrared, as with chromophore-enhanced photothermal bonding. For microsurgical repair, the opposite may pertain and in this case the precise targeting of 2-photon PDT may be exploitable.

12.5.5 Tissue Engineering Using Photodynamic Control

The low thermal damage of PDT tissue bonding has been explored by Ibusuki et al. [64] for cross-linking collagen gels as scaffolds for engineered tissues using rose bengal and riboflavin-based PDT. Subsequent cell survival in the gels was not significantly compromised, which is a critical requirement. Another approach is to use for 3-D microstructuring in biomaterials or artificial tissues or to generate controlled growth pathways in tissue engineering. This last has been demonstrated elegantly by M. Stoichet and colleagues [65], where a focused light beam photodynamically uncages a growth factor along defined channels in a gel matrix, which then directs the growth pattern of neuronal cells. The 3-D spatial precision of this technique could also be enhanced by the use of 2-photon activation. There are many other potential applications of PDT in tissue engineering and regenerative medicine that have not yet been explored.

12.6 Summary and Conclusions

This overview of strategies to PDT that are fundamentally different in some specific way(s) from PDT as it is currently widely practiced is intended to stimulate out-of-the-box thinking about how PDT might be done differently, either to overcome or circumvent limitations of standard PDT techniques or to open up new areas of application. Clearly, most of these new approaches pose substantial scientific, technological, and/or clinical challenges. It is not clear, for any of them, whether or not the potential benefit will justify the effort and possible costs required to develop them to the point of clinical utility. Some of these approaches come from observations made during investigation and development of conventional PDT methods (for example, mPDT or bone growth modulation), while others are driven by the appearance of new enabling technologies (for example, 2-γ PDT that relies on fs lasers or PMBs that are a spinoff from molecular bioimaging). Nevertheless, they do emphasize the fact that the basic concept of photodynamic therapy, namely the use of light to activate materials leading to biological changes, is far from fully explored. No doubt there will be other strategies of which we have not yet dreamt.

Acknowledgments

The author wishes to thank the following agencies for support of work illustrated here: the National Cancer Institute of Canada, the National Institutes of Heath, US (CA-43892), and the Canadian Institute for Photonic Innovations. Also, thanks to many colleagues and students in the PDT program at the Ontario Cancer Institute and to our clinical and industry collaborators.

References

[1]   Jori. G., "Photodynamic therapy of microbial infections: state of the art and perspectives," *J Environ Pathol Toxicol Oncol*, Vol. 25, 2006, pp. 505–519.

[2]   Ferrari, M., "Cancer nanotechnology: opportunities and challenges," *Nature Rev-Cancer*, Vol. 5, 2005, pp. 161–171.

[3]   Alliance for Nanotechnology of the US National Cancer Institute, website <www.nano.cancer.gov>.

[4]   Kovalev, D. and Fujii, M., "Silicon nanocrystals: photosensitizers for oxygen molecules," *Adv Mater*, Vol. 17, 2005, pp. 2531–2544.

[5]   Baba, K., et al., "New method for delivering a hydrophobic drug for photodynamic therapy using pure nanocrystal form of the drug," *Mol Pharm*, Vol. 4, 2007, pp. 289–297.

[6]   Bharali, T. J., et al., "Folate-receptor-mediated delivery of InP quantum dots for bioimaging using confocal and two-photon microscopy," *J Am Chem Soc*, Vol. 127, 2005, pp. 11347–11371.

[7]   Samia, A. C., et al., "Semiconductor quantum dots for photodynamic therapy," *J Am Chem Soc*, Vol. 125, 2003, pp. 15736–15737.

[8]   Samia, A. C., Dayal, S., Burda, C., "Quantum dot-based energy transfer: perspectives and potential for applications in photodynamic therapy," *Photochem Photobiol*, Vol. 82, 2006, pp. 617–625.

[9]   Richter, A. M., et al., "Liposomal delivery of a photosensitizer, benzoporphyrin derivative monoacid ring A (BPD), to tumor tissue in a mouse tumor model," *Photochem Photobiol*, Vol. 57, 1993, pp. 1000–1006.

[10] Wieder, M. E., et al., "Intracellular photodynamic therapy with photosensitizer-nanoparticle conjugates: cancer therapy using a 'Trojan horse'," *Photochem Photobiol Sci*, Vol. 5, 2006, pp. 727–734.

[11] Ohulchanskyy, T. Y., et al., "Organically-modified silica nanoparticles with covalently incorporated photosensitizer for photodynamic therapy of cancer," *Nano Lett*, Vol. 7, 2007, pp. 2835–2842.

[12] Zeisser-Labouébe, M., et al., "Hypericin-loaded nanoparticles for the photodynamic treatment of cancer," *Int J Pharm*, Vol. 326, 2006, pp. 174–181.

[13] Li, H., et al., "High payload delivery of optical imaging and photodynamic therapy agents to tumors using phthalocyanine-reconstituted low-density lipoprotein nanoparticles," *J Biomed Opt*, Vol. 10, pp. 041203.

[14] Li, B., et al., "Diblock Copolymer Micelles for Delivery of Hydrophobic Protoporphyrin IX for Photodynamic Therapy," *Photochem Photobiol*, Vol. 83, 2007, pp. 1505–1512.

[15] Corbin, I. R., et al., "Enhanced cancer-targeted delivery using engineered high-density lipoprotein-based nanocarriers," *J Biomed Nanotech*, Vol. 3, 2007, pp. 1–10.

[16] Gil-Thomás, J., et al., "Lethal photosensitisation of Staphylococcus aureus using a toluidine blue O-tiopronin-gold nanoparticle conjugate," *J Mater Chem*, Vol. 17, 2007, pp. 3739–3746.

[17] Reddy, G. R., et al., "Vascular targeted nanoparticles for imaging and treatment of brain tumors," *Clin Cancer Res*, Vol. 12, 2006, pp. 6677–6686.

[18] Koo, Y-E L, Photonic explorers based on multifunctional nanoparticles for biosensing and photodynamic therapy," *Appl Opt*, Vol., 46, 2007, pp. 1924–1930.

[19] Tada, D. B., "Methylene blue-containing silica-coated magnetic particles: a potential magnetic carrier for photodynamic therapy," *Langmuir*, Vol. 23, 2007, pp. 8194–8199.

[20] Cinteza, L. O., et al., "Diacyllipid micelle-based nanocarrier for magnetically-guided delivery of drugs in photodynamic therapy," *Mol Pharm*, Vol. 3, 2006, pp. 415–423.

[21] Gu, H., et al., "Synthesis and cellular uptake of porphyrin decorated iron oxide nanoparticles—a potential candidate for bimodal cancer therapy," *Chem Commun (Camb)*, Vol.14, 2005, pp. 4270–4272.

[22] Chen, W., Zhang, J., "Using nanoparticles to enable simultaneous radiation and photodynamic therapies for cancer treatment," *Nanosci Nanotech*, Vol. 6, 2006, 1159–1166

[23] Verma, S., et al., "Strategies for enhanced photodynamic effects," *Photochem Photobiol*, Vol. 83, 2007, pp. 996–1005.

[24] Trachtenberg, J., et al., "Vascular targeted photodynamic therapy with palladium-bacteriopheophorbide photosensitizer for recurrent prostate cancer following definitive radiation therapy: assessment of safety and treatment response," *J Urol*, Vol. 178, 2007, pp. 1974–1979.

[25] Sharman, W. M., van Lier, J. E., Allen, C. M., "Targeted photodynamic therapy via receptor-mediated delivery systems," *Adv Drug Deliv Rev*, Vol. 56, 2004, pp. 53–76.

[26] Schneider, R., et al., "Recent improvements in the use of synthetic peptides for a selective photodynamic therapy," *Anticancer Agents Med Chem*, Vol. 6, 2006, pp. 469–488.

[27] El-Akra, N., et al., "Synthesis of estradiol-pheophorbide a conjugates: evidence of nuclear targeting, DNA damage and improved photodynamic activity in human breast cancer and vascular endothelial cells," *Photochem Photobiol Sci*, Vol. 5, 2006, pp. 996–999.

[28] Demidova, T. N., Hamblin, M. R., "Macrophage-targeted photodynamic therapy," *Int J Immunopath Pharmacol*, Vol. 17, 2004, pp. 117–126.

[29] Embleton, M. L., et al., "Development of a novel targeting system for lethal photosensitization of novel antibiotic-resistant strains of Stapholococcus aureus," *Antimicrob Agents Chemother*, Vol. 49, 2005, pp. 3690–3696.

[30] Bisland, S. K., Singh, D., Gariepy, J., "Potentiation of chlorin e6 photodynamic activity in vitro with peptide-based intracellular vehicles," *Bioconjug Chem*, Vol. 10, 1999, pp. 982–992.

[31] Akhlynina, T. V., et al., "Nuclear targeting of chlorine e6 enhances its photosensitizing activity," *J Biol Chem*, Vol. 272, 1997, pp. 30326–30331.

[32] Mahone, K. P., et al., "Deconvolution of the cellular oxidative stress response with organelle-specific peptide conjugates," *Chem Biol*, Vol. 14, 2007, pp. 923–930.

[33] Chen, J., et al., "Protease-triggered photosensitizing beacon based on singlet oxygen quenching and activation," *J Am Chem Soc*, Vol. 126, 2004, pp. 11450–11451.

[34] Zheng, G., et al., "Photodynamic molecular beacon as an activatable photosensitizer based on protease-controlled singlet oxygen quenching and activation," *Proc Nat Acad Sci (USA)*, Vol., 2007, pp. 8989–8994.

[35] Chen, J., et al., "An mRNA-triggered photodynamic molecular beacon for the selective control of singlet oxygen quenching and activation," *Bioconj Chem*, 2008.

[36] Gabriel, D., et al., "Tailoring protease-sensitive photodynamic agents to a specific disease-associated enzyme," *Bioconjug Chem*, Vol. 18, 2007, pp. 1070–1077.

[37] Chang, E., et al., "Protease-activated quantum dot probes," *Biochem Biophys Res Comm*, Vol. 334, 2005, pp. 1317–1321.

[38] Stefflova, K., et al., "Targeted photodynamic therapy agent with built-in apoptosis sensor for in vivo near-infrared imaging of tumor apoptosis triggered by its photosensitization in situ," *Mol Imag*, Vol. 5, 2006, pp. 520–532.

[39] Karotki, A., et al., "Simultaneous Two-Photon excitation of Photofrin and its application to photodynamic therapy," *Photochem Photobiol*, Vol. 82, 2006, pp. 443–452.

[40] Khurana M., et al., " Quantitative in vitro demonstration of two-photon photodynamic therapy using Photofrin and Visudyne," *Photochem Photobiol*, 2008.

[41] Samkoe, K. S., et al., "Complete blood vessel occlusion in the chick chorioallantoic membrane using two-photon excitation photodynamic therapy: implications for treatment of wet age-related macular degeneration," *J Biomed Opt*, Vol. 12, 2007, pp. 034025.

[42] Spangler, C. W., et al., "Synthesis, characterization and preclinical studies of two-photon-activated targeted PDT therapeutic triads," *Proc Soc Photo-Instr Eng.*, Vol. 6139, 2006, pp. 61390:1–10.

[43] Collins, H., et al., "Spatially targeted blood vessel closure using sensitisers designed for two-photon excitation," in press.

[44] Kim, S., et al., "Organically modified silica nanoparticles co-encapsulating photosensitizing drug and aggregation-enhanced two-photon absorbing fluorescent dye aggregates for two-photon photodynamic therapy," *J Am Chem Soc*, Vol. 129, 2007, pp. 2669–2675.

[45] Mir, Y., Houde, D, van Lier, J. E., "Photodynamic inhibition of acetylcholinesterase after two-photon excitation of copper tetrasulfophthalocyanine," *Lasers Med Sci*, 2007, Vol. 23, 2008, pp. 19–25.

[46] Mir, Y., Houde, D, van Lier, J. E., "Two-photon absorption of copper tetrasulfophthalocyanine induces phototoxicity towards Jurkat cells in vitro," *Photochem Photobiol Sci*, Vol. 5, 2006, pp. 1024–1030.

[47] Smith, G., et al., "An efficient oxygen independent two-photon photosensitization mechanism," *Photochem Photobiol*, Vol. 59, 1994, pp. 135–139.

[48] Bisland, S. K., et al., "Metronomic photodynamic therapy as a new paradigm for photodynamic therapy: Rationale and pre-clinical evaluation of technical feasibility for treating malignant brain tumors," *Photochem Photobiol*, Vol. 80, 2004, pp. 2–30.

[49] Lilge, L., et al., "The sensitivity of normal brain and intracranially implanted VX2 tumour to interstitial photodynamic therapy," *Br J Cancer*, Vol. 73, 1996, pp. 332–343.

[50] Olivo, M., Wilson, B. C., "Mapping ALA-induced PPIX fluorescence in normal brain and brain tumour using confocal fluorescence microscopy," *Int J Oncol*, Vol. 25, 2004, pp. 37–45.

[51] Lilge, L., Portnoy, M., Wilson, B. C., "Apoptosis induced in vivo by photodynamic therapy in normal brain and intracranial tumour tissue," *Br J Cancer*, Vol. 83, 2000, pp. 1110–1117.

[52] Hirschberg, H., et al., "An indwelling brachytherapy balloon catheter: potential use as an intracranial light applicator for photodynamic therapy," *J Neurooncol*, Vol. 44, 1999, pp. 15–21.

[53] Chen, J., et al., "New technology for deep light distribution in tissue for phototherapy," *Cancer J*, Vol. 8, 2002, pp. 154–163.

[54] Moseley, H., et al., "Ambulatory photodynamic therapy: a new concept in delivering photodynamic therapy," *Br J Dermatol*, Vol. 154, 2006, pp. 747–750.

[55] "Light fantastic," *Materials World*, Vol. Aug. 2007, pp. 28–30.

[56] Zusman, E., et al., "Photodynamic therapy for epilepsy," *Proc Soc Photo-Instr Eng*, Vol. 6139, 2006, pp. 61390W,1–9.

[57] Burch, S., et al., "Photodynamic Therapy for the Treatment of Vertebral Metastases in a Rat Model of Human Breast Carcinoma," *J Orthoped Res*, Vol. 23, 2005, pp. 995–1003.

[58] Bisland, S. K., el al, "Pre-clinical in vitro and in vivo studies to examine the potential use of photodynamic therapy in the treatment of osteomyelitis," *Photochem Photobiol Sci*, Vol. 5, 2006, pp. 31–38.

[59] Bisland, S. K., et al., A new technique for physiodesis using photodynamic therapy," *Clin Orthoped Rel Res*, Vol. 461, 2007, pp. 153–161.

[60] Lucas, C., et al., "Wound healing in cell studies and animal model experiments by Low Level Laser Therapy; were clinical studies justified? a systematic review," *Lasers Med Sci*, Vol. 17, 2002, pp. 110–134.

[61] Bisland, S. K., et al., "Increased expression of mitochondrial benzodiazepine receptors following low-level light treatment facilitates enhanced protoporphyrin IX production in glioma-derived cells in vitro," *Lasers Surg Med*, Vol. 39, 2007, pp. 678–684.

[62] McNally, K. M., et al., "Photothermal effects of laser tissue soldering," *Phys Med Biol*, Vol. 44, 1999, pp. 983–1002.

[63] Johnson, S., et al., "Photochemical tissue bonding: A promising technique for peripheral nerve repair," *J Surg Res*, 2007.

[64] Ibusuki, S., et al., "Photochemically cross-linked collagen gels as three-dimensional scaffolds for tissue engineering," *Tissue Eng*, Vol. 13, 2007, pp. 1995–2001.

[65] Luo, Y., Stoichet, MS., "A photolabile hydrogel for guided three-dimensional cell growth and migration," *Nat Mater*, Vol. 3, 2004, pp. 249–253.

CHAPTER 13

PDT and Inflammation

Mladen Korbelik

13.1 Introduction

Destruction of targeted lesions by photodynamic therapy (PDT) is initiated by localized phototoxic insult triggered by generation of reactive oxygen species [1]. Therapy outcome following cancer treatment by PDT is a result of a complex contribution of the direct cancer cell killing induced by lethal photooxidative damage, effects on tumor blood vasculature and other tumor stromal elements, and elicited host response [2, 3]. The latter encompasses a regulated and integrated action of a broad spectrum of response elements mounted by the host bearing PDT-treated tumor that includes two major effector processes, inflammation, and acute phase response, and the two principal arms of immunity, innate and adaptive immune reaction. The engagement of these host response elements is responsible for the fact that the PDT, although localized treatment modality focused on the targeted lesion, has a pronounced systemic impact. This chapter will concentrate on the inflammatory response associated with PDT of solid cancerous lesions. It will be examined why and how this response is instigated, relationship with other elements of PDT-induced host response, and its impact on the therapy outcome. (Color Plate 11 schematically illustrates PDT-induced inflammatory response).

13.2 Cause and Origin

The reason for the instigation of inflammatory response manifested during and after PDT light treatment of tumor tissue is the infliction of localized oxidative stress associated with a wide range of photooxidative lesions produced rapidly in the membranes and cytoplasm of tumor cells, stroma, and vasculature [4]. This massive tumor tissue injury produced within a short time period (minutes) is in its nature not dissimilar to other physical insults (including those produced by some other types of cancer treatment like hyperthermia and cryotherapy) and is perceived by the host not much differently than a harm sustained in any part of the body. Thus this PDT-induced insult is experienced by the host as a local trauma, and as such it presents a threat to the integrity and homeostasis at the affected site. Hence, the host is provoked to intervene by launching an acute inflammatory response since this is the canonical effector process evolutionary evolved for dealing with localized injury. As a host-protecting mechanism, the acute inflammation works by first preventing the spread of tissue damage and containing the disrupted homeostasis, next eradicating the eliciting stimulus (removing the damaged/altered and dead tissue), and then promoting local healing and restoration of tissue function at the affected site [5]. The strong inflammation of targeted tumor tissue induced by PDT treatment has a critical impact on the outcome of this therapy.

The inflammation focusing on PDT-treated tumor tissue is tumor antigen non-specific process orchestrated by the innate immune system whose recognition arm is responsible for detecting the inflicted tumor-localized insult [4, 6]. The presence of such insult is revealed to the sensors of innate immune system as the appearance of "altered-self" [7]. As conceptualized by the danger model of immunity [8, 9], this alert system is called into action upon detecting alarm/danger signals from injured/distressed (i.e., PDT-treatment altered) tumor tissue. We have recently proposed that PDT used for tumor treatment is particularly effective in generating very rapidly an abundance of such endogenous danger signals [4].

13.2.1 PDT-Generated Danger Signals and Their Recognition

The sensors of innate immune system recognize danger signals by their avidity for binding specific patterns on danger signal molecules, representing highly conserved chemical structure motifs shared by damage-related self molecules or a group of invading pathogens [9]. Thus these sensors have specialized in recognizing damage-associated molecular patterns (DAMPs) such as those released from PDT treated tumor cells and acellular stromal structures or appearing on their surface. Basically, DAMP can be any molecule that is abnormally exposed, misfolded, or displayed at a wrong location, as well as a breakdown product of damaged biomolecules.

Generation of three major types of DAMPs have been implicated by tumor PDT: cell-derived molecules, extracellular matrix degradation products, and extravasated plasma proteins [7, 10]. Molecules normally contained exclusively inside cells become potent danger signals when they appear on the cell surface or become released extracellularly. A prominent example is heat shock proteins, particularly HSP70, which were shown to rapidly translocate to the cell surface after PDT and can be also released from PDT-treated cells [11]. Further PDT-induced DAMPs of this category that appear of a major importance are degradation products of cellular membranes (lysophospholipids and arachidonic acid metabolites) massively released from PDT-treated sites [12, 13]. Among other potentially relevant PDT-induced DAMPs are various intracellular molecules originating from cells rendered necrotic by PDT treatment. Since PDT can induce direct damage to extracellular matrix [14], the degradation of this tissue- supporting scaffold will liberate fragments of fibronectin, hyaluronian, collagen, and laminin that are known as danger signals [9, 15–17]. Tissue injury induced by PDT includes also the breakdown of blood vessels leading to the escape of plasma proteins normally contained only within the circulation resulting in the increased accumulation of extravasated protein such as fibrinogen in PDT-treated tumors [10]. Extravascularly localized fibrinogen, which is also recognized as a danger signal [18], appears to promote the development of host response against PDT-treated tumor since the intratumoral injection of fibrinogen after PDT treatment was found to enhance the therapeutic response [10].

DAMPs of proinflammatory danger signals such as those becoming expressed after tumor PDT treatment are detected by specialized pattern recognition receptors (PRRs) [19]. These innate immunity PRRs can be soluble, membrane-anchored, or cytoplasmic (the latter two primarily found on professional sentinel cells that include macrophages, mast cells, dendritic cells, and endothelial cells); functionally they are organized as signaling, endocytic, and opsonizing receptors [20]. Their engagement by tumor PDT-induced injury-associated DAMPs triggers the inflammatory process. Knowledge about the involvement of such PRRs in tumor PDT response is largely limited to two major representatives, complement, and Toll-like receptors, as will be elaborated below.

13.3 The Onset of Inflammation

The inductive phase of inflammation, including that induced by PDT, focuses on the vascular component of affected tissue. With vasculature nontargeting photosensitizers (such as Photofrin, m-tetrahydroxyphenylchlorin, and protoporphyrin IX induced by 5-aminolevulinic acid), the inflammatory process is predominantly initiated by signals originating from photooxidative damage produced in perivascular regions with chemotactic gradients reaching the vascular endothelium. Vasculature-targeting photosensitizers (such as benzoporphrin derivative and mono-(l)-aspartylchlorin-e$_6$) can prompt this process by inflicting photooxidative lesions directly in endothelial cells. The onset of inflammation is enacted by the conversion of vascular endothelium from a nonthrombotic nonadhesive barrier to a proadhesive surface for inflammatory cells that is permeable (leaky) for blood constituents [21, 22]. The underlying changes include (1) the vasodilatation (due to the action of arachidonic acid metabolites [23] and elevated nitric oxide production from activated nitric oxide synthase) that increases blood flow and consequently leukocyte delivery, (2) appearance on the endothelium of leukocyte adhesion molecules, (3) opening of junctions between endothelial cells, and (4) platelet activation (triggered by activating factor induced in endothelial cells by lysophosphatidylcholine) [22]. This sets the stage for the rapid and massive invasion of neutrophils into PDT-treated tumors followed by mast cells and monocytes [24–26]. The task of these inflammatory effector cells is to neutralize the focal source of danger signals by destroying the compromised tissue elements and eliminating debris as well as injured and dead cells. Damage and dysfunction of the treated tumor vasculature becomes progressively more expressed (although that depends on the type of photosensitizer used), with increasing disruption of endothelial integrity, microvascular hemorrhage, thrombosis, and microvascular collapse [27, 28]. The resulting vascular occlusion serves to "wall off" the damaged tumor tissue and in this way prevent spreading of disruption of homeostasis.

The inductive and early stages of PDT-induced acute inflammation are instigated and propagated by rapidly generated mediators independent of new gene expression. These include lysophospholipids, histamine (discharged from mast cells), arachidonic acid metabolites, complement anaphylatoxins, and members of plasma coagulation cascade [4]. The subsequent stages of inflammatory process become progressively dominated by mediators formed through upregulated gene expression (as a consequence of triggered inflammatory signaling pathways) including cytokines, chemokines, and adhesion molecules [3, 25, 26, 29, 30], as well as hormones elaborated through the activation of acute phase response [31]. Some of these mediators can be released from cells sustaining injury by direct PDT damage, but an important contribution is also made by their production in macrophages and other immune cells invading the tumor after PDT treatment [4]. Elevated serum levels of inflammatory cytokines IL-1 and TNF-α were found in PDT-treated bladder cancer patients [32], and IL-1 and IL-6 in mesothelioma patients who underwent surgery and PDT [33]. Preclinical mechanistic studies, done mostly with mouse tumor models, have identified IL-1 and IL-6 as two dominant cytokines promoting the inflammation associated with tumor PDT response [3, 25, 26, 29]. In addition to complement, the two other major plasma cascades, coagulation and fibrinolytic systems, become involved in the tumor PDT-induced inflammatory response [4, 34].

13.4   Contribution of Complement System and Toll-Like Receptor Signaling

Complement and Toll-like receptors, two essential components of innate immune system that were recently shown to closely interact in their activity [35, 36], have a critical role in the inflammatory process developing after tumor PDT. Since the recognition/initiation components of complement cascade are among the most important danger sensors of host defense and are highly effective in recognizing molecular changes associated with death and injury on autologous tissue [35, 37, 38], it is not surprising that these proteins emerge as critical for the initial recognition of the PDT insult [4, 6, 39]. The complement system translates the acquired danger information to adequate cellular response elements by either directly activating receptors of its recognition proteins (C1qR, CR3/CR4, CD91/calreticulin) or by generating C3a and C5a fragments (anaphylatoxins) that interact with their specialized receptors [35]; such events are implicated in the instigation and propagation of tumor PDT-induced inflammatory response [4, 40–43]. We have recently shown that the rapid complement activation in the vasculature of PDT-treated tumor occurring during the photodynamic illumination can be responsible with some photosensitizers for a decline in tumor oxygenation (due apparently to anaphylatoxin-mediated vasoconstriction), reflected as oxygen limitation effects preventing PDT to exert its full therapeutic potential [44]. In contrast, complement activity makes an important contribution to cell killing in PDT-treated tumors, either directly through the assembly of the terminal complement cascade components into the lytic membrane attack complex [45], or indirectly by prompting the cytocidal action of inflammatory cells and/or development of adaptive immune response [4]. Importantly, this tumoricidal capacity of complement can be successfully exploited by its amplification using complement-activating immunotherapy in conjunction with PDT [43, 46, 47].

Toll-like receptors represent a family of germline-encoded transmembrane proteins whose engagement triggers intracellular signaling pathways leading to distinct patterns of the expression of genes for cytokines and chemokines as well as their receptors, adhesion molecules and costimulatory and other proteins regulating inflammatory and immune responses [48, 49]. These receptors control the expression of more than 2,000 genes, largely by activating nuclear transcription factor NF-κB [50]. We and others have demonstrated that there is a major NF-κB activation drive initiated after PDT in treated tumors. Immunohistochemistry analysis of PDT-treated mouse SCCVII tumors revealed a uniform change in NF-κB localization in tumor cells from cytoplasmic to nuclear (corresponding with its activation) peaking at 5 hours after PDT [10]. Based on their studies, mostly done with tumor and other cells directly PDT-treated in vitro, Piette and coworkers have characterized this transcription factor as a master determinator of PDT impact on cancer cells [51]. Our evidence suggests that signals such as heat shock proteins released from cancer cells directly damaged by PDT, and recognized in particular by TLR-2 and TLR-4 on undamaged macrophages attracted to their proximity, instigate NF-κB activation in these immune cells and consequently the production of host response mediators including inflammatory cytokines and complement proteins [10, 11, 52].

13.5 Elimination of Damaged Tissue

The key phase of acute inflammatory process is the elimination of the offending source (i.e., injured tissue and debris). In the case of tumor PDT, the inflamed mass that has to be removed consists of large numbers of dead and dying cancerous and stromal cells. Also included are numerous dead neutrophils and other inflammatory cells that invaded the site after PDT and died after performing their function. A prompt and efficient disposal of all these corpses, particularly necrotic, is of essential importance because of a serious threat posed by their continuous presence for perpetuating active inflammation, impairing tissue integrity and eliciting autoimmune responses [53, 54]. The disposal of dead cells, recently named efferocytosis, is an evolutionary highly conserved process because physiologically its preservation is essential for maintenance of hemostasis [55, 56]. Although practically all types of cells have the capacity of engulfment of dying corpses, the professional phagocytes (macrophages and immature dendritic cells) are indispensable as efferocytes when the host is suddenly faced with a large burden of dead cells such as after tumor PDT. Dying cells display on their surface molecular changes (death-associated molecular patterns) that are recognized as an "eat-me" signal by efferocytes; these include molecules normally localized inside the cell appearing on the surface (phosphatidylserine, calreticulin, nucleic acids), modification of existing molecules (changed glycosylation patterns, modified carbohydrates, oxidized membrane lipids), and changes in the charge on the cell surface [38, 53, 56, 57]. For detecting "eat-me" signals on dying cells the recognition arm of innate immune system has at its disposal two types of PRRs: (1) soluble, serving as bridging molecules by opsonizing dying corpses that flags them as targets to efferocytes, and (2) membrane-anchored, functioning as phagocytic receptors on the engulfing cells [56, 57].

We have recently shown that the treatment of mouse tumor cells in vitro by PDT mediated by various photosensitizers induces in these cells a dose-dependent upregulation of serum amyloid P component (SAP) gene expression with the produced protein remaining localized to the cells [58]. The SAP gene upregulation is also evident in vivo in PDT-treated mouse tumors [31, 58]. Since SAP is one of the major bridging molecules facilitating efferocytosis (especially in the mouse) [59], these findings prompted us to propose that cells sensing they have sustained mortal injury from PDT treatment can turn on molecular programs insuring that once they are dead their elimination (facilitated by SAP) is swift and efficient. A similar idea was formulated as "paying Charon's toll" [60], a reminiscence of the mythological ferryman in the underworld who for a fee (coin placed in the mouth of the dead) transports newly departed across the river Acheron/Styx to Hades (final resting place).

As one of the key events in tumor PDT-elicited host response, efferocytosis has (in addition to securing rapid clearance of inflamed mass) a direct influence on the subsequent resolution phase of the PDT-associated inflammatory process as well as on the development of adaptive immune response against treated tumors (see below).

13.6 Engagement of Acute Phase Response

Acute phase response, an effector process mobilized by the host for utilizing the resources from the entire organism (including those distant from the local insult site) for the execution of host-protecting response [61, 62], is frequently associated with a strong inflammatory reaction and this is also the case with tumor PDT response [31, 40]. In addition to radically increased plasma levels of acute phase reactants (due to upregulated biosynthetic profile in the liver and other sites), major hallmarks of acute phase response also manifested in PDT response are the activation of hypophyseal-pituitary-adrenal hormonal axis and elevation in the levels of peripheral leukocytes (particularly neutrophils) [31, 40, 42, 45, 63]. Acute phase reactants are proteins released with the purpose to optimize and regulate the course of host-protecting reaction while minimizing the extent of detrimental inflammatory damage. A major group of acute phase reactants are complement and pentraxin proteins specialized in opsonizing dying cells to facilitate their removal; other major groups prevent the excess activity of the inflammatory enzyme cascade (proteinase inhibitors) or promote wound healing [62]. The list of acute phase reactants upregulated in mice bearing PDT-treated tumors includes complement proteins C3, ficolins A & B, and mannose-binding lectin-A, pentraxins SAP and C-reactive protein, and haptoglobin [6, 29, 31, 41]. Interestingly, HSP70 was also recently identified as acute phase reactant owing to its upregulation in the liver and spleen of the host mice following tumor PDT [64]. These proteins, made available to optimize the process of efferocytosis and inflammatory debris removal (with the exception of haptoglobin), were found to accumulate in PDT-treated tumors.

Our study has identified IL-6 and glucocorticoids as key mediators involved in the promotion of acute phase response induced by tumor PDT [31]. It has also become clear in this study that glucocorticoid hormones released in the context of acute phase response exert a major influence on the expression of various genes in PDT-treated tumors.

13.7   Downregulation of Inflammation and Healing

The acute inflammatory process is tightly regulated by multiple and overlapping mechanisms in order to prevent excessive unnecessary damage to host tissues. This includes a program insuring that its resolution is triggered without delay once the threat provoking the inflammatory response is eliminated; such a checkpoint is important for preventing the development of chronic inflammation and autoimmune disease [65]. Key resolution signals are generated by phagocytes involved in the removal of inflamed material. After engulfing apoptotic cells, macrophages switch to producing mediators that suppress inflammation and promote healing [21, 65, 66]. Important agents of this type in tumor PDT response are anti-inflammatory cytokines IL-10 and TGF-β as well as vascular endothelial growth factor (VEGF) [4, 25]. They both negatively regulate proinflammatory signaling by targeting NF-κB [67, 68] and exert other complex immunosuppressive effects, while TGF-β also promotes cell differentiation/proliferation (that replaces lost residual cells), fosters matrix production, and stimulates fibrogenic remodeling (essential in healing) [69, 70]. Increased cure rates of PDT-treated tumors seen in mice injected with antibodies blocking IL-10 and TGF-β indicate that postponing the resolution of tumor-destructive phase of PDT-induced inflammation orchestrated by these cytokines may be beneficial for therapeutic outcome [4]. Similarly, an upregulation of angiogenic factors such as VEGF and various survival factors including matrix metalloproteinases and cyclooxygenase COX-2 was detected after tumor PDT and it was demonstrated that their inhibition elevates tumor cure rates [71]. Hence, angiogenesis and stromagenesis associated with healing that follows PDT-induced inflammation expose a risk of promoting the recurrence of treated tumors in case of their incomplete eradication.

13.8   Relevance for Immune Response and Therapy Outcome

From the therapeutic endpoint, tumor PDT-associated inflammation is an important contributor relevant to both early and long-term outcome. In its role of isolating and eliminating the incapacitated tissue, inflammation becomes integrated with the tumoricidal activity of innate immune effectors amplifying PDT-instigated tumor ablation. The inflammation of tumor tissue may diverge from the course of normal tissue inflammation towards a greater expression of immune rejection mechanisms because of a more pronounced exhibition of danger signal molecules in cancerous tissue. An example is the abundance of alkyl-lipid derivatives (highly potent inflammatory/immune activators) among degradation products of membrane lipids, which reflects the predominance of alkyl ether derivatives of phospholipids and neutral lipids that are hardly detectable in the membranes of normal cells [72].

With respect to the long-term tumor cures, the tumor PDT-associated inflammation can have both positive and negative aspects. Mechanisms mobilized to prevent excessive and harmful effects of inflammation and advance healing may promote the recurrence of PDT-treated tumors (as discussed in the previous section). On the other hand, although the adaptive immune response against

PDT-treated tumors is not programmed as a part of inflammation-dominated host-protecting response, it can develop as a side-effect (analogous to autoimmune response) of incompletely controlled tumor tissue inflammation. A key factor instigating tumor antigen-specific immune response appears to be the presence of too many dead cancer cells in the PDT-treated tumor within the time window that is too short for the capacity of the available phagocytes to remove these corpses fast enough to avoid breaking immune tolerance. Moreover, dealing through inflammation with PDT-induced tumor injury can prime the innate immune system to competence in instructing the adaptive immune system to develop a response recognizing the treated tumor as its specific target.

Three major types of cellular death, necrosis, apoptosis, and autophagy are observed with PDT [73, 74]. These forms of death are interlinked because apoptotic cells can undergo secondary necrosis (which will occur if their efferocytosis is delayed by overwhelming phagocytes with a large number of corpses), while autophagy may get activated in cells destined to die by apoptosis and this will promote the expression of eat-me signals securing efficient clearance of these apoptotic cells [75]. Concurrent appearance in PDT-treated tumors of cancer cells undergoing different forms of death that are associated with different phagocytic signaling may offer complementary responses favoring the generation of "self"-reactive lymphoid populations whose targets are antigens derived from these cell corpses. Dying cells are not immunologically inert; intracellular antigens from these cells survive the phagocytic process and are effectively cross-presented to T cells [76–78]. Recent discoveries also suggest that tumor antigens emerging in the cytosol of phagocytes can gain access to MHC class II presentation pathway by autophagy [79].

Evidence supporting the relevance of death expression in PDT-treated cancer cells and the routes of their efferocytosis has recently been obtained in mouse model-based studies on whole-cell cancer vaccines generated by in vitro PDT treatment of autologous tumor cells. The results reveal that the execution of apoptotic program in vaccine cells as well as the expression of the eat-me signal phosphatidylserine promote the potency of the PDT vaccine [80], while interfering with different types of phagocytic receptors in vaccinated mice can either enhance or dampen the therapeutic impact [81].

13.9   Conclusions

Studies into the signaling pathways initiated by the inflammation that occurs after PDT will lead to further insights into the consequences of tumor cell death by apoptosis, necrosis, and autophagy, and combinations of different types of cell death. The immune response that occurs after successful PDT for cancer is now thought to play an important role in the long-term outcome of the tumor treatment. The factors that determine the strength of this immune response are therefore likely to become the subject of wider study.

Acknowledgments

This study was supported by the National Cancer Institute of Canada, with funds from the Canadian Cancer Society.

References

[1] Dougherty, T. J., et al., "Photodynamic therapy," *J. Natl. Cancer Inst.*, Vol. 90, 1998, pp. 899–905.

[2] Henderson, B. W., and Dougherty, T. J., "How does photodynamic therapy work?" *Photochem. Photobiol.*, Vol. 55, 1992, pp. 145–157.

[3] Korbelik, M., and Cecic, I., "Mechanism of tumor destruction by photodynamic therapy." In *Handbook of Photochemistry and Photobiology*, Vol. 4, pp. 39–77, H.S. Nalwa (ed.), Stevenson Ranch, CA: American Scientific Publishers, 2003.

[4] Korbelik, M., "PDT-associated host response and its role in the therapy outcome," *Lasers Surg. Med.*, Vol. 38, 2006, pp. 500–508.

[5] Galin, J .I., and Snyderman, R., *Inflammation: Basic Principles and Clinical Correlations*, Philadelphia, PA: Lippincott Williams & Wilkins, 1999.

[6] Korbelik, M., et al., "Acute phase response induced following tumor treatment by photodynamic therapy: relevance for the therapy outcome," *Proc. SPIE*, Vol. 6087, 2006, pp. 0C1–0C7.

[7] Cecic, I., et al., "Relevance of innate immunity recognition of altered self in the induction of host response associated with photodynamic therapy," *Recent Res. Devel. Cancer*, Vol. 6, 2004, pp. 153–161.

[8] Matzinger, P., "The danger model: A renewed sense of self," *Science*, Vol. 296, 2002, pp. 301–305.

[9] Seong, S.- Y., and Matzinger, P., "Hydrophobicity: An ancient damage-associated molecular pattern that initiates innate immune responses," *Nat. Rev. Immunol.*, Vol. 4, 2004, pp. 469–478.

[10] Korbelik, M., "Role of Toll-like receptors in photodynamic therapy-elicited host response," *Proc. SPIE*, Vol. 5319, 2004, pp. 87–95.

[11] Korbelik, M., Sun, J., and Cecic, I., "Photodynamic therapy-induced cell surface expression and release of heat shock proteins: Relevance for tumor response," *Cancer Res.*, Vol. 65, 2005, 1018–1026.

[12] Andrews, N. W., "Membrane repair and immunological danger," *EMBO Rep.*, Vol. 6, 2005, pp. 826–830.

[13] Agrawal, M. L., et al., "Phospholipase activation triggers apoptosis in photosensitized mouse lymphoma cells," *Cancer Res.*, Vol. 53, 1993, 5897–5902.

[14] Musser, D. A., et al., "The binding of tumor localizing porphyrins to a fibrin matrix and their effects following photoirradiation," *Res. Commun. Chem. Pathol. Pharmacol.*, Vol. 28, 1980, pp. 505–525.

[15] Beg, A. A., "Endogenous ligands of Toll-like receptors: Implications for regulating inflammatory and immune responses," *Trends Immunol.*, Vol. 23, 2002, pp. 509–512.

[16] Termeer, C., et al., "Oligosaccharides of hyaluronan activate dendritic cells via toll-like receptor 4," *J. Exp. Med.*, Vol. 195, 2002, pp. 99–111.

[17] Okamura, Y., et al., "The extra domain A of fibronectin activates Toll-like receptor 4," *J. Biol. Chem.*, Vol. 276, 2001, pp. 10229–10233.

[18] Smiley, S. T., King, J. A., and Hancock, W. W., "Fibrinogen stimulates macrophage chemokine secretion through Toll-like receptor 4," *J. Immunol.*, Vol. 167, 2001, pp. 2887–2894.

[19] Medzihtov, R., and Janeway, C. A., "Innate immunity," *N. Engl. J. Med.*, Vol. 343, 2000, pp. 338–344.

[20] Lee, M. S., and Kim, Y.- J., "Pattern-recognition receptor signaling initiated from extracellular, membrane, and cytoplasmic space," *Mol. Cells*, Vol. 23, 2007, pp. 1–10.

[21] Lentsch, A. B., and Ward, P. A., "Regulation of inflammatory vascular damage," *J. Pathol.*, Vol. 190, 2000, pp. 343–348.

[22] Pober, J. S., and Sessa, W. C., "Evolving fuctions of endothelial cells in inflammation," *Nat. Rev Immunol.*, Vol. 7, 2007, pp. 803–815.

[23] Henderson, B. W., and Donovan, J. M., "Release of prostaglandin E$_2$ from cells by photodynamic treatment in vitro," *Cancer Res.*, Vol. 49, 1989, pp. 6896–6900.

[24] Krosl, G., Korbelik, M., and Dougherty, G. J., Induction of immune cell infiltration into murine SCCVII tumor by Photofrin-based photodynamic therapy," *Br. J. Cancer*, Vol. 71, 1995, pp. 549–555.

[25] Gollnick, S. O., et al., "Altered expression of interleukin 6 and interleukin 10 as a result of photodynamic therapy in vivo," *Cancer Res.*, Vol. 57, 1997, pp. 3904–3909.

[26] Sun, J., et al., "Neutrophils as inflammatory and immune effectors in photodynamic therapy-treated mouse SCCVII tumors," *Photochem. Photobiol. Sci.*, Vol. 1, 2002, pp. 690–695.

[27] Fingar, V. H., "Vascular effects of photodynamic therapy," *J. Clin. Laser Med. Surg.*, Vol. 14, 1996, pp. 323–328.

[28] Dennis, E. J., et al., "Photodynamic therapy of cancer," *Nat. Rev. Cancer*, Vol. 3, 2003, pp. 380–387.

[29] Gollnick, S. O., et al., "Role of cytokines in photodynamic therapy-induced local and systemic inflammation," *Br. J. Cancer*, Vol. 88, 2003, pp. 1772–1779.

[30] Castano, A. P., Mroz, P., and Hamblin, M. R., "Photodynamic therapy and anti-tumor immunity," *Nat. Rev. Cancer*, Vol. 6, 2006, pp. 535–545.

[31] Korbelik, M., et al., "Acute phase response induction by cancer treatment with photodynamic therapy," *Int. J. Cancer*, Vol. 122, 2008, pp. 1411–1417.

[32] Nseyo, U. O., et al., "Urinary cytokines following photodynamic therapy for bladder cancer," *Urology*, Vol. 36, 1990, pp. 167–171.

[33] Yom, S. S., et al., "Elevated serum cytokine levels in mesothelioma patients who have undergone pleurectomy or extrapleural pneumonectomy and adjuvant intraoperative photodynamic therapy," *Photochem. Photobiol.*, Vol. 78, 2003, pp. 75–81.

[34] Ben-Hur, E., et al., "Release of clotting factors from photosensitized endothelial cells: a possible trigger for blood vessel occlusion by photodynamic therapy," *FEBS Lett.*, Vol. 236, 1988, pp. 105–108.

[35] Köhl, J., "Self, non-self, and danger: a complementary view," *Adv. Exp. Med. Biol.*, Vol. 586, 2006, pp. 71–94.

[36] Zhang, X., et al., "Regulation of Toll-like receptor-mediated inflammatory response by complement in vivo," *Blood*, Vol. 110, 2007, pp. 228–236.

[37] Nauta, A. J., Roos, A., and Daha, M. R., "A regulatory role for complement in innate immunity and autoimmunity," *Int. Arch. Allergy Immunol.*, Vol. 134, 2004, pp. 310–323.

[38] Elward, K., and Gasque, P., "Eat me" and "don't eat me" signals govern the innate immune response and tissue repair in the CNS: emphasis on the critical role of the complement system," *Mol. Immunol.*, Vol. 40, 2003, pp. 85–94.

[39] Cecic, I., and Korbelik, M., "Deposition of complement proteins on cells treated by photodynamic therapy in vitro," *J. Environ. Pathol. Toxicol. Oncol.*, Vol. 25, 2006, pp. 189–203.

[40] Cecic, I., Stott, B., and Korbelik, M., "Acute phase response-associated systemic neutrophil mobilization in mice bearing tumors treated by photodynamic therapy," *Int. Immunopharmacol*, Vol. 6, 2006, pp. 1259–1266.

[41] Cecic, I., et al., "Characteristics of complement activation in mice bearing Lewis lung carcinomas treated by photodynamic therapy," *Cancer Lett.*, Vol. 225, 2005, pp. 215–223.

[42] Cecic, I., Sun, J., and Korbelik, M., "Role of complement anaphylatoxin C3a in photodynamic therapy-elicited engagement of host neutrophils and other immune cells," *Photochem. Photobiol.*, Vol. 82, 2006, pp. 558–562.

[43] Korbelik, M., and Dougherty, G. J., "Complement activation approaches for use in conjunction with PDT for cancer treatment," *Proc. SPIE*, Vol. 5695, 2005, pp. 17–26.

[44] Cecic, I., Minchinton, A. I., and Korbelik, M., "The impact of complement activation on tumor oxygenation during photodynamic therapy," *Photochem. Photobiol.*, Vol. 83, 2007, pp. 1049–1055.

[45] Cecic, I., and Korbelik, M., "Mediators of peripheral blood neutrophilia induced by photodynamic therapy of solid tumors," *Cancer Lett.*, Vol. 183, 2002, pp. 43–51.

[46] Korbelik, M., et al., "Adjuvant treatment for complement activation increases the effectiveness of photodynamic therapy of solid tumors," *Photochem. Photobiol. Sci.*, Vol. 3, 2004, pp. 812–816.

[47] Korbelik, M., and Cooper, P. D., "Potentiation of photodynamic therapy of cancer by complement: the effect of γ-insulin," *Br. J. Cancer,* Vol. 96, 2007, pp. 67–72.

[48] Underhill, D.M., "Toll-like receptors: networking for success," *Eur. J. Immunol.*, Vol. 33, 2003, pp. 1767–1775.

[49] Chen, K., et al., "Toll-like receptors in inflammation, infection and cancer," *Int. Immunopharmacol.*, Vol. 7, 2007, pp. 1271–1285.

[50] Carmody, R. J., and Chen, Y. H., "Nuclear factor-κB: Activation and regulation during Toll-like receptor signaling," *Cell. Mol. Immunol.*, Vol. 4, 2007, 31–41.

[51] Matroule, J. -Y., Volanti, C., and Piette, J., "NF-κB in photodynamic therapy: discrepancies of a master regulator," *Photochem. Photobiol.*, Vol. 82, 2006, 1241–1246.

[52] Stott, B., and Korbelik, M., "Activation of complement C3, C5, and C9 genes in tumors treated by photodynamic therapy," *Cancer Immunol. Immunother.*, Vol. 56, 2007, 649–658.

[53] Krysko, D.V., D'Herde, K., and Vandenbeele, P., "Clearance of apoptotic and necrotic cells and its immunological consequences," *Apoptosis*, Vol. 11, pp. 1709–1726.

[54] Sauter, B., et al., "Consequences of cell death: Exposure to necrotic tumor cells, but not primary tissue cells or apoptotic cells, induces the maturation of immunostimulatory dendritic cells," *J. Exp. Med.*, Vol. 191, 2000, 423–434.

[55] deChatelineau, A. M., and Henson, P. M., "The final step in programmed cell death: phagocytes carry apoptotic cells to the grave," *Essays Biochem.*, Vol. 39, 2003, pp. 105–117.

[56] Vandivier, R. W., Henson, P. M., and Douglas, I. S., "Burying the dead. The impact of failed apoptotic cell removal (efferocytosis) on chronic inflammatory lung disease," *Chest*, Vol. 129, 2006, pp. 1673–1682.

[57] Majai, G., Petrovski, G., and Fesüs, L., "Inflammation and the apopto-phagocytic system," *Immunol. Lett.*, Vol. 104, 2006, pp. 94–101.

[58] Merchant, S., Sun, J., and Korbelik, M., "Dying cells program their expedient disposal: serum amyloid P component upregulation in vivo and in vitro induced by photodynamic therapy of cancer," *Photochem. Photobiol. Sci.*, Vol. 6, 2007, pp. 1284–1289.

[59] Roos, A., et al., "A pivotal role for innate immunity in the clearance of apoptotic cells," *Eur. J. Immunol.*, Vol. 34, 2004, pp. 921–929.

[60] Yoshimori, T., "Autophagy: paying Charon's toll," *Cell*, Vol. 128, 2007, pp. 833–836.

[61] Baumann, H., and Gauldie, J., "The acute phase response," *Immunol. Today*, Vol. 15, 1994, pp. 74–80.

[62] Gabay, C, and Kushner, I., "Acute-phase proteins and other systemic responses to inflammation," *N. Engl. J. Med.*, Vol. 340, 1999, pp. 448–454.

[63] Cecic, I., Parkins, C. S., and Korbelik, M., "Induction of systemic neutrophil response in mice by photodynamic therapy of solid tumors," *Photochem. Photobiol.*, Vol. 74, 2001, pp. 712–720.

[64] Korbelik, M., and Merchant, S., "Role of heat shock protein 70 in systemic host response induced by tumor PDT," *11th World Congress of the International Photodynamic Association,* Shanghai, China, March 28–31, 2007, abstracts pp. 190.

[65] Henson, P. M., "Dampening inflammation," *Nat. Immunology,* Vol. 6, 2005, pp. 1179–1181.

[66] Golpon, H. A., et al., "Life after corpse engulfment: Phagocytosis of apoptotic cells leads to VEGF secretion and cell growth," *FASEB J.,* Vol. 18, 2004, pp. 1716–1718.

[67] Xiao, Y. Q., et al., "Cross-talk between ERK and p38 MAPK mediates selective suppression of pro-inflammatory cytokines by transforming growth factor-β," *J. Biol. Chem.,* Vol. 277, 2002, pp. 14884–14893.

[68] Lentsch, A. B., et al.,"In vivo suppression of NF-kappa B and preservation of I kappa B alpha by interleukin-10 and interleukin-13," *J. Clin. Invest.,* Vol. 100, 1997, pp. 2443–2448.

[69] Shi, Y., and Massague, J., "Mechanisms of TGF-β signaling from cell membrane to nucleus," *Cell,* Vol. 113, 2003, pp. 685–700.

[70] O'Kane, S., and Ferguson, M. W. J., "Transforming growth factor βs and wound healing," *Int. J. Biochem. Cell Biol.,* Vol. 29, 1997, pp. 63–78.

[71] Gomer, C. J., et al., "Photodynamic therapy: combined modality approaches targeting the tumor microenvironment," *Lasers Surg. Med.,* Vol. 38, 2006, pp. 516–521.

[72] Yamamoto, N., and Ngwenya, B. Z., "Activation of mouse peritoneal macrophages by lysophospholipids and ether derivatives of neutral lipids and phospholipids," *Cancer Res.,* Vol. 47, 1987, pp. 2008–2013.

[73] Kessel, D., and Reiners Jr., J. J., "Apoptosis and autophagy after mitochondrial or endoplasmic reticulum photodamage," *Photochem. Photobiol.,* Vol. 83, 2007, pp. 1024–1028.

[74] Xue, L., et al., The death of human cancer cells following photodynamic therapy: apoptosis competence is necessary for Bcl–2 protection but not for induction of autophagy," *Photochem. Photobiol.,* Vol. 83, 2007, pp. 1016–1023.

[75] Qu, X, et al., "Autophagy gene–dependent clearance of apoptotic cells during embryonic development," *Cell,* Vol. 128, 2007, pp. 931–946.

[76] Larsson, M., Fonteneau, J.F., and Bhardwaj, N., "Dendritic cells resurrect antigens from dead cells," *Trends Immunol.,* Vol. 22, 2001, pp. 141–148.

[77] Shaif-Muthana, M., et al.,"Dead or alive: immunogenicity of human melanoma cells when presented by dendritic cells," *Cancer Res.,* Vol. 60, 2000, pp. 6441–6447.

[78] Nouri-Shirazi, M., et al., "Dendritic cells capture killed tumor cells and present their antigens to elicit tumor-specific immune responses," *J. Immunol.,* Vol. 165, 2000, pp. 3797–3803.

[79] Levine, B., and Deretic, V., "Unveiling the roles of autophagy in innate and adaptive immunity," *Nat. Rev. Immunol.,* Vol. 7, 2007, pp. 767–777.

[80] Korbelik, M., Stott, B., and Sun, J., "Photodynamic therapy-generated vaccines: relevance of tumour cell death expression," *Br. J. Cancer,* Vol. 97, 2007, pp. 1381–1387.

[81] Korbelik, M., "Photodynamic therapy-generated vaccine: therapeutic and mechanistic insights," *12th Congress of the European Society for Photobiology,* Bath, UK, September 1–6, 2007, abstracts pp. 116.

CHAPTER 14

PDT and Cellular Immunity

Paweł Mróz and Michael R. Hamblin

14.1 Introduction

The importance of the immune system in the host response against cancer has been studied for many years, but at the present time, immunotherapy of cancer is only accepted as a mainstream treatment option in a few cases. PDT has a significant effect on the immune system [1–3] that can be either immunostimulatory, or in some circumstances immunosuppressive. In this chapter we summarize the effects of PDT on the cells of the immune system and the resulting response of these cells against tumors.

There have been reports of many effects of PDT on cancer cells themselves growing in tissue culture that, if replicated in vivo, would make activation of the immune system probable after PDT treatment in patients. The combination of various PS with the appropriate activating light causes an unusual mixture of both apoptotic and necrotic cell death [4]. The balance between apoptosis and necrosis after PDT in vitro depends on several parameters including the total PDT dose (PDT dose is the product of PS concentration and light fluence), the intracellular localization of the PS, the fluence rate, the oxygen concentration, and the cell type [5]. There is an extensive body of literature that examines pathways of apoptosis—such as signaling pathways [6, 7], mitochondrial events [5] and mediators of apoptosis [8]—induced after PDT in both normal and tumor cells in tissue culture. The occurrence of apoptosis after PDT in tumors in vivo has also been demonstrated [9–11], but there have been few studies looking at in vivo clearance mechanisms of apoptotic cells after PDT of tumors.

There have been many studies examining the relationship between the mode of tumor cell death (by other methods than PDT) and the efficiency of induction of the immune response, both in vitro and in vivo [12, 13]. Although some reports show that apoptotic tumor cells are more effective than necrotic tumor cells in the induction of immune response [14, 15], there are other reports showing the opposite finding, that modes of cancer therapy that induce predominantly necrosis are actually better at activating the immune system than methods that predominantly induce apoptosis [16, 17]. In the case of necrosis, cytosolic constituents spill into the extracellular space through the damaged plasma membrane and provoke a robust inflammatory response—these products are safely isolated by the intact membranes that initially persist in apoptotic cells, which are phagocytosed by macrophages. The acute inflammation caused by PDT-induced necrosis might potentiate immunity by attracting host leukocytes into the tumor and enhancing antigen presentation as shown in Color Plate 12.

14.2 PDT and Antigen-Presenting Cells (APCs)

Antigen-presenting cells (APC) possess the unique ability to induce primary immune responses. They capture and transfer the information from the outside world to the cells of the adaptive immune system. One of their most characteristic features is the expression of the MHC class II molecules and the ability to present exogenous antigens to the T helper lymphocytes. Among professional APCs there are dendritic cells (DC), macrophages, and B lymphocytes. The following sections of this chapter will describe the role of APC in PDT mediated immune response.

14.2.1 Dendritic Cells

Dendritic cells are the key players among all APC in the process of the induction of immune response. They can effectively acquire the antigens, process them, and present in the context of MHC class II molecules. They express Toll-like receptors as well as costimulatory molecules necessary for successful DC–T cells interactions. They can travel to the lymph nodes and interact with T cells to initiate the primary immune response. Therefore, attempts have been made to understand the role and utilize the abilities of DC in the PDT mediated immunity.

14.2.1.1 Dendritic Cells and HSPs

One of the most important cellular factors induced by PDT and released from necrotic tumor cells is extracellular heat shock protein 70 (HSP70) Color Plate 11. HSP70 is effectively induced after stress, and when it remains intracellular, HSP70 chaperones unfolded proteins and prevents cell death by inhibiting the aggregation of cellular proteins [18]. These properties not only enable intracellular HSP70 to inhibit tumor cell death by apoptosis, but also promote formation of stable complexes with cytoplasmic tumor antigens that can then either be expressed at the cell surface or escape intact from dying necrotic cells to interact with antigen presenting cells and stimulate an antitumor immune response [19]. Extracellular HSP70 binds to high-affinity receptors on the surface of the APCs, leading to the activation and maturation of DCs, a process that enables the cross-presentation of the peptide antigen cargo of HSP70 by the APC to CD8 cytotoxic T-cells [20].

PDT mediated by three different PSs increased HSP70 mRNA, but only mono-L-aspartyl chlorin-e6 and tin etio-purpurin but not Photofrin increased HSP70 protein levels in mouse tumor cells in vitro and in tumors in vivo [21]. The release of HSP-bound tumor antigens that can easily be taken up by APC from PDT-induced necrotic tumor cells may therefore explain the particular efficiency of PDT in stimulating an immune response against tumors.

14.2.1.2 Dendritic Cells and PDT Generated Vaccines

A related approach that takes advantage of the immune-stimulating effects of PDT is the preparation of cancer vaccines using in vitro PDT of tumor cells growing in tissue culture. Gollnick et al. [22] compared the cancer vaccine potential of

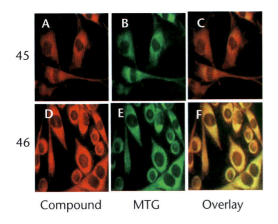

45

46

Compound   MTG   Overlay

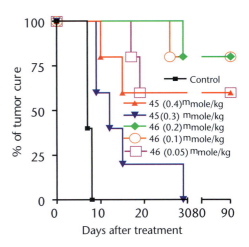

Color plate 1 In vivo photosensitzing efficacy of HPPH methyl ester 45 and the corresponding ln(III) analog 46 in C3H mice bearing RIF tumors (10 mice/group). The mice were treated with laser light (135 J/cm², 75 mW/cm², 665 nm for compund 45 and 655 nm for compound 46) at 24 hours post-injection of the drug. Control: no photosentisizer and no light exposure.

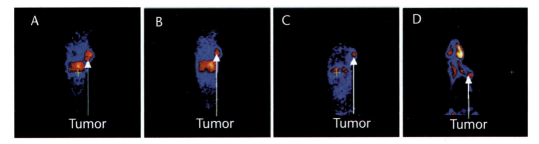

Color plate 2 Comparative (PET) images of mice bearing RIF tumors injected with ¹²⁴I-analog 4 (50 μCi) at 24 hours (A), 48 hours (B), and 72 hours (C) post-injection of the drug, and with F-18 FDG (D) at 90 minutes post-injection. (As expected from the porphyrin-based compounds, the presence of 4 was evident in some other organs, especially in liver, spleen, and intestine.) However, compared to 24 hours, better contrast was observed at 48 and 72 hours post-injection.

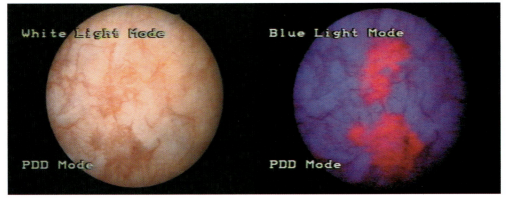

Color plate 3 The advantageous use of HAL-induced fluorescence for the diagnosis of early-stage urothelial neoplasm. The two pictures show a sequence of white-light (left) and blue-light (right) examinations of the bladder using an 8mM HAL solution after a 1-hour installation period.

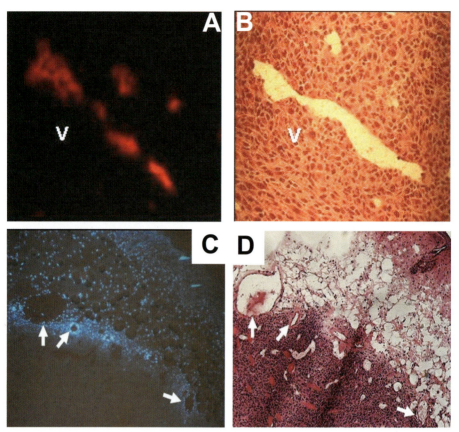

Color plate 4 Photodynamic tumor vascular targeting with photosensitizer hypericin. v = blood vessels, arrows = functional blood vessels at the tumor periphery.

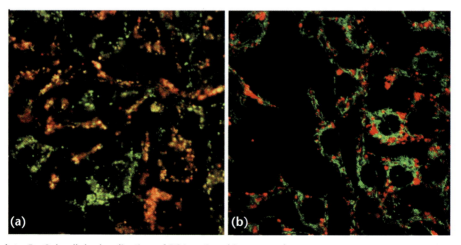

Color plate 5 Subcellular localization of BSA-ce6-mal in macrophages.

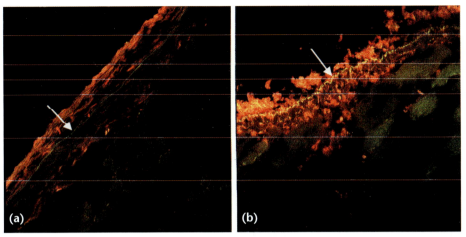

Color plate 6 Two color confocal fluorescence micrographs with 10 μm frozen sections of peritoneal wall from tumor-bearing mice at necropsy 3 hours after IP injection of (a) pl-ce6-ac, or (b) pl-ce6-PEG-ac. Images from the red channel showing ce6 fluorescence were superimposed on images from the green channel showing tissue autofluorescence. Arrows denote serosal basement membrane and bar is 100 μm. These micrographs were representative of those obtained from three independent experiments.

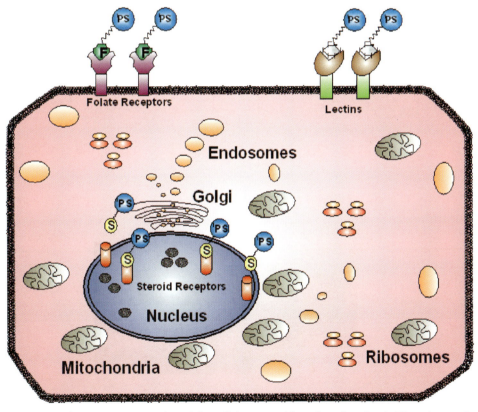

Color plate 7 Schematic representation of the cellular recognition of small molecule PS conjugates by receptors for folic acid and for lectins expressed on the cell membrane, and by steroid receptors in the nucleus.

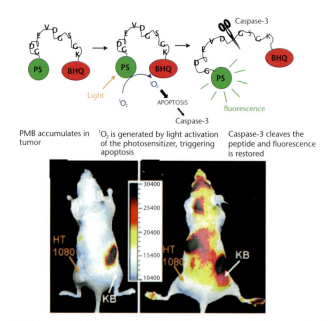

Color plate 8 The principle of PMB for reporting PDT-induced apostosis beacon (top) and fluorescence images pre (left) and 30 minutes post (right) PDT treatment using a caspase 3-cleavable beacon that is targeted to the folate receptor expressed in the target (KB) but not in the control (HT1080) tumor. (Courtesy G. Zheng: in vivo images produced from [38] with permission.)

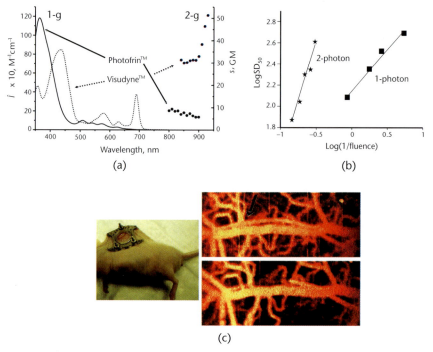

Color plate 9 Simultaneous 2-g PDT. (a) Absorption spectra of Photofrin and Visudyne, also showing the corresponding 1-g spectra (adapted from [39], with permission); (b) in vitro vascular endothelial cell kill (light fluence for 50% survival) versus inverse light fluence (log-log scales) for 1-g and 2-g activation using BPD, showing the linear and quadratic slopes, respectively; and (c) example of 2-g closure of single normal blood vessel in mouse skin in a window chamber model using systematic administration of a novel porphyrin-dimer photosensitizer (developed by Professor H. Anderson and colleagues, Oxford University, UK) and focused 100 fs pulsed laser light (arrow). The images are taken by Doppler optical coherence tomography. (Courtesy of A. Miriampillai, V. Yang, A. Vitkin, and colleagues.)

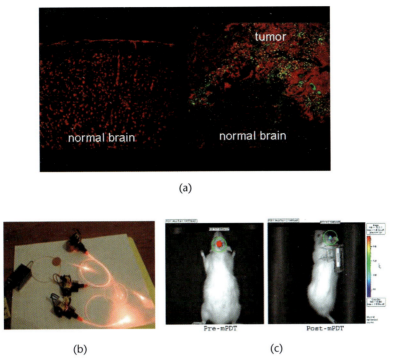

(a)

(b)   (c)

Color plate 10 *Metronomic* PDT. (a) Sections of (left) normal brain contralateral to the tumor implant and (right) intracranial brain tumor after *m*PDT with ALA, showing tumor cell-specific apoptosis (green-TUNEL stain, red-propidium iodide stain); (b) prototype fiber-coupled LED light source used for intracranial *m*PDT irradiation in rat brain tumors; and (c) an example of tumor response by bioluminescence imaging showing the reduction in viable tumor cells following *m*PDT.

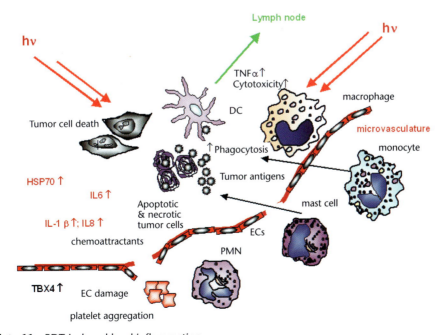

Color plate 11 PDT-induced local inflammation.

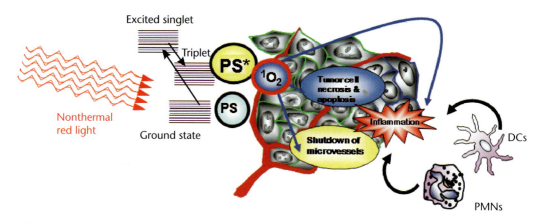

Color plate 12   Mechanisms of PDT action on tumors.

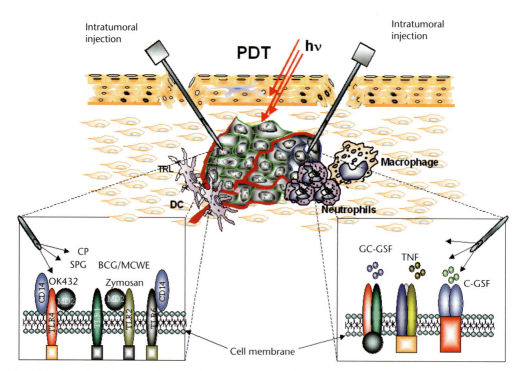

Color plate 13   Combination of PDT with immunostimulants.

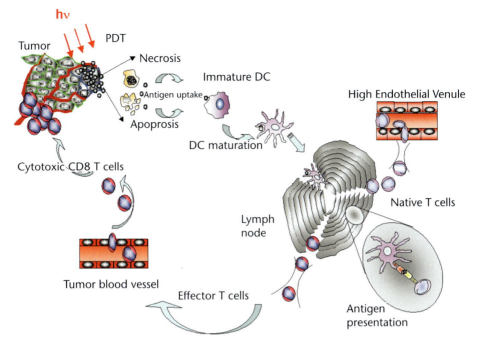

Color plate 14 PDT induces activation of antigen specific T cells.

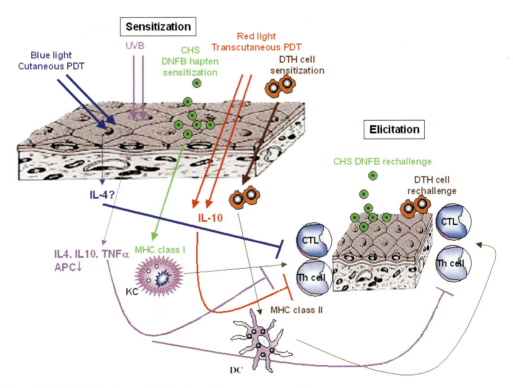

Color plate 15 Mechanism of PDT-induced immune suppression.

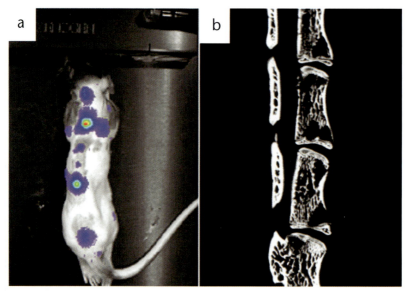

Color plate 16 (a) Spinal lesions were evident in *rnu/rnu* mice two weeks following injection of bioluminescent MT-1 cells. Imaging was conduted using the IVIS apparatus from Xenogen Corporation (Alameda, CA); and (b) osteolytic destruction of vertebrae was quantified using Micro-CT.

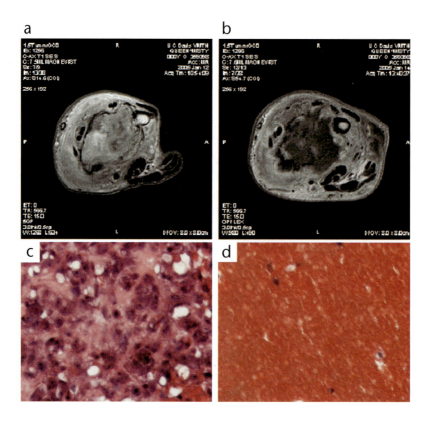

Color plate 17 T1 gadolinium-enhanced MRI axial images show: (a) osteosarcoma filling the medullary canal in a canine wrist pre-operatively followed by (b) ablation of tumor at 48 hours post-PDT. (c) Histology reveals the extensive osteoid formation and fibrin typical of high-grade osteosarcoma. (d) PDT induces hemorrhagic necrosis of the tumor with few remaining cells. Original magnification x200.

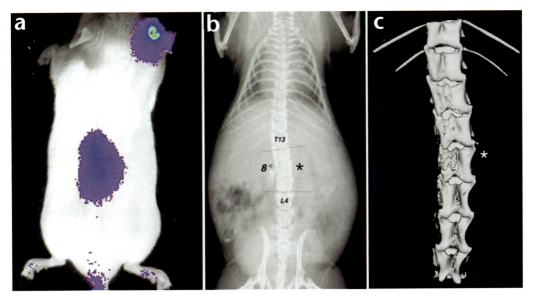

Color plate 18 (a) Increased VEGF-related bioluminescence corresponding with the area of spine targeted for PDT (two weeks post treatment). (b) Faxitron imaging reveals an 8° curve within the lumbar spine with maximal curvature at L2(*). (c) Micro-CT confirms extensive damage to the L2 vertebra consistent with curve.

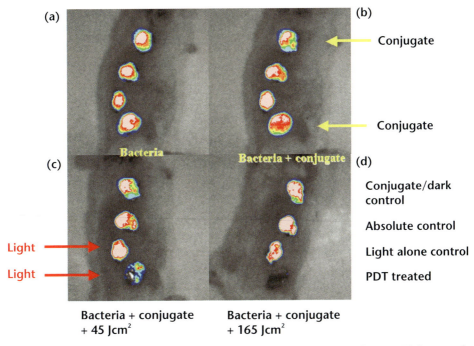

Color plate 19 Successive overlaid luminescence false color images and monochrome LED images of a mouse with four excisional wounds infected with equal numbers of *E. coli* (a). Wounds 1 (nearest tail) and 4 (nearest head) received topical application of conjugate (b). Wounds 1 and 2 (two nearest tail) were then illuminated with successive fluences (45–165 J/cm^2) of 660-nm light (c–d).

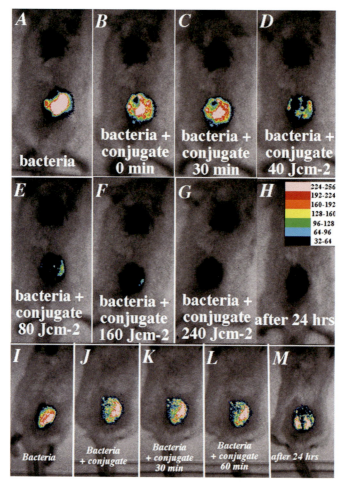

Color plate 20 Successive overlaid luminescence false color images and monochrome LED images of mice bearing an excisional wound infected with 5×10^6 luminescent *P. aeruginosa* (panels A–H). A representative mouse treated with pL-ce6 conjugate and increasing doses of light (panels I–M). A representative mouse treated with pL-ce6 and kept in the dark.

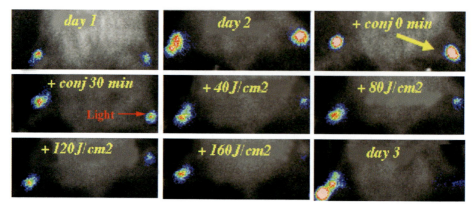

Color plate 21 Series of bioluminescence images (captured at a bit range of 2–4) from a neutropenic mouse infected on day one in both left and right hind thighs, and treated on day two with an injection of pL-ce6 into the right thigh, followed after thirty minutes by illumination of the right thigh with 660-nm light at a fluence rate of 100 mW/cm².

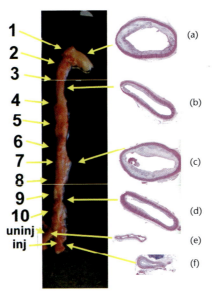

Color plate 22 Photograph of excised *en bloc* atherosclerotic aorta and iliac arteries showing numbering of segments. 1. ascending aorta; 2. aortic arch; 3–5. thoracic aorta; 6. aorta at diaphragm; 7–9. abdominal aorta; 10. aortic bifurcation, inj: right iliac artery through which balloon was introduced, uninj: normal left iliac artery. H and E sections of the typical segments obtained from the (a) aortic arch; (b) mid-thoracic noninjured site; (c) injured mid-abdominal; (d) aorta above bifurcation; (e) uninjured iliac artery; and (f) injured iliac artery.

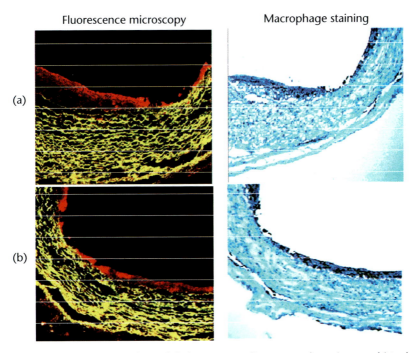

Color plate 23 Fluorescent micrographs and their corresponding macrophage immunohistochemical staining (RAM-11) in two representative segments (a and b) are shown. In the flourescent micrographs red fluorescence represents MA-ce6 uptake, whereas in RAM-11 stained images, dark blue-brown staining represents macrophages. In both sets of images, the RAM-11 staining is primarily confined to the intima. MA-ce6 uptake parallels the pattern of RAM-11 staining.

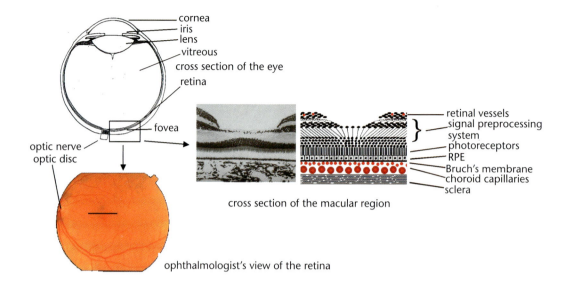

cross section of the eye

cross section of the macular region

ophthalmologist's view of the retina

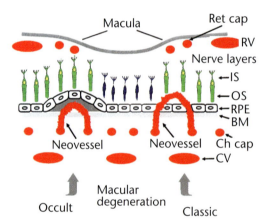

Color plate 24 A schematic cross section of the eye together with an opthamologist's view of the retina; a schematic cross section of a normal macula and a macula with choroidal neovascularization.

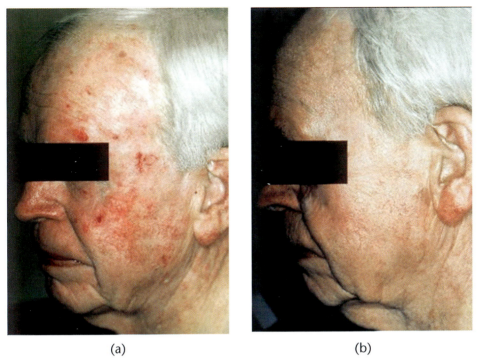

(a)   (b)

Color plate 25   (a) Before and (b) after MAL; three hours occluded; rinse saline solution; red light 37J/cm^2.

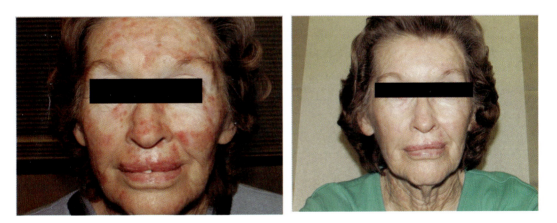

Color plate 26   (a) Before and (b) after four treatments with ALA-PDT. (Courtesy of Michael Gold, MD.)

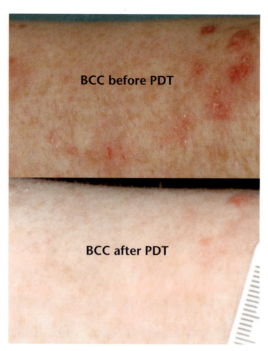

Color plate 27 Right forearm close-up of a patient with nevoid basal cell carcinoma syndrome (Gorlin Syndrome). Top photograph before the treatment; bottom photograph showing clinical improvement after 3 sessions of high dose ALA-PDT using topical 20% ALA solution. The drug was incubated for 3 hours under occlusion, and irradiated with 200 J/cm^2 at 100 mW/cm^2 of red light (635 nm, Omnilux, Phototherapeutics, Cheshire, UK). (Courtesy of R. Rox Anderson, MD, Wellman Center for Photomedicine, Massachusetts General Hospital, Boston, MA.)

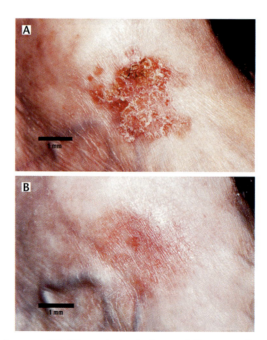

Color plate 28 Bowen's disease: a 32×25-mm lesion before and three months after a single treatment with -aminolevulinic acid photodynamic therapy. (Photo reprinted from Morton, CA, et al., "Photodynamic therapy for large or multiple patches of Bowen's disease and basal cell carcinoma," *Arch. Dermatol*, 2001; 137:319–24.)

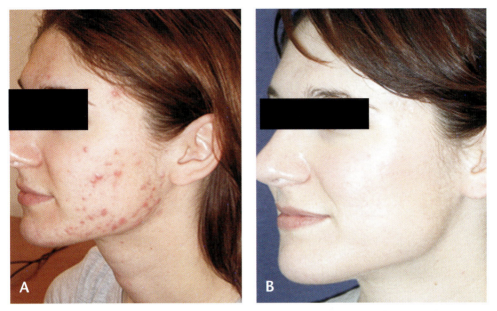

Color plate 29   (a) Before and (b) after ALA-PDT. (Courtesy of Mitchell Paul Goldman, MD.)

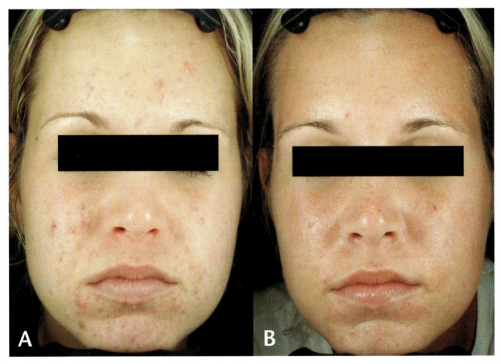

Color plate 30   (a) Before and (b) after three treatments with IPL. (Courtesy of Amy Forman Taub, MD.)

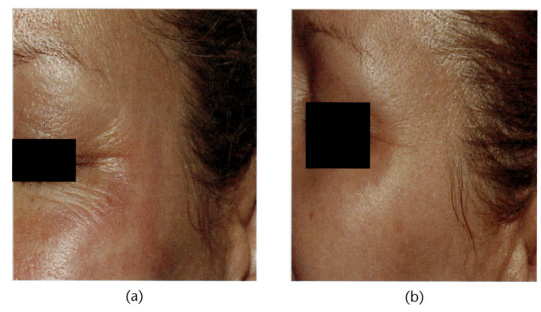

(a)   (b)

Color plate 31   (a) Before and (b) three months after three treatments of ALA-PDT with IPL. (Courtesy of Michael Gold, MD.)

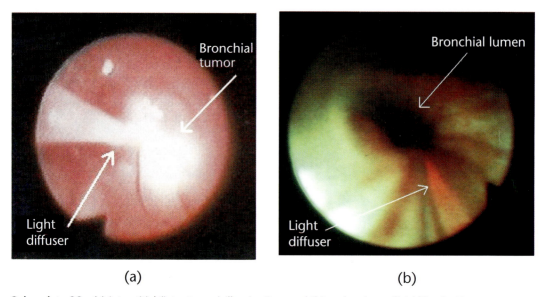

(a)   (b)

Color plate 32   (a) Interstitial (intra tumor) illumination; and (b) surface/superficial illumination.

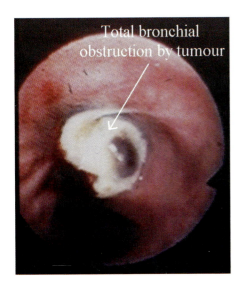

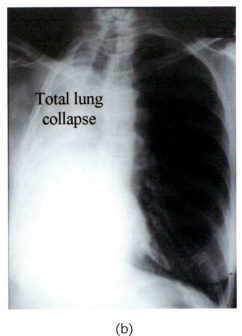

(a)   (b)

Color plate 33   (a) Bronchoscopic features of locally advanced endobronchial cancer; and (b) the chest x-ray of the above patient.

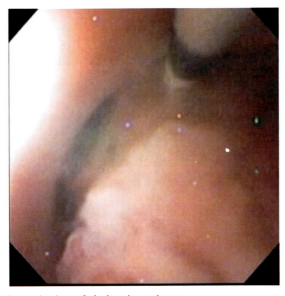

Color plate 34   Cholangioscopic view of cholangiocarcinoma.

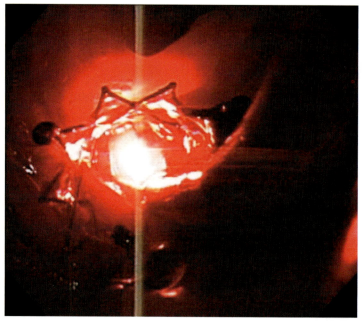

Color plate 35   Application of PDT via diffusing fiber within a metal stent in the distal bile duct.

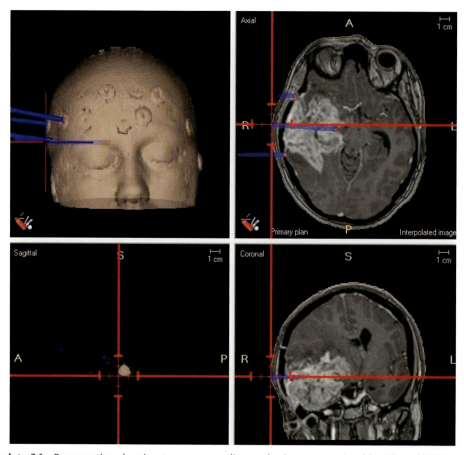

Color plate 36   Preoperative planning to remove malignant brain tumor assisted by PD and PDT.

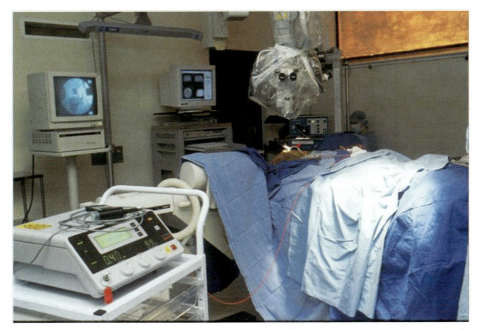

Color plate 37 The balloon diffuser, catheter, fiber-sheet, and fiber in place in a tumor cavity ready for PDT (note the image of the balloon diffuser on the fluoroscopy monitor).

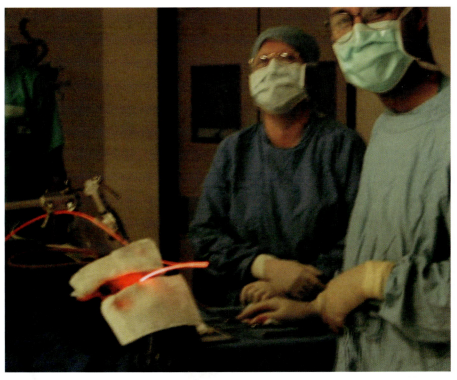

Color plate 38 A patient receiving intraoperative PDT treatment for invasive brain tumor.

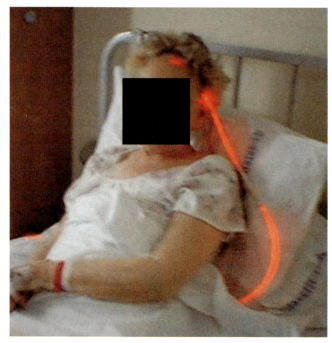

Color plate 39 A patient receiving bedside PDT tretament for invasive supratentorial tumor.

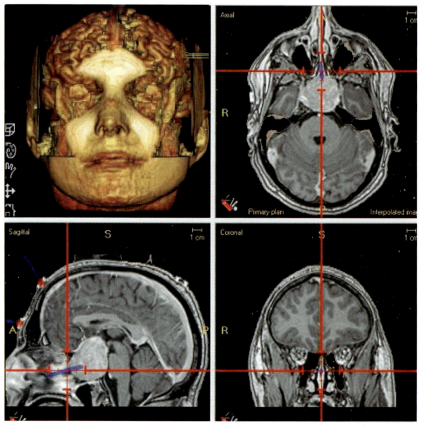

Color plate 40 Preoperative planning to remove pituitary adenoma using the transsphenoidal assisted by PD and PDT.

PDT-generated cell lysates (EMT6 and P815 tumor cells) compared to lysates generated by UV or ionizing irradiation. PDT-generated vaccines were tumor-specific, induced a cytotoxic T-cell response, and unlike the other methods of producing vaccines did not require coadministration of an adjuvant to be effective. PDT-generated lysates were able to induce phenotypic DC maturation and IL-12 expression. Korbelik and Sun [23] produced a vaccine by treating SCCVII cells with BPD-PDT and later with a lethal X-ray dose, and showed that these cells, when injected peritumorally in mice with established SCCVII tumors, produced a significant therapeutic effect, including growth retardation, tumor regression, and cures. Importantly, vaccine cells retrieved from the treatment site at 1 hour postinjection were intermixed with dendritic cells (DCs), exhibited HSP70 on their surface, and were opsonized by complement C3. This observation verifies some of the earlier findings in mouse models and in vitro.

14.2.1.3 Dendritic Cells and Toll-Like Receptor Ligands

Agents derived from microbial stimulators of innate immunity can be injected into the tumor or surrounding area before, during, or after PDT (Color Plate 13). The role of these adjuvants is to activate Toll-like receptors (TLRs) or similar pattern-recognition molecules present on macrophages and dendritic cells [24]. Combination therapy that involves the administration of immunoadjuvants (frequently potential TLR ligands) and different PDT regimens have proved effective. Myers et al. [25] combined HpD-PDT with a killed preparation of Corynebacterium parvum (CP, now Propionibacterium acnes) in a mouse model of subcutaneous bladder cancer. Administration of high dose of CP after PDT was shown to have a significantly greater effect than CP treatment before PDT. Subcutaneous mouse EMT6 tumors were treated with a single BCG administration in combination with PDT using six different PSs [26]. Regardless of the PS used, BCG significantly increased the number of cured tumors and the number of memory T cells in tumor-draining lymph nodes compared to PDT alone. PDT was combined with a single administration of Mycobacterium cell-wall extract immediately after light exposure [27] and produced significantly more long-term cures of EMT6 tumors in BALB/c mice and more tumor-infiltrating leukocytes at 22-hours post-PDT. OK-432 is a preparation derived from killed streptococcal bacteria, and when injected intratumorally 3 hours before HPD-PDT, it increased the tumor free time in mice with NRS1 tumors. OK-432 injected immediately after PDT or OK-432 alone had little effect [28]. Unpublished data from our laboratory has also shown potentiation of PDT-induced antitumor immunity against EMT6 tumors by intratumoral injection of OK432. Schizophyllan (SPG) is an example of a β-D-glucan fungal polysaccharide, which are thought to be potent inducers of humoral and cell-mediated immunity via the macrophage dectin-1 receptor [29] as well as TLR [30]. The tumor cure rate increased threefold when SPG was administered intramuscularly prior to Photofrin-PDT of mice with SCCVII, while SPG after PDT had little effect [31]. A report from Chen and colleagues [32] showed that a preparation of glycated chitosan derived from shrimp shells injected intratumorally enhanced the curative effects of Photofrin-PDT on EMT6 and Line1 lung tumors. The receptors responsible for mediating the effects of glycated chitosan are unknown.

A recent paper [33] studied the combination of intratumoral dendritic cells and PDT mediated by the chlorin-type PS, ATX-S10 Na(II) against CT26 tumors in BALB/c mice. The combination therapy produced tumor cures not seen with either treatment alone. Furthermore when mice bearing two tumors had only one treated with the combination of PDT and dendritic cells, the contralateral untreated tumor underwent regression. Tumor-specific lymphocytes were demonstrated by chromium release CTL assay and by IFN-γ production. Korbelik and Sun [34] used adoptive transfer of a human NK cell line genetically altered to produce IL-2 combined with mTHPC-PDT of subcutaneous human squamous cell carcinoma growing in SCID mice. Peritumoral or intravenous injection of cells immediately after PDT produced an improvement in the outcome of PDT, not seen with a cell line that does not produce IL-2. Comparable results were also observed in case of B16 melanoma. Golab's group [35] showed that administration of immature dendritic cells into tumors treated with Photofrin-PDT resulted in effective homing to regional and peripheral lymph nodes and stimulation of cytotoxic T lymphocytes and natural killer cells. The combination treatment produced the best tumor response and some resistance to a tumor rechallenge.

14.2.2 Macrophage Recruitment

There are reports based on in vitro data that PDT can have an effect on monocyte/macrophage and lymphocyte cell lineages. On the other hand, macrophages can be activated by low, sublethal doses of PDT [36]. Reports show that PDT-treated macrophages secrete tumor necrosis factor alpha (TNFα) [37]. PDT of a mixture of macrophages and lymphocytes produces lysophosphatidyl choline from lymphocytes that can induce expression of beta-galactosidase in B lymphocytes and together with the Neu-1 sialidase from T lymphocytes, these enzymes modified the vitamin D3-binding protein in bovine serum to yield a potent macrophage-activating factor (MAF) [38, 39]. The production of this MAF also occurs in mice where it is derived from the analogous vitamin D3-binding protein in mouse serum [39]. Evidence also indicates that macrophages can show preferential cytotoxicity towards tumor cells treated with a sublethal dose of PDT [40]. Another report [41] showed that although the tumoricidal effect of peritoneal macrophages removed from mice after PDT was unaltered, there was a reduction in natural killer (NK) cell function.

Krosl et al. [42] repeatedly injected lethally irradiated SCCVII cells genetically engineered to produce GM-CSF and demonstrated augmented antitumor effectiveness of Photofrin- and BPD-based-PDT in mice with SCCVII. The treatment with GM-CSF resulted in higher cytotoxic activity of tumor-associated macrophages against SCCVII cells.

14.2.3 B Cell Recruitment

B cells are an important part of any immune response. Therefore, it is interesting that a pubmed.org search for "photodynamic therapy and B cells/B-lymphocytes" yields no results.

14.3   PDT and other Innate Immune Cells

14.3.1   Neutrophiles

Kick et al. [43] compared IL-6 mRNA production after PDT or UVB treatment. PDT-induced IL-6 protein levels were higher and detectable earlier than after treatment with UVB. PDT-induced IL-6 expression was mediated by AP-1 and was independent of PKC activity, NF-κB, or the multiple cytokine- and second messenger-responsive element in the IL-6 promoter.

Gollnick [44] demonstrated in a BALB/c mouse model that PDT delivered to normal and tumor tissue caused marked changes in the expression of IL-6 and IL-10, but not TNFα. This group [45] also found that 2-[1-hexyloxyethyl]-2-devinyl pyropheophorbide-a (HPPH)-mediated-PDT caused neutrophil migration into the treated tumor area due to a transient and local increase in the expression of the chemokine, MIP2 (the murine equivalent of IL8), together with increased expression of the adhesion molecule E-selectin, and although increased local and systemic expression of IL-6 were found this was not necessary for neutrophil recruitment. A subsequent report [46] compared a low and a high fluence (total light energy) each delivered at a low and high fluence rate against Colo 26 murine tumor treated with HPPH. It has previously been proposed that PDT is less efficient when the light is delivered at a high fluence rate because the tissue oxygen is completely used up and cannot be supplied fast enough by the microvasculature to keep up with the photochemical consumption [47]. Oxygen-conserving low fluence rate PDT at a high fluence yielded 70% to 80% tumor cures, whereas the same fluence at the oxygen-depleting high fluence rate yielded 10 % to 15% tumor cures. High fluence at a low fluence rate led to ablation of blood vessels. The highest levels of inflammatory cytokines and neutrophilic infiltrates were measured with low fluence delivered at low fluence rate (10%–20% cures). The optimally curative PDT regimen (high fluence at low fluence rate) produced minimal inflammation. Depletion of neutrophils did not significantly change the high cure rates of that regimen but abolished curability in the maximally inflammatory regimen. These data suggest that tumor cure can be mediated by maximizing the photochemical action, but the importance of causing inflammation and neutrophil infiltration is less clear.

Sluiter et al. [48] first observed that neutrophils adhere to the microvascular wall after PDT in vivo, but PDT did not stimulate the expression of P-selectin (one of the principal adhesion molecules that bind leukocytes) by the endothelial cells (EC). The EC retracted after PDT, allowing the adherence of neutrophils by their beta 2-integrin adhesion receptors to the subendothelial matrix and this could be blocked by anti-beta2-integrin antibodies [49]. In agreement with this finding was a report describing that expression levels of the adhesion molecules ICAM-1 and VCAM-1 were downregulated on EC after PDT [50]. The administration of antirat neutrophil serum together with PDT in rhabdomyosarcoma-bearing rats completely abrogated the normal PDT-induced retardation of tumor growth [51], showing that an influx of neutrophils is required for an effective antitumor response in this model. An increase in the number of peripheral blood neutrophils was found 4 hours after PDT treatment that lasted for 24 hours. It was preceded by an increase in serum levels of IL-1β. Antigranulocyte colony-stimulating factor (G-CSF) antibodies decreased neutrophil numbers and decreased the efficacy of PDT. The reasons why neutrophils are so important in producing an effective response to PDT in some (but not absolutely all) tumor models are still uncertain.

Krosl and coworkers [52] measured cellular populations in the murine squamous cell carcinoma (SCC)VII model treated with Photofrin-PDT. They found a 200-fold increase in the number of neutrophils within 5 minutes followed immediately by an increase in the levels of mast cells, while another type of myeloid cell, most likely monocytes, invaded the tumor 2 hours after PDT. Cecic et al. [53] found that pronounced neutrophilia developed rapidly after PDT (Photofrin or mTHPC) of mice with SCCVII or EMT6 mammary carcinomas. Neutrophilia was also observed after PDT treatment of normal dorsal skin but not in the footpad of tumor-free mice. Complement inhibition completely prevented the development of PDT-induced neutrophilia. It has also been shown that blocking ICAM-1 with monoclonal antibodies reduced the number of tumor cures [54]. A marked upregulation of ICAM1 ligands CD11b/c found on neutrophils was also associated with PDT-treated tumors. IL-1β neutralizing antibodies diminished the number of cures of PDT-treated tumors. It has been found that neutrophils express MHC class II molecules, which suggests their engagement as antigen-presenting cells and involvement in the development of antitumor immune response. The same group found that IL-1β and TNF-α both acted as potent promoters of the early phase of PDT-induced neutrophilia but appear not to have a significant role in the advanced phase [55]. The data attained with blocking two other cytokines, G-CSF and IL-10, demonstrated that they are important contributors to the advanced-phase neutrophilia with no apparent influence in the early phase.

De Bruijn [56] reported that treatment of the subcutaneously (s.c.) growing rat rhabdomyosarcoma tumors with ALA-PDT resulted in a significant increase in the number of blood neutrophils during the first several days after illumination peaking at 16 and 24 hours posttreatment. They also observed that a significantly higher degree of neutrophilia could result from a twofold fractionated illumination scheme.

The reports covered above demonstrate that the acute inflammation produced by PDT and especially both a systemic and tumor-localized increase in neutrophils are of major importance in obtaining tumor cures. It is highly likely (although difficult to demonstrate) that these phenomena will also be important in the development of a memory T-cell antitumor immune response after PDT.

14.3.2 NK Cell Recruitment

In a recent report, Kabingu et al. [57] used NK cells depletion in SCID mice to assess the involvement of this cell in PDT induced immunity. Mice were injected subcutaneously and IV at the same time with EMT/6 tumor cells to establish both lung and s.c. tumors, and then the s.c. tumors alone received PDT treatment. They observed that the number of lung tumors per mouse 10 days after PDT was significantly higher in NK-depleted animals suggesting that NK participates in PDT-induced immune control of tumors. Moreover, in the absence of NK cells, SCID mice replenished with CD8+ T cells exhibited a significant increase in lung tumor number. The authors concluded that that NK cells may play important role in post-PDT activity of CD8+ T cells and control of distant nontreated metastases.

14.4 PDT and T Lymphocytes

The introduction of transplantable tumors growing in inbred mouse or rat strains that share the same MHC haplotype (syngeneic animals) and have intact immune systems has allowed the study of antitumor immunity after PDT. Canti and colleagues [58] examined the effects of PDT with the PS aluminum disulfonated phthalocyanine on the antitumor immune response in both immunosuppressed and normal mice bearing MS-2 fibrosarcomas. All mice were cured and survived indefinitely, but resistance to MS-2 rechallenge was evident only in normal surviving animals cured by PDT, while immunosuppressed surviving animals and animals cured by surgery died after tumor rechallenge. Different syngeneic murine leukemias were not rejected. These findings suggested that PDT might induce the activation of the tumor-specific cytotoxic T lymphocytes. Color Plate 14 summarizes the pathways that lead to PDT-induced activation of T cells.

14.4.1 Activation of CTLs

Indeed, the adoptive transfer of splenic T-lymphocytes from naïve BALB/c mice into SCID mice performed before PDT postponed the recurrence of treated tumors, while adoptive transfer done immediately or 7 days after PDT had no benefit. [59]. Adoptive transfer of nonadherent splenocytes (a mixture of CD4 and CD8 T cells together with some B cells, NK cells, and monocytes) from normal mice cured of EMT6 by PDT 5 weeks previously, fully restored of the curative effect of PDT on EMT6 tumors growing in SCID mice. Splenocytes obtained from donors cured by X-rays were much less effective. Depletion of specific T-cell populations from donor splenocytes indicated that CD8 CTLs had the most effect, while CD4 helper T-cells played a supportive role [60]. Analogous studies were performed by a different group [61] using PDT with the PS 2-iodo-5-ethylamino-9-diethylaminobenzo-phenothiazinium chloride.

14.4.2 Activation of Antigen-Specific CD8+ T Cells

Although PDT has been shown to efficiently engage both innate and adaptive immune responses leading to tumor rejection in various tumor models, it has never been clearly shown that PDT-mediated antitumor immunity is dependent and driven by antigen/epitope specific CD8+ T cells. A recent report from our laboratory [62] showed that BPD-mediated PDT of RIF1 tumors (poorly immunogenic) in wild-type C3H/HeN mice leads to initial tumor disappearance but not to permanent cures due to local recurrence. By contrast, when the tumors were genetically engineered to express the foreign protein, green fluorescent protein (GFP) from jellyfish, 100% cures and long-term resistance to rechallenge was obtained after PDT. PDT (but not surgical removal) induced immune recognition of the foreign GFP as a model tumor antigen. These early studies suggested that PDT induced immune response is antigen-dependent and prompted us to further study this phenomenon. In the recent project, we employed an established defined tumor antigen (DTA) β-galactosidase (β-gal) from E. coli to answer the question whether the stimulation of the immune system by PDT would be sufficient to lead to antigen-specific tumor rejection. We also asked whether PDT-mediated stimulation of antitumor immunity would be antigen/epitope-specific and therefore different in the antigen-positive and antigen-negative cancer cell lines. We employed a previously described model [63] of two colon adenocarcinoma cell lines: the CT26 wild type (CT26WT) cell line, derived from an undifferentiated carcinogen-induced colon adenocarcinoma [64], and CT26.CL25 derived from CT26WT cells that have been stably transduced with lacZ gene for bacterial β-gal using a retrovirus [65].

Vascular PDT mediated by benzoporphyrin derivative and red light cured 100% of CT26.CL25 tumors, while all CT26 wild type tumors showed local recurrence (Figure 14.1). Mice cured from CT26.CL25 were resistant to rechallenge with CT26.CL25 cells but not CT26 cells. Mice bearing two CT26.CL25 tumors, with only one treated with PDT, demonstrated robust immune response leading to regression of the distant untreated tumor in 70% of the cases. CTLs from mice cured of CT26.CL25 tumors displayed significantly more specific lysis at effector:target ratios of 25:1 and 50:1 against CT26.CL25 targets than they did against CT26WT targets (P<0.05) or irrelevant EMT6 targets (P<0.001). Likewise, lymphocytes from CT26.CL25 tumor-bearing mice also showed significantly less specific lysis against CT26.CL25 targets than did CTLs from CT26.CL25 cured mice (P<0.05). We have

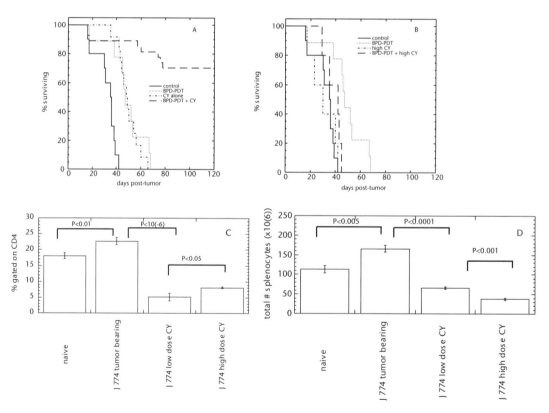

Figure 14.1 Kaplan-Meier survival curves of groups of mice that received: (A) no treatment, BPD-PDT, low dose CY and low dose CY + BPD-PDT; (B) no treatment, BPD-PDT, high dose CY and high-dose CY + BPD-PDT; (C) Percentages of CD4+FoxP3+ double positive LN cells from lymph nodes extracted from mice with or without J774 tumors 3 days post low dose CY injection; (D) Numbers of splenocytes from whole spleens removed form mice as described above.

also measured the CD8+ T cell population that binds the immunodominant peptide epitope derived from [b]-gal and restricted by MHC class I haplotype H2L[d]. DIMER X technology is a cytometry-based assay, which allows the frequency of known epitope sequence-specific CD8+ T-cells to be readily determined in a similar fashion to MHC tetramers [66]. The reagent binds a synthetic peptide epitope and is subsequently recognized by CTLs and detected by secondary antibody staining. Lymph node cells from either CT26.CL25 cured mice or CT26.CL25 tumor-bearing mice that had been incubated with DimerX loaded with TPHPARIGL peptide (β-gal peptide) were gated for size and CD8 expression ad displayed as a percentage of DIMER X positive CD8 T cell. The following negative controls were also carried out: the secondary FITC antibody was substituted for a FITC-labeled isotype control and the DimerX was not loaded with a peptide. There was a significant difference between binding of β-gal loaded DimerX by CD8-positive T cells from lymph nodes from cured mice and from tumor-bearing mice showing that PDT does indeed induce recognition of MHC class I bound β-gal peptide epitope and provides a rationale for the specific cell lysis found in the preceding section. This is the first time that this phenomenon has been clearly shown to occur after PDT, although the previous work has established that CD8+ T cells are critical to PDT-induced immunity. These data demonstrate the selectivity of PDT-induced CTLs for β-gal expressing tumor as well as the importance and PDT dependence on the tumor rejection antigen presence.

14.4.3   The Role of CD4+ T Cells in PDT

Gollnick et al. [57] demonstrated that CD4+ T cell depletion had no effect on the ability of PDT to control tumors present outside the treated area. Splenocytes transferred to SCID mice after depletion of CD4+ T cells successfully controlled the growth of tumors, while reconstitution with CD8+ T cells completely abrogated this effect. These observations were also confirmed in mice lacking CD40, a CD4+ T cells costimulatory molecule necessary for interaction with dendritic cells. The tumor growth control after PDT was not significantly different compared to wild type mice. To further elucidate the necessity of CD4+ T cells for PDT-induced immunity, they reconstituted SCID mice only with CD8+ cells and next inoculated with EMT/6 tumors. The following PDT treatment resulted in 40 days tumor-free survival and development of memory immunity demonstrated by rejection of rechallenge with intravenous administration of the same tumor.

14.5   PDT and Immunosuppression

Immunosuppression involves an act that reduces the activation or efficacy of the immune system. Immunosuppression may occur as an adverse reaction to the treatment or as a part of host protective mechanisms that control the immune response and help to restore homeostatic conditions following the onset of acute inflammation [67]. The examples of PDT being involved in both aspects of immunosuppression are described below.

14.5.1   Immunosuppressive Effects of PDT

Somewhat paradoxically, considering the discussions above, there are also several reports that PDT can induce various forms of immunosuppression [68]. These have nearly all been concerned with the suppression of the contact hypersensitivity (CHS) reaction in mice [69]. This involves application of a hapten such as dinitrofluorobenzene to skin followed by a rechallenge at a distant site, and can be suppressed for up to 28 days post-PDT, as shown in Color Plate 15.

It appears that this suppression involves systemic IL10 release in cases where the PDT illumination penetrates the skin (red light) [70], but is independent of IL10 when the PDT is confined to the skin layers (blue light) [71]. In contrast to ultraviolet B irradiation that suppresses both CHS and delayed type hypersensitivity (DTH) responses, PDT does not suppress DTH [72]. One difference between CHS and DTH is that CHS is thought to be a MHC-class I-mediated process while DTH is mediated via MHC-class II [73].

14.5.2   PDT and Regulatory T Cells

There is a growing realization that CD4+CD25+ T-regulatory cells have an important function in suppressing the immune response against multiple targets (Figure 14.2).

T regulatory cells can be efficiently depleted by a low dose of cyclophosphamide (CY), thus potentiating immunity [74], whereas high-dose CY is immunosuppressive (Figure 14.2(b, c)) [75]. Low-dose CY combined with BPD- PDT using a short drug-light interval that predominantly targeted the tumor blood vessels led to a significant number of long-term J774 reticulum cell sarcoma cures and resistance to tumor rechallenge, while either treatment alone led to 100% death from progressive tumors or metastasis [76]. Examination of lymph node cells recovered from tumor bearing mice after low-dose CY revealed that CD4+FoxP3+ T cells were reduced (Figure 14.1) [77].

14.6   Conclusion

Although PDT has been carried out in cancer patients for many years (since the 1970s), there has been remarkably little published evidence that the stimulation of antitumor immunity by PDT actually occurs in humans. There are anecdotal reports about unexpectedly long survival of patients treated with PDT for recurrent cancer. There have been two reports about immune effects in PDT of human papilloma virus lesions in patients. A report by Abdel-Hardy et al. describes the treatment of HPV-positive vulval intraepithelial neoplasia lesions with ALA-PDT. They found measured increases in immune response in responders compared with nonresponders who were likely to have loss of MHC class I in their lesions. Similar results were presented on PDT for respiratory papillomatosis [106]. A recent meeting abstract (S. O. Gollnick, personal communication) reported that patients treated with PDT for basal cell carcinoma (BCC) demonstrated a significant increase (50%–130%) in the numbers of peripheral blood T-cells that produced IFN-g when

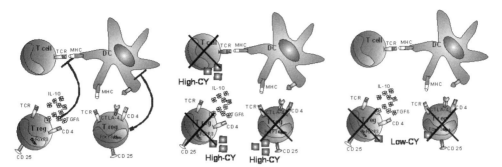

Figure 14.2 (a) Effects of cyclophosphamide on Tregs suppression. Lack of antitumor immunity is often related to impaired T-cell responses that could result from inhibition by regulatory T cells. (b) Cyclophosphamide, apart from cytotoxic effect as an alkylating chemotherapeutic agent, also has immunomodulatory effects, such as depletion of CD4+CD25+ regulatory T cells. High-dose cyclophosphamide severely decreases the numbers of all the T cells, leading to overall impaired antitumor immune reactivity. (c) In contrast, low-dose cyclophosphamide only slightly affects the numbers of T cells, while a decline in CD4+CD25+ T cell number is still profound. This allows to maintain the sufficient numbers of activated T cells that, when liberated from Tregs suppression, can actively destroy tumor targets.

they recognized the sonic hedgehog ligand, hedgehog interacting protein (HIP-1). HIP-1 has been shown to function as a tumor-associated antigen.

Further work on the determinants of immune response against tumors after PDT in experimental systems will allow some rationally designed and scientifically based recommendations for PDT regimens and combination therapies that could be tested in patients.

References

[1] Korbelik, M., "Induction of tumor immunity by photodynamic therapy.," *J. Clin. Laser Med. Surg.*, Vol. 14, 1996, pp. 329–334.

[2] van Duijnhoven, F. H., et al., "The immunological consequences of photodynamic treatment of cancer, a literature review," *Immunobiology*, Vol. 207, 2003, pp. 105–113.

[3] Canti, G., De Simone, A., and Korbelik, M., "Photodynamic therapy and the immune system in experimental oncology," *Photochem. Photobiol. Sci.*, Vol. 1, 2002, pp. 79–80.

[4] Oleinick, N. L., Morris, R. L., and Belichenko, I., "The role of apoptosis in response to photodynamic therapy: what, where, why, and how," *Photochem. Photobiol. Sci.*, Vol. 1, 2002, pp. 1–21.

[5] Castano, A. P., Demidova, T. N., and Hamblin, M. R., "Mechanisms in photodynamic therapy: part two—cellular signalling, cell metabolism and modes of cell death," *Photodiagn. Photodyn. Ther.*, Vol. 2, 2005, pp. 1–23.

[6] Agostinis, P., et al., "Regulatory pathways in photodynamic therapy induced apoptosis," *Photochem. Photobiol. Sci.*, Vol. 3, 2004, pp. 721–729.

[7] Moor, A. C., "Signaling pathways in cell death and survival after photodynamic therapy," *J Photochem Photobiol B*, Vol. 57, 2000, pp. 1–13.

[8] Plaetzer, K., et al., "Apoptosis following photodynamic tumor therapy: induction, mechanisms and detection," *Current pharmaceutical design*, Vol. 11, 2005, pp. 1151–1165.

[9] Chen, B., et al., "Photodynamic therapy with hypericin induces vascular damage and apoptosis in the RIF-1 mouse tumor model," *Int J Cancer*, Vol. 98, 2002, pp. 284–290.

[10] Kaneko, T., et al., "Detection of photodynamic therapy-induced early apoptosis in human salivary gland tumor cells in vitro and in a mouse tumor model," *Oral Oncol*, Vol. 40, 2004, pp. 787–792.

[11] Lilge, L., Portnoy, M., and Wilson, B. C., "Apoptosis induced in vivo by photodynamic therapy in normal brain and intracranial tumour tissue," *Br J Cancer*, Vol. 83, 2000, pp. 1110–1117.

[12] Magner, W. J., and Tomasi, T. B., "Apoptotic and necrotic cells induced by different agents vary in their expression of MHC and costimulatory genes," *Mol Immunol*, Vol. 42, 2005, pp. 1033–1042.

[13] Bartholomae, W. C., et al., "T cell immunity induced by live, necrotic, and apoptotic tumor cells," *J Immunol*, Vol. 173, 2004, pp. 1012–1022.

[14] Scheffer, S. R., et al., "Apoptotic, but not necrotic, tumor cell vaccines induce a potent immune response in vivo," *Int J Cancer*, Vol. 103, 2003, pp. 205–211.

[15] Shaif-Muthana, M., et al., "Dead or alive: immunogenicity of human melanoma cells when presented by dendritic cells," *Cancer Res*, Vol. 60, 2000, pp. 6441–6447.

[16] Zitvogel, L., et al., "Immune response against dying tumor cells," *Adv. Immunol.*, Vol. 84, 2004, pp. 131–179.

[17] Melcher, A., et al., "Apoptosis or necrosis for tumor immunotherapy: what's in a name?" *J. Mol. Med.*, Vol. 77, 1999, pp. 824–833.

[18] Yenari, M. A., et al., "Antiapoptotic and anti-inflammatory mechanisms of heat-shock protein protection," *Ann. N. Y. Acad. Sci.*, Vol. 1053, 2005, pp. 74–83.

[19] Korbelik, M., Sun, J., and Cecic, I., "Photodynamic therapy-induced cell surface expression and release of heat shock proteins: relevance for tumor response," *Cancer Res.*, Vol. 65, 2005, pp. 1018–1026.

[20] Todryk, S., et al., "Heat shock protein 70 induced during tumor cell killing induces Th1 cytokines and targets immature dendritic cell precursors to enhance antigen uptake," *J. Immunol.*, Vol. 163, 1999, pp. 1398–1408.

[21] Gomer, C. J., et al., "Photodynamic therapy-mediated oxidative stress can induce expression of heat shock proteins," *Cancer Res.*, Vol. 56, 1996, pp. 2355–2360.

[22] Gollnick, S. O., Vaughan, L., and Henderson, B. W., "Generation of effective antitumor vaccines using photodynamic therapy," *Cancer Res.*, Vol. 62, 2002, pp. 1604–1608.

[23] Korbelik, M., and Sun, J., "Photodynamic therapy-generated vaccine for cancer therapy," *Cancer Immunol. Immunother.*, Vol. Epub ahead of print, 2005, pp. 1–10.

[24] Takeda, K., Kaisho, T., and Akira, S., "Toll-like receptors," *Annu. Rev. Immunol.*, Vol. 21, 2003, pp. 335–376.

[25] Myers, R. C., et al., "Modulation of hematoporphyrin derivative-sensitized phototherapy with corynebacterium parvum in murine transitional cell carcinoma," *Urology*, Vol. 33, 1989, pp. 230–235.

[26] Korbelik, M., Sun, J., and Posakony, J. J., "Interaction between photodynamic therapy and BCG immunotherapy responsible for the reduced recurrence of treated mouse tumors," *Photochem. Photobiol.*, Vol. 73, 2001, pp. 403–409.

[27] Korbelik, M., and Cecic, I., "Enhancement of tumour response to photodynamic therapy by adjuvant mycobacterium cell-wall treatment," *J. Photochem. Photobiol. B*, Vol. 44, 1998, pp. 151–158.

[28] Uehara, M., et al., "Enhancement of the photodynamic antitumor effect by streptococcal preparation OK-432 in the mouse carcinoma," *Cancer Immunol. Immunother.*, Vol. 49, 2000, pp. 401–409.

[29] Taylor, P. R., et al., "The beta-glucan receptor, dectin-1, is predominantly expressed on the surface of cells of the monocyte/macrophage and neutrophil lineages," *J. Immunol.*, Vol. 169, 2002, pp. 3876–3882.

[30] Roeder, A., et al., "Toll-like receptors as key mediators in innate antifungal immunity," *Med. Mycol.*, Vol. 42, 2004, pp. 485–498.

[31]   Krosl, G., and Korbelik, M., "Potentiation of photodynamic therapy by immunotherapy: the effect of schizophyllan (SPG)," *Cancer Lett.*, Vol. 84, 1994, pp. 43–49.

[32]   Chen, W. R., et al., "Enhancement of laser cancer treatment by a chitosan-derived immunoadjuvant," *Photochem. Photobiol.*, Vol. 81, 2005, pp. 190–195.

[33]   Saji, H., et al., "Systemic antitumor effect of intratumoral injection of dendritic cells in combination with local photodynamic therapy," *Clin Cancer Res*, Vol. 12, 2006, pp. 2568–2574.

[34]   Korbelik, M., and Sun, J., "Cancer treatment by photodynamic therapy combined with adoptive immunotherapy using genetically altered natural killer cell line," *Int. J. Cancer*, Vol. 93, 2001, pp. 269–274.

[35]   Jalili, A., et al., "Effective photoimmunotherapy of murine colon carcinoma induced by the combination of photodynamic therapy and dendritic cells," *Clin. Cancer Res.*, Vol. 10, 2004, pp. 4498–4508.

[36]   Steubing, R. W., et al., "Activation of macrophages by Photofrin II during photodynamic therapy," *J. Photochem. Photobiol. B*, Vol. 10, 1991, pp. 133–145.

[37]   Evans, S., et al., "Effect of photodynamic therapy on tumor necrosis factor production by murine macrophages," *J. Natl. Cancer Inst.*, Vol. 82, 1990, pp. 34–39.

[38]   Yamamoto, N., et al., "Photodynamic immunopotentiation: in vitro activation of macrophages by treatment of mouse peritoneal cells with haematoporphyrin derivative and light," *Eur. J. Cancer*, Vol. 27, 1991, pp. 467–471.

[39]   Yamamoto, N., and Naraparaju, V. R., "Immunotherapy of BALB/c mice bearing Ehrlich ascites tumor with vitamin D-binding protein-derived macrophage activating factor," *Cancer Res.*, Vol. 57, 1997, pp. 2187–2192.

[40]   Korbelik, M., and Krosl, G., "Enhanced macrophage cytotoxicity against tumor cells treated with photodynamic therapy," *Photochem. Photobiol.*, Vol. 60, 1994, pp. 497–502.

[41]   Marshall, J. F., Chan, W. S., and Hart, I. R., "Effect of photodynamic therapy on anti-tumor immune defenses: comparison of the photosensitizers hematoporphyrin derivative and chloro-aluminum sulfonated phthalocyanine," *Photochem Photobiol*, Vol. 49, 1989, pp. 627–632.

[42]   Krosl, G., et al., "Potentiation of photodynamic therapy-elicited antitumor response by localized treatment with granulocyte-macrophage colony-stimulating factor," *Cancer Res.*, Vol. 56, 1996, pp. 3281–3286.

[43]   Kick, G., et al., "Photodynamic therapy induces expression of interleukin 6 by activation of AP-1 but not NF-kappa B DNA binding," *Cancer Res.*, Vol. 55, 1995, pp. 2373–2379.

[44]   Gollnick, S. O., et al., "Altered expression of interleukin 6 and interleukin 10 as a result of photodynamic therapy in vivo," *Cancer Res.*, Vol. 57, 1997, pp. 3904–3909.

[45]   Gollnick, S. O., et al., "Role of cytokines in photodynamic therapy-induced local and systemic inflammation," *Br. J. Cancer*, Vol. 88, 2003, pp. 1772–1779.

[46]   Henderson, B. W., et al., "Choice of oxygen-conserving treatment regimen determines the inflammatory response and outcome of photodynamic therapy of tumors," *Cancer Res.*, Vol. 64, 2004, pp. 2120–2126.

[47]   Coutier, S., et al., "Effect of irradiation fluence rate on the efficacy of photodynamic therapy and tumor oxygenation in meta-tetra (hydroxyphenyl) chlorin (mTHPC)-sensitized HT29 xenografts in nude mice," *Radiat. Res.*, Vol. 158, 2002, pp. 339–345.

[48]   Sluiter, W., et al., "Prevention of late lumen loss after coronary angioplasty by photodynamic therapy: role of activated neutrophils," *Mol. Cell. Biochem.*, Vol. 157, 1996, pp. 233–238.

[49]   de Vree, W. J., et al., "Photodynamic treatment of human endothelial cells promotes the adherence of neutrophils in vitro," *Br. J. Cancer*, Vol. 73, 1996, pp. 1335–1340.

[50]   Volanti, C., et al., "Downregulation of ICAM-1 and VCAM-1 expression in endothelial cells treated by photodynamic therapy," *Oncogene*, Vol. 23, 2004, pp. 8649–8658.

[51] de Vree, W. J., et al., "Evidence for an important role of neutrophils in the efficacy of photodynamic therapy in vivo," *Cancer Res.*, Vol. 56, 1996, pp. 2908–2911.

[52] Krosl, G., Korbelik, M., and Dougherty, G. J., "Induction of immune cell infiltration into murine SCCVII tumour by photofrin-based photodynamic therapy," *Br. J. Cancer*, Vol. 71, 1995, pp. 549–555.

[53] Cecic, I., Parkins, C. S., and Korbelik, M., "Induction of systemic neutrophil response in mice by photodynamic therapy of solid tumors," *Photochem. Photobiol.*, Vol. 74, 2001, pp. 712–720.

[54] Sun, J., et al., "Neutrophils as inflammatory and immune effectors in photodynamic therapy-treated mouse SCCVII tumours," *Photochem. Photobiol. Sci.*, Vol. 1, 2002, pp. 690–695.

[55] Cecic, I., and Korbelik, M., "Mediators of peripheral blood neutrophilia induced by photodynamic therapy of solid tumors," *Cancer Lett.*, Vol. 183, 2002, pp. 43–51.

[56] de Bruijn, H. S., et al., "Evidence for a bystander role of neutrophils in the response to systemic 5-aminolevulinic acid-based photodynamic therapy," *Photodermatol Photoimmunol Photomed*, Vol. 22, 2006, pp. 238–246.

[57] Kabingu, E., et al., "CD8+ T cell-mediated control of distant tumours following local photodynamic therapy is independent of CD4+ T cells and dependent on natural killer cells," *Br J Cancer*, Vol. 96, 2007, pp. 1839–1848.

[58] Canti, G., et al., "Antitumor immunity induced by photodynamic therapy with aluminum disulfonated phthalocyanines and laser light," *Anti-Cancer Drugs*, Vol. 5, 1994, pp. 443–447.

[59] Korbelik, M., et al., "The role of host lymphoid populations in the response of mouse EMT6 tumor to photodynamic therapy," *Cancer Res.*, Vol. 56, 1996, pp. 5647–5652.

[60] Korbelik, M., and Dougherty, G. J., "Photodynamic therapy-mediated immune response against subcutaneous mouse tumors," *Cancer Res.*, Vol. 59, 1999, pp. 1941–1946.

[61] Hendrzak-Henion, J. A., et al., "Role of the immune system in mediating the antitumor effect of benzophenothiazine photodynamic therapy," *Photochem. Photobiol.*, Vol. 69, 1999, pp. 575–581.

[62] Castano, A. P., Liu, Q., and R., H. M., "A green fluorescent protein-expressing murine tumour but not its wild-type counterpart is cured by photodynamic therapy," *Br. J. Cancer*, Vol. 94, 2006, pp. 391-397.

[63] Wang, M., et al., "Active immunotherapy of cancer with a nonreplicating recombinant fowlpox virus encoding a model tumor-associated antigen," *J Immunol*, Vol. 154, 1995, pp. 4685–4692.

[64] Brattain, M. G., et al., "Establishment of mouse colonic carcinoma cell lines with different metastatic properties," *Cancer Res*, Vol. 40, 1980, pp. 2142–2146.

[65] Wang, M., et al., "Anti-tumor activity of cytotoxic T lymphocytes elicited with recombinant and synthetic forms of a model tumor-associated antigen," *J Immunother Emphasis Tumor Immunol*, Vol. 18, 1995, pp. 139–146.

[66] Dal Porto, J., et al., "A soluble divalent class I major histocompatibility complex molecule inhibits alloreactive T cells at nanomolar concentrations," *Proc Natl Acad Sci USA*, Vol. 90, 1993, pp. 6671–6675.

[67] Belkaid, Y., "Regulatory T cells and infection: a dangerous necessity," *Nat Rev Immunol*, Vol. 7, 2007, pp. 875–888.

[68] Hunt, D. W., and Levy, J. G., "Immunomodulatory aspects of photodynamic therapy," *Expert Opin. Investig. Drugs*, Vol. 7, 1998, pp. 57–64.

[69] Musser, D. A., et al., "The anatomic site of photodynamic therapy is a determinant for immunosuppression in a murine model," *Photochem Photobiol*, Vol. 69, 1999, pp. 222–225.

[70] Simkin, G. O., et al., "IL-10 contributes to the inhibition of contact hypersensitivity in mice treated with photodynamic therapy," *J. Immunol.*, Vol. 164, 2000, pp. 2457–2462.

[71] Gollnick, S. O., et al., "IL-10 does not play a role in cutaneous Photofrin photodynamic therapy-induced suppression of the contact hypersensitivity response," *Photochem. Photobiol.*, Vol. 74, 2001, pp. 811–816.

[72] Musser, D. A., and Oseroff, A. R., "Characteristics of the immunosuppression induced by cutaneous photodynamic therapy: persistence, antigen specificity and cell type involved," *Photochem Photobiol*, Vol. 73, 2001, pp. 518–524.

[73] Ohtani, M., Kobayashi, Y., and Watanabe, N., "Gene expression in the elicitation phase of guinea pig DTH and CHS reactions," *Cytokine*, Vol. 25, 2004, pp. 246–253.

[74] North, R. J., "Cyclophosphamide-facilitated adoptive immunotherapy of an established tumor depends on elimination of tumor-induced suppressor T cells," *J. Exp. Med.*, Vol. 155, 1982, pp. 1063–1074.

[75] Zagozdzon, R., and Golab, J., "Immunomodulation by anticancer chemotherapy: more is not always better (review)," *Int. J. Oncol.*, Vol. 18, 2001, pp. 417–424.

[76] Castano, A. P., and Hamblin, M. R., "Anti-tumor immunity generated by photodynamic therapy in a metastatic murine tumor model," *Proc. SPIE*, Vol. 5695, 2005, pp. 7–16.

[77] Castano, A. P. et al., "Photodynamic therapy plus low-dose cyclophosphamide generates antitumor immunity in a mouse model," *Proc Natl Acad Sci USA*, 2008.

CHAPTER 15

Photodynamic Therapy in Bone

Stuart K. Bisland

Introduction

Recent work within our group suggests that the application of photodynamic therapy (PDT) in bone holds considerable promise for a number of key conditions specific to bone, including the treatment of primary and secondary cancers, infection, and skeletal deformity. In this chapter I will provide a synopsis of preclinical results obtained using PDT in bone that starts with an overview of the preclinical testing of PDT using liposome-formulated benzoporphyrin-derivative monoacid (BPD-MA, verteporfin) for treating human breast cancer metastases in the spine. Current treatment planning strategies, intraoperative image guidance and navigation as well as protocols for assessing posttreatment response in vivo are also discussed. Antimicrobial PDT is a growing field and Section 15.2 describes some of our work in a small animal model of osteomyelitis. Results are described for PDT treatment of Staphylococcus aureus and Pseudomonas aeruginosa cultures in vitro and in vivo that highlight the need for PDT regimens that will provide long-term management of obstinate or recurrent infections. The final section of this chapter describes some work examining the effects of PDT on endochondral bone and raises a number of interesting possibilities regarding the potential role for PDT in bone growth modulation.

15.1 Photodynamic Therapy for Spinal Metastases

15.1.1 Spinal Metastases

Almost half of all cancers reported, approximately 1.5 million new cases each year in North America alone, have the propensity to metastasize into bone, in particular the spine. Statistical review regarding the prevalence and incidence of cancers in the United States readers can be accessed online (http://www.cancer.org). Certain primary cancers; breast, prostrate, lung, and thyroid are highly metastatic to spine and account for the majority of the 100,000 patients being treated each year in North America for spinal metastases, each with varying prognoses depending on the primary tumor [1]. A study of 425 patients with spinal metastases determined a 70% survival rate at 1 year for breast cancer, 83% for prostate, 22% for lung, and 0% for gastric [2]. Irrespective of primary tumor, patients with spinal metastases are typically moribund with debilitating pain secondary to osteolysis, fractures, or nerve impingement by the lesion. The subsequent loss of ambulation can lead to conditions that dramatically impact survival, including pneumonia, bedsores, urinary tract infections, and hypercalcaemia [3–7], emphasizing the importance of quality of life for these patients. The complexity of pathways governing the behavior of cancer cells, bone cells, and progenitor cells are only being realized [8–12] and will be instrumental in the design of therapeutic strategies for the future.

15.1.2 Conventional Therapies

Medical advancements continue to prolong survival for many critically ill patients, prompting a demand for improved palliative therapies that offer maximal pain relief and functional preservation. Current conventional treatments for spinal metastases, including bisphosphonates, radiation therapy, and surgery [13–16] do little toward this goal. Treatments can be expensive and are fraught with complications. For the 10% of patients that present with epidural invasion and neurological compromise, treatment options are traditionally surgery followed by radiation, while treatment for the remaining 90% of patients that do not display neurological compromise remains controversial. Surgery can be conducted via anterior or combined anterior/posterior approach with thoracotomy and/or piecemeal excision of the tumor, and pain control is typically good with neurological recovery and continued ambulation despite the often-protracted recovery times [3–5, 7]. The risks, however, remain significant, with complication rates ranging from 20% to 30% and 1% to 9 % mortality rates at 1 month with mean mortality from 7.5 to 15.9 months [3–5, 7]. Recurrence at the surgical site is a primary cause of failure in as many as 50% of patients following intralesion resection, and preoperative radiation therapy may further increase this [16]. For patients without neurological compromise the argument for radiation therapy is often questionable due to toxicity or tumor resistance [17]. Radiation therapy also offers only partial pain relief (35%), which may be delayed and does nothing to address the bone instability and/or microfractures caused by the tumor [14, 17–19]. In fact, radiation-induced myelopathy can exacerbate instability [16]. Recurrence rates and/or failure rates are also high [19], with secondary complications related to wound dehiscence. Yet despite the poor selectivity of radiation and its related morbidity, the difficulty in defining tumor margins will ensure that preoperative radiation remains part of the standard of care. New targeted methods such as intensity modulated radiation or gamma knife radio-surgery will likely improve clinical outcome. However, the higher costs associated with these technologies currently limit availability.

15.1.3 Photodynamic Therapy

The need for improved interventional approaches for patients with advanced stage spinal metastases led us to consider photodynamic therapy. We hypothesized that placing submillimeter optical fiber(s) into diseased vertebrae would allow selective PDT-mediated tumor ablation without damaging the spinal cord. We further proposed that PDT could be used in combination with vertebroplasty or kyphoplasty to stabilize the bone. Importantly, PDT has been shown to be effective in patients who have failed radiation therapy and is not associated with resistance following repeat treatments [20, 21].

15.1.4 A Model of Human Breast Cancer Derived Spinal Metastases

To demonstrate the proof of principle, we developed a rodent model similar to that described by Engebraaten and Fodstad [22]. Human breast cancer cells, MT-1, were transfected with the luciferase gene, allowing noninvasive bioluminescence monitoring of tumor growth within the bone. A close correlation between tumor burden and bioluminescence signal was found and subsequently confirmed histologically (25). Rats typically developed lesions with quantifiable levels of bioluminescence within 10 to 14 days post intracardiac injection of 2×10^6 MT-1Luc cells (in 200 μL). Lesions were usually discretely localized to bony sites; the spine, femur, humerus, and mandible as well as other soft tissues (lung, liver, and ovaries) [23–25] (Color Plate 16).

Microcomputed tomography images revealed osteolytic degradation of rat vertebrae with mean areas of 2.92 and 2.14 mm^2 in lumbar and thoracic spine, respectively. The clinical manifestations of disease mirrored that in humans with osteolysis, cachexia, and escalating morbidity such that by day 26 postinjection, rats had to be euthanized. The effects of PDT were conclusive. In lumbar spine, an intravenous bolus injection of verteporfin (2 mg/Kg) followed 3 hours later by 690-nm light of 150J via percutaneous placement directly onto the lateral aspect of the target vertebral body, effectively ablated the tumor resulting in a 99.8% decrease in bioluminescence signal within 48 hours. Histology confirmed destruction of normal bone marrow and fat cells resulting in a dose-dependent increase in the area of effect. At 150J, the maximal mean rostal-caudal diameter of effect in lumbar spine (L2) was 13.1 $\pm$2.1 mm and 80.53 mm^2 area (mid-sagittal). The mean mid-sagittal dimensions of vertebrae were 7.1 $\pm$0.8 (rostal-caudal) by 9.4 $\pm$1.1 mm (dorsal-ventral) so treatment area typically spanned 2 to 3 vertebrae (26). Importantly, more than one third of the animals treated in the thoracic spine using the same treatment regimen became paralyzed, confirming the sensitivity of the spinal cord. Thoracic spine is an important target accounting for 70% of spinal metastic cases compared with only 20% in lumbar spine [1], and it will be important for future experiments to establish a safe, effective regimen for this region of the spine. At 3 hours postintravenous injection, Verteporfin is confined largely to the vasculature with the remainder going to liver, kidney, ovaries, and bone marrow (29). Interestingly, the amounts of Verteporfin within vertebrae containing tumor were 3.4-fold that of spinal cord at 3 hours postinjection, which further increased to 5.5-fold at 15 minutes postinjection, suggesting that 15 minutes is better. All subsequent studies were performed with this short drug-light interval. The amount of light that reaches the spinal cord in a human vertebra is expected to be orders of magnitude less than that in the rat primary due to the differences in size; nevertheless, the risk of paralysis highlights the importance of pharmacokinetics in optimizing selectivity.

15.1.5 Optical Dosimetry

Bone is naturally scattering to light, containing 58% inorganic hydroxyapatite crystals, 12% water, 25% collagen, and 5% carbohydrate. However, for dosimetry of trabecular bone it is important to consider the influence of blood and bone marrow as well. Studies to evaluate the optical properties of bone tissues have resulted in controversy with different values depending on the technique used [26–29]. Common methods of measurement include diffuse reflectance spectroscopy, which allows multiple scattering approximations based on diffusion theory or reflectance and transmittance measurements using integrating spheres [27]. The later typically involves Monte Carlo lookup tables for calculation and requires that samples be prepared as very thin (submillimeter) slices, which for trabecular bone is challenging. Nevertheless, we obtained optical properties for fresh porcine vertebrae of μa = 0.057 ±0.001 mm^{-1} and $\mu s'$ = 1.819 ±0.095 mm^{-1} at 690 nm, which were realistic when compared to those for cortical bone obtained using similar methods, μa = 0.040 ±0.002 mm^{-1}, $\mu s'$ = 2.651 ±0.053 and g = 0.925 ±0.014 nm [27]. Attenuation was reduced to 0.021 ± 0.001 following washout of residual blood. Phantoms studies representing trabecular bone and breast tumor [30] confirmed the accuracy of our measurements to within 2% error at 1.2-cm distance from the delivery fiber based on diffusion theory specific to linear diffusers [31]. Similar results were obtained in vivo [25], although tissue heterogeneity and blood pooling effects around the delivery fiber limited the reproducibility of results. Similar problems are anticipated in patients and will need to be addressed together with the dynamic changes in tissue optical properties that occur during treatment (see below).

15.1.6 PDT Dosimetry

Diffusion theory (15.1) and the finite element method can be used to calculate the fluence rate [W/cm^2] anywhere within a target volume based on tissue optical properties [31, 32]. Fluence rate integrated over treatment time provides the total fluence [J/cm^2] delivered to the tissue, which combined with the concentration of photosensitizer in each tissue type, gives the PDT dose (15.2) throughout the target volume, akin to the reciprocity principle.

$$\nabla D \cdot \nabla \mu_a \phi = 0 \tag{15.1}$$

In (15.1), diffusion theory is where D is the diffusion coefficient, $D = \left[3\left(\mu_a + \mu_s' \right) \right]^{-1}$, ϕ is the fluence rate [W/cm^2], μ_a is the absorption coefficient [cm^{-1}], and μ_s' is the reduced scattering coefficient.

$$Dose = 2.303 \varepsilon C \Phi \frac{\lambda}{1980} 10^{19} \tag{15.2}$$

where ε is the extinction coefficient of the photosensitizer [cm^{-1} (μg/g)$^{-1}$], C is the photosensitizer concentration in the tissue [μg/g], Φ is the accumulated light energy in the tissue [J/cm^2], and λ is the wavelength of the activation light [nm].

PDT dose is expressed in photons absorbed by the photosensitizer per cm^3 of tissue. Dose-volume histograms, a standard analysis tool in radiation treatment planning, yield quantitative dose statistics for individual structures, such as the percentage of tumor volume that receives a PDT dose greater or equal to the threshold dose required for tumor kill or similarly, the percentage of spinal cord volume that receives a PDT dose greater than the threshold dose required to induce spinal cord damage. By superimposing threshold dose contours onto the radiological images and comparing the actual dose received by the different anatomical structures, one can effectively determine the efficacy and safety for any given fiber placement (see below). In reality the optical environment within the tissue changes throughout the treatment and therefore so must the contour maps. Moreover, the biological response or threshold required for kill will also shift due to altered cellular metabolism and biochemistry, tissue blood flow, and oxygenation. Despite the influence of blood pooling we were able to demonstrate in porcine that 150 J/cm (150 mW/cm), 690-nm laser light 30 minutes after Verteporfin (6mg/m^2; i.v.) produces a mean radius of necrosis within bone marrow of 0.59 ±0.02 cm around the delivery fiber with a necrotic threshold of 9.3 J/cm^2 (4.3 mW/cm^2). A margin of apoptosis extending up to 2 cm out from the fiber was also evident histologically. As with previous reports in flat bone [29], we did not see any detrimental effects to the organic osteoid matrix. Indeed, prior biomechanical testing of rat vertebrae (unpublished results) confirms that PDT strengthens bone.

15.1.7   Treatment Planning

The vertebral anatomy in porcine is sufficiently similar to that of humans to provide a good model for testing a number of components specific to our treatment planning, including dosimetry, image-guided placement of optical fibers, and PDT response. Rigorous preoperative planning of the intended treatment protocol is fundamental to safety and efficacy. Treatment planning uses radiological images of the treatment site and interactive software tools to provide patient-specific prescriptions for optimized treatment. Primary components include (1) preoperative MRI/CT imaging and virtual planning, (2) intraoperative image-guidance/navigation, (3) real-time dosimetry of delivered dose with iterative adjustment to allow for changing optical properties, and (4) assessment of the biological response.

In practical terms the planning involves exporting preoperative axial CT DICOM images of target vertebra into a commercial virtual software, in our case, Mimics® software (9.0; Materialise, Ann Arbor, MI, USA), which allows segmentation of radiological images. Virtual objects, such as tumor or optical fiber, are then drawn into the vertebra. All features of the vertebra, including spinal canal, are anatomically accurate. Dose contours are projected into the virtual image using initial graph exchange specification format in order to determine the optimal fiber placement according to optical properties, PDT photosensitizer concentrations, and the sensitivities of the different tissue types to PDT (Figure 15.1). Once determined, the stereo-lithographic (STL) files of the target volume are exported into the online navigation system. The prescribed fiber position is defined in the same coordinate space as the pretreatment images, which are registered to the online navigation images through a series of fiducial markers placed onto the patient (see below). The surgeon therefore has a target to aim for when placing the actual treatment fiber. This approach is being used successfully in current clinical trials for treating prostate cancer [32]. Currently, online adjustment of delivered dose is conducted manually, although in theory biological sensors placed into the treatment zone would allow automatic feedback.

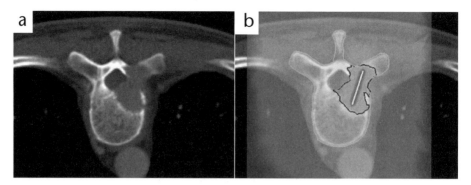

Figure 15.1 (a) CT image of target vertebra with virtual lesion embedded. (b) Fiber position within the vertebra can be optimized according to color contour maps overlaid onto the CT that show the PDT dose within the lesion and surrounding structures.

15.1.8 Image Guidance

Numerous imaging modalities, including magnetic resonance imaging, ultrasound, computer tomography (CT), and fluoroscopy, are being adapted to interventional procedures or being developed with image-guidance applications specifically in mind for surgery, interventional radiology, radiation therapy, and now photodynamic therapy. The goal is to improve the geometric precision of treatment (e.g., a scalpel, a laser, or a radiotherapeutic beam) and to move more toward minimally invasive procedures that can be conducted within diagnostic radiology. PDT in spine is no exception. Our group has developed a mobile cone beam CT [33] to provide superior guidance of optical fibers into vertebrae [34]. The current system combines an isocentric C-arm and PaxScan 4030A flat-panel detector (Varian Imaging Products, Palo Alto, CA) with servo drive for orbital motion (~178°) mounted onto a Siemens PowerMobil mobile allowing for large fields of view (15 cm axial length) and soft-tissue visualization both complimentary to its prospective use in image-guided surgery, interventional radiology, and percutaneous PDT (Figure 15.2). The detector offers real-time radiographic/fluoroscopic imaging, with rapid volume reconstruction (256×256×192) using the FDK algorithm [35]. Breakaway Imaging, LLC, (Littleton, MA) in partnership with Medtronic Inc., (Minneapolis, MN) has recently launched a new "O" arm with 360° orbital motion. A comparison to test the accuracy of cone beam CT versus conventional fluoroscopy has not been tested. For navigation we use a stereoscopic infrared camera (NDI Polaris) offering real-time acquisition (30 fps), large field of view (3 m³; depth of field 1.5-3 m), and high resolution (0.4 mm). A handheld "wand" with CT-visible fiducials is then detected by the camera and assigned a set of coordinates that define its precise location in 3-D space. Using this system we have demonstrated the feasibility of placing 0.94-mm diameter (2.5-cm diffusing) optical fibers safely into the vertebral bodies of porcine and canines via bilateral transpedicular approach.

Canine vertebrae are denser than porcine; their pedicles also project more laterally, making transpedicular approach more difficult. Nevertheless, placement was possible and moderate (200 J/cm) or high-dose PDT (500 J/cm; 250 mW/cm) within T12 vertebra 5 minutes after Verteporfin infusion (0.4 mg/Kg) resulted in lesions

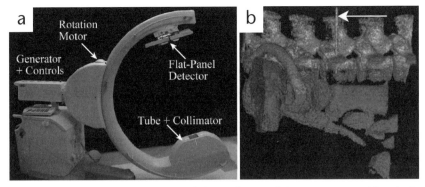

Figure 15.2 (a) A mobile cone beam CT with large, flat panel detector was used for placing fibers into the spine. (b) Rapid 3-D reconstructions of the spine and surrounding soft tissues allows for accurate intraoperative navigation.

within bone marrow and fat deposits averaging 1.1-cm diameter, slightly smaller than those in porcine [25]. MRI using contrast enhanced T1-weighted sequences provided valuable diagnostic assessment of damage at 7 days posttreatment that correlated well with histology. Enhanced signal was confined to a zone along the diffusing tip. Neurological evaluation of somato-sensory evoked potentials before, during, and after PDT confirmed sustained neurological function and standard analgesic administration provided good pain control such that animals were fully mobile the following morning after treatment. The rapid clearance of Verteporfin from blood within 30 to 60 minutes was marked by the lack of skin photosensitivity.

15.2   Photodynamic Therapy for Primary Osteosarcoma

Without a large animal model of spinal metastases with which to demonstrate efficacy, we opted to treat companion canines with large, high-grade (IIb) appendicular osteosarcoma as an alternative [36]. Seven large-breed canines with spontaneous osteosarcoma in their distal radius were MRI imaged prior to treatment. Tumors displayed necrotic centers with osteoid scarring throughout. A single 5-cm diffusing fiber was guided using fluoroscopy through the medullary cavity into the tumor. High-dose light (500 J/cm; 250 mW/cm) was delivered at 5 minutes post-Verteporfin infusion followed 48 hours later by MRI and limb amputation as part of the standard of care. Contrast-enhanced T1 sequences confirmed tumor ablation in all animals. Stereological examination revealed an average volume of effect of 14.96 cm^3 with mean medial to lateral dimensions of 3.4 cm and rostra-caudal dimensions of 5.51 cm (Color Plate 17). Importantly, similar volumes are reported for spinal lesions in clinic. Collectively this data provides definitive credence to the feasibility, efficacy, and safety of PDT treatment of lesions within the spine.

Of course it is inconceivable to assume that preclinical models can ever fully depict all of the clinical manifestations implicit to systemic disease and the practical issues of probe placement into critically ill patients with severely osteoporotic bone will no doubt prove more challenging. The true test can only be conducted in clinical trials.

15.3 Antimicrobial PDT

Antimicrobial PDT is an emerging field with more than 100 scientific manuscripts listed under the www.pubmed.gov Web site in the past 2 years. However, less than one quarter of these pertain to biofilm. Photosensitizers commonly used include cationic phenothiazines, porphyrin derivatives, merocyanine 540, and 5-aminolevulinic acid (ALA) [37, 38]. None display complete specificity for bacteria, however, but rely on charge-mediated uptake or endogenous production (see below). A clinical formulation of the phenothiazine derivative, methylene blue, Urolene blue™ is currently administered orally as an antiseptic to treat urinary tract infections as well as methemoglobinaemia or as an antidote to cyanide poisoning.

15.3.1 Bone Infection

Inflammation of bone and bone marrow following microbial contamination can be life-threatening. Infections can spread systemically in blood or locally through soft tissue following trauma, burns, or peripheral vascular disease. Secondary disease is also an important consideration and the risk of contracting skeletal infection is thought to increase up to 1,000 times in patients with diabetes or sickle cell anemia [39]. Postoperative infection is perhaps the fastest emerging causes of acute osteomyelitis with more than one million new cases of hip replacement worldwide each year [40]. Orthopedic implantations and prosthetic devices are particularly susceptible to biofilm formation derived from *Staphylococcus aureus (S. aureus)* and *Pseudomonas Aeruginosa (P. aeruginosa)*. Both strains are facultative that develop thick glycocalyx biofilm that adhere very effectively to host tissues and metallic implants, including pins and screws and prosthetic hips and joints, creating an effective barrier to antimicrobials. Biofilms are found in approximately 65% of infected patients and are highly resistant to antibiotics [41]. They comprise glycoprotein matrix that house intercommunicating microbial communities with intervening water channels for transfer of nutrients and removal of waste [41], but little is known regarding their microenvironmental oxygenation.

15.3.2 Current Strategies

Treatment of osteomyelitis currently includes surgery and parenteral antibiotics, neither of which is conducive to combat the growing number of antibiotic-resistant bacterial strains or the inherent obstinacy of bacterial biofilms and the long-term management necessary for recurring infections. There are a considerable number of reports describing small animal models of osteomyelitis spanning 40 years of research. A number of studies describe novel strategies for delivering antibiotics using biodegradable implants or beads into rat tibia or spine [42]. A common theme to most of these studies is the inability to eradicate all of the infection or prevent recurrence particularly when treating established biofilm.

We recently reported the novel application of PDT to osteomyelitis using S. aureus-biofilm-laden K wires implanted into rat tibia [43]. Using a bioluminescent strain of S. aureus we demonstrated effective treatment of biofilms grown in vivo using ALA or methylene blue. High dose, acute regimens of PDT ($75 \, J/cm^2$) resulted in transient responses, which relapsed within 48 hours after treatment. In vitro studies provided the first evidence that metronomic PDT could provide better long-term management of bacterial growth than acute PDT. Metronomic regimens of low-dose drug delivery have been adopted for chemotherapy to minimize toxicity and our group recently introduced the concept for PDT to improve selective apoptosis of brain tumors [44]. ALA is a substrate involved in heme synthesis and is well suited for metronomic delivery, with low toxicity and the option of enteral or parenteral delivery. However, gram-positive bacteria produce the less active photosensitizer, coproporphyrin III instead of protoporphyrin IX [45]. Meanwhile gram-negative strains including P. aeruginosa produce protoporphyrin IX with little coproporphyrin III. Undoubtedly, the premise that rapidly dividing cells produce more endogenous photosensitizer cannot be applied to cells in biofilm, which are largely senescent. It remains, therefore, to be confirmed whether metronomic PDT with ALA displays similar promise for in vivo models of osteomyelitis as it appears to in vitro.

15.3.3 HOT-PDT

Concurrent with these studies has been our interest in combining PDT with hyperbaric oxygen therapy (HOT) or carbogen. There is a wealth of literature describing the benefits of HOT against bacteria and previous reports confirm improved treatment of cancer using PDT in combination with HOT [46, 47]. The physiological response of host tissues and resident bacteria to HOT is not clearly understood. Oxygen under normal atmospheric pressure is poorly absorbed into tissues. HOT can facilitate improved oxygenation of tissues, improved blood flow into infected sites, and ultimately improved access for drug delivery, which may explain the synergistic effect with antibiotics [48]. Oxidative stress is likely a primary mediator, which may also involve an immunological component although the precise interaction is unclear. Bacteria are well adapted to cope with oxidative stress. S. aureus, despite lacking glutathione, and contain a family of small soluble proteins called thioredoxins encoded by *trxA* and *trxB* genes that catalyze thiol-redox reactions. TrxA and trxB are activated in response to increased thiol oxidation and disulfide bond formation promoting thioredoxin reductase-mediated quenching of reactive oxygen species in the presence of NADPH [49, 50]. P. aeruginosa meanwhile relies on catalase as well as manganese- and iron cofactored superoxide dismutases encoded by *SodA* and *SodB* genes to combat oxidative stress. Nevertheless, tumor cells like bacteria also have effective defenses against oxidative stress yet remain highly susceptible to PDT-mediated cell kill and the additional molecular oxygen proffered by HOT should enhance singlet oxygen production within the cells, although direct measurements of singlet oxygen production during HOTPDT have not been carried out thus far. So far our observations in vitro confirm that combining HOT with acute PDT using $10 \, J/cm^2$ and methylene blue can decrease the number of surviving S. aureus colonies by $>2 \log_{10}$ compared with PDT alone (61). Importantly, a similar increase in antimicrobial action was also confirmed against S. aureus biofilms using methylene blue. Recent unpublished results from our group suggest an even greater improvement combining metronomic regimens of PDT and HOT. It will be imperative for future research to discern the underlying mechanism(s) related to the improved cell kill with HOT and perhaps quantify singlet oxygen production within biofilms directly.

15.4   Bone Growth Modulation

As we grow, our cartilaginous template is replaced with bone through a process called endochondral ossification. This process normally occurs in limbs around the chronological ages of 16 in males and 14 in females. In this process mesenchymal cells within the avascular growth plate (physis) condense and mature as chondroprogenitor cells into the proliferative zone. Extracellular matrix is laid down as chondrocytes exit their proliferative phase and terminally differentiate into hypertrophic chondrocytes. The matrix provides a scaffold for vascular invasion into the physis from the adjacent metaphysis and with this newly established blood flow come preosteoblasts and mesenchymal cells that contribute to calcification of the matrix and apoptosis of the matured chondrocytes [51, 52]. Once the transition from cartilage to bone is complete closure of the physis results in growth arrest. The whole process is tightly choreographed by hypoxia-inducible factor (HIF-1α), vascular endothelial growth factor-A isoforms (VEGF$_{164}$, VEGF$_{188}$) and receptor (VEGFR1), fibroblast growth factors (FGF-2, FGF-9, FGF-18) and receptor (FGFR-3), matrix metalloproteinases (MMP-9, MMP-13), p57, bone morphogenic proteins, B-cell lymphoma-2 (bcl-2), and parathyroid hormone-related peptide [52, 53]. Disruption of this process can lead to bone growth anomalies such as limb length discrepancy (LLD) or scoliosis. Realizing that the hypoxic gradient within the physis is governing to the process of angiogenesis and bone formation we hypothesized that vascular-targeted photodynamic therapy may be able to amplify this hypoxic gradient by destroying existing vasculature outside the physis and by doing so induce proangiogenic factors like VEGF-A to accelerate the onset of ossification [54, 55]. In other words, we set out to exploit the angiogenic response following PDT as a minimally invasive, fiber-optic-based procedure to modulate bone growth [56]. This raises new and exciting possibilities of using PDT to model and potentially treat LLD or scoliosis since current approaches, including surgical osteotomy, fixation, transphyseal screw placement, or stapling are associated with serious complications related to malunion, nonunion, axial rotation infection, and protracted pain or immobility [57, 58].

To quantify the induction of VEGF-A gene following PDT in growth plates we conducted studies using immature transgenic mice that constitutively express the luciferase gene. In these mice luciferase activity is induced by a transcriptional promoter sequence specific to VEGF-A. Activation of VEGF within localized tissues results in a corresponding luciferase-mediated bioluminescence. Femoral and tibial growth plates were targeted for treatment using a 0.2-mm diameter optical fiber placed percutaneously onto the medial aspect of the lower limb facing laterally and held using a custom jig [56]. Light of varying dose was delivered 10 minutes following intravenous injection of Verteporfin to ensure vascular-targeted response [59]. A repeat dose (x2) of 10 J (50 mW output) given 3 days apart provided the most consistent calcification or closure of growth plates resulting in pronounced VEGF-mediated angiogenesis and limb growth arrest (Color Plate 18). As mice grew, the discrepancy between treated and untreated limbs averaged 9.5% ± 4.4% by 4 weeks posttreatment.

Effects were very much light dose-dependent with exaggerated limb shortening; >20% with 27J, which resulted in fracture and pronounced thickening of the growth plate following lower doses of 5 or 10J in the absence of photosensitizer. The latter observation is of particular interest as this raises the possibility of not only shortening but also lengthening limbs, although studies to substantiate this have not been completed. The significance of this become clear when we consider the current options for limb lengthening involving distraction histiogenesis and external fixation that come with formidable risks of misalignment, nonunion, nerve palsy, excruciating pain, and prolonged convalescence [60]. The psychological morbidity and financial burden to patient and government can be considerable in these cases.

A similar rationale can be applied to scoliosis, the treatment for which often requires extensive surgery resulting in placement of steel rods along length of the spine, permanently fixing the spine. There are numerous reports describing preclinical models of scoliosis such as pinealized chicken or amputation of limbs or transverse processes [61, 62]. While these do well to mimic the morphological presentation of scoliosis they offer little as to the underlying etiology and in most cases do not agree with what is currently known about the genetic predisposition of patients to idiopathic scoliosis (82). It should be noted, however, that pinealectomy reduces melatonin levels and a number of scoliosis patients with intact pineal glands have presented with reduced melatonin. Finally, melatonin is known to inhibit VEGF, so reduced levels of melatonin would tend to increase VEGF levels in a similar fashion to calmodulin, which has also been shown to be elevated in scoliosis patients [63]. These findings strengthen the argument for an angiogenic component to scoliosis.

In the early 1960s, scientists first began to investigate the preponderance of scoliosis occurring in thoracic spine and the vascular discrepancy that was known to exist between left and right sides [64]. It was concluded that disparity in the vascular supply between left and right spine during the growth period could be underlying to the etiology of scoliosis. Subsequent animal studies supported these initial hypotheses [65–67]. It is clear that if one side of the spine grows faster than the other curvature may result as wedging of the vertebrae create convexity or kyphotic curve. 3-dimensional complexity of curve may evolve as vertebrae, which possess two growth plates—one providing expansion through the rostra-caudal plane, and the other the neural central cartilage—sat dorsolaterally to the pedicles providing expansion in the axial plane [68]. An extension of this would be to suppose that like limbs, the spine might be subject to asymmetrical closure of growth plates secondary to hypoxic stress-mediated vascularization. Interestingly, in our preliminary, experiments we have demonstrated the ability to produce a modest 5° to 8° scoliotic curve in a number of mice following unilateral treatment in the lumbar spine (L1, L2) of transgenic mice (Color Plate 19). Closure to one side of the growth plate was confirmed histologically and microcomputed tomography revealed structural damage. An interesting side to this data was the histological changes to intervertebral discs. In a number of animals discs appeared to be expanded with increasing numbers of fibro-cartilaginous rings of the annulus fibrosis and notable loss of the nucleus pulposus. Immunohistochemistry revealed increased VEGF staining throughout the annulus fibrosis. The significance of this data and whether it mimics any of the histological changes evident in degenerative disc disease remains to be confirmed.

Currently, our studies do suggest a role for vascular anomaly in LLD and scoliosis and suggest that PDT is a valuable method for preclinical modeling of these conditions.

15.5   Conclusion

The application of PDT in bone opens a number of very interesting and potentially clinically important avenues for investigation. The ability to plan prior to surgery where to deliver the light in order to achieve the best possible treatment of the cancer without damaging neighboring structures, and to then execute that plan with the utmost accuracy using online navigation in the operating suite offers the kind of reassurance that clinicians must have when operating in the spine, and will go a long way in promoting clinical treatment of spinal metastases using PDT.

Osteomyelitis is a significant risk following surgery and patients with advanced stage cancers far worse than most in their ability to fight infection or endure surgical debridment or prolonged exposure to antibiotics. The potential for targeting both infection and cancer minimally invasively using PDT and perhaps even using the same photosensitizer is certainly appealing; however, it is likely that the optimal treatment regimen will differ for each ailment. The opportunity for using implantable devices that allow metronomic PDT delivery could prove highly effective against recurring infections assuming the infection has access to molecular oxygen to allow singlet oxygen generation. The same may also be true for cancers. The development of metronomic PDT for treating cancer, meanwhile, offers tremendous potential and is currently under preclinical and clinical investigation for brain cancers. Bacterial biofilms offer a particular challenge providing an effective barrier to antibiotics and photosensitizers alike, as well as to nutrients and oxygen, which will limit the photodynamic action of any photosensitizer relying on type II photooxidation. Results combining hyperbaric oxygen therapy and PDT are compelling and raise the possibility of improving PDT efficacy in poorly oxygenated infections. Nevertheless, for antimicrobial PDT to gain wider acceptance among clinicians, it is clear that new photosensitizers will have to be designed that offer improved targeting and accumulation inside bacterial cells and biofilms. Given the impending pandemic that may result as more strains become resistant to antibiotics, the pursuit of alternate strategies for treating infection should be considered one of the most important biomedical pursuits in science today. The versatility and specificity of PDT regards dosing and delivery may provide a far superior treatment and management of infection than antibiotics and minimize the risk of developing resistance as well as collateral damage to host bacteria.

Bone is a dynamic tissue, constantly changing and growing, and in the case of cancellous bone, highly conducive to the transmittance of light. The capacity to modulate bone growth using PDT toward a therapeutic end has never to our knowledge been described before. The fact that we can model limb growth arrest and create curves in the spines of rodents using PDT should allow greater understanding as to the roles of aberrant hypoxia and angiogenesis in premature growth plate closure and perhaps provide a means of correcting such anomalies without the need for painful invasive surgeries. It seems almost fitting that PDT-induced angiogenesis, while instrumental to the flurry of recent research combining anti-VEGF and PDT for treating age-related macular degeneration, should now perhaps be exploitable for another therapy. Of additional interest is the possibility that we can modulate the growth plate to expand prior to closure, thereby lengthening the bone. This would represent a major contribution to orthopedics and to the scientific community at large, galvanizing the acceptance of modern science and biophotonics into clinic.

Acknowledgments

I would like to acknowledge Drs. Shane Burch, Albert Yee, Brian Wilson, and Jeffery Siewerdsen, who are integral contributors to the ongoing research and clinical expertise related to PDT in bone here at the University Health Network in Toronto, Canada. I also wish to thank Crystal Johnson and Claudia Chien, who helped with much of the work described in this chapter.

References

[1] Walsh, G. L., et al., "Anterior approaches to the thoracic spine in patients with cancer: indications and results," *Ann Thorac Surg*, Vol. 64, 1997, pp. 1611–1618.

[2] Tatsui, H., et al., "Survival rates of patients with metastatic spinal cancer after scintigraphic detection of abnormal radioactive accumulation," *Spine*, Vol. 21, 1996, pp. 2143–2148.

[3] Bauer, H. C., and Wedin, R., "Survival after surgery for spinal and extremity metastases. Prognostication in 241 patients," *Acta Orthop Scand*, Vol. 66, 1995, pp. 143–146.

[4] Hirabayashi, H., et al., "Clinical outcome and survival after palliative surgery for spinal metastases: palliative surgery in spinal metastases," *Cancer*, Vol. 97, 2003, pp. 476–484.

[5] Klimo, P., Jr., and Schmidt, M. H., "Surgical management of spinal metastases," *Oncologist*, Vol. 9, 2004, pp. 188–196.

[6] Mercadante, S., "Malignant bone pain: pathophysiology and treatment," *Pain*, Vol. 69, 1997, pp. 1–18.

[7] Zaidat, O. O., and Ruff, R. L., "Treatment of spinal epidural metastasis improves patient survival and functional state," *Neurology*, Vol. 58, 2002, pp. 1360–1366.

[8] De Leenheer, E., et al., "Evidence of a role for RANKL in the development of myeloma bone disease," *Curr Opin Pharmacol*, Vol. 4, 2004, pp. 340–346.

[9] Hofbauer, L. C., and Schoppet, M., "Clinical implications of the osteoprotegerin/RANKL/RANK system for bone and vascular diseases," *Jama*, Vol. 292, 2004, pp. 490–495.

[10] Hormbrey, E., et al., "The relationship of human wound vascular endothelial growth factor (VEGF) after breast cancer surgery to circulating VEGF and angiogenesis," *Clin Cancer Res*, Vol. 9, 2003, pp. 4332–4339.

[11] Rajesh, L., et al., "Correlation between VEGF expression and angiogenesis in breast carcinoma," *Anal Quant Cytol Histol*, Vol. 26, 2004, pp. 105–108.

[12] Schoppet, M., Preissner, K. T., and Hofbauer, L. C., "RANK ligand and osteoprotegerin: paracrine regulators of bone metabolism and vascular function," *Arterioscler Thromb Vasc Biol*, Vol. 22, 2002, pp. 549–553.

[13] Carteni, G., et al., "Efficacy and safety of zoledronic acid in patients with breast cancer metastatic to bone: a multicenter clinical trial," *Oncologist*, Vol. 11, 2006, pp. 841–848.

[14] Faul, C. M., and Flickinger, J. C., "The use of radiation in the management of spinal metastases," *J Neurooncol*, Vol. 23, 1995, pp. 149–161.

[15] Ferris, F. D., Bezjak, A., and Rosenthal, S. G., "The palliative uses of radiation therapy in surgical oncology patients," *Surg Oncol Clin N Am*, Vol. 10, 2001, pp. 185–201.

[16] Ghogawala, Z., Mansfield, F. L., and Borges, L. F., "Spinal radiation before surgical decompression adversely affects outcomes of surgery for symptomatic metastatic spinal cord compression," *Spine*, Vol. 26, 2001, pp. 818–824.

[17] Tombolini, V., et al., "Radiation therapy of spinal metastases: results with different fractionations," *Tumori*, Vol. 80, 1994, pp. 353–356.

[18] Chow, E., et al., "Radiotherapeutic approaches to metastatic disease," *World J Urol*, Vol. 21, 2003, pp. 229–242.

[19] Ryu, S., et al., "Patterns of failure after single-dose radiosurgery for spinal metastasis," *J Neurosurg*, Vol. 101 Suppl 3, 2004, pp. 402–405.

[20] Mang, T. S., et al., "A phase II/III clinical study of tin ethyl etiopurpurin (Purlytin)-induced photodynamic therapy for the treatment of recurrent cutaneous metastatic breast cancer," *Cancer J Sci Am*, Vol. 4, 1998, pp. 378–384.

[21] Nathan, T. R., et al., "Photodynamic therapy for prostate cancer recurrence after radiotherapy: a phase I study," *J Urol*, Vol. 168, 2002, pp. 1427–1432.

[22] Engebraaten, O., and Fodstad, O., "Site-specific experimental metastasis patterns of two human breast cancer cell lines in nude rats," *Int J Cancer*, Vol. 82, 1999, pp. 219–225.

[23] Burch, S., et al., "Photodynamic therapy for the treatment of vertebral metastases in a rat model of human breast carcinoma," *J Orthop Res*, Vol. 23, 2005, pp. 995–1003.

[24] Burch, S., et al., "Multimodality Imaging for Vertebral Metastases in a Rat Osteolytic Model," *Clin Orthop Relat Res*, Vol. 454, 2007, pp. 230–236.

[25] Burch, S., et al., "Photodynamic therapy for the treatment of metastatic lesions in bone: studies in rat and porcine models," *J Biomed Opt*, Vol. 10, 2005, pp. 034011.

[26] Farrar, S. K., et al., "Optical properties of human trabecular meshwork in the visible and near-infrared region," *Lasers Surg Med*, Vol. 25, 1999, pp. 348–362.

[27] Firbank, M., et al., "Measurement of the optical properties of the skull in the wavelength range 650–950 nm," *Phys Med Biol*, Vol. 38, 1993, pp. 503–510.

[28] Flock, S. T., Wilson, B. C., and Patterson, M. S., "Monte Carlo modeling of light propagation in highly scattering tissues—II: Comparison with measurements in phantoms," *IEEE Trans Biomed Eng*, Vol. 36, 1989, pp. 1169–1173.

[29] Tauber, S., et al., "Lightdosimetric quantitative analysis of the human petrous bone: experimental study for laser irradiation of the cochlea," *Lasers Surg Med*, Vol. 28, 2001, pp. 18–26.

[30] Cerussi, A., et al., "In vivo absorption, scattering, and physiologic properties of 58 malignant breast tumors determined by broadband diffuse optical spectroscopy," *J Biomed Opt*, Vol. 11, 2006, pp. 044005.

[31] Jacques, S. L., "Light distributions from point, line and plane sources for photochemical reactions and fluorescence in turbid biological tissues. [Review] [22 refs]," *Photochem Photobiol*, Vol. 67, 1998, pp. 23–32.

[32] Weersink, R. A., et al., "Techniques for delivery and monitoring of TOOKAD (WST09)-mediated photodynamic therapy of the prostate: clinical experience and practicalities," *J Photochem Photobiol B*, Vol. 79, 2005, pp. 211–222.

[33] Rafferty, M. A., et al., "Intraoperative cone-beam CT for guidance of temporal bone surgery," *Otolaryngol Head Neck Surg*, Vol. 134, 2006, pp. 801–808.

[34] Siewerdsen, J. H., et al., "Volume CT with a flat-panel detector on a mobile, isocentric C-arm: pre-clinical investigation in guidance of minimally invasive surgery," *Med Phys*, Vol. 32, 2005, pp. 241–254.

[35] Defrise, M., Townsend, D. W., and Clack, R., "Three-dimensional image reconstruction from complete projections," *Phys Med Biol*, Vol. 34, 1989, pp. 573–587.

[36] Burch, S., et al., "Multimodality imaging strategies for vertebral metastases in a preclinical osteolytic model," submitted, Vol., 2007.

[37] Hamblin, M. R., and Hasan, T., "Photodynamic therapy: a new antimicrobial approach to infectious disease?" Vol. 3, 2004, pp. 436–450.

[38] Jori, G., et al., "Photodynamic therapy in the treatment of microbial infections: Basic principles and perspective applications," *Lasers Surg Med*, Vol. 38, 2006, pp. 468–481.

[39] Epps, C. H., Jr., et al., "Osteomyelitis in patients who have sickle-cell disease. Diagnosis and management," *J Bone Joint Surg Am*, Vol. 73, 1991, pp. 1281–1294.

[40] Fisman, D. N., et al., "Clinical effectiveness and cost-effectiveness of 2 management strategies for infected total hip arthroplasty in the elderly," *Clin Infect Dis*, Vol. 32, 2001, pp. 419–430.

[41] O'Connell, H. A., et al., "Influences of biofilm structure and antibiotic resistance mechanisms on indirect pathogenicity in a model polymicrobial biofilm," *Appl Environ Microbiol*, Vol. 72, 2006, pp. 5013–5019.

[42] An, Y. H., Kang, Q. K., and Arciola, C. R., "Animal models of osteomyelitis," *Int J Artif Organs*, Vol. 29, 2006, pp. 407–420.

[43] Bisland, S. K., et al., "Pre-clinical in vitro and in vivo studies to examine the potential use of photodynamic therapy in the treatment of osteomyelitis," *Photochem Photobiol Sci*, Vol. 5, 2006, pp. 31–38.

[44] Bisland, S. K., et al., "Metronomic photodynamic therapy as a new paradigm for photodynamic therapy: rationale and preclinical evaluation of technical feasibility for treating malignant brain tumors," *Photochem Photobiol*, Vol. 80, 2004, pp. 22–30.

[45] Nitzan, Y., et al., "ALA induced photodynamic effects on gram positive and negative bacteria," Vol. 3, 2004, pp. 430–435.

[46] Huang, Z., et al., "Hyperoxygenation enhances the tumor cell killing of photofrin-mediated photodynamic therapy," *Photochem Photobiol*, Vol. 78, 2003, pp. 496–502.

[47] Maier, A., et al., "Combined photodynamic therapy and hyperbaric oxygenation in carcinoma of the esophagus and the esophago-gastric junction," *Eur J Cardiothorac Surg*, Vol. 18, 2000, pp. 649–654; discussion 654–645.

[48] Mendel, V., Simanowski, H. J., and Scholz, H., "Synergy of HBO2 and a local antibiotic carrier for experimental osteomyelitis due to Staphylococcus aureus in rats," *Undersea Hyperb Med*, Vol. 31, 2004, pp. 407–416.

[49] Arner, E. S., and Holmgren, A., "Physiological functions of thioredoxin and thioredoxin reductase," *Eur J Biochem*, Vol. 267, 2000, pp. 6102–6109.

[50] Uziel, O., et al., "Transcriptional regulation of the Staphylococcus aureus thioredoxin and thioredoxin reductase genes in response to oxygen and disulfide stress," *J Bacteriol*, Vol. 186, 2004, pp. 326–334.

[51] Goldring, M. B., Tsuchimochi, K., and Ijiri, K., "The control of chondrogenesis," *J Cell Biochem*, Vol. 97, 2006, pp. 33–44.

[52] Kronenberg, H. M., "Developmental regulation of the growth plate," *Nature*, Vol. 423, 2003, pp. 332–336.

[53] Schipani, E., et al., "Hypoxia in cartilage: HIF-1alpha is essential for chondrocyte growth arrest and survival," *Genes Dev*, Vol. 15, 2001, pp. 2865–2876.

[54] Maes, C., et al., "Impaired angiogenesis and endochondral bone formation in mice lacking the vascular endothelial growth factor isoforms VEGF164 and VEGF188," *Mech Dev*, Vol. 111, 2002, pp. 61–73.

[55] Maes, C., et al., "Soluble VEGF isoforms are essential for establishing epiphyseal vascularization and regulating chondrocyte development and survival," *J Clin Invest*, Vol. 113, 2004, pp. 188–199.

[56] Bisland, S. K., et al., "A new technique for physiodesis using photodynamic therapy," *Clin Orthop Relat Res*, Vol. 461, 2007, pp. 153–161.

[57] Horton, G. A., and Olney, B. W., "Epiphysiodesis of the lower extremity: results of the percutaneous technique," *J Pediatr Orthop*, Vol. 16, 1996, pp. 180–182.

[58] Nouth, F., and Kuo, L. A., "Percutaneous epiphysiodesis using transphyseal screws (PETS): prospective case study and review," *J Pediatr Orthop*, Vol. 24, 2004, pp. 721–725.

[59] Bisland, S. K., et al., "A rationale for treating leg length discrepancy using photodynamic therapy," *Proc SPIE*, Vol. 5969, 2005, pp. 258–266.

[60] Aaron, A. D., and Eilert, R. E., "Results of the Wagner and Ilizarov methods of limb-lengthening," *J Bone Joint Surg Am*, Vol. 78, 1996, pp. 20–29.

[61] Machida, M., et al., "Pathologic mechanism of experimental scoliosis in pinealectomized chickens," *Spine*, Vol. 26, 2001, pp. E385–391.

[62] Thomas, S., and Dave, P. K., "Experimental scoliosis in monkeys," *Acta Orthop Scand*, Vol. 56, 1985, pp. 43–46.

[63] Cheng, J. C., et al., "Osteopenia in adolescent idiopathic scoliosis: a histomorphometric study," *Spine*, Vol. 26, 2001, pp. E19–23.

[64] Brodetti, A., and Cauchoix, J., "The vascular supply of the spine of normal and lathyric rabbits in relation to the pathogenesis of experimental scoliosis," *Clin Orthop*, Vol. 25, 1962, pp. 180–203.

[65] Crock, H. V., "The arterial supply and venous drainage of the vertebral column of the dog," *J Anat*, Vol. 94, 1960, pp. 88–99.

[66] Crock, H. V., and Goldwasser, M., "Anatomic studies of the circulation in the region of the vertebral end-plate in adult Greyhound dogs," *Spine*, Vol. 9, 1984, pp. 702–706.

[67] Crock, H. V., and Yoshizawa, H., "The blood supply of the lumbar vertebral column," *Clin Orthop Relat Res*, Vol., 1976, pp. 6–21.

[68] De Salis, J., Beguiristain, J. L., and Canadell, J., "The production of experimental scoliosis by selective arterial ablation," *Int Orthop*, Vol. 3, 1980, pp. 311–315.

CHAPTER 16

Photochemical Internalization

Kristian Berg, Anette Bonsted, Anette Weyergang, Anders Høgset, and Pål Kristian Selbo

16.1 Introduction

The major treatment modalities for cancer are still surgery, ionizing radiation, and chemotherapy. Despite substantial efforts to optimize these treatment regimens, a large number of cancer patients still die each year (e.g., approximately 550,000 per year alone in the United States). Compared with more traditional small molecular chemotherapeutics, macromolecular drugs have the potential advantage of exerting higher therapeutic specificity. These macromolecules include proteins such as ribosome-inactivating protein toxins linked to MAbs and growth factors for cell surface targeting, peptides and mRNA for vaccination, DNA for gene therapy, and oligonucleotides such as ribozymes, peptide nucleic acids (PNAs), and siRNA for gene silencing [1, 2]. The current approach to site-specific drug delivery is to attach the therapeutic agent to a carrier recognized only by the cells where the pharmacological action is desired [3]. Alternatively, in gene therapy specificity may be enhanced by tissue specific promoters for the therapeutic gene delivered to the target cells, the use of tissue specific replication of viruses, or gene silencing molecules towards genes specifically expressed in the diseased tissue [4–6]. However, there are many extracellular and intracellular barriers for these molecules to cross in order to reach the target cells, enter the cells, and reach their intracellular targets. Degradation by serum enzymes and elimination by cells of the reticuloendothelial system (RES), penetration into the target tissues through the endothelial lining, as well as transport limitations within the tissue are important hurdles to obtain sufficient biological effect of these macromolecules [7]. The delivery system for macromolecular drugs should also overcome the intracellular barriers, such as the plasma membrane, endocytic membranes, and in gene therapy, the nuclear membrane. Many of the intracellular drug-delivery methods developed are based on improved endocytic uptake and release of the therapeutic molecule from intracellular compartments, mainly endocytic vesicles, into the cytosol. However, a major limitation in the use of macromolecular therapeutics is intracellular sequestration due to low penetration through the membranes of endocytic vesicles and degradation of the drugs by lysosomal enzymes [8]. Thus, despite the improvement of specificity by means of utilizing targeting macromolecules, the limited efficacy in vivo has required increased doses resulting in dose-limiting toxicity, while the therapeutic outcome was still limited.

An alternative method to improve specificity and efficacy of therapeutic macromolecules as well as some other therapeutic agents is to utilize photosensitizing agents, which upon exposure to light induce activation of the drug. The photochemical treatment may improve the activity of the therapeutic agents and due to activation in only light-exposed areas, reduced adverse effects of the treatment may be expected. The photochemical treatment may also have a therapeutic effect by itself. The two major approaches to the use of photochemical treatment in drug and gene delivery are (1) photochemical damage of endocytic membranes and subsequent release of the drugs trapped on the inside of the vesicle (photochemical internalization (PCI)), or (2) photochemically induced polymerization, fragmentation or isomerization of the therapeutic agent or its vehicle, and in these ways activation of the drugs in the light-exposed areas [9]. The use of PCI to improve drug therapy will be discussed in this chapter with the focus on presenting the basic mechanisms and providing some experimental documentation.

16.2   Localization in Endocytic Vesicles and Cytotoxic Effects of Photosensitizers

Photodynamic therapy (PDT) is a treatment modality where a photosensitizing compound is activated by light in an oxygen-dependent manner, leading to oxidation of biomolecules in the light-exposed tissue. Porphyrins and many other structurally related photosensitizing compounds have been utilized in PDT and shown to induce cytotoxic effects on cells and tissues. The cytotoxic effects of PDT are mediated through formation of reactive oxygen species (ROS), mainly singlet oxygen ($^1O_2$). This reactive intermediate has a very short lifetime in cells (<40 ns) [10, 11]. Thus, the primary cytotoxic effect of PDT is executed during light exposure and very close to the sites of formation of $^1O_2$ (<20 nm). It is well documented that a number of photosensitizers, including di- and tetrasulfonated aluminium phthalocyanine ($AlPcS_n$), sulfonated tetraphenylporphines ($TPPS_n$), chlorine e6 derivatives (e.g., NPe_6), nile blue, uroporphyrin I, lutetium texaphyrin (LuTex), silicone phthalocyanine (Pc 4), tin ethyl etiopurpurin (SnET2), and acridine orange are partly or mainly located in endosomes and lysosomes, collectively described as endocytic vesicles, of cells in culture [12]. This is in most cases due to endocytic uptake, while in some cases the dye is a weak base and is trapped in lysosomes and acidified endosomes (Figure 16.1).

Photoimmunoconjugates, where the photosensitizers are linked to antibodies, other targeting macromolecules, or synthetic polymers may improve the specificity and efficacy of PDT [13–15]. When these conjugates are endocytosed, the photosensitizer will accumulate in endocytic vesicles as long as the conjugate is not enzymatically degraded or the photosensitizer is not able to penetrate the endocytic membranes after release from its linkage to the polymer. Light exposure of cells containing photosensitizers in their endosomes or lysosomes leads to a permeabilization of these vesicles and release of the photosensitizers into the cytosol [16]. In some cases (e.g., by using $TPPS_{2a}$ and $TPPS_1$, but not $TPPS_4$), substantial levels of lysosomal enzyme activity have been found in the cytosol after PDT, indicating that the lysosomal contents can be released into the cytosol without losing their activity [17].

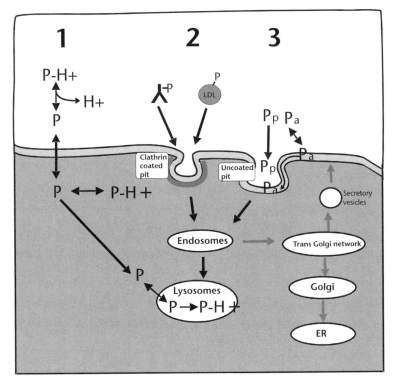

Figure 16.1 Pathways for cellular uptake of photosensitizers in endocytic vesicles.
(1) Photosensitizers that exert week base properties may penetrate through the plasma membrane and become trapped in the acidic environments such as in the late endosomes and lysosomes.
(2) Photosensitizers that are linked or associated with macromolecules (exemplified with an antibody) or particles (exemplified with LDL) may enter the cells via endocytosis. The photosenstizer may however enter the cytosol if the photosensitizer is released from its association with the macromolecule or particle and the photosensitizer is able to penetrate the cellular membranes.
(3) Photosensitizers that are highly amphiphilic or hydrophilic may not be able to penetrate a cellular membrane and will be taken up by the cell by either pinocytosis (hydrophilic photosensitizers, Pp) or adsorptive endocytosis (amphiphilic photosensitizers, Pa).

According to the "suicide bag" hypothesis postulated by de Duve, and well confirmed by others, release of lysosomal hydrolases, especially cathepsins, into the cytosol leads to apoptotic or necrotic cell death depending on the amounts of cathepsins released [18]. Some of the cathepsins are able to induce apoptosis by cleaving the cytosolic form of Bid, which is then translocated to the mitochondrial membranes, causing cytochrome c release and thereby inducing apoptosis [19]. This pathway has been shown to be activated after PDT with a lysosomally located photosensitizer [20]. However, it has been found that after photochemical rupture of lysosomes, up to 50% of lysosomal marker enzyme activity (hexosaminidase) may be released into the cytosol after doses causing only minor cell death (approximately 20%) [17]. This has been suggested to be due to a high sensitivity of cathepsins to PDT in combination with cathepsin inhibitors located in the cytosol, which can further attenuate the catalytic activity of the cathepsins [21]. Thus, cells may survive a moderate release of cathepsins into the cytosol. The substantial release of lysosomally localized enzymes into the cytosol after the photochemical treatment indicated that photoactivation of selected photosensitizing dyes may be used to release endocytosed molecules, such as therapeutic macromolecules, in a functionally intact form from endosomes and lysosomes into the cytosol as described in Figure 16.2(a) [22]. This way of improving the therapeutic effect of compounds trapped in endocytic vesicles has been named photochemical internalization and has been shown to increase the biological activity of a large variety of molecules [22].

TPPS$_{2a}$ and AlPcS2$_a$ are currently the preferred photosensitizers for use in PCI. Based on indirect evidence (e.g., [23, 24]), the preferential localization of disulfonated TPP and AlPc in endocytic vesicles seems to be as described in Figure 16.3. Amphiphilic disulfonated compounds are mainly located in the vesicular membranes while the tetrasulfonated compounds are mainly located in the matrix of the endocytic vesicle.

It was initially thought that the photosensitizer and macromolecule to be released from the endocytic compartments had to be located in the same compartments at the time of light exposure. However, it has recently been found that the photochemical treatment can be performed up to 6 to 8 hours prior to the delivery of the macromolecule without reducing the synergistic effect of the combined treatment [25]. The assumed mechanistic basis for such an observation is that newly

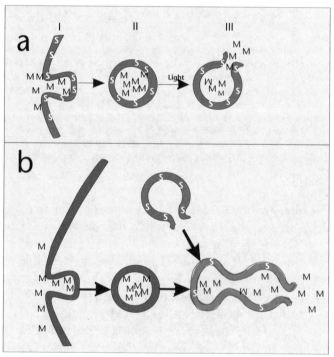

Figure 16.2 Mechanisms for PCI-induced translocation of molecules into the cytosol. (a) The photosensitizer (S) and the selected molecule (M) are endocytosed by the cells (I illustrates the invagination of the plasma membrane) and both compounds ends up in endocytic vesicles (II). When these vesicles are exposed to light, the membranes of these vesicles will be ruptured and the contents released (III). (Ia) S and M are located in the same vesicles at the time of light exposure, while in (b) S is first delivered to the cells and the cells are exposed to light (I) prior to the delivery of M (II). The damaged vesicles are assumed to fuse with vesicles formed after the photochemical treatment and containing M (III).

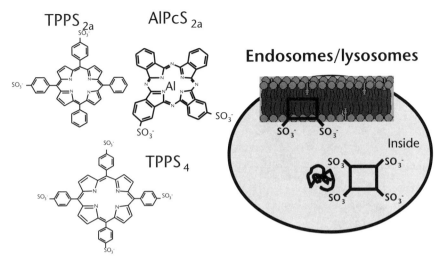

Figure 16.3   Proposed localization of sulfonated photosensitizers in endocytic vesicles. The figure shows a schematic drawing of an endocytic vesicle and drawings of the main location of a tetrasulfonated and an amphiphilic disulfonated photosensitizer (not in dimension).

formed vesicles are able to fuse with photochemically damaged vesicles and that the macromolecules are released into the cytosol after fusion of such vesicles (Figure 16.2(b)). In some cases (e.g., drug delivery by EGFR-targeting moieties), the photochemical pretreatment has not been very efficient [26, 27]. This may be due to photochemical inactivation of EGFR, which will inhibit endocytosis of the receptor [28].

16.3   Photochemical Delivery of Macromolecules

Macromolecular therapeutics includes drugs where the macromolecule itself exert a therapeutic effect as well as drugs where the macromolecule serves as a targeting moiety (Figure 16.4). Some macromolecules, such as MAbs, exert their therapeutic effect at the surface of the target cells through for example inhibition of cell signaling pathways and immune activation. MAbs can also be conjugated to moieties with extracellular activities such as radioactive compounds, immunomodulators, and prodrug-activating enzymes.

Alternatively, translocation to intracellular compartments may be required to exert the therapeutic effect and transport through the endocytic pathway is utilized to obtain cytosolic delivery of the drug. In these cases PCI may contribute to increased therapeutic efficacy and specificity. This includes macromolecules with therapeutic activities such as protein toxins, DNA for gene therapy, oligonucleotides for posttranscriptional gene silencing, peptides and mRNA for cancer vaccination, and other molecules that do not readily penetrate through the cellular membranes. The utilization of PCI to enhance the biological activities of such therapeutic macromolecules as well as to improve therapeutic specificity beyond that of the targeted macromolecules alone will be described below.

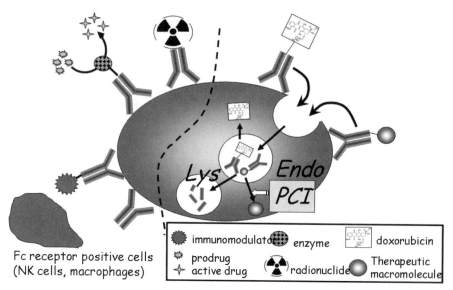

Fc receptor positive cells
(NK cells, macrophages)

immunomodulator	enzyme	doxorubicin
prodrug	radionuclide	Therapeutic
active drug		macromolecule

Figure 16.4 Schematic presentation of targeted delivery of therapeutics to cells exemplified by the use of antibodies as targeting ligand. The drugs delivered to the target cells may exert their therapeutic effect at the cell surface (left side of the dashed line) such as radionuclides, enzymes for converting a prodrug to an active drug, and immunomodulators such as cytokines and unligated antibodies for immuneactivation. Alternatively, the target of the active drug is located intracellularly (right side of the dashed line) and these substances are usually entering the cells through endocytosis. Active substances that are cleaved off their targeting moiety in the endocytic compartments and are able penetrate into the cytosol (exemplified by doxorubicin) will usually not benefit from PCI while the remaining may benefit from PCI. Endo: endosomes; Lys: lysosomes.

16.4   PCI: A Technology for Enhancing the Activity of Macromolecular Therapeutics

Macromolecules for therapeutic purposes may be divided into three groups: proteins and peptides, nucleic acids, and synthetic polymers for drug delivery and/or protection. In order for the PCI technology to induce increased translocation of therapeutic macromolecules to the cytosol, the macromolecules need to be located in endocytic vesicles at some stage in the process. It should be noted that all cells except mature erythrocytes exert the endocytic process. Thus, macromolecules will in general be endocytosed, either through receptor-mediated endocytosis, adsorptive endocytosis, or pinocytosis, and thereby become candidates for PCI.

16.4.1   Photochemical Delivery of Proteins

Protein toxins have been extensively evaluated, especially as part of immunotoxins, for use in cancer therapy as well as in graft versus host disease, bone marrow purging, autoimmune diseases, and HIV infection [29]. These protein toxins are of either bacterial or plant origin. The toxins need to enter the cytosol in order to kill the cells by inhibiting protein synthesis, either by inactivating the elongation factor 2 (EF-2) or the EF-2 binding site on the 28 S ribosome subunit. The 28S-targeting ribosome inactivating proteins (RIPs) are plant toxins that constitute either of only one polypeptide chain (A-chain, type I toxins) with enzymatic activity or in addition another targeting chain (B-chain, type II toxins, e.g., ricin) linked to the A-chain by disulfide bonds [30]. Both types of toxins are endocytosed, but while type I RIPs enter the cells through pinocytosis and are mainly degraded in the lysosomes, the type II toxins are to a higher extent able to translocate into the cytosol. Type I RIPs exert therefore a relatively low cytotoxic effect on intact cells, while the plant type II and bacterial RIPs are highly cytotoxic compounds despite the fact that all types of RIPs have the same ability to inactivate ribosomes in cell-free systems. The literature indicates that only 1 to 10 RIP molecules located in the cytosol are sufficient to kill the cell [31]. Due to the intrinsic ability of the plant type II and bacterial RIPs to undergo transmembrane translocation, these protein toxins have been most success-ful in clinical trials and the only RIP-based toxin clinically approved is based on the bacterial RIP diphtheria toxin (recombinant IL-2 truncated diphtheria toxin fusion protein (Ontak)).

The plant type II and bacterial RIPs are examples of proteins that are able to penetrate cellular membranes and therefore may not benefit from combination with PCI. This has been confirmed in case of an immunotoxin with pseudomonas exotoxin as the therapeutic agent (unpublished results). However, type I RIPs that do lack efficient membrane translocation properties are good candidates for a highly specific PCI-based activation of macromolecules and PCI has been shown to activate type I RIPs by inducing release from the endocytic vesicles both in vitro and in vivo [22, 32, 33]. Type I RIPs are relatively small proteins (e.g., gelonin, which has been frequently used in PCI, has a molecular mass of about 30 kDa, and cannot easily be used for systemic administration due to leakage through the kidneys and lack of tissue specificity) [30]. PCI of gelonin has therefore been evaluated by inject-ing gelonin intratumorally into 6- to 8-mm tumors and obtained 70% to 100% complete response of this treatment while similar photochemical treatment with intratumoral injection of saline induced 0% to 10% complete response [33, 34, unpublished data]. The in vivo studies performed on PCI of gelonin show that the depth of necrosis and effect on tumor growth was much stronger using gelonin in combination with PCI compared to using gelonin alone or the photochemical treat-ment (i.e., PDT) alone [33, 34].

16.4.2   PCI for Gene Delivery

Gene therapy is recognized as having the potential to constitute a treatment option for many different diseases [35]. However, further progress in clinical gene therapy depends on the development of methods that increase the efficacy and specificity of gene delivery [35, 36]. With most gene delivery systems the therapeutic gene is taken into the cell by endocytosis, and for many of these systems, especially nonvirus-based, the lack of efficient mechanisms for translocation of the gene out of the endocytic vesicles constitutes a major hindrance for realization of the therapeu-tic potential of the gene products.

Photochemical internalization has been studied as a gene delivery technology (reviewed in [37]) both with several nonviral [23, 38, 39] and viral vectors [40], mainly by using reporter genes such as genes encoding eGFP (enhanced green fluo-rescent protein) or β-galactosidase. Moreover, PCI treatment also enhanced the delivery, transgene expression and biological activity of therapeutic genes, such as the genes encoding HSV-tk (Herpes Simplex Virus thymidine kinase) [41], p53 [42], TRAIL [43], and IL-12 (interleukin-12) (unpublished results).

Delivery of genes to cells for therapeutic purposes requires in most cases the DNA protection from degradation and facilitation of the cellular uptake. The vehicles used for such purposes are called vectors and can be divided into chemical or nonviral and viral vectors. In addition, physical methods such as electroporation may be utilized. Some of the vectors have additional properties that facilitate escape from the endocytic vesicles into the cytosol for further transfer to the nucleus. Polyethylenimine (PEI) is an example of a nonviral vector, which in a concentration-dependent manner enhances transgene delivery into the cell cytosol. The proposed mechanism for the PEI-enhanced endosomal release of DNA is based on the "proton sponge effect," suggesting that the pK values of the amino groups of PEI are close to physiological pH and thereby cause increased accumulation of water in the acidic environment of the endocytic vesicles until they lyse. Despite the intrinsic abilities of PEI to lyse endosomes, PCI has been shown to further enhance transgene delivery of plasmid/PEI polyplexes in vitro [41]. Furthermore, a recent in vivo study showed that treatment of squamous cell carcinomas deficient in active p53 with intratumoral injection of the photosensitizer $AlPcS_{2a}$ and a plasmid expressing p53 complexed to a glycosylated PEI caused a complete tumor regression in all the transfected animals [42]. In contrast, similar PDT or PEI-p53 treatments alone did not delay tumor growth. Recently, a highly sophisticated vector design was shown by Kataoka and colleagues [44]. Their design was based on a disulfide-extended cationic peptide complexed with the plasmid. This cationic-peptide complex was mixed with a negatively charged dendrimer containing 32 carboxyl groups at the surface and a phthalocyanine photosensitizer in the core. It was shown that this complex caused efficient transfection at doses of light, causing hardly any cytotoxicity. When this vector was evaluated in the conjunctiva of rats, transgene expression was shown only in the irradiated area without any observable damage to the treated tissue. This opens up therapeutic possibilities for indications, such as monogenetic diseases, where it is important to avoid tissue damage.

Adenovirus vectors are known to be taken into cells by endocytosis and to be released from endosomes by a regulated process. This endosomal release is usually regarded as a very efficient process [45]. It is therefore somewhat surprising that PCI is able to increase the number of adenoviral tranduced cells by up to 30-fold. However, it has been documented that PCI increase the level of viral DNA in the nucleus as measured by real-time PCR and fluorescence in situ hybridization (FISH), the mRNA level of the transgene and the transgene expression. PCI with adenoviral vectors has been tested in over a dozen cell lines, and in all cases a positive effect on transduction has been observed [46]. There are also indications that PCI may enhance adeno-associated virus based treatment.

16.4.3 PCI of Antisense Molecules

Peptide nucleic acids (PNAs) are oligonucleotide mimics that can specifically hybridize to DNA or mRNA, thus inhibiting the transcription and translation of their complementary target sequences. As PNA is taken up into cells by endocytosis and tend to accumulate in endosomes, PCI is a candidate for enhancing their delivery into the cytosol. Folini and colleagues were the first to demonstrate a PCI-induced release of PNA into the cytoplasm of the cells [47]. In their approach, they used naked PNA targeting the catalytic component of human telomerase reverse transcriptase (hTERT-PNA). After photochemical treatment, cells treated with the hTERT-PNA showed a marked inhibition of telomerase activity and a reduced cell survival, which was not observed after treatment with hTERT-PNA alone. Moreover, in a direct comparison, the PCI technology proved to be more efficient to internalize the hTERT-PNA than an alternative strategy based on the HIV-Tat internalization protein. In another study, it has been shown that PCI could enhance the antisense effects (cytosolic/nuclear) of different peptide nucleic acid-peptide conjugates (Tat, Arg7, KLA) up to two orders of magnitude [48]. In addition, efficient gene silencing of the S100A4 gene by PNA delivered by PCI has also been demonstrated [49]. These results emphasize the importance of endosomal release for cellular activity of these types of drugs.

The siRNA molecules, which are the functional mediators of RNA interference, also need to enter the cytoplasm of the cells in order to be able to interrupt translation of specific proteins by inducing posttranscriptional gene silencing. PCI has been employed to facilitate the escape of siRNA molecules complexed with lipofectamine from the endocytic vesicles [50]. Combining antiepidermal growth factor receptor (EGFR) siRNA treatment with PCI resulted in a tenfold increased efficiency in knockdown of EGFR compared to siRNA treatment alone. Thus, lower doses of siRNA can be used when PCI is employed to augment its delivery. Lowering the doses of siRNA would prevent saturation of the RNAi machinery and reduce off-target effects. In addition, local light exposure of target tissue would only enhance siRNA delivery in the desired cells, which further increases the specificity of the treatment.

16.4.4   PCI: A Technology for Multilevel Specificity

As pointed out above, the main cause of treatment failures today is related to the insufficient specificity of the current cancer treatment modalities. This has paved the way for targeted macromolecular therapeutics that exerts the potential of being highly specific for the target tissue (Figure 16.4). However, as an example the use of immunotoxins for treatment of solid tumors has not been successful. This is partly due to the tumor physiology such as the long distance from the vasculature to the target cells and lack of convection due to a high interstitial pressure [51]. It has been estimated that only about 1 to 10 out of 10^5 MAb molecules may reach their targets [52]. Furthermore, the rate constant for transfer of immunotoxins from endocytic vesicles to the cytosol has in some cases been shown to be as much as 10^4-fold slower than their rate of endocytosis, indicating that release from endocytic vesicles may be a rate limiting step in the cytotoxicity of some immunotoxins [53]. Accordingly, PCI has been shown to increase the cytotoxic effect of the immunotoxin MOC31-gelonin (the MAb MOC31 binds to the EGP-2 antigen, also known as Ep-Cam and 17-1A, found on most carcinomas), Cetuximab-saporin and the affinity toxin EGF-saporin [26, 27, 54]. Similarly, EGF-coupled PEG/PEI/plasmid complexes, a transferrin-linked vector as well as an EGFR-retargeted adenovirus has been shown to improve transfection efficacy in vitro [26, 27, 38, 55, 56].

The low efficacy of macromolecular therapeutics in vivo has demanded delivery of high doses, which further leads to dose-limiting toxicity. Immunotoxins may cause dose-limiting nonspecific toxicity such as vascular leakage syndrome and hemolytic uremic syndrome [57, 58]. The nonspecific toxicity may be due to unspecific endocytic uptake of the immunotoxins. Since the access to some normal cells such as the endothelial cells is high and the therapeutic molecules often are selected for their ability to penetrate into the cytosol (e.g., pseudomonas exotoxin and diphtheria toxin), nonspecific toxicity to many normal cell types is anticipated. In addition, specific toxicity may occur due to expression of the same target antigen in the normal and the diseased cells. This is a serious problem especially in treatment of solid tumors as the immunotoxin may target vital organs. The PCI technology may therefore benefit from the use or design of therapeutic macromolecules or macromolecular complexes without an efficient intrinsic ability to penetrated cellular membranes and thereby reduce the adverse effects of the treatment, narrowing the side effects to light exposed areas (Figure 16.5). Alternatively, PCI may reduce the dose of a given drug needed to obtain therapeutic response and in this way avoid dose-limiting toxicity.

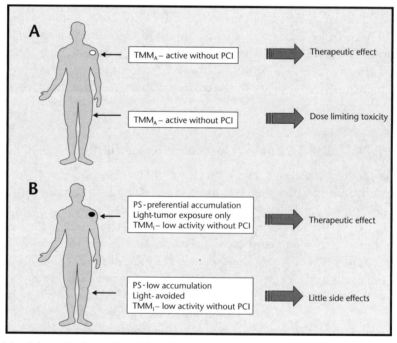

Figure 16.5 Schematic illustration of how improved specificity may be obtained with PCI. (a) Targeted macromolecules (TMM$_A$), where the therapeutic substance exerts its therapeutic function efficiently when reaching the target cells (as illustrated by the white circular area on the shoulder). These compounds may induce therapeutic effect on the target tissue, but the treatment is limited by specific or unspecific side effects. (b) In PCI, a photosensitizer (PS) with preferential accumulation in cancer tissues (dark spot on the shoulder), combined with light exposure of only the target tissue and a targeted macromolecule (TMM$_I$) with a low ability to penetrated cellular membranes or used at subtherapeutic doses induce a therapeutic effect on the target tissue. The side effects are limited since TMM$_I$ exerts little effect alone and the nontarget tissues are not exposed to light.

16.5 Conclusions

Despite a large number of new treatment modalities developed for improving therapeutic efficacy and specificity, adverse effects are still limiting factors for the therapeutic outcome in cancer patients. Photochemical activation of drugs is an attractive alternative or addition to other delivery methods that may also improve their therapeutic efficacy. The specificity of the treatment may be improved by the use of PCI since the light exposure may be focused to only the target area and by the use of drugs with low or no therapeutic effect in the absence of the photochemical treatment. Photochemical delivery of therapeutic compounds may increase the therapeutic window and thereby reduce the adverse reactions of the compounds. Photochemical drug activation and delivery by means of PCI may be considered for a large variety of clinical indications, including cancer, cardiovascular diseases, autoimmune diseases, rheumatoid arthritis, and as a delivery system for DNA vaccines.

References

[1] Yang, Z.R., et al. "Recent developments in the use of adenoviruses and immunotoxins in cancer gene therapy." *Cancer Gene Ther*, Vol. 14, No. 7, 2007, pp. 599–615.

[2] Leonetti, C., and Zupi, G. "Targeting different signaling pathways with antisense oligonucleotides combination for cancer therapy." *Curr Pharm Des*, Vol. 13, No. 5, 2007, pp. 463–470.

[3] Allen, T.M. "Ligand-targeted therapeutics in anticancer therapy." *Nat Rev Cancer*, Vol. 2, No. 10, 2002, pp. 750–763.

[4] Saukkonen, K., and Hemminki, A. "Tissue-specific promoters for cancer gene therapy." *Expert Opin Biol Therapy*, Vol. 4, No. 5, 2004, pp. 683–696.

[5] Lim,H. Y., et al. "Tumor-specific gene therapy for uterine cervical cancer using MN/CA9-directed replication-competent adenovirus." *Cancer Gene Ther*, Vol. 11, No. 8, 2004, pp. 532–538.

[6] Janowski,B. A., Hu J., and Corey D. R. "Silencing gene expression by targeting chromosomal DNA with antigene peptide nucleic acids and duplex RNAs." *Nat Protocols*, Vol. 1, No. 1, 2006, pp. 436–443.

[7] Jain, R. K. "Delivery of molecular and cellular medicine to solid tumors." *Advanced Drug Delivery Rev*, Vol. 26, No. 2–3, 1997, pp. 71–90.

[8] Cho, Y. W., Kim J. D., and Park, K. "Polycation gene delivery systems: escape from endosomes to cytosol." *J Pharm Pharmacol*, Vol. 55, No. 6, 2003, pp. 721–734.

[9] Shum, P., Kim, J. M., and Thompson, D. H. "Phototriggering of liposomal drug delivery systems." *Advanced Drug Delivery Rev*, Vol. 53, No. 3, 2001, pp. 273–284.

[10] Moan, J., and Berg, K. "The photodegradation of porphyrins in cells can be used to estimate the lifetime of singlet oxygen." *Photochem Photobiol*, Vol. 53, No. 4, 1991, pp. 549–553.

[11] Niedre, M., Patterson, M. S., and Wilson, B. C. "Direct near-infrared luminescence detection of singlet oxygen generated by photodynamic therapy in cells in vitro and tissues in vivo." *Photochem Photobiol*, Vol. 75, No. 4, 2002, pp. 382–391.

[12] Berg, K., and Moan, J. "Lysosomes and microtubules as targets for photochemotherapy of cancer." *Photochem Photobiol*, Vol. 65, No. 3, 1997, pp. 403–409.

[13] Gijsens, A., et al.. "Epidermal growth factor-mediated targeting of chlorin e6 selectively potentiates its photodynamic activity." *Cancer Res*, Vol. 60, No. 8, 2000, pp. 2197–2202.

[14] Tijerina, M., Kopeckova, P., and Kopecek, J. "Correlation of subcellular compartmentalization of HPMA copolymer-Mce6 conjugates with chemotherapeutic activity in human ovarian carcinoma cells." *Pharm Res*, Vol. 20, No. 5, 2003, pp. 728–737.

[15] del Carmen, M.G., et al. "Synergism of epidermal growth factor receptor-targeted immunotherapy with photodynamic treatment of ovarian cancer in vivo." *J National Cancer Inst*, Vol. 97, No. 20, 2005, pp. 1516–1524.

[16] Berg, K., et al. "Light induced relocalization of sulfonated meso- tetraphenylporphines in NHIK 3025 cells and effects of dose fractionation." *Photochem Photobiol*, Vol. 53, No. 2, 1991, pp. 203–210.

[17] Berg, K., and Moan, J. "Lysosomes as photochemical targets." *Int J Cancer*, Vol. 59, No. 6, 1994, pp. 814–822.

[18] Cirman, T., et al. "Selective disruption of lysosomes in HeLa cells triggers apoptosis mediated by cleavage of Bid by multiple papain-like lysosomal cathepsins." *J Biol Chem*, Vol. 279, No. 5, 2004, pp. 3578–3587.

[19] Stoka, V., et al. "Lysosomal protease pathways to apoptosis: cleavage of bid, not Pro-caspases, is the most likely route." *J Biol Chem*, 2000.

[20] Reiners, J. J., et al. "Release of cytochrome c and activation of pro-caspase-9 following lysosomal photodamage involves Bid cleavage." *Cell Death Differ*, Vol. 9, No. 9, 2002, pp. 934–944.

[21] Wilson, P. D., Firestone, R. A., and Lenard, J. "The role of lysosomal enzymes in killing of mammalian cells by the lysosomotropic detergent N-dodecylimidazole." *J Cell Biol*, Vol. 104, No. 5, 1987, pp. 1223–1229.

[22] Berg, K., et al. "Photochemical internalization: A novel technology for delivery of macromolecules into cytosol." *Cancer Res*, Vol. 59, No. 6, 1999, pp. 1180–1183.

[23] Prasmickaite, L., Hogset, A., and Berg, K. "Evaluation of different photosensitizers for use in photochemical gene transfection." *Photochem Photobiol*, Vol. 73, No. 4, 2001, pp. 388–395.

[24] Maman, N., et al. "Kinetic and equilibrium studies of incorporation of di- sulfonated aluminum phthalocyanine into unilamellar vesicles." *Biochim Biophys Acta: Bio-Membranes*, Vol. 1420, No. 1–2, 1999, pp. 168–178.

[25] Prasmickaite, L., et al. "Photochemical disruption of endocytic vesicles before delivery of drugs: a new strategy for cancer therapy." *Br J Cancer*, Vol. 86, No. 4, 2002, pp. 652–657.

[26] Weyergang, A., Selbo, P. K., and Berg, K. "Photochemically stimulated drug delivery increases the cytotoxicity and specificity of EGF-saporin." *J Control Release*, Vol. 111, No. 1–2, 2006, pp. 165–173.

[27] Yip, W. L., et al. "Targeted delivery and enhanced cytotoxicity of cetuximab-saporin by photochemical internalization in EGFR-positive cancer cells." *Mol Pharm*, Vol. 4, No. 2, 2007, pp. 241–251.

[28] Weyergang, A., Selbo, P. K., and Berg, K. "Y1068 phosphorylation is the most sensitive target of disulfonated tetraphenylporphyrin-based photodynamic therapy on epidermal growth factor receptor." *Biochem Pharm*, Vol. 74, No. 2, 2007, pp. 226–235.

[29] Thrush, G. R., et al. "Immunotoxins: an update." *Ann Rev Immunol*, Vol. 14, 1996, pp. 49–71.

[30] Barbieri, L., Battelli, M. G., and Stirpe, F. "Ribosome-inactivating proteins from plants." *Biochim Biophys Acta*, Vol. 1154, No. 3–4, 1993, pp. 237–282.

[31] Eiklid, K., Olsnes, S., and Pihl, A. "Entry of lethal doses of abrin, ricin and modeccin into the cytosol of HeLa cells." *Exp Cell Res*, Vol. 126, No. 2, 1980, pp. 321–326.

[32] Selbo, P. K., et al. "Release of gelonin from endosomes and lysosomes to cytosol by photochemical internalization." *Biochim Biophys Acta*, Vol. 1475, No. 3, 2000, pp. 307–313.

[33] Selbo, P. K., et al. "In vivo documentation of photochemical internalization, a novel approach to site specific cancer therapy." *Int J Cancer*, Vol. 92, No. 5, 2001, pp. 761–766.

[34] Dietze, A., et al., "Enhanced photodynamic destruction of a transplantable fibrosarcoma using photochemical internalisation of gelonin." *Br J Cancer*, Vol. 92, No. 11, 2005, pp. 2004–2009.

[35] Verma, I. M., and Weitzman, M. D. "Gene therapy: twenty-first century medicine." *Annu Rev Biochem*, Vol. 74 , 2005, pp. 711–738.

[36] Hacein-Bey-Abina, S., et al. "A serious adverse event after successful gene therapy for X-linked severe combined immunodeficiency." *N Engl J Med*, Vol. 348, No. 3, 2003, pp. 255–256.

[37] Høgset, A., et al. "Light directed gene transfer by photochemical internalisation." *Curr Gene Ther*, Vol. 3, No. 2, 2003, pp. 89–112.

[38] Prasmickaite, L., et al. "Role of endosomes in gene transfection mediated by photochemical internalisation (PCI)." *J Gene Med*, Vol. 2, No. 6, 2000, pp. 477–488.

[39] Høgset, A., et al. "Photochemical transfection: a new technology for light-induced, site-directed gene delivery." *Hum Gene Therapy*, Vol. 11, No. 6, 2000, pp. 869–880.

[40] Høgset, A., et al."Light-induced adenovirus gene transfer, an efficient and specific gene delivery technology for cancer gene therapy." *Cancer Gene Therapy*, Vol. 9, No. 4, 2002, pp. 365–371.

[41] Prasmickaite, L., et al., "Photochemically enhanced gene transfection increases the cytotoxicity of the herpes simplex virus thymidine kinase gene combined with ganciclovir." *Cancer Gene Therapy*, Vol. 11, No. 7, 2004, pp. 514–523.

[42] Ndoye, A., et al. "Eradication of p53-mutated head and neck squamous cell carcinoma xenografts using nonviral p53 gene therapy and photochemical internalization." *Mol Therapy*, Vol. 13, No. 6, 2006, pp. 1156–1162.

[43] Engesaeter, B. Ø., et al. "Photochemically mediated delivery of AdhCMV-TRAIL augments the TRAIL-induced apoptosis in colorectal cancer cell lines." *Cancer Biol Therapy*, Vol. 5, No. 11, 2006, pp. 1511–1520.

[44] Nishiyama, N., et al. "Light-induced gene transfer from packaged DNA enveloped in a dendrimeric photosensitizer." *Nature Materials*, Vol. 4, No. 12, 2005, pp. 934–941.

[45] Greber, U. F., et al. "Stepwise dismantling of adenovirus 2 during entry into cells." *Cell*, Vol. 75, No. 3, 1993, pp. 477–486.

[46] Engesaeter, B. Ø., et al."PCI-enhanced adenoviral transduction employs the known uptake mechanism of adenoviral particles." *Cancer Gene Therapy*, Vol. 12, No. 5, 2005, pp. 439–448.

[47] Folini, M., et al."Photochemical internalization of a peptide nucleic acid targeting the catalytic subunit of human telomerase." *Cancer Res*, Vol. 63, No. 13, 2003, pp. 3490–3494.

[48] Shiraishi, T., and Nielsen, P. E. "Photochemically enhanced cellular delivery of cell penetrating peptide-PNA conjugates." *FEBS Lett*, Vol.580, No. 5, 2006, pp. 1451–1456.

[49] Boe, S., and Hovig, E. "Photochemically induced gene silencing using PNA-peptide conjugates." *Oligonucleotides*, Vol. 16, No. 2, 2006, pp. 145–157.

[50] Oliveira, S., et al. "Photochemical internalization enhances silencing of epidermal growth factor receptor through improved endosomal escape of siRNA." *Biochim Biophys Acta*, Vol. 1768, No. 5, 2007, pp. 1211–1217.

[51] Jain, R. K. "Delivery of novel therapeutic agents in tumors: physiological barriers and strategies." *J Nat Cancer Institute*, Vol. 81, No. 8, 1989, pp. 570–576.

[52] Li, K. C., et al. "Molecular imaging applications in nanomedicine." *Biomed Microdevices*, Vol. 6, 2004, pp. 113–116.

[53] Chan, M. C., and Murphy, R. M. "Kinetics of cellular trafficking and cytotoxicity of 9.2.27-gelonin immunotoxins targeted against the high-molecular-weight melanoma-associated antigen." *Cancer Immunol Immunother*, Vol. 47, No. 6, 1999, pp. 321–329.

[54] Selbo, P. K., et al. "Photochemical internalisation increases the cytotoxic effect of the immunotoxin MOC31-gelonin." *Int J Cancer*, Vol. 87, No. 6, 2000, pp. 853–859.

[55] Bonsted, A., et al. "Photochemically enhanced transduction of polymer-complexed adenovirus targeted to the epidermal growth factor receptor." *J Gene Med*, Vol. 8, No. 3, 2006, pp. 286–297.

[56] Kloeckner, J., et al. "Photochemically enhanced gene delivery of EGF receptor-targeted DNA polyplexes." *J Drug Targeting*, Vol. 12, No. 4, 2004, pp. 205–213.

[57] Kreitman, R. J. and Pastan, I. "BL22 and lymphoid malignancies." *Best Pract Res Clin Haematol*, Vol. 19, No. 4, 2006, pp. 685–699.

[58] Pastan, I. et al. "Immunotoxin therapy of cancer." *Nat Rev Cancer*, Vol. 6, No. 7, 2006, pp. 559–565.

CHAPTER 17

Combinations of Photodynamic Therapy with Other Therapeutic Modalities

Asta Juzeniene, Mateusz Kwitniewski, and Johan Moan

17.1 Introduction

Surgery, radiotherapy (RT), and chemotherapy (CHT) are the main conventional cancer treatment modalities. They have many adverse effects, and except for surgery, they are nonselective. Thus they cannot distinguish between cancer and healthy cells properly. Consequently, healthy cells are damaged, which results in side effects. Such side effects may be severe, reducing the quality of life of the patients, compromising their ability to receive full, prescribed treatment. More selective treatment modalities, such as hyperthermia (HT), immunotherapy, photodynamic therapy (PDT), and sonodynamic therapy, have been introduced. In some cases one treatment modality cannot cure a patient because of treatment limitations and/or side effects. The use of two or more modalities of treatment (surgery, RT, CHT, immunotherapy) in combination, alternately or together, offers many advantages, and is already in clinical practice. Although PDT has been approved for several clinical applications, it appears not to be widely applied in the clinics. Efficacy of surgery, RT, CHT, HT, and sonodynamic therapy may be increased and doses and side effects lowered by combination with PDT. The combinations of PDT with other treatment modalities (Figure 17.1) will be discussed in this chapter.

17.2 Surgery Combined with PDT

Surgical treatment of a large number of solid tumors leaves residual microscopic islands of tumor cells that may lead to local recurrences. Intraoperative adjuvant PDT is intended to reduce such recurrences. A PDT photosensitizer is administered before surgery and the area is exposed to light after surgical removal of the main tumor [1]. Several reports on this technique in animal models have been published [1–4]. Momma et al. [1] reported that PDT combined with surgery gave significant local control of the primary tumor and significant reduction in distant metastases. In comparison, surgery or PDT alone gave poorer local control. PDT alone even gave a significant increase in the mean number of lung metastases. However, the relationship between PDT and risk of metastases after PDT has not been firmly established: three studies show a decrease in metastases [5–7]; two studies show an increase [1, 8].

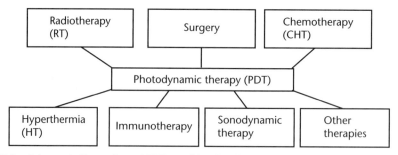

Figure 17.1 Schematic illustration of PDT combined with other treatment modalities.

The advantage of such combined treatments has been demonstrated in several clinical trials [9–15] (Table 17.1). However, one study, which was performed with Photofrin II (dihematoporphyrin ether), reported no benefit of using PDT in combination with surgery [10].

PDT is a potentially valuable adjuvant therapy in conjunction with surgery of malignant brain tumors [14–17]. The combination of fluorescence diagnosis with tumor resection may improve treatment of brain malignancies [15]. Kostron et al. reported that fluorescence guided resection followed by intraoperative PDT with Foscan significantly prolonged survival of the patients with malignant brain tumors [15].

Table 17.1 Summary of Clinical Results Obtained Using Surgery Combined with PDT

Cancer	Number of Patients	Photosensitizer	Observations	Reference
Refractory or recurrent, disseminated intraperitoneal tumors	54	Photofrin II	Safe	DeLaney et al., 1993 [18]
Colorectal carcinomas	17	Hematoporphyrin derivative (HpD)	Safe	Allardice et al., 1994 [19]
Locally recurrent rectal cancers	22	Photofrin	Safe	Harlow et al., 1995 [20]
Malignant mesotheliomas, localized low-grade carcinoid	5	mTHPC	Safe, effective	Baas et al., 1997 [9]
Malignant pleural mesotheliomas	63	Photofrin II	Ineffective	Pass et al., 1997 [10]
Gastrointestinal tract malignancies, ovarian cancers, and sarcomas	56	Photofrin	Safe	Hendren et al., 2001 [21]
Malignant brain tumors	22	mTHPC	Safe, prolonged survival	Zimmermann et al., 2001 [17]
Malignant pleural mesotheliomas	26	Foscan	Safe	Friedberg et al., 2003 [22]
Nonsmall-cell lung cancers with pleural spread	22	Photofrin	Safe, good local control, prolonged survival	Friedberg et al., 2004 [11]
Facial basal cell carcinomas	4	ALA-PpIX	Safe, effective	Kuijpers et al., 2004 [12]

Table 17.1 (continued)

Cancer	Number of Patients	Photosensitizer	Observations	Reference
Nonresectable bile duct carcinomas	8	Photofrin	Safe, prolonged survival l	Nanashima et al., 2004 [13]
Cerebral gliomas	136	HpD	Safe, prolonged survival	Stylli et al., 2005 [14]
Malignant brain tumors	26	Foscan	Safe, prolonged survival	Kostron et al., 2006 [15]

17.3   Radiotherapy (RT) Combined with PDT

Complete success of RT of cancer is limited by two main factors: the presence of hypoxic, radioresistant, and repair-proficient subpopulations of tumor cells and the adverse effects of radiation on the normal tissues at higher therapeutic doses [23]. Therefore, approaches directed toward differentially enhancing the manifestation of radiation damage in tumors and minimizing it in normal tissues would help to improve the efficacy of RT. Schwartz et al. [24], and later other groups [16, 25, 26], have demonstrated that the effect of RT can be optimized by adding hematoporphyrin derivative (HpD) or its purified form Photofrin. These drugs may under certain conditions act as radiosensitizers. However, HpD or Photofrin cause skin photosensitivity that can last for 4 weeks or more. Due to faster clearance from the body, other photosensitizers, such as 5-aminolevulinic acid-induced proto-porphyrin IX (ALA-PpIX), chlorin e6, hematoporphyrin (Hp), Zn-tetrasulphophtalocyanine, hematoporphyrin dimethyl ether (HPde), zinc phthalocyanine (ZnPC), meta-tetrahydroxyphenylchlorine (mTHPC), and indocyanine green, have been tried in combination with RT [25, 27–30]. Even though all these photosensitizers accumulated in significant amounts in the neoplastic lesions, only HPde significantly improved the response of the tumor after RT [29, 31]. The possibility to use the same chemical compound as a radiosensitizer and photosensitizer offers unique perspectives for combinations of two treatment modalities with the aim to improve the control of tumor growth. It was believed that RT could be enhanced synergistically by PDT due to (1) direct enhancement of the initial damage, (2) inhibiting cellular repair, (3) accumulating cells in a radiosensitive phase, or (4) eliminating radioresistant cells. PDT may be enhanced by RT due to (1) direct enhancement of the initial damage and (2) deeper tumor damage. However, in vitro and in vivo the experimental results show that in most cases only additive effects could be achieved by combining these two treatment modalities (Table 17.2) [16, 27, 29, 30, 32–40]. This indicates that processes leading to the cell inactivation by RT are different and independent of those of PDT. Furthermore, different studies have reported antagonistic or synergistic effects of PDT and RT [34, 37, 38, 41–43]. The discrepancy between the findings may be explained by different photosensitizers and doses, application times and intracellular localization patterns and differences in sequence of treatments. These parameters and tumor types may influence treatment outcome. For example, the

Table 17.2   Summary of Results Obtained Using RT Combined with PDT

Model	Photosensitizer	Effects	Reference
Cell lines			
Chinese hamster ovary CHO	HpD	Additive	Bellnier and Dougherty, 1986 [33]
Murine fibroblasts L929	Chloroaluminum phthalocyanine (AlPcCl)	Synergistic	Ramakrishnan et al., 1990 [41]
Murine fibroblasts L929, Chinese hamster ovary CHO K1, and human bladder carcinoma T24	HpD	Synergistic/ additive	Prinsze et al., 1992 [37]
Human colon adenocarcinoma WiDr	Photofrin II	Synergistic/ Antagonistic	Ma et al., 1993 [44]
Chinese hamster lung	HpD	Synergistic/ antagonistic	Kavarnos et al., 1994 [42]
Human colon adenocarcinoma WiDr	ALA-PpIX	Synergistic/ antagonistic	Berg et al., 1995 [43]
Human breast carcinoma	Zinc phthalocyanine (ZnPC) and mTHPC	Additive	Dobler-Girdziunaite et al., 1995 [30]
Chinese hamster fibroblasts V79	Photosan 3	Additive/ synergistic	Schnitzhofer and Krammer, 1996 [38]
Human squamous cell carcinomas V134, V175 and SCC-61	ALA-PpIX	Additive	Allman et al., 2000 [40]
Human prostate carcinoma PC-3, human prostate epithelial EPN	Indocyanine green	Additive	Colasanti et al., 2004 [27]
Mice with			
Sarcoma 180 tumors	Photofrin II	Additive/ synergistic	Graschew and Shopova, 1986 [34]
Ehrlich ascites carcinomas	HPde	Additive	Luksiene et al., 1999 [29]
Rats with			
Ethyl nitrosourea induced gliosarcomas	HpD	Additive/ synergistic	Kostron et al., 1986 [16]
Retinoblastomas	HpD	Antagonistic	Winther et al., 1988 [47]
Hamsters with			
Nonpigmented melanomas	Merocyanine MC540	Additive	Kukielczak, et al., 1999 [39]
Patients with			
Bronchogenic carcinomas	HpD	Additive	Lam et al., 1985 and 1993 [32, 48]
Retinoblastomas	HpD	Additive	Ohnishi et al., 1986 [35]
Cerebral gliomas	HpD	Additive	Kaye et al., 1987 [36]

study of Kavarnos et al. showed that only simultaneous PDT and RT gave synergistic interactions, because time intervals less than 1 minute seemed to be required for the effective involvement of the "fast reparation system" [42]. The work of Ma et al. demonstrated the importance of light and radiation exposure doses [44].

Historically, DNA has been considered to be the main target for radiation therapy. However, this DNA-centric model has been questioned because cell killing and

DNA damage diverge [45]. Such pathways include membrane-dependent signaling and bystander responses (when cells respond not to direct radiation exposure but to the radiation of effects on their neighboring cells) [45]. This focus may be important when attempting to predict the consequences of combined therapies involving RT and PDT. Membrane-dependent signaling pathways may sometimes be important for both RT and PDT. HpD and Photofrin localize in many intracellular compartments, including cell membranes (due to their impurities [46]), but HPde is mostly localized in the cell membrane [31]. They also act as radiosensitizers. This hypothesis needs to be checked with other photosensitizers which localize in plasma membrane. Sequence and dose of the treatments may also play important roles.

17.4   Chemotherapy (CHT) Combined with PDT

Clinical trials clearly show that concomitant RT and CHT significantly improve local control in a variety of advanced solid tumors [49]. The combination of RT and CHT demonstrates independent cell-killing effects. RT is aimed at controlling the primary tumor, while CHT is intended to eradicate distant metastases. The addition of conventional CHT to PDT may enhance the local effects of PDT and give effects on malignant tissue outside the PDT treated area. It may enable reduction of the doses of photosensitizer and chemotherapeutic drug required, thus diminishing undesirable side effects. The combination of PDT with CHT has been applied in many experimental studies and in three clinical trials (Table 17.3). The combination of PDT and CHT may act positively (additive or synergistic interaction) [50–53] or negatively (antagonistic interaction) [50, 54–56]. The interaction depends on the sequence and the time interval between the two treatments, the type of drugs used, the dose of the treatments and the type of tumor treated [56, 57].

Almost all solid tumors have hypoxic and anoxic regions [58]. Furthermore, PDT itself will reduce oxygen concentrations due to photochemical oxygen consumption [59] or vascular damage [60]. Hypoxic tumors are resistant to PDT [61–63]. This resistance can be partially overcome by applying bioreductive drugs, which generate cytotoxic metabolites depending on the availability of oxygen in tissue. Combinations of HpD or Photofrin II mediated PDT and the bioreductive drug misonidazole were reported for the first time in 1986 [61, 64]. Gonzalez et al. found that administration of misonidazole 20 minutes prior to or after light exposure increased tumor growth delay or even cured the treated rats [64]. Graschew and Shopova obtained similar results, and found that the simultaneous application of misonidazole and light exposure increased the therapeutic effect [61]. Bioreductive drugs may reduce the inhibition of PDT caused by acute or chronic hypoxia [61]. Similar conclusions were drawn by Winther et al. [47]. Combination of other bioreductive drugs like nitroimidazole or mitomycin C with PDT were found to be more effective than these therapies alone [65, 66].

The effect of disulphonated aluminum phthalocyanine-mediated PDT and bioreductive drug nitroimidazole RSU1069 and its prodrug RB6145 was investigated using RIF-1 experimental murine tumor model [67]. The increase in tumor regrowth time in the presence of the bioreductive drugs was greatest if the time between giving the photosensitizer and light exposure was shorter than one hour.

Table 17.3   Summary of Results Obtained Using CHT Combined with PDT

Model	Photosensitizer	Cytotoxic Drug	References
Cells			
Mouse lymphocytic leukemia L1210	Hp	Phenylalanine mustard, actinomycin D	Creekmore and Zaharko, 1983 [51]
Raji or Lewis lung carcinoma	HpD	Adriamycin, methotrexate	Cowled et al., 1987 [54]
Human cervical adenocarcinoma HeLa S3	Photofrin II	Adriamycin, mitomycin C, 5-fluorouracil, vinblastine	Dima et al., 1990 [66]
Human gastric adenocarcinoma MGc 80-3	HpD	Vincristine, mitomycin, bleomycin A5, 5-fluorouracil	Niu, 1992 [69]
Human malignant mesothelioma H-MESO-1	Photofrin II	Adriamycin	Brophy and Keller, 1992 [87]
Human colon adenocarcinoma WiDr	Photofrin II	Mitomycin C	Ma et al., 1993 [53]
Human glioma C6	HpD	MX2, a Morpholino Anthracycline	Kabuto et al., 1995 [102]
Human ovarian carcinoma OVCAR-3	Meso-chlorin e6 monoethylene diamine	Adriamycin	Peterson et al., 1995 [88]
Human leukemia K562	Aluminum phthalocyanine tetrasulfonate (AlPcS4)	Etoposide	Gantchev et al., 1996 [103]
Human bladder carcinoma J82, mitomycin C-resistant J82/MMC	ALA-PpIX	Mitomycin C	Data et al., 1997 [74]; French et al., 2004 [76]
Human breast adenocarcinoma MCF-7	Indocyanine green	Cisplatin	Crescenzi et al., 2004 [83]
Human bladder carcinoma J82, human normal urothelial cells UROtsa	Porphyrin–platinum conjugates	Cisplatin, oxaliplatin	Lottner et al., 2004 [84]
Human prostate carcinoma LNCaP	ALA-PpIX	Methotrexate	Sinha et al., 2006 [104]
Mice			
Lewis lung carcinoma	HpD	Adriamycin, methotrexate, cyclophosphamide, thiotepa, vincristine, and 5-fluorouracil	Cowled et al., 1987 [54]
Radiation-induced fibrosarcoma (RIF-1) and murine mammary carcinoma EMT-6	HpD	Cisplatin, doxorubicin	Nahabedian et al., 1988 [56]
Walker 256 carcinosarcoma	HpD	Adriamycin	Edell and Cortese, 1988 [86]
Solid Ehrlich carcinoma	Hp	Nitroimidazole	Konig et al., 1989 [65]
Murine transitional cell carcinoma (MBT-2)	Photofrin II	Thiotepa, adriamycin, mitomycin C	Cho et al., 1992 [50]
IPDT and RIF-1 tumors	Photofrin	Mitomycin C, indoloquinone EO9	Baas et al., 1994 [70]
RIF-1 tumors	HpD	Misonidazole, pimonidazole, metronidazole, nimorazole, RB6145, RSU1069, SR4233, mitomycin-C, RB90740.	Bremmer et al., 1994 [68]

Table 17.3 (continued)

Model	Photosensitizer	Cytotoxic Drug	References
Human colon adenocarcinoma WiDr	Photofrin	Mitomycin C	Ma et al., 1995 [71]
RIF-1 tumors	mTHPC, BCA	Mitomycin C	Van Geel et al., 1995 [72]
CaD2 mammary carcinomas	TPPS2a	Vincristine, taxol	Ma et al., 1996 [55]
RIF-1 tumors	Photofrin	Mitomycin C	Baas et al., 1996 [105]
Mammary adenocarcinoma	ALA-PpIX	Adriamycin	Casas et al., 1997 [89]
L1210 leukemia and P388 lymphoma	AlS2Pc	Adriamycin, cisplatin	Canti et al., 1998 [81]
Carcinoma epidermoides LL of the lung	Photohem	Adriamycin	Streckyte et al., 1999 [90]
OVCAR-3 carcinoma	Meso-chlorin e6 monoethylene diamine	HPMA copolymer-bound adriamycin	Shiah et al., 2000 [92]
RIF-1 tumors	Hypericin	Mitomycin C	Chen et al., 2003 [75]
Mouse squamous cell carcinoma NR-S1	Photofrin	Cisplatin	Uehara et al., 2006 [85]
Rats			
Colon carcinoma CC531	Photofrin	Mitomycin C	Veenhuizen et al., 1996 [73]
Patients			
Advanced cardiac cancers	HpD	UFT (tegafur and uracil) and mitomycin C	Jin et al., 1992 [52]
Recurrent superficial bladder cancer	ALA-PpIX	Mitomycin C	Skyrme et al., 2005 [77]
Advanced esophagocardiac carcinoma	PSD-007	5-fluorouracil	Zhang et al., 2007 [106]

This is due to a greater vasculature damage (and therefore a more prominent tumor hypoxia) being achieved when the light exposure occurs when the photosensitizer is still in the tumor vasculature [67]. The antitumor effect of nine bioreductive drugs (misonidazole, pimonidazole, metronidazole, nimorazole, RB6145, RSU1069, SR4233, mitomycin-C, or RB90740) used in combination with PDT was compared. It was concluded that RSU1069, RB6145 and mitomycin-C showed the best effect in combination with PDT [68]. Mitomycin C also induced an effect when given alone [68]. Several more studies have been carried out to examine the effect of mitomycin C in combination with PDT [50, 53, 68–76]. In all experimental studies mitomycin C enhanced the antitumor response of PDT and was selected for clinical trials in combination with PDT. In total 144 patients with advanced cardiac cancers were treated with HpD-mediated PDT, CHT, or PDT combined with CHT [52]. A combination of UFT (tegafur and uracil) and mitomycin C was used as standard CHT. A better treatment outcome was observed in patients treated with PDT and CHT than in patients treated with PDT or CHT alone [52]. Another clinical study involving 24 patients with recurrent superficial bladder cancer showed that combination therapy with sequential mitomycin C and ALA-PDT is safe, well tolerated, and effective [77].

The three platinum-containing drugs cisplatin, carboplatin, and oxaliplatin are classified as DNA alkylating agents and used to treat several types of cancer [78].

High-dose platinum-based therapy is accompanied by a set of severe toxic side effects [79] and tumor resistance [80]. Cisplatin combined with PDT has been investigated in vitro and in vivo [56, 81–85]. Low doses of cisplatin itself were ineffective, but in combination with PDT, it had a significant antitumor effect. Low doses of cisplatin may be as effective as currently used high doses if appropriately combined with PDT, and toxic effects on normal host tissues can be reduced [81, 83, 85].

Another effective drug in combination with PDT is adriamycin (doxorubicin) [50, 54, 66, 81, 86–90]. PDT combined with adriamycin may act synergistically [86–88] or antagonistically [54, 56], depending on the treatment sequences, treatment doses, and tumor types. The mechanism of interaction between PDT and adriamycin is not clear. Potentiation of PDT with HpD by adriamycin may be related to the fact that both of them act on mitochondria, and both form reactive oxygen species [90].

High doses of adriamycin, like of many other chemotherapeutic drugs, can cause suppression of bone marrow, and lead to mouth ulcers, sensitivity to sunlight, damage to heart muscle, and so forth [91]. Covalent binding of low molecular weight drugs to water-soluble polymer carriers offers a potential method to enhance the specificity of drug action and to reduce the drug concentration. N-(2-hydroxypropyl)methacrylamide (HPMA) copolymer was designed as an anticancer drug carrier [92]. HPMA copolymer-bound adriamycin gave marked advantages over free adriamycin [93]. HPMA copolymer-bound adriamycin and PDT with mesochlorin e6 acted synergistically in the treatment of ovarian cancer cells [93].

Tubulin is also a sensitive target to PDT [94, 95]. Combinations of PDT with HpD or TPPS2a and microtubule inhibitors, like vincristine or taxol, gave enhanced antitumor effects [55, 69].

Changes in cellular transport of a number of compounds occur after treatment with porphyrins and light [96, 97]. A 300% enhancement of short-term actinomycin D uptake as a result of photodynamic injury was reported by Kessel [98]. In order to explore the implications of the reported enhanced drug uptake, Creekmore and Zaharko [51] used actinomycin D in combination with Hp and red light. Actinomycin D (dactinomycin) is a well-known antibiotic of the actinomycin group that exhibits antibacterial and antitumor activity, which binds to DNA and inhibits transcription [99]. Enhanced uptake of toxic drugs by PDT led to additive or slightly synergistic toxic effects. It was already demonstrated in 1965 that actinomycin D may act as a fluorochrome and a photodynamic agent: Cells stained with actinomycin D exhibited a weak brownish fluorescence of nuclear material, and visible light in the presence of actinomycin D inactivated Venezuelan equine encephalitis virus [100]. Later it was found that actinomycin D binds to both double-stranded and single-stranded DNA, and such binding greatly enhances photodamage of DNA [101]. Radicals of superoxide anions and actinomycin D (absorption maximum in 440–460 nm region) were identified as important intermediates in the photodynamic process [101]. However, actinomycin D has not yet been used as a photosensitizer for PDT or in combination with PDT and other photosensitizers.

17.5   Hyperthermia (HT) Combined with PDT

In the 19th century, HT was already considered to be of therapeutic value in cancer treatment [107]. Studies on cell cultures and experimental tumors in animals in the 1970s demonstrated that tumor cells may be more sensitive to heat than normal cells [108]. HT can selectively kill chronically hypoxic, nutritionally deficient or with a low pH tumor cells in comparison with normal cells [108]. Furthermore, heat preferentially kills cells in the S phase, which is known to be resistant to RT [108].

Christensen et al. [109] and Waldow et al. [110, 111] were the first to use HT in combination with PDT in 1984. Since then, additive as well as synergistic interactions between PDT and HT have been demonstrated in several in vitro and in vivo studies (Table 17.4). The sequence and time interval between treatments are important [112–114]. Antagonistic or additive effects have been found when heat is given before PDT, while synergistic effects have been observed when PDT is given before HT [114, 115]. The reason for the low potentiating effect of HT (temperature above $44°$ C) given before PDT may be related to shutdown of blood vessels after HT. This may lead to the tumor tissue deoxygenation. The mechanisms of the synergistic interaction of PDT and postirradiation HT are not yet completely understood. PDT and HT may act on similar targets. Therefore, both therapies induce direct cell damage, protein inactivation, injury of repair system, activation of immune system, expression of heat-shock proteins, damage of microvasculature in tumors, and so forth [116]. It is known that PDT requires oxygen, while HT selectively inactivates hypoxic cells. Tumor cells become more sensitive to HT after PDT, because PDT leads to more acidic and at the same time more hypoxic conditions in the tumor.

Table 17.4   Summary of Results Obtained Using HT Combined with PDT

Model	Photosensitizer	Effects	References
Cells			
Human cervix carcinoma NHIK 3025	HPD	Synergistic	Christensen et al., 1984 [109]
EMR-6 mammary carcinoma	Photofrin II	Synergistic/ Additive	Mang and Dougherty, 1985 [113]
Squamous cell carcinoma, malignant melanoma, nonmalignant kidney cells	N,N'-Bis(2-ethyl-1,3-dioxylene) -kryptocyanine (EDKC)	Synergistic/ Additive	Oseroff et al., 1987 [117]
Mmouse lymphocytic leukemia L1210	HpD	Synergistic/ Additive	Miyoshi et al., 1988 [118]
Murine L929 fibroblasts	HpD	Additive	Boegheim et al., 1989 [119]
Normal skin fibroblasts, HT-1080 fibrosarcoma cells, squamous cell carcinoma SCC-25, malignant melanoma	AlPcS4	Synergistic/ Additive	Glassberg et al., 1991 [120]
Human skin fibroblast	Photosan 3	Additive	Krammer and Heidegger, 1996 [121]
Chinese hamster ovary CHO	Aluminum phthalocyanine chloride (AlPc)	Synergistic/ Additive	Rasch et al., 1996 [122]
Human skin fibroblasts	Photosan 3	Synergistic/ Additive	Krammer and Heidegger, 1996 [121]

Table 17.4 (continued)

Model	Photosensitizer	Effects	References
Wild-type (H69) and cisplatin-resistant mutant (H69/CDDP) human small cell lung cancer cells	Merocyanine 540	Synergistic/ Additive	Tsujino et al., 2001 [123]
Mice			
SMT-F mammary carcinoma	HpD	Synergistic	Waldow et al., 1984 [110]
RIF tumors	Photofrin II	Synergistic/ Anta-gonistic	Henderson et al., 1985 [115]
Ehrlich ascites	HpD	Synergistic/ Additive	Hau, 1990 [124]
Spontaneous mammary tumor (SMT-F)	Photofrin II	Synergistic	Mang, 1990 [125]
Squamous cell carcinoma	Hp oligomer	Synergistic	Matsumoto et al., 1990 [126]
Mammary carcinoma	Photofrin II	Synergistic/ Additive	Chen et al., 1996 [114]
NR-S1 carcinoma	Hp oligome	Synergistic/ Additive	Uehara et al., 1996 [127]
RIF-1	Hypericin	Synergistic	Chen et al., 1999 [128]
Human and rat glioma spheroids	ALA-PpIX	Synergistic	Hirschberg et al., 2004 [129]
Osteosarcoma	ALA-PpIX	Synergistic	Yanase et al., 2006 [130]
Rats			
Murine tumor rhabdomyosarcoma, type R-1	HpD	Synergistic/ Additive	Levendag et al., 1988 [131]
Liver tumor	ALA-PpIX	Synergistic/ Additive	Liu et al., 1997 [132]

17.6   Sonodynamic Therapy Combined with PDT

A new approach, so-called sonodynamic therapy, was introduced in the 1970s [133]. The goal was to overcome the limited tissue penetrating ability of light in PDT. Sonodynamic therapy is based on synergistic interactions of ultrasound and certain chemical compounds, sonosensitizers. Ultrasound of certain frequencies can penetrate deeply into tissues. It can be focused into a small region where the sonosensitizer can be activated. Drugs such as Photofrin, Photofrin II, Hp, zinc, and chloroaluminum phthalocyanines and PpIX can act not only as photosensitizers but also as sonosensitizers [134, 135].

Ultrasound acts on biological material in two ways: thermal and nonthermal processes. Thermal effects occur when the ultrasound energy is absorbed and transformed into heat. The thermal effects depend on the absorption and dissipation of the ultrasound energy. Nonthermal mechanisms can be classified as mainly shear stress and cavitation. Shear stress includes mechanical pressure, force, and fluid jet streaming on cellular membrane induced by ultrasound waves. Collapse of cavitation bubbles leads to the formation of radicals. In spite of the experimental proof of the sonodynamic effects, attempts to elucidate its action mechanisms have been so far unsuccessful [133].

An advantage of combining sonodynamic therapy and PDT is that the same drug can be used as a sonosensitizer and a photosensitizer, and deeper tumors can be treated at the same time. Only one experimental study has been reported on PDT combined with sonodynamic therapy [136]. The combination of PDT and ultrasound using either pheophorbide-a derivative PH-1126 or gallium porphyrin analogue ATX-70 resulted in significantly improved inhibition of tumor growth (additive effect) as compared to single treatments. Moreover, the median survival of tumor-bearing mice period given after PDT combined with sonodynamic therapy was significantly larger than that after single treatments. Histological changes revealed that combination therapies may induce tumor necrosis 2 to 3 times deeper than the single modalities do. The combination of PDT and sonodynamic therapy may be useful for treatment of nonsuperficial or nodular tumors, but further research is needed to understand the mechanisms behind it and to exploit them.

17.7   Other Methods Combined with PDT

PDT induces vasculature damage that initiates a physiological cascade of responses, including platelet aggregation, release of vasoactive molecules, leukocyte adhesion, increase in vascular permeability, and vessel constriction [60]. Since vascular endothelium may be damaged by PDT, it was thought that drugs affecting vasculature could modify the outcome of PDT. However, vasoactive drugs, as noradrenaline, propranolol, hydralazine, and phenoxybenzamine, either had no effect or inhibited the cytotoxicity of PDT [137]. Verapamil, a calcium channel blocker and a vasodilator, potentiated the action of PDT [137, 138], whereas other calcium channel blockers, such as diltiazem and nifedipine, had no effect [137].

PDT acts on tumor microenvironment. Angiogenesis and inflammation may follow [139]. These reactions are emerging as important determinants of PDT responsiveness [139, 140]. The relationship between PDT and angiogenesis was first documented by Gomer and colleagues [141]. Their studies in mice indicate that Photofrin-mediated PDT increased expression of hypoxia-inducible factor-1 alpha (HlF-1α), and also increased protein levels of the HIF-1 target gene, VEGF, in tumors [140–142]. Since tumor recurrence due to neovascularization can occur after PDT, the use of antiangiogenic compounds was proposed to improve PDT responsiveness [141]. The addition of antiangiogenic agents targeting VEGF, such as IM862, EMAP-II, Avastin, SU6668, or SU5416, enhanced the therapeutic efficacy of PDT with Photofrin or hypericin in mice [141–143]. Inhibitors of angiogenic-associated growth factor receptor tyrosine kinases, PD166285 and PD173074, also displayed potent antiangiogenic, and prolonged the duration of anti-tumor response to Photofrin-mediated PDT [144].

Cyclooxygenase-2 (COX-2) is an inducible enzyme involved in producing prostaglandins and other eicosanoids in inflammatory reaction and other pathologic processes. Increased expression of COX-2 has been found in several types of cancer (colon, breast, prostate, pancreas, and Barrett's oesophagus) and appears to control many cellular processes [145]. Inhibition of COX-2 influences angiogenesis, apoptosis, and metastatic potential, and can even increase the effect of RT [146]. One of the explanations for tumor recurrences after PDT may be that PDT is an efficient inducer of biologically active COX-2 expression [147, 148]. The combination of PDT with COX-2 inhibitors NS-398, rofecoxib, nimesulide, or celecoxib enhanced PDT responsiveness in vitro and in vivo [140, 147–151]. The sequences of the treatments are important: COX-2 inhibitors given alone or before PDT did not influence the therapeutic efficacy of the treatment [148], but their administration after PDT gave a significant improvement in long-term tumor-free survival [147, 148, 150]. COX-2 inhibition enhanced PDT-mediated apoptosis in vitro and decreased expression of angiogenic and inflammatory factors in treated tumors [150].

Degradation of extracellular matrix is crucial for growth, invasion, and metastasis of malignant tumor and angiogenesis. Matrix metalloproteinases (MMPs) are the family of zinc-dependent neutral endopeptidases collectively capable of degrading essentially all matrix components. Elevated levels of MMPs can be detected in tumor tissue or in serum of patients with advanced cancer, and their role as prognostic indicators in cancer has been widely examined [152, 153]. MMPs are involved in the early steps of tumor growth formation, including stimulation of cell proliferation and modulation of angiogenesis [153]. Certain MMP inhibitors may limit tumor growth [152, 153]. Therefore, the role of Photofrin-mediated PDT in eliciting expression of MMPs alone or in combination with a MMP inhibitor was investigated [140, 154]. Ferrario et al. documented increased protein expression of MMP-1, MMP-3, MMP-8, and MMP-9 in tumor after PDT [154]. Administration of a synthetic MMP inhibitor, Prinomastat, significantly improved PDT-mediated tumor response without affecting normal skin photosensitization [154].

Much work has been performed with the aim to enhance photocytotoxic reactions. The reactions of surviving cancer cells, as well as of normal host cells, are important elements for PDT outcome. PDT activates a variety of stress related genes and cell signaling pathways [140, 148, 155]. A deeper understanding of the molecular responses during PDT may help in choosing efficient combination therapies and in improving cancer responsiveness. Wong et al. investigated 29 kDa C/EBP homologous protein (CHOP), 78 kDa glucose regulated protein (GRP-78), and 70 kDa heat shock stress protein (HSP-70) expression patterns following PDT [156]. Porphyrin-mediated PDT induced expression of CHOP and GRP-78, but not of HSP-70, while NPe6-mediated PDT induced protein expression of HSP-70, but did not activate CHOP or GRP-78 expression. Molecular responses-induced by PDT depend on the intracellular localization of the photosensitizer and on the initial photodamage. It is of clinical interest to determine if PDT responsiveness can be changed modifying CHOP activity by different inhibitors [156].

PDT may change the VEGF level, which can lead to enhanced or decreased tumor growth and formation of metastasis. Lisnjak et al. found that the application of ALA-PDT resulted in reduced rate of metastatic spreading and decreased VEGF level (twofold) in blood serum of mice with Lewis lung carcinoma, and in morphologic alterations of the vascular system in tumor tissue [157]. On the other hand, another study showed that subcurative PDT in an orthotopic model of prostate cancer increased VEGF secretion (twofold) and more animals got lymph node metastases [8]. Antiangiogenic treatment in combination with PDT was proposed.

The authors found that a combination of PDT and an antiangiogenic agent, TNP-470, administered in the appropriate sequence, was more effective in controlling local tumor growth and metastases as well as in reducing disease-related toxicities [8].

Recombinant human tumor necrosis factor alpha (rHuTNF–α) or an antivascular drug 5, 6-dimethylxanthenone-4-acetic acid (DMXAA) have been also used to boost PDT [158, 159]. Such a combined therapy allowed reduction of the dose of photosensitizer or therapeutic light to be made without any loss in treatment efficiency. Lowering the drug dose may result in a decrease of side effects associated with PDT or DMXAA therapy. Systemic injection of TNF-α is highly toxic [160], while DMXAA induces TNF-α production mainly in tumors [161]. This makes the treatment more tolerable using PDT with DMXAA.

PDT is a strong activator of VEGF, MMP, and COX-2 derived prostaglandins in tumor microenvironments. These findings should inspire clinical trials to evaluate combination procedures involving PDT and VEGF, COX-2, or MMP inhibitors.

C225, a humanized murine monoclonal antibody (mAb) directed against the epidermal growth factor receptor (EGFR), was introduced by del Carmen et al. [162] as adoptive immunotherapy for benzoporphyrin derivative-based PDT. Synergistic enhancement of survival was observed, and the treatment was well tolerated. This finding indicates that combinations of PDT and immunotherapy with monoclonal antibodies may be easily introduced in clinical practice, since different mAb-based drugs are commercially available.

Abnormal tumor microvasculature and anemia are major causes for development of tumor hypoxia, which has been linked to treatment resistance, tumor progression, and poor prognosis [163]. Anemia is a common complication of cancer and its treatments, such as CHT and RT [164], and possibly PDT [21]. Anemia affects the outcome of CHT and RT negatively [164]. The influence of anemia on PDT outcome has not been studied in patients yet. PDT is mediated by oxygen-dependent photochemical reactions, and the oxygen concentration in the tissue is of critical importance for PDT outcome (PDT is less efficient in hypoxia and is completely inefficient in anoxia [62, 63]). Golab et al. studied the influence of CHT-induced anemia on PDT outcome in mice for the first time [165]. They found that anemia can influence the therapeutic effectiveness of PDT negatively and showed that erythropoietin, a regulator of red blood cell growth and differentiation, can improve PDT outcome [165]. Erythropoietin treatment alone had no effect on the growth rate of the investigated tumors. Combinations of anemia treatment by erythropoietin or other agents and PDT merit further clinical investigations [165].

Singlet oxygen is the most important reactive oxygen species in PDT for most photosensitizers [166]. Other reactive oxygen species, such as superoxide anion, hydrogen peroxide and hydroxyl radical, may also be generated during PDT [167]. Indications of increased generation of superoxide anion in cancer cells exposed to PDT has been published [167]. However, the influence of superoxide anion in photocytoxicity is not clear, because cells are able to scavenge this reactive oxygen species. Golab et al. found that superoxide dismutases, antioxidative enzymes, protect tumor cells from lethal damage induced by PDT [168]. The influence of superoxide dismutase inhibitors like sodium diethyldithiocarbamate, catalase (hydroxyl amine and 3, amino 1,2,4-triazole) and 2-methoxyestradiol in photosensitization was tested [168, 169]. Sodium diethyldithiocarbamate and catalase augmented Photofrin II mediated cutaneous photosensitization [169]. 2-methoxyestradiol, combined with Photofrin-mediated PDT, produced synergistic antitumor effects in vitro and in vivo [168]. Reduction of the superoxide dismutase activity by inhibitors may be an effective treatment modality to potentiate PDT [168, 169].

A low pH value of most tumors may play a role for the selective tumor uptake of photosensitizers [170]. Several studies have demonstrated that glucose administration lowers the tumor pH and enhances the tumor uptake of photosensitizers, and thereby increases phototoxicity [171]. Moreover, many other approaches (iontophoresis [172], electroporation [173], ultrasound [174], electromagnetic fields [175], and administration of aspirin [176]) are used in combination with PDT to increase drug delivery.

ALA-PDT efficiency may be increased by combinations with inhibitors of energy metabolism, like lonidamine and levamisole [177], with modulators of heme synthesis (iron chelators [178, 179]) and with differentiation-promoting hormone vitamin D [180].

17.8 Conclusions

In summary, combination of PDT with other therapeutic modalities may give considerable improvement of treatment efficiency over monotherapy alone. Unfortunately, the number of investigations is limited. Most experiments have been done with animals and cell lines. Well-designed clinical trials are needed to translate evidences into clinical practice guidelines.

Acknowledgments

We thank the Norwegian Cancer Society (Kreftforeningen) for financial support.

References

[1] Momma, T., et al., "Photodynamic therapy of orthotopic prostate cancer with benzoporphyrin derivative: local control and distant metastasis," *Cancer Res.*, Vol. 58, No. 23, 1998, pp. 5425–5431.

[2] Abulafi, A. M., et al., "Adjuvant intraoperative photodynamic therapy in experimental colorectal cancer using a new photosensitizer," *Br. J. Cancer*, Vol. 84, No. 3, 1997, pp. 368–371.

[3] van Hillegersberg R., et al., "Adjuvant intraoperative photodynamic therapy diminishes the rate of local recurrence in a rat mammary tumour model," *Br. J. Cancer*, Vol. 71, No. 4, 1995, pp. 733–737.

[4] Davis, R. K., et al., "Intraoperative phototherapy (PDT) and surgical resection in a mouse neuroblastoma model," *Lasers Surg. Med.*, Vol. 10, No. 3, 1990, pp. 275–279.

[5] Gomer, C. J., Ferrario, A., and Murphree, A. L., "The effect of localized porphyrin photodynamic therapy on the induction of tumour metastasis," *Br. J. Cancer*, Vol. 56, No. 1, 1987, pp. 27–32.

[6] Rousset, N., et al., "Effects of photodynamic therapy on adhesion molecules and metastasis," *J. Photochem. Photobiol. B*, Vol. 52, No. 1–3, 1999, pp. 65–73.

[7] Canti, G., et al., "Antitumor immunity induced by photodynamic therapy with aluminum disulfonated phthalocyanines and laser light," *Anticancer Drugs*, Vol. 5, No. 4, 1994, pp. 443–447.

[8] Kosharskyy, B., et al., "A mechanism-based combination therapy reduces local tumor growth and metastasis in an orthotopic model of prostate cancer," *Cancer Res.*, Vol. 66, No. 22, 2006, pp. 10953–10958.

[9] Baas, P., et al., "Photodynamic therapy as adjuvant therapy in surgically treated pleural malignancies," *Br. J. Cancer*, Vol. 76, No. 6, 1997, pp. 819–826.

[10] Pass, H. I., et al., "Phase III randomized trial of surgery with or without intraoperative photodynamic therapy and postoperative immunochemotherapy for malignant pleural mesothelioma," *Ann. Surg. Oncol.*, Vol. 4, No. 8, 1997, pp. 628–633.

[11] Friedberg, J. S., et al., "Phase II trial of pleural photodynamic therapy and surgery for patients with non-small-cell lung cancer with pleural spread," *J. Clin. Oncol.*, Vol. 22, No. 11, 2004, pp. 2192–2201.

[12] Kuijpers, D. I., et al., "Photodynamic therapy as adjuvant treatment of extensive basal cell carcinoma treated with Mohs micrographic surgery," *Dermatol. Surg.*, Vol. 30, No. 5, 2004, pp. 794–798.

[13] Nanashima, A., et al., "Adjuvant photodynamic therapy for bile duct carcinoma after surgery: a preliminary study," *J. Gastroenterol.*, Vol. 39, No. 11, 2004, pp. 1095–1101.

[14] Stylli, S. S., et al., "Photodynamic therapy of high grade glioma—long term survival," *J. Clin. Neurosci.*, Vol. 12, No. 4, 2005, pp. 389–398.

[15] Kostron, H., Fiegele, T., and Akatuna, E., "Combination of FOSCAN(R) mediated fluorescence guided resection and photodynamic treatment as new therapeutic concept for malignant brain tumors," *Med. Laser Appl.*, Vol. 21, No. 4, 2006, pp. 285–290.

[16] Kostron, H., et al., "The interaction of hematoporphyrin derivative, light, and ionizing radiation in a rat glioma model," *Cancer*, Vol. 57, No. 5, 1986, pp. 964–970.

[17] Zimmermann, A., Ritsch-Marte, M., and Kostron, H., "mTHPC-mediated photodynamic diagnosis of malignant brain tumors," *Photochem. Photobiol.*, Vol. 74, No. 4, 2001, pp. 611–616.

[18] DeLaney, T. F., et al., "Phase I study of debulking surgery and photodynamic therapy for disseminated intraperitoneal tumors," *Int. J. Radiat. Oncol. Biol. Phys.*, Vol. 25, No. 3, 1993, pp. 445–457.

[19] Allardice, J. T., et al., "Adjuvant intraoperative photodynamic therapy for colorectal carcinoma: a clinical study," *Surg. Oncol.*, Vol. 3, No. 1, 1994, pp. 1–10.

[20] Harlow, S. P., et al., "Intraoperative photodynamic therapy as an adjunct to surgery for recurrent rectal cancer," *Ann. Surg. Oncol.*, Vol. 2, No. 3, 1995, pp. 228–232.

[21] Hendren, S. K., et al., "Phase II trial of debulking surgery and photodynamic therapy for disseminated intraperitoneal tumors," *Ann. Surg. Oncol.*, Vol. 8, No. 1, 2001, pp. 65–71.

[22] Friedberg, J. S., et al., "A phase I study of Foscan-mediated photodynamic therapy and surgery in patients with mesothelioma," *Ann. Thorac. Surg.*, Vol. 75, No. 3, 2003, pp. 952–959.

[23] Libshitz, H. I., et al., "Radiation change in normal organs: an overview of body imaging," *Eur. Radiol.*, Vol. 6, No. 6, 1996, pp. 786–795.

[24] Schwartz, S., Absolon, K., and Vermund, H., "Some relationships of porphyrins, X-rays, and tumors," *Univ. Minn. Med. Bull.*, Vol. 27, 1955, pp. 7–13.

[25] Schaffer, M., et al., "Photofrin as a specific radiosensitizing agent for tumors: studies in comparison to other porphyrins, in an experimental in vivo model," *J. Photochem. Photobiol. B*, Vol. 66, No. 3, 2002, pp. 157–164.

[26] Kulka, U., et al., "Photofrin as a radiosensitizer in an in vitro cell survival assay," *Biochem. Biophys. Res. Commun.*, Vol. 311, No. 1, 2003, pp. 98–103.

[27] Colasanti, A., et al., "Combined effects of radiotherapy and photodynamic therapy on an in vitro human prostate model," *Acta Biochim. Pol.*, Vol. 51, No. 4, 2004, pp. 1039–1046.

[28] Schaffer, M., et al., "Radiation therapy combined with photofrin or 5-ALA: effect on Lewis sarcoma tumor lines implanted in mice. Preliminary results," *Tumori*, Vol. 88, No. 5, 2002, pp. 407–410.

[29] Luksiene, Z., Kalvelyte, A., and Supino, R., "On the combination of photodynamic therapy with ionizing radiation," *J. Photochem. Photobiol. B*, Vol. 52, No. 1–3, 1999, pp. 35–42.

[30] Dobler-Girdziunaite, D., et al., "The combined use of photodynamic therapy with ionizing radiation on breast carcinoma cells in vitro," *Strahlenther. Onkol.*, Vol. 171, No. 11, 1995, pp. 622–629.

[31] Luksiene, Z., Juzenas, P., and Moan, J., "Radiosensitization of tumours by porphyrins," *Cancer Lett.*, Vol. 235, No. 1, 2006, pp. 40–47.

[32] Lam, S., et al., "Combined photodynamic therapy and radiotherapy in the treatment of obstructive endobronchial tumors." In *Photodynamic Therapy of Tumours and Other Diseases*, pp. 321–324, G. Jori and C. Perria (eds.), Padova: Libreria Progetto Editore, 1985.

[33] Bellnier, D. A. and Dougherty, T. J., "Haematoporphyrin derivative photosensitization and gamma-radiation damage interaction in Chinese hamster ovary fibroblasts," *Int. J. Radiat. Biol. Relat Stud. Phys. Chem. Med.*, Vol. 50, No. 4, 1986, pp. 659–664.

[34] Graschew, G. and Shopova, M., "Photodynamic therapy and -irradiation of tumours: Effect of tumour-cell reoxygenation," *Lasers Med. Sci.*, Vol. 1, No. 3, 1986, pp. 193–195.

[35] Ohnishi, Y., Yamana, Y., and Minei, M., "Photoradiation therapy using argon laser and a hematoporphyrin derivative for retinoblastoma—a preliminary report," *Jpn. J. Ophthalmol.*, Vol. 30, No. 4, 1986, pp. 409–419.

[36] Kaye, A. H., Morstyn, G., and Brownbill, D., "Adjuvant high-dose photoradiation therapy in the treatment of cerebral glioma: a phase 1-2 study," *J. Neurosurg.*, Vol. 67, No. 4, 1987, pp. 500–505.

[37] Prinsze, C., et al., "Interaction of photodynamic treatment and either hyperthermia or ionizing radiation and of ionizing radiation and hyperthermia with respect to cell killing of L929 fibroblasts, Chinese hamster ovary cells, and T24 human bladder carcinoma cells," *Cancer Res.*, Vol. 52, No. 1, 1992, pp. 117–120.

[38] Schnitzhofer, G. M. and Krammer, B., "Photodynamic treatment and radiotherapy: combined effect on the colony-forming ability of V79 Chinese hamster fibroblasts," *Cancer Lett.*, Vol. 108, No. 1, 1996, pp. 93–99.

[39] Kukielczak, B., Romanowska, B., and Bryk, J., "Gamma radiation and MC540 photosensitization of melanoma in the hamster's eye," *Melanoma Res.*, Vol. 9, No. 2, 1999, pp. 115–124.

[40] Allman, R., Cowburn, P., and Mason, M., "Effect of photodynamic therapy in combination with ionizing radiation on human squamous cell carcinoma cell lines of the head and neck," *Br. J. Cancer*, Vol. 83, No. 5, 2000, pp. 655–661.

[41] Ramakrishnan, N., et al., "Post-treatment interactions of photodynamic and radiation-induced cytotoxic lesions," *Photochem. Photobiol.*, Vol. 52, No. 3, 1990, pp. 555–559.

[42] Kavarnos, G., Nath, R., and Bongiorni, P., "Visible-light and X irradiations of Chinese hamster lung cells treated with hematoporphyrin derivative," *Radiat. Res.*, Vol. 137, No. 2, 1994, pp. 196–201.

[43] Berg, K., et al., "Combined treatment of ionizing radiation and photosensitization by 5-aminolevulinic acid-induced protoporphyrin IX," *Radiat. Res.*, Vol. 142, No. 3, 1995, pp. 340–346.

[44] Ma, L., Iani, V., and Moan, J., "Combination therapy: photochemotherapy; electric current; and ionizing radiation. Different combinations studied in a WiDr human colon

adenocarcinoma cell line," *J. Photochem. Photobiol. B*, Vol. 21, No. 2–3, 1993, pp. 149–154.

[45] Prise, K. M., et al., "New insights on cell death from radiation exposure," *Lancet Oncol.*, Vol. 6, No. 7, 2005, pp. 520–528.

[46] Peng, Q., Moan, J., and Nesland, J. M., "Correlation of subcellular and intratumoral photosensitizer localization with ultrastructural features after photodynamic therapy," *Ultrastruct. Pathol.*, Vol. 20, No. 2, 1996, pp. 109–129.

[47] Winther, J., Overgaard, J., and Ehlers, N., "The effect of photodynamic therapy alone and in combination with misonidazole or X-rays for management of a retinoblastoma-like tumour," *Photochem. Photobiol.*, Vol. 47, No. 3, 1988, pp. 419–423.

[48] Lam, S., et al., "Combined photodynamic therapy using Photofrin and radiotherapy versus radiotherapy alone in patients with inoperable obstructive nonsmall-cell bronchogenic carcinoma," *Proc. SPIE*, Vol. 1616, 1993, pp. 20–28.

[49] Bartelink, H., Schellens, J. H., and Verheij, M., "The combined use of radiotherapy and chemotherapy in the treatment of solid tumours," *Eur. J. Cancer*, Vol. 38, No. 2, 2002, pp. 216–222.

[50] Cho, Y. H., Straight, R. C., and Smith, J. A., Jr., "Effects of photodynamic therapy in combination with intravesical drugs in a murine bladder tumor model," *J. Urol.*, Vol. 147, No. 3, 1992, pp. 743–746.

[51] Creekmore, S. P. and Zaharko, D. S., "Modification of chemotherapeutic effects on L1210 cells using hematoporphyrin and light," *Cancer Res.*, Vol. 43, No. 11, 1983, pp. 5252–5257.

[52] Jin, M. L., et al., "Combined treatment with photodynamic therapy and chemotherapy for advanced cardiac cancers," *J. Photochem. Photobiol. B*, Vol. 12, No. 1, 1992, pp. 101–106.

[53] Ma, L. W., et al., "Potentiation of photodynamic therapy by mitomycin C in cultured human colon adenocarcinoma cells," *Radiat. Res.*, Vol. 134, No. 1, 1993, pp. 22–28.

[54] Cowled, P. A., Mackenzie, L., and Forbes, I. J., "Pharmacological modulation of photodynamic therapy with hematoporphyrin derivative and light," *Cancer Res.*, Vol. 47, No. 4, 1987, pp. 971–974.

[55] Ma, L. W., et al., "Enhanced antitumour effect of photodynamic therapy by microtubule inhibitors," *Cancer Lett.*, Vol. 109, No. 1–2, 1996, pp. 129–139.

[56] Nahabedian, M. Y., et al., "Combination cytotoxic chemotherapy with cisplatin or doxorubicin and photodynamic therapy in murine tumors," *J. Natl. Cancer Inst.*, Vol. 80, No. 10, 1988, pp. 739–743.

[57] Ma, L. W. and Moan, J., "Developments in photodynamic therapy in combination with other treatment modalities," *Recent Research Develop Photochem Photobiol*, Vol. 2, 1998, pp. 65–83.

[58] Weinmann, M., Belka, C., and Plasswilm, L., "Tumour hypoxia: impact on biology, prognosis and treatment of solid malignant tumours," *Onkologie*, Vol. 27, No. 1, 2004, pp. 83–90.

[59] Foster, T. H., et al., "Oxygen consumption and diffusion effects in photodynamic therapy," *Radiat. Res.*, Vol. 126, No. 3, 1991, pp. 296–303.

[60] Krammer, B., "Vascular effects of photodynamic therapy," *Anticancer Res.*, Vol. 21, No. 6B, 2001, pp. 4271–4277.

[61] Graschew, G. and Shopova, M., "Hypoxia, misonidazole and hyperthermia in photodynamic therapy of tumours," *Lasers Med. Sci.*, Vol. 1, No. 3, 1986, pp. 181–186.

[62] Henderson, B. W. and Fingar, V. H., "Relationship of tumor hypoxia and response to photodynamic treatment in an experimental mouse tumor," *Cancer Res.*, Vol. 47, No. 12, 1987, pp. 3110–3114.

[63] Moan, J. and Sommer, S., "Oxygen dependence of the photosensitizing effect of hematoporphyrin derivative in NHIK 3025 cells," *Cancer Res.*, Vol. 45, No. 4, 1985, pp. 1608–1610.

[64] Gonzalez, S., et al., "Treatment of Dunning R3327-AT rat prostate tumors with photodynamic therapy in combination with misonidazole," *Cancer Res.*, Vol. 46, No. 6, 1986, pp. 2858–2862.

[65] Konig, K. and Bockhorn, V., "The effect of nitroimidazole and photochemotherapy on solid Ehrlich carcinomas," *Radiobiol. Radiother. (Berl)*, Vol. 30, No. 6, 1989, pp. 535–539.

[66] Dima, V. F., et al., "Studies of the effects of associated photodynamic therapy and drugs on macromolecular synthesis of tumoral cells grown in vitro," *Arch. Roum. Pathol. Exp. Microbiol.*, Vol. 49, No. 2, 1990, pp. 155–175.

[67] Bremner, J. C., et al., "Increasing the effect of photodynamic therapy on the RIF-1 murine sarcoma, using the bioreductive drugs RSU1069 and RB6145," *Br. J. Cancer*, Vol. 66, No. 6, 1992, pp. 1070–1076.

[68] Bremner, J. C., et al., "Comparing the anti-tumor effect of several bioreductive drugs when used in combination with photodynamic therapy (PDT)," *Int. J. Radiat. Oncol. Biol. Phys.*, Vol. 29, No. 2, 1994, pp. 329–332.

[69] Niu, M. Y., "[Effect of combined use of chemotherapeutic agents and hematoporphyrin derivative (HPD) on human gastric cancer cell line in vitro]," *Zhonghua Zhong. Liu Za Zhi.*, Vol. 14, No. 1, 1992, pp. 70–72.

[70] Baas, P., et al., "Enhancement of interstitial photodynamic therapy by mitomycin C and EO9 in a mouse tumour model," *Int. J. Cancer*, Vol. 56, No. 6, 1994, pp. 880–885.

[71] Ma, L. W., et al., "Anti-tumour activity of photodynamic therapy in combination with mitomycin C in nude mice with human colon adenocarcinoma," *Br. J. Cancer*, Vol. 71, No. 5, 1995, pp. 950–956.

[72] van Geel, I. P., et al., "Mechanisms for optimising photodynamic therapy: second-generation photosensitisers in combination with mitomycin C," *Br. J. Cancer*, Vol. 72, No. 2, 1995, pp. 344–350.

[73] Veenhuizen, R. B., et al., "Intraperitoneal photodynamic therapy of the rat CC531 adenocarcinoma," *Br. J. Cancer*, Vol. 73, No. 11, 1996, pp. 1387–1392.

[74] Datta, S. N., et al., "Effect of photodynamic therapy in combination with mitomycin C on a mitomycin-resistant bladder cancer cell line," *Br. J. Cancer*, Vol. 76, No. 3, 1997, pp. 312–317.

[75] Chen, B., et al., "Potentiation of photodynamic therapy with hypericin by mitomycin C in the radiation-induced fibrosarcoma-1 mouse tumor model," *Photochem. Photobiol.*, Vol. 78, No. 3, 2003, pp. 278–282.

[76] French, A. J., et al., "Investigation of sequential mitomycin C and photodynamic therapy in a mitomycin-resistant bladder cancer cell-line model," *BJU Int.*, Vol. 93, No. 1, 2004, pp. 156–161.

[77] Skyrme, R. J., et al., "A phase-1 study of sequential mitomycin C and 5-aminolaevulinic acid-mediated photodynamic therapy in recurrent superficial bladder carcinoma," *BJU Int.*, Vol. 95, No. 9, 2005, pp. 1206–1210.

[78] Kelland, L., "Broadening the clinical use of platinum drug-based chemotherapy with new analogues. Satraplatin and picoplatin," *Expert. Opin. Investig. Drugs*, Vol. 16, No. 7, 2007, pp. 1009–1021.

[79] Galanski, M. and Keppler, B. K., "Searching for the magic bullet: anticancer platinum drugs which can be accumulated or activated in the tumor tissue," *Anticancer Agents Med Chem.*, Vol. 7, No. 1, 2007, pp. 55–73.

[80] Rabik, C. A. and Dolan, M. E., "Molecular mechanisms of resistance and toxicity associated with platinating agents," *Cancer Treat. Rev.*, Vol. 33, No. 1, 2007, pp. 9–23.

[81] Canti, G., et al., "Antitumor efficacy of the combination of photodynamic therapy and chemotherapy in murine tumors," *Cancer Lett.*, Vol. 125, No. 1–2, 1998, pp. 39–44.

[82] Nonaka, M., Ikeda, H., and Inokuchi, T., "Effect of combined photodynamic and chemotherapeutic treatment on lymphoma cells in vitro," *Cancer Lett.*, Vol. 184, No. 2, 2002, pp. 171–178.

[83]   Crescenzi, E., et al., "Photodynamic therapy with indocyanine green complements and enhances low-dose cisplatin cytotoxicity in MCF-7 breast cancer cells," *Mol. Cancer Ther.*, Vol. 3, No. 5, 2004, pp. 537–544.

[84]   Lottner, C., et al., "Combined chemotherapeutic and photodynamic treatment on human bladder cells by hematoporphyrin-platinum(II) conjugates," *Cancer Lett.*, Vol. 203, No. 2, 2004, pp. 171–180.

[85]   Uehara, M., Inokuchi, T., and Ikeda, H., "Enhanced susceptibility of mouse squamous cell carcinoma to photodynamic therapy combined with low-dose administration of cisplatin," *J. Oral Maxillofac. Surg.*, Vol. 64, No. 3, 2006, pp. 390–396.

[86]   Edell, E. S. and Cortese, D. A., "Combined effects of hematoporphyrin derivative phototherapy and adriamycin in a murine tumor model," *Lasers Surg. Med.*, Vol. 8, No. 4, 1988, pp. 413–417.

[87]   Brophy, P. F. and Keller, S. M., "Adriamycin enhanced in vitro and in vivo photodynamic therapy of mesothelioma," *J. Surg. Res.*, Vol. 52, No. 6, 1992, pp. 631–634.

[88]   Peterson, C. M., et al., "Isobolographic assessment of the interaction between adriamycin and photodynamic therapy with meso-chlorin e6 monoethylene diamine in human epithelial ovarian carcinoma (OVCAR-3) in vitro," *J. Soc. Gynecol. Investig.*, Vol. 2, No. 6, 1995, pp. 772–777.

[89]   Casas, A., et al., "Enhancement of aminolevulinic acid based photodynamic therapy by adriamycin," *Cancer Lett.*, Vol. 121, No. 1, 1997, pp. 105–113.

[90]   Streckyte, G., et al., "Effects of photodynamic therapy in combination with Adriamycin," *Cancer Lett.*, Vol. 146, No. 1, 1999, pp. 73–86.

[91]   Gewirtz, D. A., "A critical evaluation of the mechanisms of action proposed for the antitumor effects of the anthracycline antibiotics adriamycin and daunorubicin," *Biochem. Pharmacol.*, Vol. 57, No. 7, 1999, pp. 727–741.

[92]   Shiah, J. G., et al., "Antitumor activity of N-(2-hydroxypropyl) methacrylamide copolymer-Mesochlorine e6 and adriamycin conjugates in combination treatments," *Clin. Cancer Res.*, Vol. 6, No. 3, 2000, pp. 1008–1015.

[93]   Peterson, C. M., et al., "HPMA copolymer delivery of chemotherapy and photodynamic therapy in ovarian cancer," *Adv. Exp. Med. Biol.*, Vol. 519, 2003, pp. 101–123.

[94]   Berg, K. and Moan, J., "Photodynamic effects of Photofrin II on cell division in human NHIK 3025 cells," *Int. J. Radiat. Biol. Relat Stud. Phys. Chem. Med.*, Vol. 53, No. 5, 1988, pp. 797–811.

[95]   Sporn, L. A. and Foster, T. H., "Photofrin and light induces microtubule depolymerization in cultured human endothelial cells," *Cancer Res.*, Vol. 52, No. 12, 1992, pp. 3443–3448.

[96]   Moan, J. and Christensen, T., "Cellular uptake and photodynamic effect of hematoporphyrin," *Photochem. Photobiophys.*, Vol. 2, 1981, pp. 291–299.

[97]   Dubbelman, T. M., De Goeij, A. F., and Van, S. J., "Protoporphyrin-induced photodynamic effects on transport processes across the membrane of human erythrocytes," *Biochim. Biophys. Acta*, Vol. 595, No. 1, 1980, pp. 133–139.

[98]   Kessel, D., "Effects of photoactivated porphyrins at the cell surface of leukemia L1210 cells," *Biochemistry*, Vol. 16, No. 15, 1977, pp. 3443–3449.

[99]   Koba, M. and Konopa, J., "Actinomycin D and its mechanisms of action," *Postepy Hig.Med Dosw.(Online.)*, Vol. 59, 2005, pp. 290–298.

[100]   Zhdanov, V. M. and Yershov, F. I., "Photodynamic and fluorochromic properties of the antibiotic actinomycin D," *J. Cell. Physiol.*, Vol. 65, No. 3, 1965, pp. 433–434.

[101]   Pan, J. X., et al., "Photodynamic action of actinomycin D: an EPR spin trapping study," *Biochim. Biophys. Acta*, Vol. 1527, No. 1–2, 2001, pp. 1–3.

[102]   Kabuto, M., et al., "Antitumor effect of MX2, a new morpholino anthracycline against C6 glioma cells and its combination effect with photodynamic therapy in vitro," *No To Shinkei*, Vol. 47, No. 10, 1995, pp. 969–973.

[103] Gantchev, T. G., Brasseur, N., and van Lier, J. E., "Combination toxicity of etoposide (VP-16) and photosensitisation with a water-soluble aluminium phthalocyanine in K562 human leukaemic cells," *Br. J. Cancer*, Vol. 74, No. 10, 1996, pp. 1570–1577.

[104] Sinha, A. K., et al., "Methotrexate used in combination with aminolaevulinic acid for photodynamic killing of prostate cancer cells," *Br. J. Cancer*, Vol. 95, No. 4, 2006, pp. 485–495.

[105] Baas, P., et al., "Enhancement of photodynamic therapy by mitomycin C: a preclinical and clinical study," *Br. J. Cancer*, Vol. 73, No. 8, 1996, pp. 945–951.

[106] Zhang, N. Z., et al., "Photodynamic therapy combined with local chemotherapy for the treatment of advanced esophagocardiac carcinoma," *Photodiagn. Photodyn. Ther.*, Vol. 4, No. 1, 2007, pp. 60–64.

[107] Issels, R., et al., "Hyperthermia in cancer research. Historical development, current status of research, future perspectives and differentiation from alternative medical procedures," *Versicherungsmedizin*, Vol. 41, No. 2, 1989, pp. 48–53.

[108] Connor, W. G., et al., "Prospects for hyperthermia in human cancer therapy. Part II: implications of biological and physical data for applications of hyperthermia to man," *Radiology*, Vol. 123, No. 2, 1977, pp. 497–503.

[109] Christensen, T., Wahl, A., and Smedshammer, L., "Effects of haematoporphyrin derivative and light in combination with hyperthermia on cells in culture," *Br. J. Cancer*, Vol. 50, No. 1, 1984, pp. 85–89.

[110] Waldow, S. M., Henderson, B. W., and Dougherty, T. J., "Enhanced tumor control following sequential treatments of photodynamic therapy (PDT) and localized microwave hyperthermia in vivo," *Lasers Surg. Med.*, Vol. 4, No. 1, 1984, pp. 79–85.

[111] Waldow, S. M. and Dougherty, T. J., "Interaction of hyperthermia and photoradiation therapy," *Radiat. Res.*, Vol. 97, No. 2, 1984, pp. 380–385.

[112] Waldow, S. M., Henderson, B. W., and Dougherty, T. J., "Potentiation of photodynamic therapy by heat: effect of sequence and time interval between treatments in vivo," *Lasers Surg. Med.*, Vol. 5, No. 2, 1985, pp. 83–94.

[113] Mang, T. S. and Dougherty, T. J., "Time and sequence dependent influence of in vitro photodynamic therapy (PDT) survival by hyperthermia," *Photochem. Photobiol.*, Vol. 42, No. 5, 1985, pp. 533–540.

[114] Chen, Q., et al., "Sequencing of combined hyperthermia and photodynamic therapy," *Radiat. Res.,* Vol. 146, No. 3, 1996, pp. 293–297.

[115] Henderson, B. W., et al., "Interaction of photodynamic therapy and hyperthermia: tumor response and cell survival studies after treatment of mice in vivo," *Cancer Res.*, Vol. 45, No. 12 Pt. 1, 1985, pp. 6071–6077.

[116] Wust, P., et al., "Hyperthermia in combined treatment of cancer," *Lancet Oncol.*, Vol. 3, No. 8, 2002, pp. 487–497.

[117] Oseroff, A. R., Ohuoha, D., and Ara, G., "Mild hyperthermia synergistically enhances killing of malignant cells by the cationic photosensitizer EDKC: implications for a "selective photohyperthermic therapy," *Proc. SPIE*, Vol. 847, 1987, pp. 11–14.

[118] Miyoshi, N., et al., "The effect of hyperthermia on murine leukaemia cells in combination with photodynamic therapy," *Int. J. Hyperthermia*, Vol. 4, No. 2, 1988, pp. 203–209.

[119] Boegheim, J. P., et al., "Damaging action of photodynamic treatment in combination with hyperthermia on transmembrane transport in murine L929 fibroblasts," *Biochim. Biophys. Acta*, Vol. 979, No. 2, 1989, pp. 215–220.

[120] Glassberg, E., et al., "Hyperthermia potentiates the effects of aluminum phthalocyanine tetrasulfonate-mediated photodynamic toxicity in human malignant and normal cell lines," *Lasers Surg. Med.*, Vol. 11, No. 5, 1991, pp. 432–439.

[121] Krammer, B. and Heidegger, W., "Investigation of the combined effect of photodynamic cell treatment and hyperthermia by transmembrane resting potential measurement of human skin fibroblasts," *Bioelectrochem. Bioenerg.*, Vol. 39, No. 1, 1996, pp. 109–113.

[122] Rasch, M. H., et al., "Synergistic interaction of photodynamic treatment with the sensitizer aluminum phthalocyanine and hyperthermia on loss of clonogenicity of CHO cells," *Photochem. Photobiol.*, Vol. 64, No. 3, 1996, pp. 586–593.

[123] Tsujino, I., Anderson, G. S., and Sieber, F., "Postirradiation hyperthermia selectively potentiates the merocyanine 540-sensitized photoinactivation of small cell lung cancer cells," *Photochem. Photobiol.*, Vol. 73, No. 2, 2001, pp. 191–198.

[124] Hau, D. M., Chang, H., and Hsu, H. Y., "Effects of hyperthermia and photodynamic therapy on BALB/c mice bearing subcutaneous tumors," *Proc. Natl. Sci. Counc. Repub. China B*, Vol. 14, No. 1, 1990, pp. 20–26.

[125] Mang, T. S., "Combination studies of hyperthermia induced by the neodymium: yttrium-aluminum-garnet (Nd:YAG) laser as an adjuvant to photodynamic therapy," *Lasers Surg. Med.*, Vol. 10, No. 2, 1990, pp. 173–178.

[126] Matsumoto, N., et al., "Combination effect of hyperthermia and photodynamic therapy on carcinoma," Arch. Otolaryngol. Head Neck Surg., Vol. 116, No. 7, 1990, pp. 824–829.

[127] Uehara, M., Inokuchi, T., and Sano, K., "Experimental study of combined hyperthermic and photodynamic therapy on carcinoma in the mouse," *J. Oral Maxillofac. Surg.*, Vol. 54, No. 6, 1996, pp. 729–736.

[128] Chen, B., et al., "Synergistic effect of photodynamic therapy with hypericin in combination with hyperthermia on loss of clonogenicity of RIF-1 cells," *Int. J. Oncol.*, Vol. 18, No. 6, 2001, pp. 1279–1285.

[129] Hirschberg, H., et al., "Enhanced cytotoxic effects of 5-aminolevulinic acid-mediated photodynamic therapy by concurrent hyperthermia in glioma spheroids," *J. Neurooncol.*, Vol. 70, No. 3, 2004, pp. 289–299.

[130] Yanase, S., et al., "Synergistic interaction of 5-aminolevulinic acid-based photodynamic therapy with simultaneous hyperthermia in an osteosarcoma tumor model," *Int. J. Oncol.*, Vol. 29, No. 2, 2006, pp. 365–373.

[131] Levendag, P. C., et al., "Interaction of interstitial photodynamic therapy and interstitial hyperthermia in a rat rhabdomyosarcoma—a pilot study," *Int. J. Radiat. Oncol. Biol. Phys.*, Vol. 14, No. 1, 1988, pp. 139–145.

[132] Liu, D. L., et al., "Tumour vessel damage resulting from laser-induced hyperthermia alone and in combination with photodynamic therapy," *Cancer Lett.*, Vol. 111, No. 1–2, 1997, pp. 157–165.

[133] Milowska, K., "Ultrasound—mechanisms of action and application in sonodynamic therapy," *Postepy Hig. Med Dosw.(Online.)*, Vol. 61, 2007, pp. 338–349.

[134] Yumita, N. and Umemura, S., "Sonodynamic therapy with photofrin II on AH130 solid tumor. Pharmacokinetics, tissue distribution and sonodynamic antitumoral efficacy of photofrin II," *Cancer Chemother. Pharmacol.*, Vol. 51, No. 2, 2003, pp. 174–178.

[135] Liu, Q., et al., "Comparison between sonodynamic effect with protoporphyrin IX and hematoporphyrin on sarcoma 180," *Cancer Chemother. Pharmacol.*, Vol. 60, No. 5, 2007, pp. 671–680.

[136] Jin, Z. H., et al., "Combination effect of photodynamic and sonodynamic therapy on experimental skin squamous cell carcinoma in C3H/HeN mice," *J. Dermatol.*, Vol. 27, No. 5, 2000, pp. 294–306.

[137] Cowled, P. A. and Forbes, I. J., "Modification by vasoactive drugs of tumour destruction by photodynamic therapy with haematoporphyrin derivative," *Br. J. Cancer*, Vol. 59, No. 6, 1989, pp. 904–909.

[138] Purkiss, S. F., Grahn, M. F., and Williams, N. S., "Haematoporphyrin derivative—photodynamic therapy of colorectal carcinoma, sensitized using verapamil and adriamycin," *Surg. Oncol.*, Vol. 5, No. 4, 1996, pp. 169–175.

[139] Gollnick, S. O., et al., "Role of cytokines in photodynamic therapy-induced local and systemic inflammation," *Br. J. Cancer*, Vol. 88, No. 11, 2003, pp. 1772–1779.

[140] Gomer, C. J., et al., "Photodynamic therapy: combined modality approaches targeting the tumor microenvironment," *Lasers Surg. Med.*, Vol. 38, No. 5, 2006, pp. 516–521.

[141] Ferrario, A., et al., "Antiangiogenic treatment enhances photodynamic therapy responsiveness in a mouse mammary carcinoma," *Cancer Res.*, Vol. 60, No. 15, 2000, pp. 4066–4069.

[142] Ferrario, A. and Gomer, C. J., "Avastin enhances photodynamic therapy treatment of Kaposi's sarcoma in a mouse tumor model," *J. Environ. Pathol. Toxicol. Oncol.*, Vol. 25, No. 1–2, 2006, pp. 251–259.

[143] Zhou, Q., et al., "Enhancing the therapeutic responsiveness of photodynamic therapy with the antiangiogenic agents SU5416 and SU6668 in murine nasopharyngeal carcinoma models," *Cancer Chemother. Pharmacol.*, Vol. 56, No. 6, 2005, pp. 569–577.

[144] Dimitroff, C. J., et al., "Anti-angiogenic activity of selected receptor tyrosine kinase inhibitors, PD166285 and PD173074: implications for combination treatment with photodynamic therapy," *Invest New Drugs*, Vol. 17, No. 2, 1999, pp. 121–135.

[145] Sarkar, F. H., et al., "Back to the future: COX-2 inhibitors for chemoprevention and cancer therapy," *Mini. Rev. Med Chem.*, Vol. 7, No. 6, 2007, pp. 599–608.

[146] Giercksky, K. E., "COX-2 inhibition and prevention of cancer," *Best Pract. Res. Clin. Gastroenterol.*, Vol. 15, No. 5, 2001, pp. 821–833.

[147] Ferrario, A., et al., "Cyclooxygenase-2 inhibitor treatment enhances photodynamic therapy-mediated tumor response," *Cancer Res.*, Vol. 62, No. 14, 2002, pp. 3956–3961.

[148] Makowski, M., et al., "Inhibition of cyclooxygenase-2 indirectly potentiates antitumor effects of photodynamic therapy in mice," *Clin. Cancer Res.*, Vol. 9, No. 14, 2003, pp. 5417–5422.

[149] Akita, Y., et al., "Cyclooxygenase-2 is a possible target of treatment approach in conjunction with photodynamic therapy for various disorders in skin and oral cavity," *Br. J. Dermatol.*, Vol. 151, No. 2, 2004, pp. 472–480.

[150] Ferrario, A., et al., "Celecoxib and NS-398 enhance photodynamic therapy by increasing in vitro apoptosis and decreasing in vivo inflammatory and angiogenic factors," *Cancer Res.*, Vol. 65, No. 20, 2005, pp. 9473–9478.

[151] Harvey, E. H., et al., "Killing tumor cells: the effect of photodynamic therapy using mono-L-aspartyl chlorine and NS-398," *Am. J. Surg.*, Vol. 189, No. 3, 2005, pp. 302–305.

[152] Coussens, L. M., Fingleton, B., and Matrisian, L. M., "Matrix metalloproteinase inhibitors and cancer: trials and tribulations," *Science*, Vol. 295, No. 5564, 2002, pp. 2387–2392.

[153] Vihinen, P., la-aho, R., and Kahari, V. M., "Matrix metalloproteinases as therapeutic targets in cancer," *Curr. Cancer Drug Targets*, Vol. 5, No. 3, 2005, pp. 203–220.

[154] Ferrario, A., et al., "The matrix metalloproteinase inhibitor prinomastat enhances photodynamic therapy responsiveness in a mouse tumor model," *Cancer Res.*, Vol. 64, No. 7, 2004, pp. 2328–2332.

[155] Oleinick, N. L. and Evans, H. H., "The photobiology of photodynamic therapy: cellular targets and mechanisms," *Radiat. Res.*, Vol. 150, No. 5 Suppl, 1998, pp. S146–S156.

[156] Wong, S., et al., "CHOP activation by photodynamic therapy increases treatment induced photosensitization," *Lasers Surg. Med*, Vol. 35, No. 5, 2004, pp. 336–341.

[157] Lisnjak, I. O., et al., "Effect of photodynamic therapy on tumor angiogenesis and metastasis in mice bearing Lewis lung carcinoma," *Exp. Oncol.*, Vol. 27, No. 4, 2005, pp. 333–335.

[158] Bellnier, D. A., et al., "Treatment with the tumor necrosis factor-alpha-inducing drug 5,6-dimethylxanthenone-4-acetic acid enhances the antitumor activity of the photodynamic therapy of RIF-1 mouse tumors," *Cancer Res.*, Vol. 63, No. 22, 2003, pp. 7584–7590.

[159] Seshadri, M., et al., "Tumor vascular response to photodynamic therapy and the antivascular agent 5,6-dimethylxanthenone-4-acetic acid: implications for combination therapy," *Clin. Cancer Res.*, Vol. 11, No. 11, 2005, pp. 4241–4250.

[160] Mocellin, S., et al., "Tumor necrosis factor, cancer and anticancer therapy," *Cytokine Growth Factor Rev.*, Vol. 16, No. 1, 2005, pp. 35–53.

[161] Joseph, W. R., et al., "Stimulation of tumors to synthesize tumor necrosis factor-alpha in situ using 5,6-dimethylxanthenone-4-acetic acid: a novel approach to cancer therapy," *Cancer Res.*, Vol. 59, No. 3, 1999, pp. 633–638.

[162] del Carmen, M. G., et al., "Synergism of epidermal growth factor receptor-targeted immunotherapy with photodynamic treatment of ovarian cancer in vivo," *J Natl. Cancer Inst.*, Vol. 97, No. 20, 2005, pp. 1516–1524.

[163] Vaupel, P., Thews, O., and Hoeckel, M., "Treatment resistance of solid tumors: role of hypoxia and anemia," *Med Oncol.*, Vol. 18, No. 4, 2001, pp. 243–259.

[164] Hurter, B. and Bush, N. J., "Cancer-related anemia: clinical review and management update," *Clin. J. Oncol. Nurs.*, Vol. 11, No. 3, 2007, pp. 349–359.

[165] Golab, J., et al., "Erythropoietin restores the antitumor effectiveness of photodynamic therapy in mice with chemotherapy-induced anemia," *Clin. Cancer Res.*, Vol. 8, No. 5, 2002, pp. 1265–1270.

[166] Weishaupt, K. R., Gomer, C. J., and Dougherty, T. J., "Identification of singlet oxygen as the cytotoxic agent in photoinactivation of a murine tumor," *Cancer Res.*, Vol. 36, No. 7 PT 1, 1976, pp. 2326–2329.

[167] Sharman, W. M., Allen, C. M., and van Lier, J. E., "Role of activated oxygen species in photodynamic therapy," *Methods Enzymol.*, Vol. 319, 2000, pp. 376–400.

[168] Golab, J., et al., "Antitumor effects of photodynamic therapy are potentiated by 2-methoxyestradiol. A superoxide dismutase inhibitor," *J. Biol. Chem.*, Vol. 278, No. 1, 2003, pp. 407–414.

[169] Athar, M., et al., "In situ evidence for the involvement of superoxide anions in cutaneous porphyrin photosensitization," *Biochem. Biophys. Res. Commun.*, Vol. 151, No. 3, 1988, pp. 1054–1059.

[170] Moan, J., Smedshammer, L., and Christensen, T., "Photodynamic effects on human cells exposed to light in the presence of hematoporphyrin. pH effects," *Cancer Lett.*, Vol. 9, No. 4, 1980, pp. 327–332.

[171] Peng, Q., Moan, J., and Cheng, L. S., "The effect of glucose administration on the uptake of photofrin II in a human tumor xenograft," *Cancer Lett.*, Vol. 58, No. 1–2, 1991, pp. 29–35.

[172] Rhodes, L. E., et al., "Iontophoretic delivery of ALA provides a quantitative model for ALA pharmacokinetics and PpIX phototoxicity in human skin," *J. Invest Dermatol.*, Vol. 108, No. 1, 1997, pp. 87–91.

[173] Fang, J. Y., et al., "Enhancement of topical 5-aminolaevulinic acid delivery by erbium:YAG laser and microdermabrasion: a comparison with iontophoresis and electroporation," *Br. J. Dermatol.*, Vol. 151, No. 1, 2004, pp. 132–140.

[174] Ma, L., et al., "Production of protoporphyrin IX induced by 5-aminolevulinic acid in transplanted human colon adenocarcinoma of nude mice can be increased by ultrasound," *Int. J. Cancer*, Vol. 78, No. 4, 1998, pp. 464–469.

[175] Pang, L., et al., "Photodynamic effect on cancer cells influenced by electromagnetic fields," *J. Photochem. Photobiol. B*, Vol. 64, No. 1, 2001, pp. 21–26.

[176] Stern, S. J., et al., "Effect of aspirin on photodynamic therapy utilizing chloroaluminum sulfonated phthalocyanine (CASP)," *Lasers Surg. Med*, Vol. 12, No. 5, 1992, pp. 494–499.

[177] Shevchuk, I., et al., "Effects of the inhibitors of energy metabolism, lonidamine and levamisole, on 5-aminolevulinic-acid-induced photochemotherapy," *Int. J. Cancer*, Vol. 67, No. 6, 1996, pp. 791–799.

[178] Hanania, J. and Malik, Z., "The effect of EDTA and serum on endogenous porphyrin accumulation and photodynamic sensitization of human K562 leukemic cells," *Cancer Lett.*, Vol. 65, No. 2, 1992, pp. 127–131.

[179] Berg, K., et al., "The influence of iron chelators on the accumulation of protoporphyrin IX in 5-aminolaevulinic acid-treated cells," *Br. J. Cancer*, Vol. 74, No. 5, 1996, pp. 688–697.

[180] Ortel, B., et al., "Differentiation-specific increase in ALA-induced protoporphyrin IX accumulation in primary mouse keratinocytes," *Br. J. Cancer*, Vol. 77, No. 11, 1998, pp. 1744–1751.

CHAPTER 18

Photodynamic Therapy in Treatment of Infectious Diseases: Basic Aspects and Mechanisms of Action

Michela Magaraggia and Giulio Jori

18.1 Introduction

Infectious diseases of microbial origin are increasingly spreading worldwide owing to a multiplicity of factors, such as the emergence of microbial strains against which traditional therapeutic approaches are poorly effective, the rise in the number of transplanted, HIV, or advanced cancer patients where infections are often intractable, greater likelihood of infections propagation as a consequence of global travel between developed and developing countries and the constant expansion of poverty areas. The treatment of such diseases by the topical or systemic administration of antibiotics, which was originally believed to drastically reduce their impact on human health, is encountering serious limitations:

- The development of resistance to many classes of antibiotics exhibited by a large number of microbial cells has been observed even in nosocomial environments and can lead to severe morbidity and possibly lethal effects [1]. Typical examples are represented by methicillin-resistant *Staphylococcus aureus* (MRSA) and vancomycin-resistant enterococci [1]. A vancomycin-resistant MRSA strain, which had acquired the enterococcal vanA gene, has been recently isolated [2, 3].
- The often excessive or inappropriate prescription of antibiotics even in countries with an advanced medical care, coupled with the failure of some patients to complete their treatment regimen.
- The truly large variety of strategies adopted by microorganisms to potentiate their degree of resistance to the action of antibiotics, including the generation of mutants deficient in specific porin channels, encoding of proteins that prevent the influx of potentially dangerous chemicals, reinforced production of systems promoting an active efflux of drugs, and thickening of the outer wall, especially at the level of the peptidoglycan layer [4].
- The broad differences in structure and organization displayed by microbial cells, including the presence of a finely structured outer wall in fungi and bacteria whose biochemical composition and permeability to chemicals can appreciably change for different classes, the formation of biofilms, and the

complex life cycle typical of protozoa, which can exist in either a trophic feeding state or a resting and resistant cystic stage. In particular, cysts are characterized by the presence of a wall consisting of tightly packed fibrillar systems, known as the exocyst and the endocyst, which are often osmotically inextensible. Some important details are specified in Table 18.1.

As a consequence, it has so far proven very difficult to identify a comprehensive, efficacious, and reliable methodology based on antibiotics to adequately addressing the problem of microbial infections. The need to find alternative antimicrobial therapeutic agents prompted the testing of novel approaches, such as the use of bacteriophages to treat local or systemic diseases caused by Vibrio vulnificus [5] or the synthesis of peptides antagonizing Pseduomonas aeruginosa [6].

Photodynamic therapy (PDT) is attracting increasing attention as a modality with favorable properties for the treatment of localized infections caused by a wide spectrum of microbial pathogens, including those that are recalcitrant to antibiotic therapies [7–10].

In actual fact, present evidence suggests that a suitable choice of the photosensitizer dose and irradiation conditions for the treatment of infectious diseases allows one to overcome most of the drawbacks which severely limit the success of antibiotic-based therapeutic strategies [9]. The approaches that are presently under consideration involve the administration of the photosensitizing agent in the infected lesions through topical application, spray formulations, or instillation, followed by irradiation of the photosensitizer-loaded area with full spectrum visible light or selected intervals of visible wavelengths. Thus, several laboratories are actively engaged in the definition of PDT protocols that cause a marked drop in the population of microbial pathogens, as well as the destruction of the associated virulence factors [11], with a parallel minimal damage to the perilesional districts of the host tissue, as well as a low risk of inducing undesired systemic effects.

Table 18.1   Selected Structural and Physicochemical Features of Microbial Cells

Microbial Class	Thickness	Outer Wall Chemical Composition	Permeability
Gram(+)-bacteria	20–80 nm	Ca. 100 peptidoglycan layers traversed by negatively charged lipoteichoic/teichuronic acids anchored in the membrane	Macromolecules with up to 60,000 MW can cross to the plasma membrane
Gram(-)-bacteria	10–15 nm layer in addition to the Gram(+)-bacteria wall	As mentioned for Gram(+)-bacteria with an extra envelope including proteins with porin functions, lipopolysaccharide trimers, and lipoproteins	Relatively hydrophilic compounds with <700 MW can diffuse through the porin channels
Yeasts	variable	Mixture of glucan, mannan, chitin, and lipoproteins	Intermediate between Gram(+) and Gram(-) -bacteria
Protozoa (trophic stage)	–	absent	–
Protozoa (cystic stage)	300 nm per layer	2 or 3 layers constituted by fibrous material (largely cellulose) with an interdispersed amorphous substance	Very low owing to the osmotically inextensible endocyst wall

18.2   Photodynamic Inactivation of Microbial Cells: The Photosensitizer

18.2.1   Photophysical Processes

Photodynamic sensitizers are known [12] to carry out their cytotoxic action via two reaction mechanisms, as illustrated in the following scheme:

$$
\begin{array}{lll}
\text{Sens} + h\nu & \rightarrow {}^1\text{Sens} & \text{absorption} \\
{}^1\text{Sens} & \rightarrow {}^3\text{Sens} & \text{intersystem crossing} \\
{}^3\text{Sens} + {}^3O_2 & \rightarrow \text{Sens}^{\cdot +} + O_{2\cdot -} & \text{type I pathway} \\
{}^3\text{Sens} + {}^3O_2 & \rightarrow \text{Sens} + {}^1O_2 & \text{type II pathway}
\end{array}
$$

where Sens, ^{1}Sens, and ^{3}Sens represent the ground state, the first excited singlet state and, respectively, the lowest excited triplet state of the photosensistizer; $^3O_2$ and $^1O_2$ are the ground state (a triplet) and, respectively, the first excited singlet state of molecular oxygen (singlet oxygen).

The type I reaction pathway involves electron transfer from the photogenerated lowest excited triplet state of the photosensitizer to a substrate with the consequent formation of radical species. Most frequently, the electron acceptor is represented by oxygen, which is ubiquitous in biological systems, hence, the process leads to the initial formation of the superoxide anion $O_{2\cdot -}$, which can be further converted to the highly reactive OH$^{\cdot}$ radical through the Fenton reaction, especially in the presence of Fe^{2+} ions [13]. The alternative type II mechanism is based on electronic energy transfer from the photosensitizer triplet state to a suitable substrate; once again, most frequently, the photosensitizer triplet interacts in a diffusion-controlled process with ground state oxygen, which is thus promoted to the hyperreactive singlet oxygen ($^1O_2$). The latter process is facilitated by the large concentration (in the millimolar range) of oxygen in many cell/tissue compartments, as well as by the small energy gap (22.5 kcal/mole) between the ground and first excited singlet state of oxygen, which is lower than the energy level of most triplet photosensitizers.

It is generally assumed [14] that the $^1O_2$-involving pathway plays a predominant role in the photosensitized inactivation of microbial cells. This would require the generation of the $^1O_2$ species in close proximity of or even inside the cells owing to the property of this oxygen derivative to efficiently react with a large variety of cellular targets (see Table 18.2), which precludes its diffusion over significant distances from its generation site [15]. As a consequence, only photosensitizers that closely interact with the outer wall have been shown to inactivate Gram-negative bacteria upon illumination with visible light [8, 9, 16] and the photokilling of both Gram-positive and Gram-negative bacteria is modulated by the addition of quenchers (e.g., histidine, sodium azide) or enhancers (e.g., D_2O) of $^1O_2$ lifetime [17]. However, the question is not completely settled: thus, Escherichia coli underwent an extensive photoinactivation even though the photosensitizer was physically separated from the bacterial cells [18]; Valduga et al. [19] demonstrated that $^1O_2$ can diffuse in a water-saturated atmosphere over distances as large as 1 to 1.5 mm from its generation site to kill E. coli after damaging some plasma membrane proteins of the bacterial cells. Therefore, the possible contribution of type I mechanisms

Table 18.2   Typical Biological Targets of Photodynamic Processes

Cell Constituent	Photosensitive Sites	Functional Group	Typical Photoproducts
Nucleic acids	Guanosine	Purine	Hydroxy, ketone derivatives
Proteins	Methionine	Thioether	Sulfoxide
	Cysteine	Thiol	Disulfide, sulphonates
	Tryptophan	Indole	Kynurenine, hydroxy-indoles
	Histidine	Imidazole	Ketone derivatives
	Tyrosine	Phenol	Quinones, melanin-type polymeric material
Lipids	Unsaturated lipids, steroids	C-C double bond	Endoperoxides, allylic hydroperoxides

to the overall photoprocess cannot be ruled out: the formation of the radical anion of Al(III)-tetrasulphonated-phthalocyanine bound to bacterial cells was unequivocally observed by fast spectroscopic techniques [20]; this is in agreement with the observation that OH radical scavengers exert a protective role in the photoinactivation of E. coli mediated by xanthene and acridine dyes [21].

18.2.2 Properties of an Antimicrobial Photodynamic Agent

The choice of an efficient photosensitizer for the treatment of microbial infections is driven by the peculiar features of the different classes of pathogens that are responsible for the specific disease. Thus, while the relatively leaky three-dimensional organization of the outer wall that is characteristic of Gram-positive bacteria and fungi raises less strict requirements with regard to the physicochemical properties of the photosensitizer molecule, the low porosity and the exclusion at 600 to 700 Dalton exhibited by the outer wall of Gram-negative bacteria and cystic protozoa often inhibit any significant photosensitized inactivation of the two latter microorganisms. The relatively large and often hydrophobic molecules of the most frequently used photodynamic sensitizers cannot reach the sites in the plasma membrane or the cytoplasm whose integrity is critical for bacterial cell survival [22]. As a consequence, a large variety of photosensitizing agents have proven to induce an extensive decrease in the survival of Gram-positive bacteria and fungi upon irradiation with visible light [7, 8]. On the other hand, several porphyrins or phthalocyanines, such as hematoporphyrin and the tetrasulphonated derivatives, which act efficiently toward Gram-positive bacteria or tumor cells, display no significant phototoxicity against Gram-negative bacteria. That the lack of permeability of the outer wall is responsible for such an inefficient process is demonstrated by the finding that even Gram-negative bacteria, such as E. coli or Pseudomonas aeruginosa, become photosensitive when the irradiations are carried out after addition of external wall-permeabilizing agents. For example, the introduction of the nonapeptide polymixin B into the incubation medium of a suspension of Gram-negative bacterial cells results in an expansion of the outer leaflet, so that the photosensitizer molecules can diffuse through the peptidoglycan layers to partition in endocellular sites where the photogenerated reactive oxygen species can cause lethal damage [23, 24]. A second approach involves the addition of a metal chelator, such as ethylenediamino tetraacetic acid (EDTA), to the bacterial cell suspension; this provokes the removal of the Mg^{2+} and Ca^{2+} ions that neutralize the large number of negative charges present at the surface of the bacterial cells, thereby causing the onset of electrostatic repulsion and the reorganization of the native architecture of the outer wall into a less compact overall structure [25]. The consequent release of a substantial fraction (up to 50%) of the liposaccharides from the outer wall again allows the loading of the plasma membrane by the photosensitizer and the photoinduced killing of Gram-negative bacteria, such as E.coli and Krebsiella pneumoniae.

Even though the above described strategies open the way to the treatment of a broad number of microbial infections, including those caused by a heterogeneous flora, it would be highly preferable in view of clinical applications to develop photosensitizers that show an efficient antimicrobial action without the need of added chemicals. In the last decade of the previous century, the latter goal was achieved by the development of photosensitizing agents that are positively charged at physiological pH values. Thus, it was independently discovered by three laboratories that cationic dyes belonging to the classes of phenothiazines [26], porphyrins [27], and phthalocyanines [28] can directly promote the photoinactivation of Gram-negative bacteria upon irradiation under mild experimental conditions. The use of cationic photosensitizers also results in an enhanced inactivation efficiency of Gram-positive bacteria, as well as in an extensive killing of parasitic protozoa in both the trophozoitic and cystic stages [29, 30]. In particular, the photodynamic treatment inhibits both the conversion of the active feeding trophozoite into cysts and the excystment process [31].

As shown in Table 18.3, an extensive inactivation of a broad spectrum of pathogens can be achieved by a protocol involving short photosensitizer-cell incubation times and low fluence rates and light fluences. Typically, by choosing the parameters indicated in the Table 18.3, the exposure to light of cultures involving ca. 10^8 cells/ml induces a 5 to 6 log drop in the survival [14–16]. The possibility to use short incubation times is a consequence of the fast electrostatic interaction occurring between the cationic functional groups in the photosensitizer molecule and the negatively charged teichuronic and lipoteichoic acids located in the outer wall of bacterial and fungal cells (Table 18.1). The prolongation of the incubation

Table 18.3 Typical Protocol for an Efficient And Selective Photosensitized Inactivation of Microbial Pathogens*

Property	Optimal Values
Photosensitizing agent	Positively charged phenothiazines, meso-substituted porphyrins, peripherally substituted phthalocyanines
Enhancing structural factors	Increase in hydrophobicity by addition of hydrocarbon chains (C>10); combination with cationic polypeptides or liposomes
Preirradiation incubation time	5–30 minutes
Incubation medium	Presence of large amounts of serum proteins reduces the photoinactivation efficiency
Photosensitizer dose	0.1–5 μM
Fluence rate	<50 mW/cm^2
Light fluence (irradiation time)	<10 J/cm^2

*The pathogens include Gram-(+) and Gram-(-) bacteria, mycoplasmas, fungi, and parasitic protozoa in the vegetative or cystic stage.

time from 5 to 60 minutes brings about no detectable increase in the amount of cell-bound photosensitizer [32]. This feature plays a key role in determining the selectivity of antimicrobial PDT in in vivo systems, since incubation times as short as a few minutes do not allow an appreciable accumulation of polycyclic aromatic compounds by human or higher animal cells, especially when low photosensitizer concentrations are utilized [33]. In actual fact, the red light irradiation of both a wild and a methicillin-resistant (MRSA) strain of Staphylococcus aureus in the presence of <2 μM concentrations of a tetracationic Zn(II)-phthalocyanine causes about a 5-log decrease in the bacterial population with a negligible phototoxic effect on two typical constituents of potential host tissues, namely HT-1080 fibroblasts and HaCaT keratinocytes (Figure 18.1).

Only when larger doses of phthalocyanine are utilized, an important photoinduced killing of the two human cell lines takes place. The histograms shown in Figure 18.2 also emphasize that PDT is very effective toward a pathogen, such as MRSA, which is quite difficult to be treated by the currently available therapeutic procedures, and is the cause of significant morbidity and even mortality in infected patients [34].

This finding is in full agreement with previous reports [7, 10, 22] indicating that the sensitivity of most bacteria to photodynamic processes is independent of their antibiotic resistance spectrum.

While positively charged derivatives of phenothiazines, porphyrins, and phthalocyanines are at present most frequently used for the photoinactivation of a

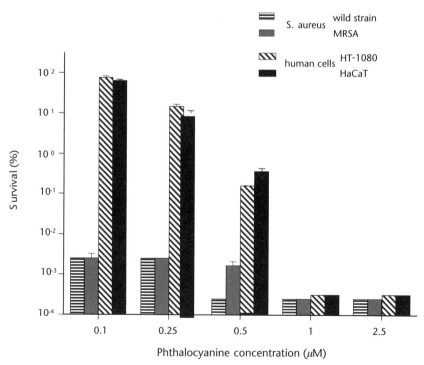

Figure 18.1 Survival of S. aureus cells, fibroblasts, and keratinocytes upon 5 minutes of irradiation with 600 to 700 nm (50 mW/cm^2) after 5 minutes of dark incubation with 0.1- to 2.5-μM tetracationic phthalocyanine in phosphate-buffered saline.

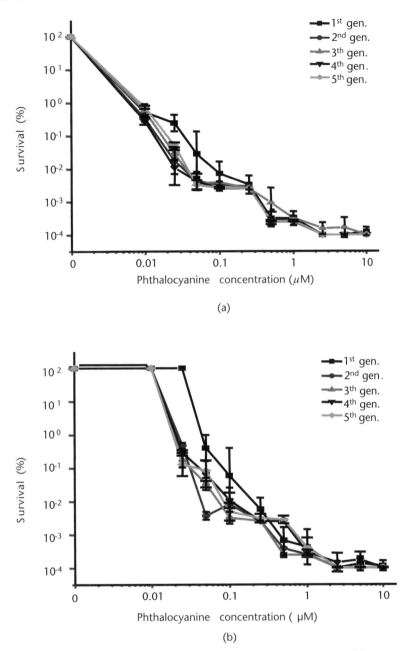

Figure 18.2   Survival of S. aureus cells upon 5 minutes of irradiation of (a) a wild strain and (b) a meticillin-resistant strain with 600- to 700-nm light (50 mW/cm^2) after 5 minutes of dark incubation with 0.01- to 10-μM tetracationic phthalocyanine.

variety of pathogens, as indicated in Table 18.3, it is now becoming apparent that other kinds of cationic dyes can act as broad spectrum antimicrobial photosensitizers (e.g., the Se-containing analogues of phenothiazines ("selenazinium" derivatives) have been recently shown [35] to induce the extensive killing of mycobacteria both in vitro and in in vivo models). On the other hand, even fullerenes where a nitrogen atom, which has been made cationic by quaternarization, protrudes from the C60 core were found to display a significant photocytocidal action against Gram-negative bacteria [36].

Several observations suggest that cationic photosensitizers are accumulated by Gram-negative bacterial cells through the self-promoted uptake pathway similar to what has been demonstrated to occur for cationic peptides [37]. This would involve the displacement of divalent cations from the surface of the outer layer, followed by disruption of the barrier properties typical of this structural element owing to their bulky and amphiphilic nature; no similar action occurs on eukaryotic cells, which usually are characterized by the presence of positively charged lipids and a relatively low number of anionic moieties [38]. Thus, the incubation of E. coli in the dark with a tetra-cationic Zn(II)-phthalocyanine increased the sensitivity of the bacterial cells to the action of hydrophobic, rather than hydrophilic, antibiotics and promoted a larger uptake of radiolabeled protoporphyrin IX [39]. Additionally, upon illumination, the close proximity of the photosensitizer to potentially sensitive targets in the outer wall could cause an initial photooxidative damage of selected constituents of the outer membrane (e.g., lipoproteins), thereby further contributing to the alteration of the compact native structure [32].

The key role played by the interaction between the cationic photosensitizer and the negatively charged cell surface of several microbial cells in modulating the efficiency of the photosensitization process is further confirmed by the finding that the incorporation of the porphyrin into either electrically neutral liposomal vesicles completely prevents the photoinactivation of Gram-negative bacteria, independently of the fact that the liposomes are in a fluid (dimiristoyl-phosphatidylcholine, DMPC) or quasi-solid (dipalmitoyl-phosphatidylcholine, DPPC) state at the physiological temperature of 37°C [40]. Under these conditions, the porphyrin is embedded within the phospholipid bilayer, hence it cannot undergo an ionic bonding with the bacterial cell [32]. On the other hand, when the cationic porphyrin is delivered to an aqueous suspension of E. coli cells via positive liposomes (N-[1-(2,3-dioleoyloxy)propyl]-N,N,N-trimethylammonium methylsulphate, DOTAP), the efficiency of cell killing is appreciably enhanced as compared with the free photosensitizer [40, 41].

While most cationic photosensitizers act on a large variety of pathogens, selected structural features can be introduced into their molecule in order to enhance their photoantimicrobial activity (see Table 18.3). Specific approaches that have given satisfactory results include:

- Improving the photophysical properties of the antimicrobial photosensitizer. Thus, the replacement of one sulfur atom in the tricyclic aromatic skeleton of phenothiazines by one selenium atom is accompanied by a greater photosensitizing activity, in particular towards Gram-positive or Gram-negative bacteria [42], as well as against intracellular parasites [43]. This has been ascribed to the heavy atom effect induced by Se, which results in a higher quantum yield of triplet state generation, hence in a sustained production of cytotoxic ROS.
- Optimization of the disorganizing effect of the photosensitizer on the outer wall. The photokilling of fungi and bacteria is actually enhanced by a moderate increase in the hydrophobicity of the photosensitizer molecule. Thus, Reddi et al. [44] studied the photocydal activity of a number of

meso-substituted tetra(N-alkyl-pyridyl)porphyrins against MRSA and E. coli and observed that the extent of photoinduced cell killing increased upon replacing one N-methyl moiety by longer hydrocarbon chains. Maximal efficiency was found upon introduction of one N-tetradecyl group, leading to a >6-log decrease in cell survival after about a 5-minute irradiation at a fluence rate of 50 mW/cm^2. Further elongation of the hydrocarbon chain to 18 or 22 carbon atoms was accompanied by a drop in the overall photosensitizing activity, due to the aggregation of the porphyrin and the consequent shorter lifetime of the photosensitizer excited states. The hydrocarbon chain appears to act as an arm that partitions into lipid domains of the external wall because of its hydrophobicity, thus interfering with the set of intermolecular forces that stabilize this highly ordered protective structure [45, 46]. Similarly, the replacement of two methyl groups in N,N-dialkyl-phenothiazines by two butyl chains yields a very active photoantimicrobial agent, which is now under clinical trials for the disinfection of chronic ulcers [47, 48]. The photoinactivation efficiency can be additionally optimized by inserting a spacer (e.g., a propoxy bridge) between the tetrapyrrolic macrocycle and the cationic centers, which imparts a greater flexibility and facilitates the proper orientation of the positive charges toward the anionic groups at the outer wall surface [49].

• Conjugation of the photosensitizer with a polycationic moiety, such as poly-lysine [9], poly-ornithine [50], and poly-ethyleneimine [51]. The polypeptide can both alter the permeability of the outer membrane and fulfill the requirement for the presence of positive charges, thus eliminating the need of a cationic photosensitizer. In actual fact, a neutral photosensitizing agent, such as chlorin e6, which had been bound to a polypeptide chain composed by 20 lysyl residues, caused an extensive killing of selected oral pathogens upon red light illumination [52]. These findings were confirmed by the irradiation of oral pathogens in the presence of blood [53], and subsequently extended to conjugates between poly-lysine and another neutral photosensitizer, namely 9-acetoxy-tetramethyl-porphycene for the photosensitized inactivation of yeasts, Gram-positive, and Gram-negative bacteria [54]. Subsequent investigations pointed out that the length of the poly-lysine chain appreciably modulates the bactericidal action of both porphycenes and chlorin e6 [55, 56]. Present evidence suggests that the use of polypeptides containing at least 20 poly-lysines is essential to achieve an optimal disinfecting action.

Porphyrins and their analogues, such as chlorins and phthalocyanines, offer unique possibilities for studying the relationships between the chemical structure and photoantimicrobial activity since their molecules can be modified by suitable synthetic strategies at different levels, including the introduction of substituents in the peripheral positions of the tetrapyrrole or tetraazaisoindole macrocycle, the coordination of metal ions with the central nitrogen atoms, and the addition of ligands to the axial positions of the metal ions [57, 58]. In most cases, the nature and number of such substituents have a limited influence on the photophysical properties of the parent compound. On the other hand, the nature of the added moieties can appreciably affect the kinetics and efficiency of photosensitizer binding with microbial cells, as well as its distribution among the subcellular compartments [16, 46]. A major role is played by the balance between hydrophilic and hydrophobic properties, which is frequently modulated by the number of charged functional groups in the photosensitizer molecule: this parameter is especially important for enhancing the photocytocidal activity toward a specific class of pathogens. Thus, tetra- to octa-cationic porphyrins and phthalocyanines are particularly efficient against Gram-negative bacteria, probably because the larger number of positive substituents promotes a tighter binding with the surface array of negative charges in the bacterial cell. On the contrary, in the case of Gram-positive bacteria and yeasts, optimal results are obtained by using amphiphilic photosensitizing agents (e.g., dicationic porphyrins having the two positively charged functions bound to two adjacent pyrrole rings) [32, 59].

So far, the most convenient compromise for the photodynamic treatment of infections involving a heterogeneous microbial flora appears to be represented by the use of tetracationic derivatives, such as the 2(3),9(10),16(17),23(24)-tetratrimethylammoniumphenoxy-Zn(II)-phthalocyanine [60], or dicationic derivatives, such as the 3,7-bis(N,N-dibutylamino)phenotiazin-5-ium bromide [48], which are presently being proposed for clinical trials of infectious diseases.

18.3   Photodynamic Inactivation of Microbial Cells: The Target

18.3.1   Photosensitized Inactivation of Bacteria

The data shown in Table 18.4 point out that a typical Gram-positive bacterium, namely Enterococcus seriolicida, is efficiently inactivated upon red light irradiation using either a tetra-anionic (TPPS$_4$) or a tetra-cationic (T$_4$MPyP) porphyrin. The positively charged meso-substituted porphyrin displays a greater phototoxicity, as discussed in detail in the previous paragraphs. On the other hand, the negatively charged TPPS$_4$ is ineffective toward the Gram-negative E. coli even after relatively long light exposure times, and the use of a cationic porphyrin, such as T$_4$MPyP, is necessary in order to induce a significant decrease in the survival of this bacterium.

Table 18.4   Decrease (Expressed in Log) in Survival of a Typical Gram-Positive (E. seriolicida) and Gram-Negative (E. coli) Bacterium Irradiated (600–700 nm, 40 mW/cm^2) in the Presence of 5-μM Porphyrin after 5 Minutes of Dark Incubation

Photosensitizer	Irradiation Time (Min)		
	1	5	10
Enterococcus seriolicida			
TPPS$_4$	0.0	3.7	4.5
T$_4$MPyP	2.3	4.9	5.8
Escherichia coli			
TPPS$_4$	0.0	0.2	0.2
T$_4$MPyP	1.9	3.1	4.5

Cell density = 10^8 cells/ml
TPPS$_4$ = meso-tetra(4-sulphonato-phenyl)porphine
T$_4$MPyP = meso-tetra(4-N-methyl-pyridyl)porphine

On the basis of the available evidence, the eventual death of photosensitized bacterial cells can be described by a stepwise mechanism:

1. *Fast interaction of the cationic photosensitizer with the negatively charged (largely carboxylate) groups on the surface of the outer wall.* This process is completed within a few minutes of incubation since the binding is of electrostatic nature.

2. *Dark-or photo-induced enhancement of the permeability of the outer wall.* The increased permeability is the consequence of the displacement of the naturally present Mg^{2+} and Ca^{2+} ions by the cationic photosensitizers, which have about two orders of magnitude larger affinity, as well as of steric hindrance generated by the bulky aromatic macrocycles. The close proximity of the photosensitizer to the constituents of the outer wall can also induce the photooxidative modification of selected proteins, which in turn causes a series of more pronounced alteration of various structural elements. In actual fact, electrophoretic analysis of the outer membrane proteins in T_4MPyP-photosensitized E. coli showed an extensive modification of some protein bands in the 14- to 20- and 25- to 30-kDa ranges [61].

3. *Translocation of the photosensitizer to the cytoplasmic membrane.* The leaky outer wall allows the penetration of the photosensitizer across the periplasmic space to reach the plasma membrane, which becomes the main binding site at least of predominantly hydrophobic dyes, such as porphyrins and other tetrapyrrolic derivatives [7, 8, 60]. Thus, subcellular distribution studies in both S. aureus and E. coli photosensitized by T_4MPyP showed that the amount of porphyrin associated with the protoplast increased as the irradiation proceeded [32, 62].

4. *Photoxidative modification of multiple targets in the plasma membrane of the bacterial cell.* The short lifetime of the photogenerated reactive intermediates produced upon visible light irradiation explains the repeated observations indicating that the plasma membrane is involved in the primary stages of the photoinactivation process [9, 10, 33]. The main evidence supporting this conclusion can be summarized as follows:

   · Selected plasma membrane proteins undergo an extensive cross-linking at a rate that is comparable with the rate of photoinduced cell death in the case of phenothiazine [63] or porphyrin [61] photosensitization of various bacterial strains. Thus, SDS-PAGE electrophoresis of plasma membrane proteins in photosensitized E. coli showed a gradual attenuation of specific bands associated with transport proteins upon increasing the light exposure [61].

   · Typical plasma membrane marker enzymes such as NADH, succinate, and lactate dehydrogenases were extensively inactivated in the very early stages of the photoprocess, namely before a marked reduction in cell survival could be observed (Figure 18.3). Similarly, several membranous proteins underwent an extensive cross-linking in the early stages of Porphyromonas gingivalis inactivation photosensitized by methylene blue [63].

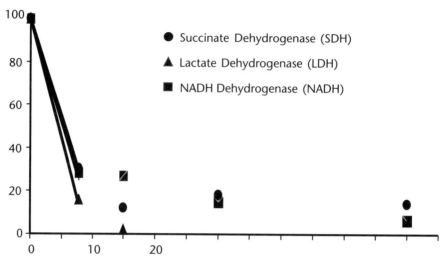

Figure 18.3 Loss of enzymic activities in S. aureus upon irradiation (600–700 nm, 50 mW/cm^2) after 5 minutes incubation with 1 μM tetracationic phthalocyanine.

- Loss of clonogenicity in photosensitized bacteria was found to be closely correlated with the leakage of intracellular contents, including a collapse of K+ and ionic balance [64].
- Confocal fluorescence microscopy studies with phthalocyanine-treated bacterial cells clearly showed [10] that the photosensitizer is located at the level of the plasma membrane prior to irradiation and diffuses into inner subcellular districts only after several minutes of exposure to light. This pattern of irradiation-dependent changes in the subcellular distribution is in agreement with the observation that DNA damage occurs at later stages of the overall photoprocess and is not directly correlated with cell death. Thus, Deinococcus radiodurans, which possesses an efficient DNA repair system, was shown to be readily killed by photodynamic processes [65]; analogously, no alteration of plasmidial DNA extracted from extensively photoinactivated E. coli cells was detected [61]. However, caution must be taken before general conclusions are drawn, since recent findings suggest that photoinactivation of E. coli upon irradiation in the presence of tetra-meso(N-methyl-pyridyl)porphine is primarily dependent on damage of genomic DNA [66].

5. *Inhibition of cell growth and cell death* is eventually caused by the photoinduced impairment of various cell functions and metabolic processes.

The mechanisms that control the photoinduced killing of bacterial cells justify the lack of mutagenic effects observed by several investigators [9, 16]. At the same time, the multitarget nature of membrane photodamage is in agreement with the inability of the bacterial cells to repair the photoinduced modifications, as well as with the lack of selection of photoresistant species [23, 56]. Thus, up to five consecutive generations of extensively (>90%) photoinactivated MRSA cells exhibited an essentially identical sensitivity to the photosensitizing action of a tetracationic Zn(II)-phthalocyanine (G. Jori, C. Fabris, M. Soncin, unpublished results). The latter finding represents a major advancement of PDT in comparison with antibiotic treatment of bacterial infections, since it allows the repetition of the photodynamic treatment when multiple therapeutic sessions are required. Moreover, investigations presently in progress in our laboratory indicate that the sensitivity of partially photoinactivated S. aureus cells to a number of antibiotics that act by different mechanisms is essentially identical for control bacteria, that have not being subjected to photosensitization, and bacterial strains exposed to one or five consecutive phototherapeutic treatments (see Table 18.5).

Most in vitro studies of bacteria photosensitization have so far been performed by using cell monolayers or, more frequently, cell suspensions. However, the indications provided by this wide body of investigations appear to be of general validity, since bacterial cells were found to be readily photoinactivated when they grow as biofilms [67], or at different stages of development, even though cells in the stationary phase of growth seem to be less susceptible to photodynamic inactivation than the corresponding cells in the logarithmic phase [7, 45]. Moreover, Demidova and Hamblin [68] demonstrated that even Bacillus spores can be killed upon irradiation with selected phenothiazines. Thus, PDT appears to be potentially useful for the treatment of a large variety of pathologies and infectious diseases of bacterial origin.

18.3.2   Photosensitized Inactivation of Yeasts

Yeasts and fungi constitute a group of rather disparate eukaryotic organisms, which are also protected by a relatively thick external wall, whose permeability properties are fairly similar with those typical of Gram-positive bacteria. As a consequence, the susceptibility of yeasts to the action of photodynamic sensitizers is less dependent on structural factors as compared with Gram-negative bacteria and the stepwise scheme previously detailed for the photosensitized inactivation of bacteria obtains also for this class of pathogens [45, 46]. Thus, negatively charged dyes, such as hematoporphyrin [69] or eosin Y [70], are taken up by Saccharomyces cerevisiae and photosensitize an extensive killing of this micro-organism. Similar results were

Table 18.5   Effect of Selected Antibiotics on a Wild (ATCC) and Methicillin-Resistant (MRSA) Strain of S. aureus

Antibiotics	MIC μm/ml)					
	S. aureus wild			S. aureus MRSA		
	(A)	(B)	(C)	(A)	(B)	(C)
Cephalotin	0.25	0.12	0.25	4.00	4.00	4.00
Vancomycin	2.10	2.00	2.30	3.50	3.50	3.70
Erythromycin	4.25	4.25	4.25	3.50	3.00	3.50
Tetracyclin	0.55	0.50	0.50	0.50	0.50	0.25
Chloramphenicol	8.40	8.40	8.40	64.00	64.00	64.00
Riphampicin	0.03	0.03	0.03	0.55	0.53	0.55

MIC (minimal inhibitory concentration): minimal concentration of antibiotic yielding a 3 log decrease in cell survival.
A: Untreated control cells.
B: Cells exposed to one phototreatment.
C: Cells from five consecutive generations that had been exposed to one phototreatment (about 90% inactivation), restabilized, and reirradiated.

obtained upon treatment of Candida albicans with visible light after incubation with Photofrin [71], rose bengal [72], or subcellular Al(III)-tetrasulphonated phthalocyanine [73]. However, also in the case of yeasts, cationic photosensitizers appear to be markedly more active than their neutral or anionic counterparts [46, 74].

Extensive mechanistic studies have been focused on C. albicans, a fungus that commonly colonizes the epithelial surfaces of the body, with the oropharyngeal cavity and the vaginal tract as primary sites [75]. An overall examination of the available literature information points out that:

- The initial photoinduced damage of specific constituents of the external wall facilitates the passage of the photodynamic agent to deeper districts, thereby inducing a greater cytotoxic effect [73].
- The cytoplasmic membrane represents the main target of yeast photosensitization, as suggested by the altered electrophoretic mobility of selected membrane proteins, as well as by the loss of membrane-typical transport and barrier properties [76, 77].
- The involvement of the genetic material in the photoprocess occurs at later stages, as suggested by the essentially identical levels of 2-deoxy-guanosine, the most important product of DNA photooxidation, in unirradiated and extensively photoinactivated yeast cells [78].
- Both early (i.e., formed for less than 6 hours) and mature (i.e., formed for longer than 40 hours) biofilms of C. albicans displayed a high sensitivity to porphyrin photosensitization; the efficacy of the photodynamic treatment was at least comparable with that observed for most effective antifungal formulations in current use [79].
- The main strategies commonly adopted by Candida and other fungi to develop resistance against drugs, such as enzymatic modification of the cytotoxic agent or induction of drug efflux pumps, were found to be not operative in the case of photodynamic processes [79]. As mentioned for bacteria, the lack of selection of PDT-resistant yeast strains can be ascribed to the multiplicity of targets at the level of the cytoplasmic membrane.

The brief exposure time (incubation + irradiation) and the low photosensitizer concentrations required to mediate a marked decrease in yeast survival emphasizes the possibility to define effective treatment regimes for fungal diseases by means of photodynamic approaches that will result in minimal damage to the surrounding host tissue. These findings provide a rationale for the development of PDT as an adjunctive or alternative mode of therapy against candidiasis or similar pathologies. In particular, the observation that the protocols leading to optimal antibacterial and antifungal effects are very similar could be especially useful in clinical practice since cutaneous and mucocutaneous mycoses are frequently superinfected by bacteria and may represent one important advantage of PDT with respect to standard anti-fungal chemotherapeutic approaches, which often have no or poor antibacterial activity [72].

18.3.3 Photosensitized Inactivation of Parasitic and Pathogenic Protozoa

A truly large number of parasitic protozoa are associated with hosts by different kinds of interactions, living as endobionts or endocytobionts; in particular, several protozoa are widely recognized etiologic agents of fatal infections for humans. The intestinal-dwelling Entamoeba histolytica, Giardia intestinalis, and Balantidium coli are so closely adapted to humans and other animals that they are unable to exist outside the host except as resistant cystic stages, which are responsible for infection transmission. Some parasitic protozoa are digenetic with alternating generations in two different hosts and often exhibit complex structural and functional changes in the different phases of existence. Thus, the malarian parasites, Plasmodium spp., have one form during the invasion of the mammalian host and different forms during part of their growth in the insect host. Some have become adapted to invade specialized cells of animals such as erythrocytes (Plasmodium), and the wandering cells of the immune system (Leishmania, Trypanosoma). The free-living soil and freshwater amoebae Naegleria fowleri, Acanthamoeba spp., and Balamuthia mandrillaris, can become highly pathogenic and are responsible for opportunistic and nonopportunistic infections, which can be lethal or invalidating, such as granulomatous amoebic encephalitis, cutaneous and nasopharyngeal infections in immunocompromised individuals, and amoebic keratitis (Acanthamoeba spp.) in immunocompetent individuals [80]. The general pattern of the life cycle of amoebic protozoa involves a trophic or feeding stage alternating with a resting cystic stage, which is highly resistant to biocides. Such a variety and complexity of life cycles often makes it problematic to define an adequate therapeutic protocol. Furthermore, the treatment of these organisms is associated with some risk due to the activation of dormant cysts, which can lead to patient relapse following apparently effective treatment [81].

The photosensitized inactivation of Colpoda inflata, a soil- and freshwater-dwelling ciliate used as a model of a protozoan developing a cystic stage, and the free-living opportunistic A. palestinensis, gave very positive results. Hence, PDT could play a useful role for the treatment of diseases caused by parasitic protozoa. Thus, a cationic porphyrin bearing four meso-N-methyl-pyridyl peripheral substituents at 1- to 10-μM concentrations, upon visible light irradiation, induced extensive photodamage and inhibition of excystment to produce vegetative cells [29]. The phototoxic activity was significantly enhanced by the replacement of at least one methyl group with a decyl or tetradecyl hydrocarbon chain. Analogously, a tetracationic Zn(II)-phthalocyanine proved to efficiently inactivate cultures of A. palestinensis in both the cystic and vegetative stages upon illumination with 600- to 700-nm light [30, 31]. The two forms exhibited a comparable level of photosensitivity as a function of the photosensitizer concentration; however, cysts required a significantly longer irradiation time in order to achieve a similar degree of inactivation. A phthalocyanine dose as low as 0.5 μM, followed by irradiation with red light for 20 minutes, induced a 50% inhibition of excystment in vegetative cells after the addition of fresh culture medium. Fluorescence microscopy studies [30] indicated that the phthalocyanine is largely localized in the contractile vacuole in unirradiated cells, but gradually diffuses throughout the cell volume in the photosensitized samples. On the other hand, in the A. palestinensis cysts the tetracationic phthalocyanine appears to readily cross the external wall, in spite of its relatively large molecular weight, and to localize in various subcellular sites, including the double cystic wall or some organelles. After irradiation, the distribution pattern was very similar; however, many cysts were clearly devoid of any residual fluorescence, possibly owing to a redistribution and release of cellular content and photosensitizer into the medium.

The high degree of photosensitivity displayed by A. palestinensis in both vegetative and cystic stages emphasizes the promising role of phototreatments based on cationic phthalocyanines to disinfect waters, which are contaminated by different pathogenic amoebae.

Merocyanine 540, cationic phthalocyanines, and lipophilic pheophorbide derivatives have also been shown to induce an extensive photoinactivation of blood-borne pathogens, such as the erythrocyte parasites Plasmodium falciparum and Babesia divergens [82, 83]. The inactivation of P. falciparum was also achieved by the photodynamic action of porphyrin-type intermediates of heme-cycle derived from 5-amino-levulinic acid [84]. The sensitivity of such parasites to photodynamic treatment has been exploited for their elimination from blood bank samples. Trypanosoma cruzi, a kinetoplastid protozoan responsible of Chagas' disease, could be eliminated in the blood by means of crystal violet and light-enhanced free radical formation [85]. Different phthalocyanines inactivated the trypomastigote forms of T. cruzi in fresh frozen plasma and red blood concentrates [86]. The efficiency of the photoprocess was significantly higher in the case of cationic phthalocyanines in agreement with their larger endocellular accumulation. The use of relatively mild irradiation conditions guarantees against any significant parallel damage to normal blood constituents. Ultrastructural analysis of treated parasites suggested that mitochondria are a primary target of this photodynamic process.

The trypanosomatid Leishmania donovani infantum, an intracellular parasite of monocytes and macrophages responsible of the visceral leishmaniasis was highly sensitive to photoinactivation by means of a DNA-intercalating flexible photosensitizer (i.e., thiopyrylium) [86]. Leishmaniasis is transmitted by blood-sucking females of the sand fly vector, in which Leishmania parasites exist as extracellular motile promastigote in the alimentary tract. Upon entry into a mammalian host, the parasites reside in the phagolysosomes of mononuclear phagocytes or macrophages, wherein they replicate as nonmotile amastigotes. As a consequence, PDT has been recently used to also treat cutaneous leishmaniasis, which appears to avoid the well-documented development of drug resistance in chemotherapy of this disease [87–89].

Another promising field of PDT application against parasitic protozoa concerns the treatment of subfoveal choroidal neovascularization associated with retinochoroiditis of Toxoplasma gondii origin. In this connection, a newly synthesized monocarboxylic porphyrin derivative, usually termed benzoporphyrin derivative and known under the commercial name of Verteporfin, was found to yield important curative effects; the photodynamic treatment appears to be effective and safe even in young adults and children [90].

18.4 Conclusions

The growing diffusion of antibiotic-resistant microbial strains and the consequent increased risk of the outbreak of hard-to-treat epidemic diseases make it essential to identify novel therapeutic approaches, which can act on both wild and multidrug resistant microorganisms. The problem is aggravated by the escalating number of immunocompromised patients undergoing organ transplantation and HIV/AIDS patients who are frequently attacked by infective agents, such as intestinal protozoa. Even though the application of PDT in the field of localized infectious diseases is still at an experimental stage, this therapeutic modality appears to be endowed with several potentially favorable properties, since it is characterized by a high level of safety, an efficient activity against a large variety of pathogens while most conventional antimicrobials show activity toward one or two pathogen types, and the possibility to repeat the treatment in case of insufficient response or recurrences. The latter feature is related with the low probability for PDT to promote the onset of repair or mutagenic processes. The possibilities of clinical applications of antimicrobial PDT are reinforced by the very promising results that are being obtained in studies involving suitable animal models, as well as by the encouraging reports of initial clinical trials [47, 89].

References

[1]   Cookson, B. D., "The emergence of mupirocin resistance: a challenge to infection control and antibiotic prescription practice," *J. Antimicrob. Chemother.*, Vol. 41, 1998, pp. 11–18.

[2]   Cunha, B. A., "Antibiotic resistance: control strategies," *Crit. Care Clinic*, Vol. 14, 1998, pp. 309–327.

[3]   Al-Masaudi, S. B., N. J. Day, and A. D. Russell, "Antimicrobial resistance and gene transfer in Staphylococcus aureus," *J. Appl. Bacteriol.*, Vol. 70, 1991, pp. 279–290.

[4]   Pfeltz, R. F., et al., "Characterization of passage-selected vancomycin-resistant Staphylococcus aureus strains of diverse parental backgrounds," *Antimicrob. Agents Chemoter.*, Vol. 44, 2000, pp. 294–303.

[5]   Cerveny, K. E., et al., "Phage therapy of local and systemic disease caused by Vibrio vulnificus in iron-dextran-treated mice," *Infect. Immun.*, Vol. 23, 2002, pp. 6251–6262.

[6]   Sajjan, U. S., et al., "P-113D, an antimicrobial peptide active against Pseduomonas aeruginosa, retains activity in the presence of sputum from cystic fibrosis patients," *Antimicrob. Agents Chemother.*, Vol. 45, 2001, pp. 3437–3444.

[7]   Wainwright, M., "Photodynamic antimicrobial chemotherapy," *J. Antimicrob. Chemother.*, Vol. 42, 1998, pp. 13–28.

[8]   Jori, G., and S. B. Brown, "Photosensitised inactivation of microorganisms," *Photochem. Photobiol. Sci.*, Vol. 3, 2004, pp. 403–405.

[9]   Hamblin, M. R., and T. Hasan, "Photodynamic therapy: a new antimicrobial approach to infectious disease?," *Photochem. Photobiol. Sci.*, Vol. 3, 2004, pp. 436–450.

[10]   Jori, G., et al., "Photodynamic therapy in the treatment of microbial infections: basic principles and perspective applications," *Lasers Surg. Med.*, Vol. 38, 2006, pp. 468–481.

[11]   Komerick, N., M. Wilson, and S. Poole, "The effect of photodynamic action on two virulence factors of Gram-negative bacteria," *Photochem. Photobiol.*, Vol. 62, 1995, pp. 184–189.

[12] Ochsner, M., "Photophysical and photobiological processes in the photodynamic therapy of tumors," *J. Photochem. Photobiol., B:Biol.*, Vol. 39, 1997, pp. 1–18.

[13] Sawyer, D. T., and J. S. Valentine, "Photoassisted Fenton degradations in natural polyelectrolyte microshells," *Accs. Chem. Res.*, Vol. 14, 1981, pp. 393–399.

[14] Jori, G., "Photodynamische therapie in der mikrobiologie." In: *Klinische Fluoreszenzdiagnostik und Photodynamische Therapie*, pp. 360–371, R.- M. Szeimies, D. Jocham and M. Landthaler (eds.), Berlin: Blackwell Verlag, 2003.

[15] Redmond, R. W., and J. N. Gamlin, "A compilation of singlet oxygen yields from biologically relevant molecules," *Photochem. Photobiol.*, Vol. 70, 1999, pp. 391–475.

[16] Jori, G., "Photodynamic therapy of microbial infections: state-of-the-art and perspectives," *J. Env. Path. Tox. Oncol.*, Vol. 25, 2006, pp. 505–519.

[17] Nitzan, Y., H. M. Wexler, and S. M. Firegold, "Inactivation of anaerobic bacteria by various photosensitising porphyrins and hemin," *Curr. Microbiol.*, Vol. 29, 1994, pp. 126–131.

[18] Dahl, T.A., W. R. Midden, and P. E. Hartman, "Comparison of killing of Gram-negative and Gram-positive bacteria by pure singlet oxygen," *J. Bacteriol.*, Vol. 171, 1989, pp. 2188–2194.

[19] Valduga, G.,et al., "Effect of extracellularly generated singlet oxygen on Gram-positive and Gram-negative bacteria," *J. Photochem. Photobiol., B: Biol.*, Vol. 21, 1993, pp. 81–86.

[20] Laia, C. A. T., et al., "Photoinduced charge-transfer reactions between tetrasulfonated aluminium phthalocyanine and methyl viologen," *Photochem. Photobiol. Sci.*, Vol. 2, 2003, pp. 555–562.

[21] Martin, J. P., and N. Lorgsdam, "The role of oxygen radicals in dye-mediated photodynamic effects in Escherichia coli," *J. Biol. Chem.*, Vol. 262, 1997, pp. 7213–7219.

[22] Malik, Z., H. Ladan, and Y. Nitzan, "Photodynamic inactivation of Gram-negative bacteria: problems and possible solutions," *J. Photochem. Photobiol., B: Biol.*, Vol. 14, 1992, pp. 262–266.

[23] Nitzan, Y., et al., "Inactivation of gram-negative bacteria by photosensitized porphyrins," *Photochem. Photobiol.*, Vol. 55, 1992, pp. 89–96.

[24] Nitzan, Y., A. Balzam-Sudakevitz, and H. Ashkenazi, "Eradication of Acinetobacter baumannii by photosensitized agents in vitro," *J. Photochem. Photobiol., B:Biol.*, Vol. 42, 1998, pp. 211–218.

[25] Bertoloni, G., et al., "Photosensitizing activity of water- and lipid-soluble phthalocyanines on Escherichia coli," *FEMS Microbiol. Lett.*, Vol. 59, 1990, pp. 149–155.

[26] Wilson, M., et al., "Bacteria in supragingival plaque samples can be killed by low power laser light in the presence of a photosensitizer," *J. Appl. Bacteriol.*, Vol. 78, 1995, pp. 569–574.

[27] Merchat, M., et al., Meso-substituted cationic porphyrins as efficient photosensitizers of Gram-positive and Gram-negative bacteria," *J. Photochem. Photobiol., B:Biol.*, Vol. 32, 1996, pp. 153–157.

[28] Minnock, A., et al., "Photoinactivation of bacteria: use of a cationic water-soluble zinc-phthalocyanine to photoinactivate both Gram-negative and Gram-positive bacteria," *J. Photochem. Photobiol., B:Biol.*, Vol. 32, 1996, pp. 159–164.

[29] Kassab, K., et al., "Photosensitization of Colpoda inflata cysts by meso-substituted cationic porphyrins," *Photochem. Photobiol. Sci.*, Vol. 1, 2002, pp. 560–564.

[30] Ferro, S., et al, "Photosensitised inactivation of Acanthamoeba palestinensis in the cystic stage," *J. Applied Microbiol.*, Vol. 101, 2006, pp. 206–212.

[31] Kassab, K., et al., "Phthalocyanine-photosensitized inactivation of a pathogenic protozoan Acanthamoeba palestinensis," *Photochem. Photobiol. Sci.*, Vol. 2, 2003, pp. 668–672.

[32] Merchat, M., et al., "Studies on the mechanism of bacteria photosensitization by meso-substituted cationic porphyrins," *J. Photochem. Photobiol., B:Biol.*, Vol. 35, 1996, pp. 149–157.

[33]   Soncin, M., et al., "Approaches to selectivity in the Zn(II)-phthalocyanine- photosensitized inactivation of wild-type and antibiotic-resistant Staphylococcus aureus," *Photochem. Photobiol. Sci.*, Vol. 1, 2002, pp. 815–819.

[34]   Smith, T. L., et al., "Emergence of vancomycin resistance in Staphylococcus aureus: glycopeptide-intermediate Staphylococcus aureus working group," *New England J. Med.*, Vol. 340, 1999, pp. 493–501.

[35]   O'Riordan, K., et al., "Real-time fluorescence monitoring of phenothiazinium photosensitizers and their anti-mycobacterial photodynamic activity against Mycobacterium bovis BCG in in vitro and in vivo models of localized infection," *Photochem. Photobiol. Sci.*, Vol. 6, 2007, pp. 1117–1123.

[36]   Tegos, G. P., et al., "Cationic fullerenes are effective and selective antimicrobial photosensitizers," *Chemistry Biol.*, Vol. 12, 2005, pp. 1127–1135.

[37]   Boman, H. G., "Peptide antibiotics: holy or heretic grails of innate immunity?" *Scand. J. Immunol.*, Vol. 43, 1996, pp. 475–482.

[38]   Falla, T. J., D. N. Karunaratne, and R. E. Hancock, "Mode of action of the antimicrobial peptide indolicidin," *J. Biol. Chem.*, Vol. 271, 1996, pp. 19298–192303.

[39]   Minnock, A., et al., "Mechanism of uptake of a cationic water-soluble pyridinium zinc phthalocyanine across the outer membrane of Escherichia coli," *Antimicrob. Agents Chemother*, Vol. 44, 2000, pp. 522–527.

[40]   Ferro, S., et al., "Inactivation of methicillin-resistant Staphylococcus aureus (MRSA) by liposome-delivered photosensitising agents," *J. Photochem. Photobiol., B:Biol.*, Vol. 83, 2006, pp. 98–104.

[41]   Ferro, S., et al., "Efficient photoinactivation of methicillin-resistant Staphylococcus aureus by a novel porphyrin incorporated into a poly-cationic liposome," *Int. J. Biochem. Cell Biol.*, Vol. 39, 2007, pp. 1026–1034.

[42]   Tegos, G. P., and M. R. Hamblin, "Phenothiazinium antimicrobial photosensitizers are substrates of bacterial multidrug resistance pumps," *Antimicrob. Agents Chemother.*, Vol. 50, 2006, pp. 196–203.

[43]   Akilov, O. E., et al., "The role of photosensitizer molecular charge and structure on the efficacy of photodynamictherapy against Leishmania Parasites," *Chem. Biol.*, Vol. 13, 2006, pp. 839–847.

[44]   Reddi, E., Met al., "Photophysical properties and antibacterial activity of meso-substituted cationic porphyrins," *Photochem. Photobiol.*, Vol. 75, 2002, pp. 462–470.

[45]   Maisch, T., et al., "Antibacterial photodynamic therapy in dermatology," *Photochem. Photobiol. Sci.*, Vol. 3, 2004, pp. 907–917.

[46]   Jori, G., and O. Coppellotti, "Inactivation of pathogenic microorganisms by photodynamic techniques: mechanistic aspects and perspective applications," *Anti-Infective Agents in Medicinal Chemistry*, Vol. 6, 2007, pp. 119–131.

[47]   Brown, S. B., "Clinical studies using antimicrobial PDT," *Proc. 11th Congress of the International Photodynamic Association*, Shanghai, China, Mar. 28–31, 2007, p. 51.

[48]   Brown, S. B., et al., "A double-blinded, randomised, placebo controlled clinical trial to determine whether PDT using the phenothiazinium salt, PPA 904 can reduce bacterial load in chronic leg ulcers and chronic diabetic foot ulcers," *Proc. 12th Congress of the European Society for Photobiology,* Bath, UK, Sept. 1–6, 2007, p. 118.

[49]   Caminos, D.A., M. B. Spesia, and E. N. Durantini, "Photodynamic inactivation of Escherichia coli by novel meso-substituted porphyrins by 4-(3-N,N,N-trimethylammoniumpropoxy)phenyl and 4-(trifluoromethyl)phenyl groups," *Photochem Photobiol Sci.*, Vol. 5, 2006, pp. 56–65.

[50]   Hancock, R. E., and P. G. Wong, "Compounds which increase the permeability of the Pseudomonas aeruginosa outer membrane," *Antimicrob. Agents Chemother.*, Vol. 26, 1984, pp. 48–52.

[51] Helander, I. M., et al., "Polyethyleneimine is an effective permeabilizer of gram-negative bacteria," *Microbiology*, Vol. 143, 1997, pp. 3193–3199.

[52] Soukos, S. N., M. R. Hamblin, and T. Hasan, "The effect of charge on cellular uptake and phototoxicity of polylysine-chlorin e6 conjugates," *Photochem. Photobiol.*, Vol. 65, 1997, pp. 723–729.

[53] Rovaldi, C. R., et al., "Photoactive porphyrin derivative with broad spectrum activity against oral pathogens in vitro," *Antimicrob. Agents Chemother.*, Vol. 44, 2000, pp. 3364–3367.

[54] Polo, L., et al., "Polylysine-porphycene conjugates as efficient photosensitizers for the inactivation of microbial pathogens," *J. Photochem. Photobiol., B: Biol.*, Vol. 59, 2000, pp. 152–158.

[55] Hamblin, M. R., et al., "Polycationic photosensitizer conjugates: effects of chain length and Gram classification on the photodynamic inactivation of bacteria," *J. Antimicrob. Chremother.*, Vol. 49, 2002, pp. 941–951.

[56] Lauro, F., et al., "Photoinactivation of bacterial strains involved in periodontal diseases sensitised by porphycene-polylysine conjugates," *Photochem. Photobiol. Sci.*, Vol. 1, 2002, pp. 468–470.

[57] Sessler, J. L., and S. J. Weghorn, *Expanded, Contracted and Isomeric Porphyrins*, Amsterdam: Elsevier, 1997.

[58] Moser, F. H., and Thomas, A. L., *The Phthalocyanines, Vol. I*, Boca Raton: CRC Press, 1997.

[59] Caminos, D. A., and E. N. Durantini, "Synthesis of asymmetrically meso-substituted porphyrins bearing amino groups as potential cationic photodynamic agents," *J. Porphyrins Phthalocyanines*, Vol. 9, 2005, pp. 334–342.

[60] Jori, G., and G. Roncucci, "Photodynamic therapy in microbial infections," *Adv. Clin. Exp. Med.*, Vol. 15, 2006, pp. 421–426.

[61] Valduga, G., et al., "Photosensitization of wild and mutant strains of Escherichia coli by meso-tetra(N-methyl-4-pyridyl)porphine," *Biochem. Biophys. Res. Comm.*, Vol. 256, 1999, pp. 84–88.

[62] Bertoloni, G., et al., "Photosensitizing activity of water- and lipid-soluble phthalocyanines on prokaryotic and eukaryotic microbial cells," *Microbios*, Vol. 71, 1992, pp. 33–46.

[63] Bhatti, M., et al., "Identification of photolabile outer membrane proteins of Porphyromonas gingivalis" *Curr. Microbiol.*, Vol. 43, 2001, pp. 96–99.

[64] Malik, Z., et al., "Collapse of K+ and ionic balance during photodynamic inactivation of leukemic cells, erythrocytes and Staphylococcus aureus," *Int. J. Biochem.*, Vol. 25, 1993, pp. 1399–1406.

[65] Schafer M., C. Schmitz, and G. Horneck, "High sensitivity of Deinococcus radiodurans to photodynamically produced singlet oxygen," *Int. J. Radiat. Biol.*, Vol. 74, 1998, pp. 249–253.

[66] Salmon-Divon M., Y. Nitzan, and Z. Malik, "Mechanistic aspects of Escherichia coli photodynamic inactivation by cationic tetra-meso(N-methyl-pyridyl)porphine," *Photochem. Photobiol. Sci.*, Vol. 3, 2004, pp. 423–429.

[67] Wilson M., "Susceptibility of oral bacterial biofilms to antimicrobial agents," *J. Med. Microbiol.*, Vol. 44, 1996, pp. 79–87.

[68] Demidova T. N., and M. R. Hamblin, "Photodynamic inactivation of Bacillus spores, mediated by phenothiazinium dyes," *Appl. Environ. Microbiol.*, Vol. 71, 2005, pp. 6918–6925.

[69] Sharma, R. K., and V. Jain, "Effects of 2-deoxy-D-glucose on the photosensitisation-induced bioenergetic changes in Saccharomyces cerevisiae as observed by in vivo NMR spectroscopy," *Indian J. Biochem. Biophys.*, Vol. 31, 1994, pp. 36–42.

[70] Cohn, G. E., and H. Y. Tseng, "Photosensitised inactivation of yeast sensitised by eosin Y," *Photochem. Photobiol.*, Vol. 26, 1977, pp. 465–474.

[71]   Bliss, J. M., et al., "Susceptibility of Candida species to photodynamic effects of Photofrin," *Antimicrob. Agents Chemother.*, Vol. 48, 2004, pp. 2000–2006.

[72]   Lazarova, G., "Effect of glutathione on rose bengal-photosensitised yeast damage," *Microbios*, Vol. 75, 1993, pp. 39–43.

[73]   Bertoloni, G., et al., "Photosensitising activity of water- and lipid–soluble phthalocyanines on prokaryotic and eukaryotic microbial cells," *Microbios*, Vol. 71, 1992, pp. 33–46.

[74]   Wilson M., and N. Mia, "Lethal photosensitisation of bacteria in subgingival plaque samples from patients with Chronic Periodontitis, *J. Oral Pathol. Med.*, Vol. 22, 1993, pp. 354–357.

[75]   Calderone, R. A., *Candida and candidiasis*, Washington, DC: ASM Press, 2002

[76]   Paardekopper, M., et al., "Photodynamic treatment of yeast cells with the dye toluidine blue: all-or-none loss of plasma membrane barrier properties," *Biochim. Biophys. Acta*, Vol. 1108, 1992, pp. 86–90.

[77]   Paardekopper, M., et al., "The effect of photodynamic treatment of yeast with the sensitiser chloroaluminum phthalocyanine on various cellular parameters," *Photochem. Photobiol.*, Vol. 62, 1995, pp. 561–567.

[78]   Lazarova, G., and H. Tashiro, "Protective effect of amphotericin B against lethal photodynamic treatment in yeast," *Microbios*, Vol. 82, 1995, pp. 187–196.

[79]   Chabrier-Rosello, Y., et al., "Sensitivity of Candida albicans germ tubes and biofilms to Photofrin-mediated phototoxicity," *Antimicrob. Agents Chemother.*, Vol. 49, 2005, pp. 4288–4295.

[80]   Marciano-Cabral, F., and G. Cabral, "Acanthamoeba spp. as agents of disease in humans," *Clin. Microbiol. Rev.*, Vol. 16, 2003, pp. 273–307.

[81]   Schuster, F. L., and G. S. Visvesvara, "Opportunistic amoebae: challenges in prophylaxis and treatment," *Drug. Resist. Update*, Vol. 7, 2004, pp. 41–51.

[82]   Lustigman, S., and E. Ben-Hur, "Photosensitised inactivation of Plasmodium falciparum in human red cells by phthalocyanines," *Transfusion*, Vol. 36, 1996, pp. 543–546.

[83]   Grellier, P., et al., "Photosensitized inactivation of Plasmodium falciparum and Babesia divergens – infected erythrocytes in whole blood by lipophilic pheophorbide derivatives," *Vox Sang.*, Vol. 72, 1997, pp. 211–220.

[84]   Berg, K., "Mechanisms of cell damage in photodynamic therapy." In *Fundamental Basis of Phototherapy*, pp. 181–207, H. Honigsmann, G. Jori and A. Young (eds.), Milano, Italy: OEMF, 1996.

[85]   Docampo, R., et al., "Light-enhanced free radical formation and trypanocidal action of gentian violet (crystal violet)," *Science*, Vol. 220, 1983, pp. 1292–1295.

[86]   Gottlieb, P., et al., "Inactivation of Trypanosoma cruzi: trypomastigote forms in blood components with a psoralen and UV-A light," *Photochem. Photobiol.*, Vol. 63, 1996, pp. 562–565.

[87]   Gardlo, K., et al., "Photodynamic therapy of cutaneous leishmaniasis. A promising new therapeutic modality," *Hautarzt*, Vol. 55, 2004, pp. 381–383.

[88]   Asilian, A., and M. Davami, "Comparison between the efficacy of photodynamic therapy and topical paromomycin in the treatment of Old World cutaneous leishmaniasis: a placebo-controlled, randomized clinical trial," *Clin. Exp. Dermatol.*, Vol. 31, 2006, pp. 634–637.

[89]   Akilov, O. E., et al., "Photodynamic therapy for cutaneous leishmaniasis: the effectiveness of topical phenothiaziniums in parasite eradication and Th1 immune response stimulation," *Photochem. Photobiol. Sci.*, Vol. 6, 2007, pp. 1067–1075.

[90]   Ruiz-Moreno, J. M., et al., "Photodynamic therapy and high dose intravitreal triamcinolone to treat exudative age-related macular degeneration: 1-year outcome," *Retina*, Vol. 26, 2006, pp. 602–612.

[91]   Gad F., et al., "Targeted photodynamic therapy of established soft-tissue infections in mice," *Photochem. Photobiol. Sci.*, Vol. 3, 2004, pp. 451–458.

CHAPTER 19

Photodynamic Therapy for Infectious Disease

Michael R. Hamblin and Stanley B. Brown

19.1   Introduction

The increasing occurrence of multiantibiotic-resistant microbes has led to the search for alternative methods of killing pathogens and treating infections. Photodynamic therapy (PDT) uses the combination of nontoxic dyes and harmless visible light to produce reactive oxygen species that can kill mammalian and microbial cells. There were many reports of photodynamic inactivation (PDI) of various species of bacterial and fungal cells as well as viruses over the years between the discovery of antimicrobial PDI in 1904 and 1990. In the 1990s it was observed that fundamental differences in susceptibility to PDT exist between Gram (+) and Gram (–) bacteria. This was explained by differences in their morphology: the Gram (+) cytoplasmic membrane is surrounded by a layer of only peptidoglycan and lipoteichoic acid that is relatively porous, while Gram (–) bacteria have a somewhat more intricate, nonporous cell wall structure consisting of an inner cytoplasmic membrane and an outer membrane, which are separated by the peptidoglycan-containing periplasm. It was discovered that in general, neutral or anionic PS molecules are efficiently bound to and mediate the photodynamic inactivation (PDI) of Gram (+) bacteria [1], but they are not able to photoinactivate Gram negative bacteria. The latter can be achieved by employing several different techniques. It is possible to use agents that are capable of increasing the permeability of the cell outer membrane such as polymyxin B nonapeptide [2], or EDTA [3] together with traditional PSs. Alternatively, one can use a PS molecule with an intrinsic positive charge [4, 5], or polycationic PS conjugates formed from polymers such as polylysine [6–9]. Several studies have shown that antibiotic-resistant bacteria are as susceptible to PDI as their naïve counterparts [10, 11]. The nature of the PDI-induced damage that involves oxidative modification of vital cellular constituents, suggests that bacteria will not easily be able to develop resistance mechanisms and one study has shown that resistance to PDI does not occur [8].

The demonstration of efficient PDI of multiple classes of microorganisms, together with concern about rapidly increasing emergence of antibiotic resistance among pathogenic bacteria, has suggested that PDT may be a useful tool to combat infectious disease [12]. Nonetheless, there are several limitations. Because the delivery of visible light is almost by definition a localized process, PDT for infections is likely to be applied exclusively to localized disease, as opposed to systemic infections such as bacteremia. The key issues to be addressed with PDT are the effectiveness of the treatment in destroying sufficient numbers of the disease-causing pathogens; selectivity of the PS for the microbes, thus avoiding an unacceptable degree of PDT damage to host tissue in the area of infection; and the avoidance of regrowth of the pathogens from a few survivors in the time following the treatment.

In this chapter we will cover the following topics:

- A literature survey of in vivo experiments in which PDT has been used in animal models of infection;
- A summary of experiments undertaken in the Hamblin laboratory using PDT of infections caused by bioluminescent bacteria in mouse models;
- A literature survey of clinical trials and applications of PDT for infectious disease in humans.

19.2 PDT in Animal Models of Infection

19.2.1 PDT for Bacterial Infections

An early report of PDT being used to treat a bacterial infection in an animal model was presented in 1994. Berthiaume et al. [13] evaluated the efficacy of antibody-targeted photolysis to kill bacteria in vivo using specific antibacterial photosensitizer (PS) immunconjugates. After infecting the dorsal skin in mice with *P. aeruginosa*, both specific and nonspecific tin (IV) chlorin e6-monoclonal antibody conjugates were injected at the infection site. After a 15-minute incubation period, the site was exposed to 630-nm light with a power density of 100 mW/cm^2 for 1,600 seconds. Irradiation resulted in a greater than 75% decrease in the number of viable bacteria at sites treated with a specific conjugate, whereas normal bacterial growth was observed in animals that were untreated or treated with a nonspecific conjugate.

Wong and coworkers [14] reported on PDT of wound infections in mice caused by the highly invasive Gram-negative bacterium *Vibrio vulnificus* that is responsible for human opportunistic infections; 53% (10 of 19) of mice treated with 100 μg of toluidine blue O (TBO) per mL and exposed to broad-spectrum red light (150 J/cm^2 at 80 mW/cm^2) survived, even though systemic septicemia had been established with a bacterial inoculum 100 times the 50% lethal dose. In vitro PDT severely damaged the cell wall, killing the cells and also reduced cell motility and virulence.

PDT has also been used to treat animal models of dental infections. In the first study [15], *Porphyromonas gingivalis* (one of the major causative organisms of periodontitis) was subjected to PDT on the buccal mucosa of the maxillary molars of rats. When 25 μL of a *P. gingivalis* suspension (10^{10} CFU/mL in RTF) was combined with 1mg/mL of TBO and 48J of 630-nm laser light, there were no viable bacteria. On histological examination, no adverse effect of photosensitization on the adjacent tissues was observed. In a further group of animals, after time was allowed for the disease to develop in controls, the rats were killed and the level of maxillary molar alveolar bone was assessed. The bone loss in the animals treated with light and TBO was found to be significantly less than that in the control groups.

In another study [16], beagle dogs were infected with *P. gingivalis* and *Fusobacterium nucleatum* in all subgingival areas. PDT was tested with two photosensitizers, chlorine e6 and BLC1010 combined with a diode laser at 662-nm and a power of 0.5 W. After infection, clinical signs of gingival inflammation, including an increase of redness and bleeding on probing (BOP) were observed. Microbiological monitoring before and after treatment was performed using polymerase chain reaction (PCR). PDT caused a significant reduction in the clinical inflammation signs of redness and BOP, compared to the controls (laser only and no treatment). Furthermore, PDT with chlorine e6 caused a significant reduction in *P. gingivalis*-infected sites, whereas there was a lack in suppression after PDT with BLC1010. F. nucleatum could hardly be reduced with chlorine e6, and only to a certain extent with BLC 1010 and laser only.

A recent study [17] investigated whether PDT has a role to play in treatment of tuberculosis. TB therapy is currently hindered by prolonged antibiotic regimens and the emergence of significant (and sometimes extreme) drug resistance. PDT may be effective in curtailing *Mycobacterium tuberculosis* in discrete anatomical sites in the most infectious phase of pulmonary TB. To demonstrate experimental proof of principle, PDT was tested in an in vivo mouse model using *M. bovis* (BCG). A new three-dimensional collagen gel was employed as an infectious site for BCG, subcutaneously inserted, to induce specifically localized granuloma-like lesions in mice. When a benzoporphyrin derivative was utilized as the PS, exposure to light killed extracellular and intracellular BCG in significant numbers. Collagen scaffolds containing BCG inserted in situ in BALB/c mice for 3 months mimicked granulomatous lesions and demonstrated a marked cellular infiltration upon histological examination, with evidence of caseating necrosis and fibrous capsule formation. When 105 BCG were present in the in vivo-induced granulomas, a significant reduction in viable mycobacterial cells was demonstrated in PDT-treated granulomas compared to those of controls.

A study by Bisland et al. [18] investigated whether PDT had a role to play in treating osteomyelitis produced by implanting bacteria coated wires in the rat tibia. This study is covered in detail in Chapter 16 in the present volume.

19.2.2 PDT for Fungal Infections

There has been one report of PDT in a mouse model of infection with *Candida albicans*. Teichert et al. [19] used methylene blue (MB)-mediated PDT to treat oral candidiasis in an immunosuppressed murine model, mimicking what is found in human patients. SCID mice were inoculated orally with *C. albicans* by swab three times a week for a 4-week period. On treatment day, mice were cultured for baseline fungal growth and received a topical oral cavity administration of 0.05 mL MB solution at concentrations ranging from 250 to 500 μg/mL. After 10 minutes the mice were recultured and underwent illumination with 664-nm diode laser light with a cylindrical diffuser. After PDT the mice were cultured again for CFU/mL and then killed, and their tissue harvested for histopathology. Results indicated an MB dose-dependent effect and concentrations of 450 and 500 μg/mL totally eradicated *C. albicans* from the oral cavity (an almost 3-log reduction in CFU).

19.2.3   PDT for Parasite Infection

Two reports have looked at PDT in animal models of Leismaniasis. The motivation for doing this was the appearance of multiple reports that ALA-PDT could be a useful treatment for clinical cases of old-world cutaneous Leishmaniasis. Since it is well known that Leishmania parasites do not possess the appropriate biosynthetic enzymes necessary to transform the precursor molecule ALA to the PS PPIX [20], the mechanism of how ALA-PDT could improve Leismaniasis lesions was investigated [21, 22]. Following in vitro coincubation of *Leishmania major* with 0.1 μM ALA, the intracellular PpIX concentration remained at the basal level, whereas after coincubation with 0.1 μM exogenous PPIX, the intracellular PPIX level was 100-fold higher. No differences in ALA-derived PPIX levels were detected between Leishmania-infected and noninfected J774.2 cells, and PDT did not demonstrate any parasiticidal effects on amastigotes. In contrast, in vivo topical ALA-PDT, performed on a murine CL model, resulted in significant reductions of the parasite loads and vigorous tissue destruction. After ALA-PDT, a dramatically decreased percentage of macrophages and increased levels of interleukin-6 were observed in the infected skin. The clinical outcome observed with ALA-PDT is therefore likely the result of unspecific tissue destruction accompanied by depopulation of macrophages rather than direct killing of parasites.

19.2.4   PDT for Viral Infection

There is one report that is relevant to PDT of viral infection in a mouse model. Stevenson et al. [23] investigated the ability of hypericin to protect mice from splenomegaly resulting from infection with Friend leukemia virus (FLV). FLV-induced splenomegaly was not prevented or ameliorated in mice injected with 100-μg hypericin, either mixed with the FLV inoculum or administered 1 day later either under normal laboratory light or in the dark. These results contradict previous findings. Both hypericin and rose bengal, however, inactivated the FLV inoculum at low doses (<11 μg), provided that the mixture was illuminated for 1 hour under a normal fluorescent desk lamp. This procedure protected mice completely from FLV-induced splenomegaly. They concluded that for FLV illumination of hypericin with the virus is absolutely required for hypericin's antiviral (virucidal) effects.

19.3   PDT of Bioluminescent Bacterial Infections in Mice

As can be seen from the reports summarized in Section 19.2, in vivo studies of PDT on infection models are relatively rare. One of the reasons for this is probably the difficulty in monitoring the development of an infection in animal models and its response to treatment. Standard microbiological techniques used to follow infections in animal models frequently involve sacrifice of the animals, removal of the infected tissue, homogenization, serial dilution, plating, and colony counting. These assays use a large number of animals, are time consuming, and often are not statistically reliable.

In order to facilitate the noninvasive monitoring of animal models of infection, we have developed a procedure that uses bioluminescent genetically-engineered bacteria and a light-sensitive imaging system to allow real-time visualization of infections. When these bacteria are treated with PDT in vitro, the loss of luminescence parallels the loss of colony-forming ability. We have developed several mouse models of localized infections that can be followed by bioluminescence imaging [24].

19.3.1 Bioluminescent Imaging for Infectious Disease

Various living organisms are able to emit light [25]. The enzymes involved in this process, named luciferases, are oxygenases that utilize molecular oxygen to oxidize a substrate (luciferin), with the formation of a product molecule in an electronically excited state that emits the light. Several different luciferases and substrates from a diversity of marine and terrestrial organisms are known, many with different colors of emission [25].

Bacterial luciferases are heterodimeric and use oxygen, long-chain fatty aldehydes (e.g., decanal) and reduced flavin mononucleotide (FMNH2) as substrates to produce a blue-green light (emission peak at 490 nm) [25]. In both marine and terrestrial bioluminescent bacteria, a five genes operon (luxCDABE) encodes the luciferase and biosynthetic enzymes (for the synthesis of the aldehyde substrate) necessary for light production. luxA and B encode the alpha and beta subunits of the luciferase, with luxC, D, and E encoding proteins for aldehyde production [26]. The lux operon from P. luminescens is ideally suited for the study of pathogens in mammalian animal models as the enzyme retains significant activity at 37° C [27].

The detection of light from small animals containing bioluminescent cells can be achieved using a CCD-based imaging system. These systems consist of a light-tight chamber in which the animal subjects are placed, a sensitive CCD camera to detect the light emitted and a computer controller to acquire the image and allow analysis of the data. Typically, a grayscale reference image of the animal is acquired under weak illumination, and then the bioluminescent signal is captured in complete darkness. This process may take from a few seconds to several minutes, depending on the brightness of the bioluminescent signal, the depth within the tissue from which it arises, and the sensitivity of the detector. The signal intensity is then represented as a pseudocolor image and superimposed on the grayscale reference image. The magnitude of the signal can then be measured from specified regions of the animals using a "region of interest" function.

BLI can be used either to track the course of an infection or monitor the efficacy of antimicrobial therapies. Small animals are routinely used to model both human infections and the effects of antibiotics against pathogens. The use of pathogens that have been engineered to express luciferase and imaging of their location and cell number have streamlined these studies and refined these animal models, as the necessity to sacrifice the animals to access the data has essentially been eliminated. Bacterial pathogenesis appeared to be unaffected by the presence of the luciferase genes, and bioluminescence can be detected throughout the study period in animals. Further, the intensity of the bioluminescence measured from the living animal correlated well with the bacterial burden subsequently determined by standard protocols

[28–30]. Subsequent studies have used transposon-mediated integration of the luciferase operon into the bacterial chromosome to improve stability and to create strains that remain bioluminescent in the absence of drug selection. This means that reduction of luminescence from sites of infection in animals can be attributed to reduction of bacterial numbers rather than loss of plasmids.

19.3.2 PDT of Nonlethal *E. coli* Wound Infection

We initially used the Gram-negative species *Escherichia coli* that had been transformed by electroporation with a plasmid, pCGSL1, containing the entire *P. luminescens* lux operon [31], which also confers resistance to ampicillin (carbenicillin) on the bacteria. BLI was carried out using a low-light imaging system (Hamamatsu photon-counting camera). The luminescence image was presented as a false-color image superimposed on top of the grayscale reference image. We used a molecular construct covalently formed between poly-L-lysine chains and the PS chlorin(e6) as a microbial-targeted PS. We have previously shown [6, 7, 32] that these pL-ce6 conjugates are highly effective in mediating the PDI of both Gram-positive and Gram-negative bacteria. Their positive charges help them to bind to the negatively charged bacteria and their polycationic nature enables them to penetrate the outer membrane of Gram-negative cells by disturbing the structure of the lipopolysaccharide layers. The macromolecular nature of these conjugates gives a temporal selectivity for bacteria over mammalian cells as the latter take them up by the time-dependent process of endocytosis, while they bind rapidly to bacteria. The size of the pL chain was on average 160 lysine residues (range 137–173) and there was an average of 6 ce6 molecules (range 5–7) attached per polypeptide chain. For the light source for PDT we used a 660-nm diode laser providing up to 1W of light through an SMA coupled fiber and lens that could provide a uniform spot ranging from 1 to 3 cm in diameter

We initially sought to establish the animal model of infection by inoculating bioluminescent *E. coli* into an excisional wound on the mouse [33]. Five million CFU from a mid-log culture in 50 μL gave a sufficiently bright luminescence signal from the wound to allow at least two logs of signal reduction to be accurately followed. Bioluminescence lasted for 1 day in a wound made on the back of a mouse, but the next day the wounds had lost on average 90% of the original luminescence signal and mice survived these infections well.

Since the wound infection with *E. coli* DH5α was found to be self-limiting (i.e., this particular strain of *E. coli* is noninvasive) [34], it allowed the use of each mouse as its own control to follow wound healing with four wounds per mouse. The effect of topical application of pL-ce6 conjugate and successive applications of 660-nm light is presented in a series of overlaid luminescence (false-color) and grayscale reference images (Color Plate 20). This data was obtained from a mouse in which bacteria were inoculated in all wounds; 30 minutes later conjugate was added to wounds 1 (nearest head) and 4 (nearest tail), and after another 30 minutes wounds 3 and 4 were illuminated with red light. Therefore wound 1 was the dark control with conjugate, wound 2 was the absolute control, wound 3 was the light alone control, and wound 4 was PDT treated. The fluence rate was 100 mW/cm^2 and mice were imaged after 7.5 minutes and again after 27.5 minutes corresponding to the delivery of 45 and 165 J/cm², respectively. Topical application of a targeted polycationic PS conjugate followed by illumination led to a 99% reduction in luminescence as measured by the imaging software (Figure 19.1). We observed that PDT of infected wounds did not lead to any inhibition of wound healing and there was an indication that the PDT-treated wounds actually healed somewhat faster relative to the other control wounds but this was not statistically significant.

The lack of host tissue phototoxicity may have been due to the macromolecular pL-ce6 demonstrating temporal selectivity for bacteria compared to mammalian due to a combination of the topical delivery method together with the large molecular weight of the conjugate and the relatively short incubation time.

19.3.3 PDT of Lethal Pseudomonas aeruginosa Wound Infections in Mice

In order to test PDT in a more clinically relevant infection model, we used a potentially fatal *P. aeruginosa* wound infection [35]. We used a bioluminescent derivative of strain 180 (ATCC 19660) that has been shown to be invasive and leads to development of fatal sepsis after intraperitoneal injection in rats [36]. Mice with single dorsal excisional wounds infected with 5×10^6 CFU (LD50 was approximately 200,000 CFU) of bioluminescent *P. aeruginosa* quickly developed an illness consistent with systemic sepsis. They lost weight, had ruffled coats, and developed progressive inactivity leading to a moribund condition and death occurred between 24 to 60 hours after infection. The pL-ce6 conjugate was added as 50-μL of a 200-μM ce6 equivalent concentration and spread evenly throughout the surface of the wound and was retained by the edges of the wound to prevent the liquid running off. It was necessary to give the conjugate at least 30 minutes to bind to and pene-

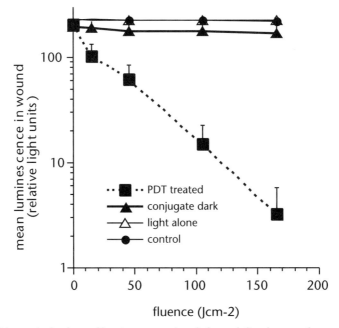

Figure 19.1 Mean pixel values of luminescence signals from defined areas of wounds measuring 1,200 pixels determined by image analysis. Data points are means of values from the corresponding wound on six mice per group and bars are SD.

trate the bacteria in order to see effective loss of luminescence after illumination with 660-nm light.

As can be seen from a set of luminescence images from a representative mouse shown in Color Plate 21, PDT produced a fluence-dependent loss of luminescence until only a trace remained after 240 J/cm² had been delivered (40 minutes illumination). When the mouse was imaged the next day all traces of luminescence had gone (panel 3H). There was a drop in luminescence seen shortly after applying the conjugate in the dark (Color Plate 21B and J), but this did not decrease further after 30 minutes of incubation (Color Plate 21C and K) or indeed after 60 minutes of incubation (Color Plate 21L), approximately equal to the time for illumination of the PDT wounds. Infected wounds left untreated or treated with illumination alone showed a rise in luminescence signal (up to twofold, Figure 19.2(a)), presumably due to

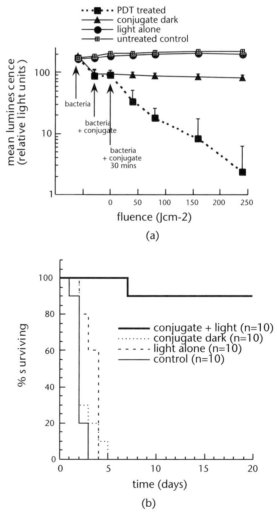

Figure 19.2 (a) Mean pixel values of bioluminescence signals from defined areas measuring 1,200 pixels covering infected wounds determined by image analysis. The four groups comprise untreated control, light-alone control, dark conjugate control, and PDT treated. Data points are means of values from the wounds on 10 mice per group and bars are SD. (b)Kaplan-Meier survival plot for the four groups of mice described in (a).

growth of the bacteria in the nutrient-rich medium of the wound. There was significant luminescence present in control wounds until death occurred 2 to 4 days later (Figure 19.2(b)). All the mice in the three control groups (untreated, light alone, and dark conjugate) died within a period of 5 days infection. By contrast, 90% of the mice treated with PDT survived, as seen in Figure 19.2(b). These mice appeared to suffer from some symptoms of bacterial infection (weight loss, ruffled fur, and inactivity) similar to those mice who received a sublethal dose of bacteria described above. They recovered quickly however, and by 5 days after infection were regaining weight and moving normally.

19.3.4 PDT of Established Soft-Tissue Infections in Mice

The previous experiments were carried out on animals whose wounds were recently contaminated with relatively large numbers of CFU. It is unlikely that patients would present for treatment under these circumstances. A more realistic and clinically relevant model would consist of inoculation of a smaller number of bacteria and then allowing the infection to grow and become established in tissue over time. A second major consideration was that the previous experiments used an infection model where the bacteria were relatively near the surface of the tissue in an excisional wound. In real life, the bacteria could be beneath the surface of the skin or tissue either because they had already invaded or because they were on skin or clothing that had been forcibly introduced into a penetrating wound such as those caused by gunshot. Since the penetration of visible light (even red light) into tissue is limited, we questioned whether PDT could be used to treat an infection where the bacteria had been allowed to multiply several hundred-fold and were some distance beneath the skin surface.

For this experiment, we used a strain of stable bioluminescent *S. aureus* (mouse pathogenic strain 8325-4), injecting 1 million log-phase CFU into the mouse thigh muscle (2-mm deep) [37]. The mice had previously been rendered temporarily neutropenic by pretreatment with cyclophosphamide. We used a model in which the mice developed two equivalent infections, one in each hind thigh in order to allow each mouse to have a PDT-treated infection and a control untreated infection and act as its own control. Twenty-four hours after infection the bioluminescence had increased dramatically as the bacteria had multiplied within the infected tissue (Color Plate 22). The pL-ce6 conjugate ($50\,\mu$L) at a concentration of 1-mM ce6 equivalent was injected into the infected area, resulting in a visible green coloration noticeable beneath the skin. This allowed a judgment to be made about the uniformity of the PS distribution within the infection. Light (660 nm) was delivered to the infection as a spot on the skin about 8-mm in diameter centered on the infected area. There was a slight reduction in bacterial bioluminescence observed immediately after the conjugate was injected into the infection. Luminescence was further reduced after the 30-minute incubation period in the dark. When illumination was commenced there was a light-dose dependent decrease in luminescence after each 40-J/cm^2 increment of red light (Figure 19.3). A typical mouse treated with injection of conjugate into the right infected thigh, followed by illumination of this thigh as described previously, is shown in Figure 19.3.

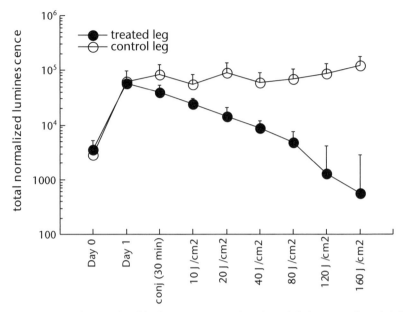

Figure 19.3 Mean total normalized bioluminescence values from left (untreated) and right (PDT treated) thighs of five mice infected in both thighs. Bars are SEM.

After 160 J/cm^2 had been delivered, the bioluminescence of the treated infected legs had been reduced by >99% compared to the untreated contralateral legs. However, 4 out of 5 of these treated legs suffered a recurrence of the bioluminescence on succeeding days (data not shown).

19.3.5   PDT for Burn Infections

We used PDT mediated by meso-mono-phenyl-tri(N-methyl-4-pyridyl)-porphyrin (PTMPP) to treat burn wounds in mice with established *Staphylococcus* aureus infections [38]. The third-degree burn was caused by application of two steel blocks to an elevated skin fold on the mouse back, and burns were infected with 10^9 CFU of bioluminescent *S. aureus*. PDT was applied after 1 day of bacterial growth by adding 500-μM PTMPP dissolved in a 25% aqueous DMSO solution to the wound followed by illumination with red light and periodic BLI of the mice. More than 98% of the bacteria were eradicated after a light dose of 210 J/cm^2 in the presence of PTMPP. However, bacterial regrowth was observed. The treatment needs to be optimized to reduce wound damage and prevent recurrence.

19.4   Clinical Studies in Antimicrobial PDT

Until recently, there were very few reported clinical studies using antimicrobial PDT, in spite of the wide range of potential applications and the clear need for new approaches to treatment of infections and disease with microbial involvement. As already stated, it should be emphasized that, under currently available light administration regimes, treatment is limited to local disease. For the most part, though not exclusively, this is equivalent to treatment of microorganisms that are superficial or at least may be accessed by topical application of photosensitizer. Nevertheless, the range of potential applications is large and includes colonization/infections in the following:

- Dental conditions (e.g., in periodontal disease);
- Acute wounds of various kinds, (e.g., burns, trauma, and surgical);
- Chronic wounds of various kinds (e.g., diabetic foot ulcers, venous leg ulcers, and pressure sores);
- Parasitic lesions (e.g., cutaneous Leishmaniaisis);
- Carriers of Staphylococcus (including MRSA) (e.g., in the nose);
- *Helicobacter pylori* in the gastrointestinal system;
- Acne vulgaris;
- Superficial skin conditions such as erythrasma.

The substantial literature on photodynamic inactivation of viruses, especially as it relates to blood products, is not considered here.

A number of case reports in the above areas have appeared but there have been few reports of rigorous, controlled clinical trials. In the periodontal area, research has been led by Wilson and coworkers, who have recently published a report on a randomized trial for treatment of periodontal disease by PDT compared to scaling and root planning. In 33 subjects with moderate to advanced periodontal disease, randomized to PDT alone, PDT plus scaling and root planing, or scaling and root planing alone, while it was not possible to demonstrate bacterial reduction, the clinical assessments showed advantages of combining scaling and root planing with PDT over scaling and root planing alone [39]. In an as-yet-unpublished study, the first of its kind, a phase IIa randomized, blinded, placebo-controlled, trial in 32 patients with chronic venous leg ulcers and chronic diabetic foot ulcers showed a strongly significant reduction in bacterial load following treatment with PDT using a phenothiazinium salt (S. B. Brown, personal communication).

In a case study of a 72-year-old woman with a chronic, recalcitrant venous ulceration, it has been shown that twice-weekly treatment with ALA-PDT reduced the bacterial load, which correlated with significant improvement in the ulcer [40].

Photoeradication of *Helicobacter pylori* has been the subject of two clinical reports. This is a common, Gram-negative organism implicated in the development of peptic ulcers and gastric neoplasms [41]. In 13 *Helicobacter pylori* positive volunteers, Wilder-Smith and colleagues showed that exposure to oral ALA and either 410-nm laser or white light resulted in up to 85% of subjects with complete eradication at 4 hours postirradiation. The second report by Ganz and colleagues was not based on PDT but on application of blue light alone and showed that up to 99% reduction in the bacterial levels could be achieved [42]. In view of this data, it is not clear to what extent the eradication seen in the earlier study is due to a PDT effect over and above a possible light-alone effect.

Erythrasma is a skin condition caused by superficial infection by *Corynebacterium minutissimum* and is characterized by fluorescence under a Wood's lamp, due to the presence of endogenous porphyrins [43]. Darras-

Vercambre and coworkers treated 13 patients with erythrasma by illumination with broadband red light at 80 J/cm^2. As a result of the treatment, three patients experienced a complete recovery and in most other cases, there was a reduction in the extent of lesions (mean 29% reduction after one treatment).

Many studies have demonstrated the potential of PDT to inactivate fungal organisms (usually Candida) in vitro, but this remains to be converted into effective clinical application. A review by Calzavara-Pinton et al. [44] summarizes the literature and includes a clinical study [45]. The latter enrolled nine patients with interdigital mycosis of the feet. Treatment included application of 20% ALA cream under an occlusive dressing followed 4 hours later by 75 J/cm^2 of broadband red light. Clinical and microbiological efficacy was observed in four patients after a single treatment and two patients after four treatments. However, the remission was only maintained in two patients.

Treatment of cutaneous Leishmaniasis by PDT is an attractive possibility. Some clinical studies have been reported though mostly with small patient numbers or single-patient case reports [46–48]. In every case the photosensitizing agent has been ALA or Metvix (ALA methyl ester). A study in 2003 compared Metvix PDT and paromomycin in 10 lesions in a 35-year-old man [46]. Five lesions treated with PDT and two of the paromomycin-treated lesions gave a complete clinical response and became clinically and histologically Leishmania-free. The three lesions treated with paomomycin were then subsequently treated with PDT and all responded. Ten months after therapy, there was no recurrence. In a subsequent study, ALA-PDT was applied in five patients with weekly treatments for 4 weeks [47]. Direct smears of the lesions showed no amastigotes after one or two sessions. Four months after treatment cosmetic results were reported as excellent and there were no signs of clinical recurrence. A more extensive study [48] was recently reported in 60 patients who were randomized to equal groups to receive weekly topical ALA-PDT (Group 1), twice-daily topical paromomycin (Group 2), and placebo (Group 3) respectively for 4 weeks in each case. At the end of the study, complete improvement was seen in 29 of 31 (93.5%), 14 of 34 (41.2%), and 4 of 30 lesions (13.3%) in groups 1, 2, and 3, respectively (P<0.001). At the same time point, 100%, 64.7%, and 20% of the lesions had parasitological cure in group 1, 2, and 3, respectively (P<0.001).

Acne vulgaris is a complex dermatological condition with four key pathological components: abnormal keratinization, increased sebum production, colonization by the bacterium *Propionibacterium acnes*, and development of inflammation [49]. Photodynamic therapy can potentially intervene to decrease sebum production (by damaging sebocytes) or by reducing levels of *P. acnes*. In practice it is difficult to delineate the PDT effects, but it is assumed that killing of *P. acnes* is an important contributing factor in the efficacy of PDT in this condition. Many clinical studies of PDT in acne treatment have been reported. Most of the early studies were uncontrolled, but interest in this field is increasing and well-controlled trials are now being reported. All show some success with ALA and Metvix and there are now excellent recent reviews dealing with the subject [49–51]. There is therefore considerable optimism that PDT will provide solutions to treatment of this disease, especially in difficult-to-treat patients with moderate to severe acne vulgaris. However, with the drugs used to date (ALA and Metvix), pain remains an issue, with some patients withdrawing from treatment because of adverse side effects, and further trials are in progress to optimize the approach.

19.5 Conclusion

PDT for infectious disease is likely to be a growing clinical application. With the increasing international concern about multidrug-resistant bacteria, and the specter of infectious diseases that have become untreatable by antibiotics constantly discussed by the popular media, alternative antimicrobial therapies have become a hot topic. The rapid bacterial killing typical of PDT and the unlikelihood of bacteria developing resistance to PDT suggests that PDT should be at the forefront of new therapies for infectious disease.

References

[1] Malik, Z., Ladan, H., and Nitzan, Y., "Photodynamic inactivation of Gram-negative bacteria: problems and possible solutions," *J Photochem Photobiol B*, Vol. 14, 1992, pp. 262–266.

[2] Nitzan, Y., et al., "Inactivation of gram-negative bacteria by photosensitized porphyrins," *Photochem Photobiol*, Vol. 55, 1992, pp. 89–96.

[3] Bertoloni, G., et al., "Photosensitizing activity of water- and lipid-soluble phthalocyanines on Escherichia coli," *FEMS Microbiol Lett*, Vol. 59, 1990, pp. 149-155

[4] Merchat, M., Bertolini, G., and Giacomini, P., "Meso-substituted cationic porphyrins as efficient photosensitizers of gram-positive and gram-negative bacteria," *J Photochem Photobiol B*, Vol. 32, 1996, pp. 153–157.

[5] Minnock, A., et al., http://www.ncbi.nlm.nih.gov/sites/entrez?Db=pubmed&Cmd= ShowDetailView&TermToSearch=8622179&ordinalpos=24&itool=EntrezSystem2.PEn trez.Pubmed.Pubmed_ResultsPanel.Pubmed_RVDocSum, "Photoinactivation of bacteria. Use of a cationic water-soluble zinc phthalocyanine to photoinactivate both gram-negative and gram-positive bacteria," *J Photochem Photobiol B.*, Vol. 32, 1996, pp.159–164.

[6] Hamblin, M. R., et al., "Polycationic photosensitizer conjugates: effects of chain length and Gram classification on the photodynamic inactivation of bacteria," *J Antimicrob Chemother*, Vol. 49, 2002, pp. 941–951.

[7] Soukos, N. S., et al., "Targeted antimicrobial photochemotherapy," *Antimicrob Agents Chemother*, Vol. 42, 1998, pp. 2595–2601.

[8] Lauro, F. M., et al., "Photoinactivation of bacterial strains involved in periodontal diseases sensitized by porphycene-polylysine conjugates," *Photochem Photobiol Sci*, Vol. 1, 2002, pp. 468–470.

[9] Rovaldi, C. R., et al., "Photoactive porphyrin derivative with broad-spectrum activity against oral pathogens In vitro," *Antimicrob Agents Chemother*, Vol. 44, 2000, pp. 3364–3367.

[10] Wilson, M., and Yianni, C., "Killing of methicillin-resistant Staphylococcus aureus by low-power laser light," *J Med Microbiol*, Vol. 42, 1995, pp. 62–66.

[11] Wainwright, M., et al., "Photobactericidal activity of phenothiazinium dyes against methicillin-resistant strains of Staphylococcus aureus," *FEMS Microbiol Lett*, Vol. 160, 1998, pp. 177–181.

[12] Hamblin, M. R., and Hasan, T., "Photodynamic therapy: a new antimicrobial approach to infectious disease?" *Photochem Photobiol Sci*, Vol. 3, 2004, pp. 436–450.

[13] Berthiaume, F., et al., "Antibody-targeted photolysis of bacteria in vivo," *Biotechnology*, Vol. 12, 1994, pp. 703–706.

[14] Wong, T. W., et al., "Bactericidal effects of toluidine blue-mediated photodynamic action on Vibrio vulnificus," *Antimicrob Agents Chemother*, Vol. 49, 2005, pp. 895–902.

[15] Komerik, N., et al., "In vivo killing of Porphyromonas gingivalis by toluidine blue-mediated photosensitization in an animal model," *Antimicrob Agents Chemother*, Vol. 47, 2003, pp. 932–940.

[16] Sigusch, B. W., et al., "Efficacy of photodynamic therapy on inflammatory signs and two selected periodontopathogenic species in a beagle dog model," *J Periodontol*, Vol. 76, 2005, pp. 1100–1105.

[17] O'Riordan, K., et al., "Photoinactivation of Mycobacteria in vitro and in a new murine model of localized Mycobacterium bovis BCG-induced granulomatous infection," *Antimicrob Agents Chemother*, Vol. 50, 2006, pp. 1828–1834.

[18] Bisland, S. K., et al., "Pre-clinical in vitro and in vivo studies to examine the potential use of photodynamic therapy in the treatment of osteomyelitis," *Photochem Photobiol Sci*, Vol. 5, 2006, pp. 31–38.

[19] Teichert, M. C., et al., "Treatment of oral candidiasis with methylene blue-mediated photodynamic therapy in an immunodeficient murine model," *Oral Surg Oral Med Oral Pathol Oral Radiol Endod*, Vol. 93, 2002, pp. 155–160.

[20] Sah, J. F., et al., "Genetic rescue of Leishmania deficiency in porphyrin biosynthesis creates mutants suitable for analysis of cellular events in uroporphyria and for photodynamic therapy," *J Biol Chem*, Vol. 277, 2002, pp. 14902–14909.

[21] Akilov, O. E., et al., "Parasiticidal effect of delta-aminolevulinic acid-based photodynamic therapy for cutaneous leishmaniasis is indirect and mediated through the killing of the host cells," *Exp Dermatol*, Vol. 16, 2007, pp. 651–660.

[22] Kosaka, S., et al., "A mechanistic study of delta-aminolevulinic acid-based photodynamic therapy for cutaneous leishmaniasis," *J Invest Dermatol*, Vol. 127, 2007, pp. 1546–1549.

[23] Stevenson, N. R., and Lenard, J., "Antiretroviral activities of hypericin and rose bengal: photodynamic effects on Friend leukemia virus infection of mice," *Antiviral Res*, Vol. 21, 1993, pp. 119–127.

[24] Demidova, T. N., et al., "Monitoring photodynamic therapy of localized infections by bioluminescence imaging of genetically engineered bacteria," *J Photochem Photobiol B.*, Vol. 81, 2005, pp. 15–25.

[25] Hastings, J. W., "Chemistries and colors of bioluminescent reactions: a review," *Gene*, Vol. 173, 1996, pp. 5–11.

[26] Meighen, E. A., "Molecular biology of bacterial bioluminescence," *Microbiol Rev*, Vol. 55, 1991, pp. 123–142.

[27] Meighen, E. A., "Bacterial bioluminescence: organization, regulation, and application of the lux genes," *FASEB J*, Vol. 7, 1993, pp. 1016–1022.

[28] Rocchetta, H. L., et al., "Validation of a noninvasive, real-time imaging technology using bioluminescent escherichia coli in the neutropenic mouse thigh model of infection," *Antimicrob Agents Chemother*, Vol. 45, 2001, pp. 129–137.

[29] Francis, K. P., et al., "Monitoring bioluminescent Staphylococcus aureus infections in living mice using a novel luxABCDE construct," *Infect Immun*, Vol. 68, 2000, pp. 3594–3600.

[30] Francis, K. P., et al., "Visualizing pneumococcal infections in the lungs of live mice using bioluminescent Streptococcus pneumoniae transformed with a novel gram-positive lux transposon," *Infect Immun*, Vol. 69, 2001, pp. 3350–3358.

[31] Frackman, S., Anhalt, M., and Nealson, K. H., "Cloning, organization, and expression of the bioluminescence genes of Xenorhabdus luminescens," *J Bacteriol*, Vol. 172, 1990, pp. 5767–5773.

[32] Gad, F., et al., "Effects of growth phase and extracellular slime on photodynamic inactivation of gram-positive pathogenic bacteria," *Antimicrob Agents Chemother*, Vol. 48, 2004, pp. 2173–2178.

[33] Hamblin, M. R., et al., "Rapid control of wound infections by targeted photodynamic therapy monitored by in vivo bioluminescence imaging," *Photochem Photobiol,* Vol. 75, 2002, pp. 51–57.

[34] Busch, N. A., et al., "A model of infected burn wounds using Escherichia coli O18:K1:H7 for the study of gram-negative bacteremia and sepsis," *Infect Immun*, Vol. 68, 2000, pp. 3349–3351.

[35] Hamblin, M. R., et al., "Optical monitoring and treatment of potentially lethal wound infections in vivo," *J Infect Dis*, Vol. 187, 2003, pp. 1717–1726.

[36] Milligan, R. C., Rust, J., and Rosenthal, S. M., "Gamma globulin factors protective against infections from Pseudomonas and other organisms," *Science*, Vol. 126, 1957, pp. 509–511.

[37] Gad, F., et al., "Targeted photodynamic therapy of established soft-tissue infections in mice," *Photochem Photobiol Sci*, Vol. 3, 2004, pp. 451–458.

[38] Lambrechts, S. A., et al., "Photodynamic therapy for Staphylococcus aureus infected burn wounds in mice," *Photochem Photobiol Sci*, Vol. 4, 2005, pp. 503–509.

[39] Anderson, R., et al., "Treatment of periodontal disease by photodisinfection compared to scaling and roort planing," *J Clin Dent*, 18, 2007, pp. 34–38.

[40] Clayton, T. H., and Harrison, P. V., "Photodynamic therapy for infected leg ulcers," *Br J Dermatol*, Vol. 156, 2007, pp. 384–385.

[41] Wilder-Smith, C. H., et al., "Photoeradication of Helicobacter pylori using 5-aminolevulinic acid: preliminary human studies," *Lasers Surg Med*, Vol. 31, 2002, pp. 18–22.

[42] Ganz, R. A., et al., "Helicobacter pylori in patients can be killed by visible light," *Lasers Surg Med*, Vol. 36, 2005, pp. 260–265.

[43] Darras-Vercambre, S., et al., "Photodynamic action of red light for treatment of erythrasma: preliminary results," *Photodermatol Photoimmunol Photomed*, Vol. 22, 2006, pp. 153–156.

[44] Calzavara-Pinton, P. G., Venturini, M., and Sala, R., "A comprehensive overview of photodynamic therapy in the treatment of superficial fungal infections of the skin," *J Photochem Photobiol B*, Vol. 78, 2005, pp. 1–6.

[45] Calzavara-Pinton, P. G., et al. "Photodynamic therapy of interdigital mycoses of the feet with topical application of 5-aminolevulinic acid," *Photodermatol. Photoimmunol Photomed*, Vol. 20, 2004, 144–147.

[46] Sohl, S., Kauer, F., Paasch, U., and Simon, J. C. "Photodynamic treatment of cutaneous leishmaniasis." *J Dtsch Dermatol Ges*, Vol. 5, 2007, 128–130.

[47] Ghaffarifar, F., et al. "Photodynamic therapy as a new treatment for cutaneous Leishmaniasis," *East Mediterr Health J*, Vol. 12, 2006, 902–908.

[48] Asilian, A., and Davami, M. "Comparison between the efficacy of photodynamic therapy and topical paromomycin in the treatment of Old World cutaneous leishmaniasis: A placebo-controlled, randomized clinical trial," *Clin Exp Dermatol*, Vol. 31, 2006, 634–637.

[49] Wiegell S. R, and Wulf, H. C. "Photodynamic therapy of acne vulgaris using methyl aminolaevulinate: a blinded, randomized, controlled trial," *Br J Dermatol*, Vol. 154, 2006, 969–976.

[50] Gold, M. "Acne and PDT: new techniques with lasers and light sources," *Lasers Med Sci*, Vol. 22, 2007, 67–72.

[51] Bhardwaj, S. S., Rohrer, T. E., and Arndt, K. "Lasers and light therapy for acne vulgaris," *Semin Cutaneous Med Surg*, Vol. 24, 2005, 107–112.

CHAPTER 20

PDT for Cardiovascular Disease

Ana P. Castano and Michael R. Hamblin

20.1 Introduction

Cardiovascular disease is the world's leading cause of death and morbidity. One of the most important manifestations of cardiovascular disease is atherosclerosis, which can occur in either coronary or peripheral arteries. Until relatively recently, the common understanding of the natural progression of atherosclerotic lesions was defined as continuous accumulation of foam cells, cholesterol and calcium crystals, and fibroproliferative tissue in the form of growing stenotic plaques that gradually reduce the cross-sectional luminal area available for blood flow. The danger of plaque progression was previously considered mainly due to progressive luminal narrowing with eventual slowing of flow, culminating in thrombosis. The prevailing belief about the culprit plaque was "the smaller, the better." This has proved to be an incomplete picture. Atherosclerosis is no longer considered as a simple buildup of fat leading to progressive narrowing of the arterial wall. Instead plaque is an active collection of cells (mainly macrophages and smooth muscle cells) arising where the endothelial layer is injured or as a response to chronic infection. It was suggested that plaque rupture followed by occlusive thrombosis as the underlying mechanism for the majority of sudden cardiac deaths, particularly in young men. Myocardial infarction frequently develops on lesions with preexisting noncritical stenoses, and therefore cast a shadow of doubt over the value of angiography in prediction of myocardial infarction and future acute coronary events. "Vulnerable plaque" is a useful term that should include various types of high-risk plaques predisposing patients to develop acute thrombotic coronary syndrome/death.

It has been observed for many years that PSs such as those commonly employed for PDT tend to specifically accumulate in the plaques in the arterial wall that are the hallmark of atherosclerosis. This preferential accumulation has led to suggestions that intravascular PDT could be employed as a therapeutic option. If a PS could be delivered either systemically or locally into the affected artery, and an intravascular catheter fitted with a diffusing tipped fiber was subsequently introduced into a vascular access point and threaded down to the affected lesion, then illumination with the appropriate wavelength light may kill the pathogenic cells within the plaque, and produce a therapeutic benefit.

Whether the most appropriate application of PDT in arteries is to reduce obstructive plaque, prevent restenosis occurring after other interventions (angioplasty or stent placement), or to prevent the rupture of "vulnerable plaques" occurring and leading to coronary thrombosis and myocardial infarction still remains to be established. This chapter will cover the relevant PDT studies on an in vitro level and applications of PDT to several animal models of cardiovascular diseases, as well as the limited number of clinical trials of PDT in cardiovascular disease.

20.2   Cardiovascular PDT In Vitro

The cells involved in cardiovascular disease are as follows: endothelial cells that line the inside of all blood vessels and can regrow after injury in order to recoat the vessel wall and allow smooth blood flow; smooth muscle cells that provide contractility in arteries and can also grow after injury, in some cases leading to recurrent blockages in the artery known as intimal hyperplasia, fibroblasts that produce collagen and are components of fibrous plaques, macrophages that are thought to be a major culprit cell type in atherogenesis and in the vulnerable inflamed plaque; lymphocytes and other inflammatory cell types. There have been some in vitro studies on how these cell types behave after incubation with various PSs followed by in vitro illumination.

Vascular smooth muscle cells (VSMCs) were cultured from long saphenous veins and restenotic lesions removed during revision coronary and peripheral vein graft surgery [1]. Cultured VSMCs were incubated with Photofrin at doses of 0 to 5 μg/ml for 48 hours, and then exposed to 4 J/cm^2 of polychromatic light. Cells were minimally affected by either Photofrin alone, but PDT was severely toxic to cells derived from saphenous veins as well as 264.7 cells derived from restenotic lesions.

Fluorescence microscopy of RAW macrophages and human vascular smooth muscle cells revealed time-dependent uptake of motexafin lutetium [2]. PDT with 732-nm light (2 J/cm^2) impaired cellular viability and growth. Depletion of intracellular glutathione potentiated and the addition of antioxidant N-acetylcysteine attenuated cell death, suggesting that the intracellular redox state influences motexafin lutetium action. PDT was associated with the loss of mito-chondrial membrane potential, mitochondrial release of cytochrome c, and caspase activation. PDT promoted phosphatidylserine externalization and induced apoptotic DNA fragmentation

Our laboratory devised a technology to specifically target PSs to macrophages [3]. This approach involves covalently attaching the PS to a macromolecule that is specifically recognized by cell surface receptors expressed on macrophages, and by only illuminating the diseased artery wall resulting in localized and specific destruction of macrophages. This concept is graphically illustrated in Figure 20.1.

In this case we used specific ligands of scavenger receptors such as maleylated albumin. Scavenger receptors are expressed mainly on mature macrophages [4]. Class A scavenger receptor (SRA) is an appropriate target for macrophage-specific PDT. Some of the natural function of SRA include phagocytosis of bacteria and other pathogens, phagocytosis of apoptotic cells, phagocytosis of senescent red blood cells, endocytosis of oxidized low-density lipoprotein, and advanced glycation endproduct-modified proteins, and calcium-independent adhesion. The SRA is a multidomain trimeric transmembrane protein and has a high capacity to internalize ligands, and therefore investigators have explored the possibility of preparing cova-

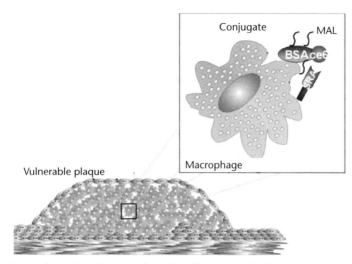

Figure 20.1   Macrophage targeting in vulnerable atherosclerotic plaque.

lent conjugates between SRA ligands and various drugs to produce macrophage targeted therapy. The precise structural motifs that lead to SRA recognition of ligands are complex and incompletely understood and their function has been referred to as "molecular flypaper". After initial binding, the ligands are rapidly internalized and are routed to lysosomes for degradation by proteases and other lysosomal enzymes. When PSs are joined to ligands of the scavenger receptor, cellular accumulation is enhanced because the SRA is high capacity and leads to efficient degradation of endocytosed molecules in lysosomes, thus releasing the possibly more photoactive free PS.

Our molecular construct designed to target the SRA is bovine serum albumin to which three molecules of the PS chlorin (e6) have been covalently attached via amide bond formation between the carboxyl groups on the tetrapyrrole and the epsilon amino groups of lysine residues in the protein. To further increase the affinity of this molecule to macrophage SRA we further modify the protein amino groups by maleylation to give BSA-ce6-mal. The high degree of selectivity of this SRA-targeted PS conjugates for macrophages have been shown in Chapter 11. In the next section we will describe the use of BSA-ce6-mal to target macrophages in atherosclerosis

de Vries et al. [5] incorporated the PS aluminum phthalocyanine chloride (AlPc) into oxidized LDL. Macrophages (RAW 264.7) were incubated with various concentrations of OxLDL-AlPc for different periods. After illumination of the cells with red light, cytotoxicity was observed that was dependent on the time of illumination and incubation. In the presence of the polyanion polyinosinic acid, a specific ligand for scavenger receptors, no cytotoxicity could be observed.

20.3   Studies on Ex Vivo Arteries

Machida et al. [6] compared the site of hematoporphyrin (HP) accumulation with changes in the HP fluorescence spectrum in ex vivo atheromatous plaques and in a liposome control model, using a microscope equipped with a spectrometer. Wavelength shifts of the two peaks of HP fluorescence (F1, 620 nm; and F2, 640-690 nm) were monitored, and the integrated F2/F1 ratio was calculated as a measure of HP fluorescence. The F1 peak is characteristic of a predominantly aqueous site. The ratio reflects selective changes in the distribution and overcrowding of HP molecules in the limited space of the artificial membrane model. Compared with a normal artery, the atherosclerotic lesions showed an increase in the area of HP fluorescence, increased fluorescence intensity, a red shift of the HP fluorescence spectrum, and an increased F2/F1 ratio. The F2/F1 ratio of the membranous structures was markedly greater in the cores of the fibrous plaques than in the other plaques. The F1 peak showed increased intensity in the atheromatous plaque core, whereas in hydrophilic fibrous regions, such as the cap of the plaque, the intensity of the F1 peak was lower than in the core region. HP aggregation was observed in damaged cells and in water surrounded by lipid in the atheromatous core. Gonschior et al. [7] also looked at human plaques and normal arteries incubated with 2.5- and 5-μg HPD/ml cell culture medium. Fluorescence intensity was concentration-dependent, with 80% of the maximal uptake reached at 1 hour. A preferential uptake of HPD was measured in arteriosclerotic as compared to normal vessel segments (primary lesion: fluorescence-ratio of 3:1 at 1 hour; restenosed lesion: fluorescence-ratio of 4:1 at 1 hour).

Delettre et al. [8] incubated human atheromatous aorta segments with solutions of various purified dicarboxylic porphyrins including hematoporphyrin (HP) and hydroxyethylvinyldeuteroporphyrin (HVD), and Photofrin. Selective labeling of the atheroma was shown by macroscopic and microscopic observations of the characteristic porphyrin fluorescence associated with the atheromatous plaques. The time dependence of the uptake, monitored by absorption spectrophotometry or by high-performance liquid chromatography, was inferred from the disappearance of the porphyrins in the incubation medium. Significant binding was observed in the absence of albumin or serum proteins. The uptake of HP was less than that of the more hydrophobic compounds HVD or Photofrin when these porphyrins were used alone. The presence of albumin or serum drastically reduces atheroma labeling. Some competition between HP and HVD for binding sites is also seen.

Hsiang et al. [9] incubated samples of atherosclerotic human femoral and popliteal arteries were with BPD (1, 5, 10, 20, 30, and 40 μg/mL) for 1 hour. Chemical extraction and spectrofluorimetry showed a dose-dependent increase in BPD uptake. In addition, three miniswine were rendered atherosclerotic and given BPD 2.0 mg/kg intravenously. The concentration of BPD-MA in miniswine aorta was 93 to 190 ng/g and the plaque/normal ratio was 1.7–3.5. For miniswine iliac arteries, the [BPD-MA] was 60–178 ng/g and the plaque/normal ratio was 1.1–3.3.

Bialy et al. incubated [10] specimens of human aorta and coronary arteries with mono-l-aspartyl chlorin e6 and then washed out the PS. They noted a very strong red fluorescence of chlorin e6 originating from lipid-rich plaque. The ratio of chlorin e6 red fluorescence (660 nm) to green autofluorescence centered at 515 nm was highest at the atheromatous samples, followed by calcified and normal ones.

20.4   PDT for Atherosclerosis In Vivo

The studies in this section use different animal models of atherosclerosis, different arteries, and some focus mainly on the potential of PDT agents to mediate fluorescence or even scintigraphic detection of atherosclerosis, while other studies are more concerned with the potential therapeutic effects of PDT. We will classify the studies on PDT for atherosclerosis in animal models by the different PS used.

20.4.1   Photofrin or Hematoporphyrin

The first studies in the 1980s used mainly hematoporphyrin derivative (HpD) or sometimes hematoporphyrin (HP) itself. In 1983, Spears and colleagues showed [11] selective uptake of HPD into experimental atheromatous plaques in the aorta 48 hours after IV injection in rabbits and monkeys that had been maintained on high fat/cholesterol diets. A subsequent study [12] found HpD accumulation in both sterile and infected (Staphylococcus and Streptococcus) valvular vegetations in rabbit hearts. They went on [13] to obtain specimens containing atheromatous plaques from patients undergoing surgical vascular procedures, and incubated in autologous oxygenated blood at 37° C with HpD for 2 hours. On exposure to ultraviolet light, porphyrin fluorescence was noted throughout each plaque, whereas adjacent plaque-free tissue showed no fluorescence. Three types of arterial lesions (induced by a high-cholesterol diet, catheters, or balloon injury) were studied in rabbits. Each lesion fluoresced selectively with the same intensity whether hematoporphyrin derivative exposure was performed in vitro or in vivo. Studies by Hsiang et al. [14] have underscored the affinity of porphyrin derivatives for diseased arterial wall in rabbits and miniswine. They found maximal drug concentration in the intimal surface layers, diminishing radially into the media [15].

Another early study [16] injected HpD (10 mg/kg) into atherosclerotic rabbits. Subsequently intravascular 636-nm laser radiation was delivered to either the thoracic aorta or the aortic arch. A total of 32 to 288 J of laser energy was delivered through a 300-mu quartz fiber. All rabbits that received in vivo HPD had red fluorescence of their aortas when placed under ultraviolet light. The pattern of fluorescence corresponded precisely to the pattern of atheroma. In segments that received PDT, light microscopic examination revealed an accumulation of smooth muscle cells at the intimal surface. Assessment of treated thoracic aortic segments revealed quantitative and qualitative differences compared with control segments. In the arch-treated segments, however, no changes were seen.

Neave et al. [17] induced atherosclerotic plaques in abdominal aortas of rabbits. At 8 weeks, Photofrin II 5 mg/kg was injected intravenously followed by sacrifice of the animal, fluorescence microscopy, and quantitative assay of porphyrin in the plaque-containing aortas at 1, 12, 24, 48, and 72 hours. Photofrin II was taken up preferentially by the plaque, with the highest plaque to normal wall ratio occurring at 48 hours. Intravascular PDT with a 630-nm light source of the pair of plaques was treated while the other served as a control. Animals were killed at 2, 4, and 6 weeks. The 6-week specimens showed the most dramatic reduction in plaque in comparison to controls. Vever-Bizet et al. induced atherosclerotic lesions in normal and Watanabe rabbits by atherogenic diet and stripping of aorta endothelium. The rabbits were injected with Photofrin II and sacrificed 2 days later. Atheromatous aorta (as well as normal aorta from control animals) were characterized by their fluorescence emission peaks at 631 and 694 nm. The excitation spectrum shows a strong band at 394 nm and weaker bands at 446, 504, 536, and 574 nm. Although no fluorescence of normal aorta can be seen by visual inspection, emission with a maximum at 626 nm was detected by spectrofluorimetry. Normal phase high-performance liquid chromatography analysis of extracts from atheroma and control aorta was also carried out. The specific labeling of atheroma involves mainly protoporphyrin, hematoporphyrin, and also minor components of Photofrin II that are accumulated. Wong and colleagues [18] used ^{111}In-labeled HPD in rabbits with plaques surgically induced in the abdominal aorta, and found selective uptake over normal blood vessels averaging 0.01% ID/g tissue. Normal aorta and thoracic artery concentrated an average of 0.0026% ID/g, which is less than the mean blood activity of 0.0034% ID/mL. In hypercholesteremic rabbits, the mean plaque segment to normal blood vessels ratio was 4:1 (range 2 to 9:1) sufficiently high to permit plaque delineation in the scintigram. Prevosti et al. [19] also studied normal and atherosclerotic rabbits after injection of 2.5 mg/kg. In plaque from atherosclerotic rabbits given HpD, there was a broad spectral peak at 632 nm not seen in control groups. Similar studies were done by Okunaka et al. [20].

Katoh and colleagues [21] injected rabbits with plaques in the abdominal aorta with 5 mg/kg of HpD and 24 hours later, 120 J of intravascular 630-nm light was delivered at two different fluence rates. In PDT treated arteries at 7 days most intimal cells and endothelial cells had become necrotic and disappeared, and a loss of intima was observed. No such changes were found in control groups. Hsiang and colleagues [22] induced aorto-iliac atherosclerosis in Yucatan miniswine, weighing between 25 and 35 kg by a combination of balloon endothelial injury and dietary supplementation with 2% cholesterol and 15% lard for 7 weeks. Pigs were injected with 2.5 mg/kg Photofrin and treated with 120J of 630 nm light through an intravascular, cylindrical, diffusing fiberoptic probe. Seven miniswine had an increase in luminal diameter, but five had no increase. Microscopy demonstrated a broad range of features in treated vessels, including areas with re-endothelialization and regions of platelet and blood cell adherence with absent or abnormal endothelium. In a subsequent study in the same model, they compared different light doses (60, 120, and 240 J/cm^2) in surgically exposed aortae [23]. The percentage intimal thickness 36.7, 9.1, and 6.4 for the three energy densities, respectively. Although both 120 and 240 J/cm^2 energy densities produced significant reduction in atheroma, considerable damage to the underlying media was also observed in the 240 J/cm2 group.

20.4.2 Mono-L-Aspartyl Chlorin e6

Mono-L-aspartyl chlorin e6, a chlorophyll-a derivative (LS11, MACE), subsequently referred to here as Npe6, is a second generation PS currently in advanced-stage clinical trials for PDT. It is a PS that exhibits chemical purity, absorption at 664-nm wavelength. It is a potent photosensitizing agent in the mouse, it binds mainly to mouse plasma high-density lipoproteins (HDL) and albumin, with only 1% bound to LDL [24]. It has been shown that Npe6 enters the cell through endocytosis [25], and when photoactivated destroys lysosomes [26].

Hayashi et al. were the first [27] to report that Npe6 injected intravenously (0.5 mg/kg) into cholesterol-fed atherosclerotic rabbits localized in plaques. Transadventitial spectrofluorimetry with a dual real-time imaging system and a flexible endoscopic catheter and a pulsed excimer dye laser demonstrated a peak at 675 nm, with no fluorescence in aortic segments free of atheroma. It was also noted that the intensity of the specific peak of the spectrum detected from outside a vessel was closely related to the depth of atheromatous lesions, as determined by histological analysis. An in vivo study revealed good correlation between the peak intensity (which could vary with the amount of NPe6 accumulated in the tissue) measured laparoscopically from outside the abdominal aorta and the peak intensity measured angioscopically from inside the abdominal aorta. A second study [28] used 2 mg/kg of Npe6 in the same animal model and a epifluorescence stereoscope system to visualize several brightly illuminated branching small coronary arteries were observed clearly against the dark heart surface. A fluorescence micrograph of the coronary artery, at which orange-red fluorescence was seen through the epifluorescence stereoscope, showed that the atheromatous plaques emitted orange-red fluorescence.

These authors went on [29] to use the same model (Npe6 2 mg/kg) to test extravascular illumination (100 or 200 J/cm^2) of a plaque through the adventitia of the abdominal aorta. An area of 1-cm diameter was irradiated just below the celiac artery or the renal artery bifurcation, at which the atherosclerotic plaque was observed. The irradiated portion of the aorta could be recognized 7 days after treatment. After treatment, all atherosclerotic rabbits received a normal diet. Fourier transform infrared (FTIR) microspectroscopy was used 7 days after PDT to show a marked decrease in the peak intensity in the treated atheroma related to the carbonyl ester bond with no concomitant increase in the intensity of the peaks related to free cholesterol, suggesting the depletion of cholesterol esters in the atheromas after PDT.

20.4.3   Motexafin Lutetium (Lutetium Texaphyrin)

Texaphyrins are new PSs and are synthetic expanded macrocycles that are water-soluble with long wavelength absorption peaks in the near-infrared region of the spectrum [30]. They are thought to bind with circulating lipoproteins to form LDL-PS complexes in plasma, facilitating uptake into atheroma [31]. They localize both in cancerous lesions and in atheromatous plaque. Incorporation of a diamagnetic lanthanide, lutetium, into the texaphyrin molecule yields a potent PDT agent that is activated by tissue-penetrating NIR light (732 nm). In addition, motexafin lutetium fluoresces at 750 nm; endogenous chromophores do not emit light at 750 nm. Hence, in vivo real-time imaging of target structures is feasible, thus facilitating clinical diagnosis and treatment planning. Similarly, the related, paramagnetic gadolinium texaphyrin might facilitate MRI of atheromatous vascular disease [32].

Hayase et al. [33] administered motexafin lutetium (Lu-Tex) intra-arterially in rabbits with bilateral iliac atherosclerosis caused by balloon injury and high-cholesterol diet. Fluorescence spectral imaging and chemical extraction techniques were used to measure Lu-Tex levels (40x control iliac atheroma) within the atheroma and adjacent normal tissue. Intravascular PDT was performed 15 minutes following Lu-Tex administration (180 J/cm fiber at 200 mW/cm fiber) and 2 weeks post-PDT, vessels were harvested and stained with hematoxylin and eosin (H&E) and RAM11 (macrophages). Plaque area in the treated segments was significantly lower than in the nontreated contralateral lesions. No medial damage was observed. Quantitative analysis using RAM11-positive cells revealed significant reduction of macrophages in treated lesions in both the intima and in media compared to untreated contralateral segments.

20.4.4 Scavenger Receptor-Targeting

As mentioned previously we have employed a scavenger-receptor targeted approach via BSA-ce6-mal to deliver PSs to macrophages in atherosclerotic plaque. We reported [34] on the ability of this conjugate to localize in macrophage-rich atherosclerotic plaques in vivo. Both the conjugate and the free PS ce6 were studied after injection into New Zealand White rabbits that were rendered atherosclerotic by a combination of aortic endothelial injury and cholesterol feeding. Rabbits were sacrificed at 6 and 24 hours after injection and intravascular fluorescence spectroscopy was carried out by fiber-based fluorimetry in intact blood-filled arteries. Surface spectrofluorimetry of numbered excised aortic segments (Color Plate 23) together with injured and normal iliac arteries was carried out, and quantified ce6 content by subsequent extraction and quantitative fluorescence determination of the arterial segments and also of nontarget organs. There was good agreement between the various techniques for quantifying ce6 localization, and high contrast between arteries from atherosclerotic and normal rabbits was obtained. Fluorescence correlated with the highest burden of plaque in the aorta and the injured iliac artery (Figure 20.2).

The highest accumulation in plaques is obtained using MA-ce6 at 24 hours. Free ce6 gave better accumulation at 6 hours compared to 24 hours. The liver, spleen, lung, and gall bladder had the highest uptake in nontarget organs.

A subsequent report [35] used the same animal model and the BSA-ce6-mal conjugate at the 24-hour time point and showed by comparison of red fluorescence confocal microscopy and immunohistochemical analysis of the specimens (Color Plate 24) that there was a significant correlation between MA-ce6 uptake and RAM-11 macrophage staining (Figure 20.3), and an inverse correlation between MA-ce6 uptake and α-actin smooth muscle cell staining. The high specificity of the macrophage localization suggests that this technology could be used to identify those plaques with high macrophage content and which are therefore most likely to rupture.

20.4.5 Miscellaneous PSs

Allison et al. [36] compared the plasma distribution and arterial accumulation of a BPD, in spontaneous atherosclerotic lesions of the Watanabe heritable hyperlipidemic (WHHL) rabbit and induced lesions of the balloon-injured, choles-

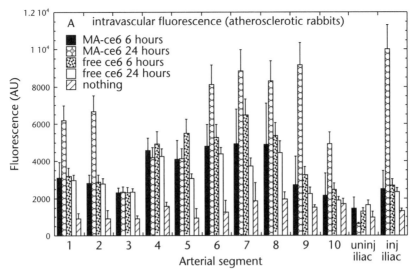

Figure 20.2   Mean intravascular fluorescence signal (in arbitrary units) for arterial segments gathered by fiber pullback in atherosclerotic rabbits. Values are means of triplicate determinations at each segment from six rabbits, and bars are SEM.

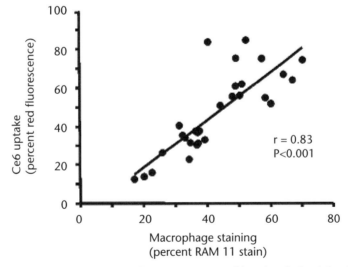

Figure 20.3   Comparison of MA-ce6 uptake versus Immnunohistochemical staining. There was a significant correlation between MA-ce6 uptake and RAM-11 staining (R=0.83, p<0.001).

terol-fed New Zealand white (NZW) rabbit. Liposome-based formulations were compared to freshly isolated native low-density lipoprotein (LDL) and acetylated-LDL (Ac-LDL) as delivery vehicles for BPD. Although the delivery vehicle influenced plasma distribution immediately postinjection, BPD subsequently partitioned according to the plasma concentration of the lipoproteins. BPD demonstrated a selective accumulation in atherosclerotic tissue. Preassociation with LDL and Ac-LDL enhanced accumulation of BPD in atherosclerotic tissue when compared with normal artery (mean ratios of 2.8 and 4.1 were achieved, respectively).

Saito and colleagues [37] injected the pheophorbide-a derivative PH-1126 at 1 mg/kg into cholesterol-fed atherosclerotic rabbits. Twenty-four hours later, PH-1126 selectively accumulated in atherosclerotic plaques. Then, atherosclerotic lesions in the upper thoracic aorta were treated by irradiation with a krypton ion laser at 647 nm. At 6 hours after PDT, the treated aorta was examined by scanning electron microscopy. Numerous teardrop-shaped cells were observed on the endothelial surface of the plaque irradiated at a total energy of 100 J/cm². These cells may be foam cells from the intimal layer of atherosclerotic plaque that were expelled into the aortic lumen.

20.5   PDT for Prevention and Treatment of Intimal Hyperplasia

Intimal hyperplasia is the thickening of the *tunica intima* of a blood vessel as a complication of a reconstruction procedure or angioplasty. The animal and clinical studies of intimal hyperplasia during the last two decades have documented over and over again that it is a universal response to injury and a complication of all forms of arterial reconstruction including bypass graft.

Although pathological remodeling (a decrease in overall arterial cross-sectional area) is a more important mechanism for luminal narrowing in vessels treated by balloon angioplasty, intimal hyperplasia followed by stenosis or restenosis is the principal cause for failure in vein and synthetic grafts and in stented atherosclerotic arteries. Restenosis affects about 20% to 30% of coronary and other small arterial reconstructions, and the treatment of restenosis is generally further vascular reconstruction.

The arterial wall thickens and the lumen narrows because vascular smooth muscle cells (SMCs) accumulate in the intima and secrete matrix proteins. It is known from animal studies that SMCs are derived from adventitial cells and blood-borne stem cells as well as populations of SMCs in and around the zone of injury. The migration of these cells from one tissue compartment to another followed by proliferation in the intima are required for intimal thickening and are regulated by factors released from thrombus (thrombin, PDGF), inflammatory cells (TNFα, IL1β), or the vascular wall cells themselves (basic FGF, TGFβ, etc.). The growth and migratory factors as well as critical intracellular signaling pathways represent logical targets for pharmacological blockade and the prevention of intimal hyperplasia. Approaches to prevention include adjuvant pharmacology (taxol and rapamycin), radiation, and PDT.

In the case of PDT studies, various reports have used PDT to prevent IH from occurring (usually a few days after injury) or to treat already established IH by treating several weeks after arterial injury. Another experimental variable is whether the light was delivered externally to the artery after it was exposed by cutdown in small animals, or whether the light was delivered intravascularly by a fiber-optic catheter advanced through the blood vessels to the injured region in larger animals. A third variable in these studies is whether the PS was injected systemically in the whole circulation, or infused locally into the injured arterial segment by a porous balloon device. Since there are a substantial number of animal studies of PDT for IH, we will classify them by PS used.

20.5.1   Chloroaluminum-Sulfonated Phthalocyanine

One of the first reports by Ortu et al. described the use of PDT to inhibit intimal hyperplasia using [38] chloroaluminum-sulfonated phthalocyanine (CASPc, 5 mg/kg IV) and a rat model of IH after balloon catheter injury to the left common carotid artery. Twenty minutes after drug injection, the distal left common carotid artery was irradiated externally under saline after a cutdown with 675-nm laser light (100 J/cm^2 at 100 mW/cm^2). At sacrifice 14 days after injury the cross-sectional areas of the neointima were significantly lower in PDT-irradiated segments versus the laser-only controls. There was histological absence of medial smooth muscle cells or inflammatory cells, but no other structural injury was identified. These authors went on to show [39] that CASPc had selectivity for IH with 60% lower uptake and retention of CASPc by normal arterial tissue as compared to arteries with IH; the difference became more pronounced at 24 hours. A third study [40] looked at long-term effects in this model and found that the anti-IH effect of PDT lasted as long as 16 weeks. There was complete reendothelialization of the intima by 4 weeks.

Using the same PS, LaMuraglia et al. [41] showed that PDT could also inhibit restenosis in reversed external jugular vein bypass grafts of the common carotid artery in rats. Medial areas and percent of stenoses were also significantly less in PDT than in controls, but longitudinal sections within 2 mm of the anastomoses did not demonstrate a difference between PDT and control. They proposed that the artery may be the source of proliferating smooth muscle cells that contribute to the anastomotic vein graft IH. Next, the entire rat common carotid artery was balloon-injured to induce IH, whereas only the cervical segment below the bifurcation was subjected to PDT [42]. PDT resulted in complete local depletion of medial SMC, which was associated with a lack of IH until 2 weeks. However, at 4 and 16 weeks there was significant IH in PDT-treated arteries despite a lack of medial SMC repopulation. A wave of IH progression over the acellular media was observed in these arteries, migrating from the injured non-PDT-treated area. The treatment field should therefore include the whole of the injured area and some normal artery as well. However, a different group carried out similar experiments [43] on balloon-injured carotid arteries of rabbits with CASPc and external illumination and found no benefit of PDT to inhibit restenosis, and only a temporary benefit in treating already established restenosis.

The previous experiments were all carried out with a preparation (CASPc) containing a mixture of degrees of sulfonation, but Nyamekye et al. used [44] the pure compound aluminum disulphonated phthalocyanine (AlS2Pc) in balloon-injured rat carotids. AlS2Pc fluorescence intensity increased with increasing dosage, with maximal fluorescence in the arterial media at 30 minutes. After laser irradiation (50 J/cm^2, 675 nm), PDT produced medial cell depletion at 3 days that persisted for 6 months and completely inhibited IH at 2 and 4 weeks. Inhibition of IH was partial after 6 to 26 weeks (51% of untreated level).

20.5.2   Photofrin

Hsiang et al. [22, 45] found a benefit of Photofrin PDT in rabbits with balloon-injured abdominal aortas after intravascular illumination with a diffusing fiber attached to an argon-pumped dye laser. They also reported selective uptake of Photofrin in IH aortic segments [14]. This group went on to use a model of IH in the abdominal aortae of swine created by a combination of fat-supplemented diet and balloon catheter injury prior to PDT [46]. They found a reduction in IH that lasted for up to 6 months. However, Eton et al. [47] found that no beneficial effect was obtained in the same model of IH, using Photofrin as the PS.

Usui et al. [48] injected HPD into Japanese white rabbits with balloon injury in the common iliac artery. Twenty-four hours later, intravascular Hg-Xe flash-lamp illumination was carried out immediately 3, 7, or 14 days postinjury. Slight, uniform HPD accumulation was observed in the injured media immediately after the balloon injury, and throughout the entire media and the neointima on day 7. On day 14, HPD accumulation had diminished in the media and increased in the intima, and on day 28 no HPD remained in the media. In the 0D- or 3D-PDT groups, no inhibition of intimal hyperplasia was observed. In contrast, there was significant inhibition of intimal hyperplasia in the 7D- and 14D-PDT groups.

Gonschior et al. compared the local delivery of Photofrin with the systemic delivery [49]. A catheter with a porous balloon enabled local application of Photofrin II in rabbits and pigs (5 ml of 2.5 mg/ml) or systemically (5 mg/kg i.v.). After systemic application there was an increase of Photofrin II after a 4-hour period as judged by fluorescence microscopy of arterial segments. In contrast, a maximum concentration of Photofrin II was measured immediately after local application and found to be decreasing over a period of 4 hours. The intima showed the higher uptake of HPD after local versus systemic application, and higher than the media and the adventitia. In subsequent studies in pigs [50, 51], they used their local PS delivery system to inhibit restenosis in a unidirectional arterial injury. An inflammatory and myoproliferative response was observed after injury in vessels from control groups, while in the PDT group the myoproliferative response was significantly reduced.

Local PDT was used to prevent neointimal hyperplasia after stenting [52]. Slotted tube stents were placed with 16 atmospheres in porcine femoral arteries with the external diameter to match the diameter at 10 atmospheres. Animals were randomly allocated to Group 1 (stenting only); or Group 2 with stenting, local delivery of a PS (5-mg Photofrin), and subsequent exposure to light (PDT, 100 J). Fourteen days later, all vessels were excised, fixed, and processed for histology. Tissue hyperplasia was observed after stenting in vessels from Group 1. In Group 2 with PDT, the myoproliferative response was significantly reduced. Tissue hyperplasia after stenting was effectively suppressed by PDT.

20.5.3   Monoaspartyl Chlorin (e6)

Japanese workers have used the PS known as monoaspartyl chlorin e6, (MACE, Npe6, taloporphin, or LS11) to treat balloon-injured rabbits arteries and demonstrated that a significant inhibition of intimal hyperplasia occurs at 14 days after PDT [53]. In a longer-term study [54], they carried out vascular PDT with talaporfin sodium-inhibited intimal hyperplasia following balloon distension injury to the carotid artery in rabbits. Talaporfin, 5.0 mg/kg, was delivered systemically immediately after balloon injury and the injury site was externally irradiated with 50 J/cm^2 of 664-nm diode laser light after 30 minutes. Thirty minutes after talaporfin administration, drug fluorescence was found only in the balloon-injured carotid artery wall. At 3 days, no smooth muscle cells were seen in the media of the PDT-treated arterial segments. Intimal hyperplasia developed progressively in the untreated balloon-injured segments; however, in the segments treated with PDT, intimal hyperplasia was markedly suppressed until 25 weeks and the media was repopulated by smooth muscle cells without macrophages.

20.5.4 Benzoporphyrin Derivative

Adili et al. [55] delivered BPD-MA locally into balloon-injured rat common carotid arteries that were pressurized at 400 mm Hg for 2 minutes, and irradiated with 690-nm laser light at a fluence of 100 J/cm^2. Pressurization with BPD resulted in complete penetration of the intima and media and was associated with relatively high tissue, but almost no detectable serum BPD concentrations. After 9 days, PDT-treated arteries displayed a significantly lower number of smooth muscle cells in the arterial wall than balloon-injured or saline-pressurized arteries, and no intimal hyperplasia. At 21 days, IH after PDT was significantly reduced as compared with balloon-injured or saline-pressurized arteries. In a subsequent study [56], these authors compared low-dose PDT (0.5 μg/mL BPD and 50 J/cm^2) resulted in incomplete cell eradication and significant IH at 2 weeks. Irradiation with 100 J/cm^2 at the same BPD concentration completely eradicated the cells in the artery wall at 24 hours but still led to IH at 2 weeks. However, 25 μg/mL BPD at 100 J/cm^2 resulted in total cell eradication at 24 hours and inhibition of IH at 2 weeks. In contrast, high-dose PDT with 25 μg/mL BPD and 200 J/cm^2 led to thrombus development and vascular occlusion at 24 hours. This data, demonstrating the effects of increasing PDT dose on injured arteries, emphasize the critical importance of appropriate PDT dosimetry for the inhibition of IH.

Turnbull and colleagues [57] tested the hypothesis that BPD could exert inhibitory effects on smooth muscle cell (SMC) proliferation in rabbit aortic intimal injuries in the absence of light stimulation. A small (20%) but significant decrease in viability of human smooth muscle cells was noted for BPD-MA concentrations above 15 μg/mL. This was an all-or-none phenomenon with no further decrease in viability at higher concentrations. Treatment with BPD-MA was also carried out in vivo using a balloon injury model of intimal hyperplasia in rabbit aortas. No statistically significant difference was seen in the amount of intimal hyperplasia that developed in any of the five groups.

20.5.5 5-Aminolevulinic Acid

As discussed previously in this volume, 5-ALA is not itself a photosensitizer, but is converted in vivo into the photoactive metabolite, protoporphyrin IX (PPIX). Following systemic ALA administration, PPIX shows a dose- and time-dependent increase in the intima, media, and adventitia of the arterial wall. The drug can be given by mouth, and skin photosensitivity is limited to 24 to 48 hours [58]. Side effects at the clinical dose of 60 mg/kg are few, although they do include mild nausea and a transient rise in liver transaminases. PPIX has a convenient absorption peak at 635 nm in the red part of the visible spectrum.

Nyamekye et al. [59] injected ALA (20–200 mg/kg) into healthy and balloon-injured carotid artery rats and found arterial media fluorescence increased in a dose-dependent manner. Rats received external laser illumination (50 J/cm^2, 630 nm) 30 to 90 minutes after sensitization. PDT produced a dose-dependent cellular depletion in the treated arterial segment at 3 days, and this was complete with 100 and 200 mg/kg of ALA. At 14 days, the media remained acellular, although the endothelial lining had regenerated. In the balloon-injured arteries, PDT produced complete inhibition of intimal hyperplasia at both 14 and 28 days. In noninjured pigs that had received [60] 120 mg/kg ALA, intravascular 630-nm light was delivered via a 4-mm transparent percutaneous transluminal angioplasty balloon inflated so as to occlude flow, but not distend the external iliac artery. Fluorescence peaked in the adventitia, intima, and medial layers at 1.5, 4, and 6 hours, respectively. PDT at both 3 and 14 days produced VSMC depletion compared with controls.

Another study in rabbits [61] used ALA 60 mg/kg, 3 hours prior to endovascular illumination of the iliac artery (635 nm at 50 J/cm^2) either immediately before or after deployment of an oversized (3-mm diameter) stent. PDT treated arteries showed almost complete medial cell ablation when light was delivered before stent deployment with little effect when illumination followed stent deployment. Four weeks after PDT, the neointimal areas were lower in the light before stent group compared to the other groups. They went on to study [62] intravascular PDT with ALA in balloon-injured iliac or coronary arteries in juvenile White-Landrace cross-bred pigs. Compared with control injured vessels, PDT-treated, balloon-injured coronary arteries had a larger lumen, larger area within the external elastic lamina, and smaller area of neointimal hyperplasia 28 days after intervention. Similar trends, but with smaller differences, were seen in the iliac arteries.

20.5.6 Miscellaneous PSs

Heckenkamp et al. [63] delivered the phenothiazinium dye methylene blue locally into balloon-injured rat carotid arteries and used external illumination with 100 J/cm^2 of 660 nm. No IH developed in PDT-treated arteries compared with untreated controls. Arterial injury resulted in an increase of versican and procollagen type I messenger RNA (mRNA) in the adventitia and neointima. In the repopulating cells of the adventitia after PDT, there was a significant decrease in versican mRNA but not in procollagen type I mRNA.

Waksman [64] reported on the use of intracoronary PhotoPoint PDT with a new PS MV0611 (indium chloride methyl pyropheophorbide) in the overstretch balloon and stent porcine models of restenosis. Pigs were injected with 3 mg/kg of MV0611 systemically 4 hours before a light diffuser (25–30-mm length) centered within a proprietary modified percutaneous transluminal coronary angioplasty-type balloon was inserted into the coronary artery over a flexible 0.014-inch guidewire. The diffuser was connected to a 2.5W diode-pumped solid-state laser, which delivered light in the visible spectrum at 532 nm to activate MV0611, localized to the arterial wall. The total light fluence of 125 J/cm^2 at an irradiance of 250 mW/cm^2 was delivered in

10 to 12 equal fractionations in the artery to cover the injured area. Serial sections of vessels were processed 14 days after treatment showed that PDT significantly reduced intimal thickness in both BI and stented arteries. PDT increased luminal area by about 60% within arteries. Complete reendothelialization was observed by immunohistochemical and gross histological analyses in all PDT and control arteries.

Nagae et al. [65] used a scavenger receptor-targeted conjugate (BSA-ce6-mal) similar to the one described previously to target IH. Arterial wall injury was produced by a balloon catheter pulled through the abdominal aorta of the rat and 2 weeks after injury compounds were injected. Fluorescence of BSA-ce6-mal was higher for IH lesions as compared to control areas. An argon-pumped dye laser was used to deliver 20 J/cm^2 and 40 J/cm^2 4 hours later. Cell numbers were significantly reduced by PDT in the BSA-ce6-mal injected group versus the free ce6.

20.6 Cardiovascular PDT in Clinical Trials

Although there have been a large number of animal studies of PDT for both restenosis and atherosclerosis (covered in preceding sections), we are aware of only three clinical studies. The first in 1999 was by Jenkins et al. [66] and investigated the role of adjuvant ALA-mediated PDT following femoral percutaneous transluminal angioplasty (PTA). Eight PTAs were studied in seven patients (two women) with a median age of 70 who had previously undergone conventional angioplasty at the same site that resulted in symptomatic restenosis or occlusion between 2 and 6 months. Each patient was sensitized with oral 5-aminolaevulinic acid 60 mg/kg, 5 to 7 hours before the procedure. Following a second femoral angioplasty, up to 50 J/cm^2 red light (635 nm) was delivered to the angioplasty site via a laser fiber within the angioplasty balloon. All patients tolerated the procedure well and were rendered asymptomatic throughout the study interval. All vessels remained patent and no lesion attained the duplex definition of restenosis. The median peak systolic velocity ratio (PSVR) across stenotic segments was 4.7 before angioplasty, 1.1 at 24 hours, and 1.4 at 6 months after intervention ($P = 0.04$ compared with preoperative value). A later paper [67] extended the followup of these patients to 4 years post-PDT with overall very good continuing long-term outcomes.

The second study used the texaphyrin PS, Antrin, or motexafin lutetium [68]. Patients had symptomatic claudication and objectively documented peripheral arterial insufficiency (an ankle/brachial index (ABI) of 0.85 in at least one lower extremity, either at rest or after treadmill exercise, or an ipsilateral toe pressure of 60 mm Hg.) Photoangioplasty of a single atherosclerotic lesion was performed in the external iliac, common femoral, or superficial femoral artery. Many patients had multisegmental disease; the illuminated lesion was chosen on the basis of accessibility and was not necessarily the most flow-limiting stenosis. In the first phase the drug dose was escalated, by patient cohort, from 1 to 5 mg/kg at a constant 732-nm light fluence of 400 J/cm fiber. In the second phase a combination of escalating drug and light dosages was used. The former ranged from 2 to 4 mg/kg; light fluences of 500, 625, and 781 J/cm fiber, respectively, were used. Each patient received a single dose of drug and light. Twenty-four hours before photoangioplasty, the patient received a single intravenous dose of motexafin lutetium. Angiography was performed on day 1. Iliofemoral arterial dimensions were measured with the QCA Plus System and intravascular ultrasonography (IVUS) was performed before intervention. A fiberoptic catheter was coaxially positioned under fluoroscopic guidance. Laser light energy was delivered through a 3-cm diffuser fiber for 941 seconds at the predetermined fluence rate. Angiographic and IVUS reevaluations were performed either on day 14 or on day 28. Therapy was well tolerated throughout and the infrequent side effects were limited to transient paresthesias and minor, self-limited cutaneous eruptions. The median change in arterial stenosis was 24.0% less, and the standardized classification of clinical outcomes (based on the Rutherford-Becker classification) for the patients at followup showed improvement in 29 (62%), no change in 17 (36%), and moderate worsening in 1 (2%).

A second phase I trial [69] looked at drug and light dose-escalation of motexafin lutetium (MLu) and intravascular illumination in subjects with coronary artery disease undergoing percutaneous coronary intervention and stent deployment. The therapeutic changes were achieved without documented adverse vascular responses or any treatment limiting phototoxicity after doses of 1 to 5 mg/kg of Antrin and a flexible optical fiber (0.018-inch OD), with a distal active illumination length of 30 or 50 mm from which light emission was circumferential and uniform, was delivered under fluoroscopic guidance through a Transit catheter (2.5F). Light at a wavelength of 732 6 nm was produced by a diode laser. Illumination lasted 12 minutes, after which the laser fiber was removed and stent deployment was followed. The timing of PT relative to MLu administration (18 to 24 hours after) was chosen to allow MLu clearance from plasma, thus minimizing circulating MLu that could impede light delivery to the vessel wall.

20.7 Conclusions

The market for drugs and devices to combat cardiovascular disease is one of the world's biggest medical opportunities. In the past decades, balloon angioplasty followed by application of first bare-metal stents, and subsequently drug-eluting stents have each in turn been hailed as the latest panacea for atherosclerosis and restenosis [70]. However, despite the large numbers of patients treated with each of these devices, problems still remain. In the case of bare-metal stents, in-stent restenosis remains a problem [71], and in the case of drug-eluting stents, late thrombosis events are becoming problematic [72]. Can PDT play a role in these markets? Considering the large amount of money available for these types of products the possibility must exist. Another application in which PDT may have a role to play is in the problem of "vulnerable plaque" discussed previously. Here the therapeutic aim is not to remove or ablate the plaque in order to allow blood flow to be reestablished, but rather to reduce the dangerous inflammatory elements in the plaque that allow rupture and thrombosis to occur. The stabilization of these TCFA lesions may be particularly suited to PDT as PSs may selectively target the inflammatory cells such as macrophages.

References

[1]   Sobeh, M. S., et al., "Photodynamic therapy in a cell culture model of human intimal hyperplasia," *Eur. J. Vasc. Endovasc. Surg.*, Vol. 9, 1995, pp. 463–468.

[2]   Chen, Z., et al., "Photodynamic therapy with motexafin lutetium induces redox-sensitive apoptosis of vascular cells," *Arterioscler. Thromb. Vasc. Biol.*, Vol. 21, 2001, pp. 759–764.

[3]   Demidova, T. N., and Hamblin, M. R., "Macrophage-targeted photodynamic therapy," *Int. J. Immunopathol.Pharmacol.*, Vol. 17, 2004, pp. 117–126.

[4]   van Berkel, T. J., et al., "Scavenger receptors: friend or foe in atherosclerosis?" *Curr Opin Lipidol*, Vol. 16, 2005, pp. 525–535.

[5]   de Vries, H. E., et al., "Oxidized low-density lipoprotein as a delivery system for photosensitizers: implications for photodynamic therapy of atherosclerosis," *J. Pharmacol. Exp. Ther.*, Vol. 289, 1999, pp. 528–534.

[6]   Machida, M., et al., "Fluorescence spectroscopic and histochemical analysis using hematoporphyrin as a microenvironmental probe for atherosclerotic change in the human aorta," *Lab Invest*, Vol. 79, 1999, pp. 733–745.

[7]   Gonschior, P., et al., "Uptake and distribution of hematoporphyrin derivatives (HPD) in arteriosclerotic and normal vessel segments," *Z Kardiol*, Vol. 80, 1991, pp. 435–440.

[8]   Delettre, E., et al., "In vitro uptake of dicarboxylic porphyrins by human atheroma. Kinetic and analytical studies," *Photochem Photobiol*, Vol. 54, 1991, pp. 239–246.

[9]   Hsiang, Y. N., et al., "In vitro and in vivo uptake of benzoporphyrin derivative into human and miniswine atherosclerotic plaque," *Photochem. Photobiol.*, Vol. 57, 1993, pp. 670–674.

[10] Bialy, D., et al., "In vitro photodynamic diagnosis of atherosclerotic wall changes with the use of mono-l-aspartyl chlorin e6. A preliminary report," *Kardiol Pol*, Vol. 59, 2003, pp. 293–301.

[11] Spears, J. R., et al., "Fluorescence of experimental atheromatous plaques with hematoporphyrin derivative," *J Clin Invest*, Vol. 71, 1983, pp. 395–399.

[12] Spokojny, A. M., et al., "Uptake of hematoporphyrin derivative by valvular vegetations in experimental infective endocarditis," *Circulation*, Vol. 72, 1985, pp. 1087–1091.

[13] Spokojny, A. M., et al., "Uptake of hematoporphyrin derivative by atheromatous plaques: studies in human in vitro and rabbit in vivo," *J Am Coll Cardiol*, Vol. 8, 1986, pp. 1387–1392.

[14] Hsiang, Y., et al., "Assessing Photofrin uptake in atherosclerosis with a fluorescent probe: comparison with photography and tissue measurements," *Lasers Surg Med*, Vol. 13, 1993, pp. 271–278.

[15] Vincent, G. M., et al., "Presence of blood significantly decreases transmission of 630 nm laser light," *Lasers Surg Med*, Vol. 11, 1991, pp. 399–403.

[16] Litvack, F., et al., "Effects of hematoporphyrin derivative and photodynamic therapy on atherosclerotic rabbits," *Am. J. Cardiol.*, Vol. 56, 1985, pp. 667–671.

[17] Neave, V., et al., "Hematoporphyrin uptake in atherosclerotic plaques: therapeutic potentials," *Neurosurgery*, Vol. 23, 1988, pp. 307–312.

[18] Wong, D. W., et al., "Scintigraphic detection of atherosclerotic plaques in rabbits with 111In-labeled hematoporphyrin derivative," *Int J Rad Appl Instrum B*, Vol. 16, 1989, pp. 511–517.

[19] Prevosti, L. G., et al., "Laser-induced fluorescence detection of atherosclerotic plaque with hematoporphyrin derivative used as an exogenous probe," *J Vasc Surg*, Vol. 7, 1988, pp. 500–506.

[20] Okunaka, T., et al., "Hematoporphyrin derivative uptake by atheroma in atherosclerotic rabbits: The spectra of fluorescence from hematoporphyrin derivative demonstrated by an excimer dye laser," *Photochem Photobiol*, Vol. 46, 1987, pp. 769–775.

[21] Katoh, T., et al., "In vivo intravascular laser photodynamic therapy in rabbit atherosclerotic lesions using a lateral direction fiber," *Lasers Surg. Med.*, Vol. 20, 1997, pp. 373–381.

[22] Hsiang, Y. N., et al., "Photodynamic therapy for atherosclerotic stenoses in Yucatan miniswine," *Can. J. Surg.*, Vol. 37, 1994, pp. 148–152.

[23] Hsiang, Y. N., Todd, M. E., and Bower, R. D., "Determining light dose for photodynamic therapy of atherosclerotic lesions in the Yucatan miniswine," *J. Endovasc. Surg.*, Vol. 2, 1995, pp. 365–371.

[24] Kessel, D., Whitcomb, K. L., and Schulz, V., "Lipoprotein-mediated distribution of N-aspartyl chlorin-E6 in the mouse," *Photochem Photobiol*, Vol. 56, 1992, pp. 51–56.

[25] Roberts, W. G., and Berns, M. W., "In vitro photosensitization I. Cellular uptake and subcellular localization of mono-L-aspartyl chlorin e6, chloro-aluminum sulfonated phthalocyanine, and photofrin II," *Lasers Surg Med*, Vol. 9, 1989, pp. 90–101.

[26] Roberts, W. G., Liaw, L. H., and Berns, M. W., "In vitro photosensitization II. An electron microscopy study of cellular destruction with mono-L-aspartyl chlorin e6 and photofrin II," *Lasers Surg Med*, Vol. 9, 1989, pp. 102–108.

[27] Hayashi, J., et al., "Transadventitial localisation of atheromatous plaques by fluorescence emission spectrum analysis of mono-L-aspartyl chlorin e6," *Cardiovasc Res*, Vol. 27, 1993, pp. 1943–1947.

[28] Hayashi, J., et al., "Direct visualization of atherosclerosis in small coronary arteries using the epifluorescence stereoscope," *Cardiovasc Res*, Vol. 30, 1995, pp. 775–780.

[29] Hayashi, J., Saito, T., and Aizawa, K., "Change in chemical composition of lipids accumulated in atheromas of rabbits following photodynamic therapy," *Lasers Surg. Med.*, Vol. 21, 1997, pp. 287–293.

[30] Young, S. W., et al., "Lutetium texaphyrin (PCI-0123): a near-infrared, water-soluble photosensitizer," *Photochem Photobiol*, Vol. 63, 1996, pp. 892–897.

[31] Chou, T. M., et al., "Photodynamic therapy: applications in atherosclerotic vascular disease with motexafin lutetium," *Catheter Cardiovasc Interv*, Vol. 57, 2002, pp. 387–394.

[32] Miller, R. A., et al., "Motexafin gadolinium: a redox active drug that enhances the efficacy of bleomycin and doxorubicin," *Clin Cancer Res*, Vol. 7, 2001, pp. 3215–3221.

[33] Hayase, M., et al., "Photoangioplasty with local motexafin lutetium delivery reduces macrophages in a rabbit post-balloon injury model," *Cardiovasc Res*, Vol. 49, 2001, pp. 449–455.

[34] Tawakol, A., et al., "Photosensitizer delivery to vulnerable atherosclerotic plaque: comparison of macrophage-targeted conjugate versus free chlorine(e6)," *J Biomed Opt*, Vol. 11, 2006, pp. 21008.

[35] Tawakol, A., et al., "Intravascular detection of inflamed atherosclerotic plaques with a scavenger receptor-targeted fluorescent photosensitizer," *Photochem Photobiol Sci*, 2007.

[36] Allison, B. A., et al., "Delivery of benzoporphyrin derivative, a photosensitizer, into atherosclerotic plaque of Watanabe heritable hyperlipidemic rabbits and balloon-injured New Zealand rabbits," *Photochem Photobiol*, Vol. 65, 1997, pp. 877–883.

[37] Saito, T., et al., "Scanning electron microscopic analysis of acute photodynamic therapy for atherosclerotic plaques of rabbit aorta by using a pheophorbide derivative," *J Clin Laser Med Surg*, Vol. 14, 1996, pp. 1–6.

[38] Ortu, P., et al., "Photodynamic therapy of arteries. A novel approach for treatment of experimental intimal hyperplasia," *Circulation*, Vol. 85, 1992, pp. 1189–1196.

[39] LaMuraglia, G. M., et al., "Chloroaluminum sulfonated phthalocyanine partitioning in normal and intimal hyperplastic artery in the rat. Implications for photodynamic therapy," *Am J Pathol*, Vol. 142, 1993, pp. 1898–1905.

[40] LaMuraglia, G. M., et al., "Photodynamic therapy inhibition of experimental intimal hyperplasia: acute and chronic effects," *J Vasc Surg*, Vol. 19, 1994, pp. 321–329; discussion 329–331.

[41] LaMuraglia, G. M., et al., "Photodynamic therapy of vein grafts: suppression of intimal hyperplasia of the vein graft but not the anastomosis," *J Vasc Surg*, Vol. 21, 1995, pp. 882–890; discussion 889–890.

[42] Statius van Eps, R. G., et al., "Importance of the treatment field for the application of vascular photodynamic therapy to inhibit intimal hyperplasia," *Photochem Photobiol*, Vol. 67, 1998, pp. 337–342.

[43] Eton, D., et al., "Photodynamic therapy. Cytotoxicity of aluminum phthalocyanine on intimal hyperplasia," *Arch Surg*, Vol. 130, 1995, pp. 1098–1103.

[44] Nyamekye, I., et al., "Inhibition of intimal hyperplasia in balloon injured arteries with adjunctive phthalocyanine sensitised photodynamic therapy," *Eur J Vasc Endovasc Surg*, Vol. 11, 1996, pp. 19–28.

[45] Hsiang, Y., et al., "Preventing intimal hyperplasia with photodynamic therapy using an intravascular probe," *Ann Vasc Surg*, Vol. 9, 1995, pp. 80–86.

[46] Hsiang, Y. N., Crespo, M. T., and Todd, M. E., "Dosage and timing of Photofrin for photodynamic therapy of intimal hyperplasia," *Cardiovasc Surg*, Vol. 3, 1995, pp. 489–494.

[47] Eton, D., et al., "Cytotoxic effect of photodynamic therapy with Photofrin II on intimal hyperplasia," *Ann Vasc Surg*, Vol. 10, 1996, pp. 273–282.

[48] Usui, M., et al., "Photodynamic therapy for the prevention of intimal hyperplasia in balloon-injured rabbit arteries," *Jpn Circ J*, Vol. 63, 1999, pp. 387–393.

[49] Gonschior, P., et al., "Selective hematoporphyrin derivative (HMD) application in arterial vessels using a porous balloon catheter results in equivalent levels as compared to high-dose systemic administration," *Z Kardiol*, Vol. 80, 1991, pp. 738–745.

[50] Gonschior, P., et al., "Local photodynamic therapy reduces tissue hyperplasia in an experimental restenosis model," *Photochem Photobiol*, Vol. 64, 1996, pp. 758–763.

[51] Gonschior, P., et al., "Endovascular catheter-delivered photodynamic therapy in an experimental response to injury model," *Basic Res Cardiol*, Vol. 92, 1997, pp. 310–319.

[52] Valassis, G., et al., "Local photodynamic therapy reduces tissue hyperplasia after stenting in an experimental restenosis model," *Basic Res Cardiol*, Vol. 97, 2002, pp. 132–136.

[53] Nagae, T., et al., "Endovascular photodynamic therapy using mono-L-aspartyl-chlorin e6 to inhibit Intimal hyperplasia in balloon-injured rabbit arteries," *Lasers Surg Med*, Vol. 28, 2001, pp. 381–388.

[54] Wakamatsu, T., et al., "Long-term inhibition of intimal hyperplasia using vascular photodynamic therapy in balloon-injured carotid arteries," *Med Mol Morphol*, Vol. 38, 2005, pp. 225–232.

[55] Adili, F., et al., "Photodynamic therapy with local photosensitizer delivery inhibits experimental intimal hyperplasia," *Lasers Surg Med*, Vol. 23, 1998, pp. 263–273.

[56] Adili, F., Statius van Eps, R. G., and LaMuraglia, G. M., "Significance of dosimetry in photodynamic therapy of injured arteries: Classification of biological responses," *Photochem Photobiol*, Vol. 70, 1999, pp. 663–668.

[57] Turnbull, R. G., et al., "Benzoporphyrin derivative monacid ring A (Verteporfin) alone has no inhibitory effect on intimal hyperplasia: In vitro and in vivo results," *J Invest Surg*, Vol. 13, 2000, pp. 153–159.

[58] Webber, J., Kessel, D., and Fromm, D., "Side effects and photosensitization of human tissues after aminolevulinic acid," *J Surg Res*, Vol. 68, 1997, pp. 31–37.

[59] Nyamekye, I., et al., "Photodynamic therapy of normal and balloon-injured rat carotid arteries using 5-amino-levulinic acid," *Circulation*, Vol. 91, 1995, pp. 417–425.

[60] Jenkins, M. P., et al., "Intra-arterial photodynamic therapy using 5-ALA in a swine model," *Eur J Vasc Endovasc Surg*, Vol. 16, 1998, pp. 284–291.

[61] Pai, M., et al., "Inhibition of in-stent restenosis in rabbit iliac arteries with photodynamic therapy," *Eur J Vasc Endovasc Surg*, Vol. 30, 2005, pp. 573–581.

[62] Jenkins, M. P., et al., "Reduction in the response to coronary and iliac artery injury with photodynamic therapy using 5-aminolaevulinic acid," *Cardiovasc Res*, Vol. 45, 2000, pp. 478–485.

[63] Heckenkamp, J., et al., "Local photodynamic action of methylene blue favorably modulates the postinterventional vascular wound healing response," *J Vasc Surg*, Vol. 31, 2000, pp. 1168–1177.

[64] Waksman, R., et al., "Intracoronary photodynamic therapy reduces neointimal growth without suppressing re-endothelialisation in a porcine model," *Heart*, Vol. 92, 2006, pp. 1138–1144.

[65] Nagae, T., et al., "Selective targeting and photodynamic destruction of intimal hyperplasia by scavenger-receptor mediated protein-chlorin e6 conjugates," *J Cardiovasc Surg (Torino)*, Vol. 39, 1998, pp. 709–715.

[66] Jenkins, M. P., et al., "Clinical study of adjuvant photodynamic therapy to reduce restenosis following femoral angioplasty," *Br J Surg*, Vol. 86, 1999, pp. 1258–1263.

[67] Mansfield, R. J., et al., "Long-term safety and efficacy of superficial femoral artery angioplasty with adjuvant photodynamic therapy to prevent restenosis," *Br J Surg*, Vol. 89, 2002, pp. 1538–1539.

[68] Rockson, S. G., et al., "Photoangioplasty for human peripheral atherosclerosis: Results of a phase I trial of photodynamic therapy with motexafin lutetium (Antrin)," *Circulation*, Vol. 102, 2000, pp. 2322–2324.

[69] Kereiakes, D. J., et al., "Phase I drug and light dose-escalation trial of motexafin lutetium and far red light activation (phototherapy) in subjects with coronary artery disease undergoing percutaneous coronary intervention and stent deployment: procedural and long-term results," *Circulation*, Vol. 108, 2003, pp. 1310–1315.

[70] Saia, F., Marzocchi, A., and Serruys, P. W., "Drug-eluting stents. The third revolution in percutaneous coronary intervention," *Ital Heart J*, Vol. 6, 2005, pp. 289–303.

[71] Kivela, A., and Hartikainen, J., "Restenosis related to percutaneous coronary intervention has been solved?" *Ann Med*, Vol. 38, 2006, pp. 173–187.

[72] Stone, G. W., et al., "Safety and efficacy of sirolimus- and paclitaxel-eluting coronary stents," *N Engl J Med*, Vol. 356, 2007, pp. 998–1008.

CHAPTER 21

Photodynamic Therapy for Neovascular Eye Diseases: Past, Present, and Future

Hubert van den Bergh and Jean-Pierre Ballini

21.1 Introduction

Age-related macular degeneration (AMD) is the main cause of significant loss of vision in the Western world [1–3] for people over 50 years old. AMD is most prevalent in the elderly, which is the fastest growing population group in the developed world [2, 4]. Poorly regulated leaking blood vessels of the choroid (choroidal neovessels or CNV) represent only about 15% of all AMD cases, but this wet or neovascular AMD causes nearly all rapid and extensive loss of vision [1, 5, 6].

21.2 The Pathogenesis of Wet AMD

Details of the etiology of CNV associated with AMD are not yet very well established [7–9]. The disease can often progress quite rapidly, as shown by the Macular Photocoagulation Study Group [10–13] where less than 3% of the patients entering the observation period were unable to read, and this percentage progressed to more than 10% after 3 months of observation. Nearly half the patients could no longer read 2 years into this study. Color Plate 24 shows schematically a cross section of the eye (a) together with an ophthalmologist's view of the retina (b), a schematic cross section of a normal macula (c), and a macula with CNV (d). In Color plate (d), a layer of photoreceptors is shown above the single layer of cells called the retinal pigment epithelium (RPE). Blood supply to the retina occurs via retinal vessels close to the interface between the retina and the vitreous, and choroidal vessels, which are situated below the RPE and Bruch's membrane (BM). Vision would be strongly hampered if retinal vessels, which absorb and scatter light, grew above the macula, as this is the region where high resolution and color vision are mostly located. The very central part of this region (foveola, about $200\,\mu$m in diameter) contains about 200,000 cones per mm^2 [14]. Hence, this very active region of the human body is supplied to a large extent with oxygen and nutrients from the choroidal blood supply below the RPE and BM.

Nonvascular (dry) AMD is characterized by lipidic deposits containing lipofuscin in and under the RPE. These are called drusen and show up as yellowish spots upon visual inspection of the retina (Figure 21.1).

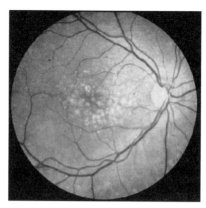

Figure 21.1 Image of the retina showing yellow drusen.

It has been suggested [15] that the material of these deposits comes, at least in part, from reduced RPE enzyme activity that causes the outer segments of the photoreceptors to be only partially digested with increasing age [15, 16]. These outer segments are highly layered structures containing the pigment Rhodopsin, which is 11-cis retinal linked to the protein opsin. They have to be shed occasionally due to a small degree of unavoidable photooxidation, which accompanies the vision process. As this dry form of the disease progresses, and the size of the drusen and the thickness of Bruch's membrane increase, central vision may start to blur, and one may start to suffer from metamorphopsia (i.e., apparent perception of changes in form, contour, or size). Unfortunately, this slow nonneovascular form of the disease may progress further to the neovascular form of AMD. It has been suggested that the lack of oxygen in the neural retina, caused in part by the lipidic deposits that inhibit oxygen transport across the RPE and Bruch's membrane from the choriocapillaries, starts a biochemical cascade induced by the hypoxic stress. This includes an increased production of the protein HIF-1α [17], which leads to the release of proangiogenic factors, including vascular endothelial growth factor-A (VEGF-A). Thus it is interesting to note that it is originally hyperoxidative stress in the photoreceptors, which in the end leads to retinal hypoxia, which in turn initiates angiogenesis.

The VEGF-A released [17] by the oxidative stress may now bind to the receptors VEGFR-1 and VEGFR-2 located on the surface of the choroidal endothelial cells that line the interior of these choriocapillaries [18, 19]. This in term causes the release of proteins in the cytoplasm of these cells; that is, cytokines, including matrix metalloproteinases, which cause the breakdown of the basement membrane of the choriocapillary. The VEGF-A binding to the VEGFR's 1 and 2, possibly with the aid of other factors, also causes the proliferation of endothelial cells. These then migrate and form buds of lots of endothelial cells stacked up on top of one another, so that tubes are formed on the wall of the choriocapillary from which finally new vessels sprout. Before these new vessels mature, with the help of pericites and an extracellular layer of connective tissue, they are quite leaky. This is also in part due the changes wrought by VEGF-A among others in the tight junctions between the endothelial cells of the choroidal capillaries, thus enhancing leakage. These new vessels may penetrate Bruch's membrane and the RPE, which makes them easily detectable in fluorescein angiography ("classical" membranes), or they may remain below these highly pigmented layers that absorb and diffuse the light used to excite and record this fluorescence ("occult" membranes). The leakage of blood serum from the CNV into the retina can then lead to macular edema, and even to macular detachment, which are often visible in optical coherence tomography (OCT). Both of these can lead to the loss of visual acuity. Other vascular endothelial growth factors are known (B, C, D, and E) but these seem to have a less dominant role in the formation of the choroidal neovasculature. The messenger RNA responsible for the VEGF protein can be spliced at various points leading to different numbers of amino acids in the VEGF-A sequence (121, 165, 189 and 206) [20, 21]. Plasmid cleavage can lead to further isoforms (VEGF-A 110). As the various isoforms do or do not contain certain binding sites, this observation is essential when one wants to try to block individual isoforms with a particular antibody.

21.3   Types of AMD

For the purpose of treating the disease of AMD optimally it can be essential, at least in some modes of action, to classify its type, stage, and location according to a number of observations. Above we have mentioned the yellow patches called drusen observable on the retina. Another important factor is the number, the size, the location, and the confluence of these drusen; other observables are the position of the CNV either in the center of the retina or close to it (i.e., subfoveal, juxtafoveal, or extrafoveal), and the appearance of the leaking CNV in fluorescein angiography as classic (early hyperfluorescence with sharp borders) or occult (later leakage with poorly defined borders, which is more difficult to observe). A mixture of both classic and occult CNV is also possible and this is either defined as "predominantly classic" or "minimally classic," depending on the areas of these components representing more or less than 50% of the lesion area (Figure 21.2).

21.4   Detection of AMD

As in many diseases, early detection of AMD followed by its precise diagnosis and treatment at an early stage of disease development will in general give a better chance for a good treatment outcome. Often patients may observe themselves a loss of vision, or a distortion of their central vision. If the disease does not affect the lead eye, such detection may fall at a much later point in time. This may be particularly unfortunate as the presence of AMD in one eye implies a significant probability of finding it in the other eye after a number of years (about 40% in 5 years). The tiles in your bathroom or the so-called Amsler grid (a pattern of vertical and horizontal crossed straight lines) can also be used to detect the distortion, the blurring, or even the absence of these lines, possibly indicating the presence of an edema that may be caused by the disease (i.e., CNV due to AMD). Loss of visual acuity as measured by the old Snellen chart (named after Dutch ophthamologist Herman Snellen, 1834–1908) or the newer Early Treatment of Diabetic Retinopathy Study (ETDRS) chart [22, 23], will result in the best-corrected visual acuity in a quite reproducible

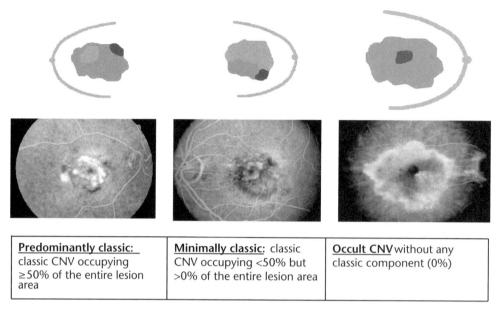

Predominantly classic: classic CNV occupying ≥50% of the entire lesion area	**Minimally classic:** classic CNV occupying <50% but >0% of the entire lesion area	**Occult CNV** without any classic component (0%)

Figure 21.2 Predominantly classic: classic CNV occupying ≥50% of the entire lesion; minimally classic: classic CNV occupying <50% but >0% of the entire lesion area. Occult CNV without any classic component (0%) area. Classic (light gray), occult (medium gray), and blood (dark gray) components.

way (Figure 21.3). This again is a good way of quantifying vision and its loss or gain with time.

Fundus photography with different cameras and colors permits accurate observation of the macula's surface. Fluorescence angiography measures the luminescence of either fluorescein or indocyanine green (ICG) in the retina as a function of time after the injection. Typically 0.5g of fluorescein is injected i.v. and fluorescence images at ~520 nm are recorded on a CCD camera with excitation at ~480 nm. Hyperfluorescence of fluorescein can indicate leaking blood vessels. ICG is strongly bound to albumin and is not seen to leak extensively, however, it gives supplementary information on the deeper lying blood vessels due to its excitation/emission near 800 nm. Finally, optical coherence tomography (OCT) is a newer method based on interferometry that allows for fairly high-resolution observation of refractive index changes associated with the (normally) quite layered structure of the retina. It permits measurement of the retinal structure in some depth. Typically, retinal thickness changes due to macular edema can be measured quantitatively in order to follow up on the effectiveness of the treatment of the leakiness associated with wet AMD, either by PDT or other methods.

21.5   Previous Treatments of Exudative (Wet) AMD

Several treatments for exudative (i.e., neovascular) AMD have been tested that have not lead to very satisfactory outcomes.

- Radiation therapy [24], where vision loss could not be presented in a consistent way.

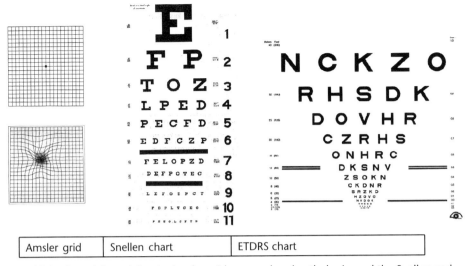

| Amsler grid | Snellen chart | ETDRS chart |

Figure 21.3 From left to right: An Amsler grid—normal and pathologic, and the Snellen and ETDRS charts.

- Surgery is a second option. The surgical removal of the neovasculature can in principle be done with limited damage to the overlying layers [25]; however, rather high rates of recurrence and significant side effects were observed. Another interesting attempt was the translocation of the macula, by rotating the retina around the optic nerve so that a still healthy part was substituted geometrically for the diseased part of the central vision. This is quite a delicate operation and was never proven to be effective in an appropriate clinical trial [26].

- Thermal laser photocoagulation. Thermal laser destruction of CNV associated with AMD was extensively tested and reported on by the Macular Photocoagulation Study Group [11–13, 27, 28]. Due to the type of laser pulse used the thermal photocoagulation goes hand in hand with significant damage to the neighboring photoreceptors and neural retina. This can result in a blind or dark spot in the visual field (scotoma). A high degree of recurrence ($\geq 50\%$) was observed in the 5-year observation period, and recurrence of for instance the juxtafoveal lesions (i.e., lesions with posterior border closer than 200 μm to the center of the foveal avascular zone) often reoccurred on the foveal side of the lesion [25]. Consequently, this treatment can be applied only for slowing down the development of the disease in a very small fraction of wet AMD patients, and can hardly be recommended as a first treatment choice.

21.6 Photodynamic Therapy for AMD

21.6.1 History and Principles

The history and principles of photodynamic therapy for treating choroidal neovasculature (CNV) associated with age-related macular degeneration have been recently reviewed [29–33]. PDT with verteporfin (Visudyne®) was really the first approved therapy for treating the subfoveal lesions. In this sense PDT changed everything for both patients and ophthalmologists, as legal blindness was no longer necessarily the main outcome of this devastating disease, and several hundreds of thousands of eyes have now been treated and saved from blindness by this modality since the year 2000. The compound also known as benzoporphyrin derivative monoacid ring A (BPD-MA) is shown in Chapter 2 (structure of BPD-MA). BPD-MA administrated in liposomal formulation (Visudyne) [34–37]. The compound as injected consists of two regioisomers, each of which is a racemic mixture of two enantiomers (i.e., it is not a pure compound).

One might note that several other compounds, among which tin-etiopurpurin and Lutetium texaphyrin were tested in phase I-II clinical trials, but failed to reach the market. At present, other compounds are being developed in the hope to end up with an even higher treatment selectivity. This implies less damage induced by PDT in the surroundings of the CNV, and in particular less closure of the normal choriocapillaries. One example of this is the creation of a conjugate between BPD-MA and a peptide that binds selectively to endothelial cell receptors that are up–regulated in CNV, such as the VEGF receptor 2 [38].

For PDT of subfoveal CNV, freshly made up verteporfin solution, which is reconstituted from the lyophilized drug, is intravenously injected over a 10-minute period. Fifteen minutes after the start of the perfusion, the excitation light is applied to the retina from a diode laser at a wavelength of 689 nm. To do this in a well-controlled way, the irregularly shaped output of the diode laser is injected into a multimode optical fiber, which homogenizes the beam. The distal end of the fiber, which is a nearly perfectly homogeneously illuminated circle, is then imaged on the retina, in the form of a circular spot of variable size, employing an adjustable lens system and a slit lamp. The treatment beam is coaxial with a much weaker targeting beam at about 630 nm. This targeting beam has the same beam size and divergence as the treatment beam, thus permitting targeting of the diseased part of the retina. The target area, which includes the leaky CNV, is designated by fluorescein angiography. Generally one takes the greatest linear diameter of the lesion and adds a couple of hundred microns at each end to define the optimal size of the circular laser beam spot. Irradiation is via a planar-concave (mainster) contact lens placed on the eye. The fluence rate at the retina is adjusted to be 600 mW/cm^2, which is delivered over 83 seconds, giving a fluence of 50 J/cm^2.

21.6.2 Selectivity in PDT of CNV

There are multiple aspects of the selectivity in the angioocclusion of CNV in AMD by photodynamic therapy. In the first place we have the selectivity of vascular damage and the subsequent blood flow stasis. This selectivity is inherent in the short time interval between the drug injection and the light application (i.e., 15 minutes after the start of the intravenous injection of the Visudyne, when the 83-second irradiation takes place, most of the drug that is in the retina is still within the blood vessels, and more specifically, on or in the endothelial cells lining the CNV that are to undergo the angioocclusion. Thus the main photodynamic effect takes place in the endothelium being irradiated. A second possible reason for the "selective" angioocclusion of the targeted CNV became evident in the phase I/II trials that were done during the development of Visudyne. Indeed in the early clinical tests in Lausanne we actually did Visudyne angiography. What we observed in these experiments was that the retinal vessels will empty of Visudyne fluorescence significantly faster than the choroidal vessels. Thus at the time of irradiation, the retinal capillaries appear to have much less drug in them than the CNV and choroidal vessels in general (Figure 21.4).This may well imply a significant level of protection of the retinal capillaries.

Note that occlusion of the retinal capillaries must be avoided at all costs because it leads to immediate and heavy loss of visual acuity. This was also shown in the phase I/II studies. A third possible reason for the selectivity in the closure of CNV is that retinal capillaries are protected by the blood retinal barrier, which signifies among others tighter junctions between endothelial cells and hence probably more resistance to PDT. The CNV on the contrary are new and leaky vessels with presumably still somewhat weak junctions between the endothelial cells, and not yet significant reinforcement of the capillary walls by pericytes and connective tissue (i.e., the CNV should be relatively prone to PDT induced angioocclusion). A fourth reason for the more or less selective angioocclusion of the CNV that is often invoked, is that these rapidly growing neovessels tend to have a relatively high activity of LDL receptors on their endothelium. The injected verteporfin, which is a fairly lipophilic drug, upon breakup of the liposomal carriers is transferred to a significant extent to LDL. Thus the rapidly proliferating CNV endothelium may selectively be loaded with verteporfin, as has been effectively shown in rabbit eye neovessels [39].

Finally, another reason for the selective angioocclusion of the CNV by PDT may be a lower level of tissue molecular oxygen in the region of the retinal vessels as compared to the choroid. The latter might be inferred from measurements in the pig's eye [40].

21.6.3 PDT-Induced Angioocclusion Process

The PDT-induced angioocclusion process starts with the light-drug interaction that generates the reactive intermediates that damage, among others, different sites in and on the endothelium. Schematically, this process, which could eventually even lead to apoptosis, is shown somewhat simplified in the biochemical cascade of Figure 21.5.

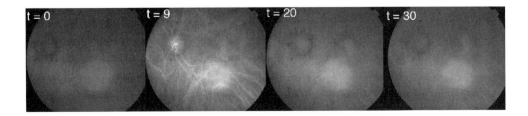

Figure 21.4 Visudyne, fluorescence angiography showing that the retinal vessels empty faster than the CNV membrane and the choroidal vessels (time in minutes).

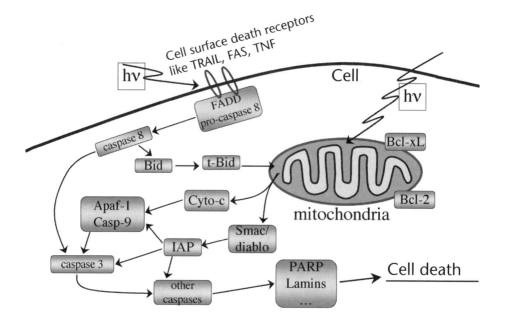

Figure 21.5 Biochemical cascade induced by PDT (adapted from van den Bergh [32]).

It has been shown [41–43] that in such a process the cytoskeleton of the endothelial cells can be damaged, which leads to shrinking and rounding of these cells. This in turn may cause rupture of the more or less tight junctions between the CNV's endothelial cells. To demonstrate the rupture of the tight junctions in the endothelium, we injected a pig with a photosensitizer, after which one of the eyes was irradiated (PDT); the other eye was not irradiated. Both eyes were then enucleated and stained with occludine (a stain for tight junctions) before histopathological investigation. The results are shown in Figure 21.6, and clearly demonstrate the breakup of the tight junctions in the eye with PDT [44].

This breakup of the tight endothelial junctions (Figures 21.6(b) and Figure 21.7(b) is followed by the release of von Willebrand factor (vWF). vWF is a glycoprotein, which is present among others in the endothelial cells and the subendothelium. One of its functions is related to the adhesion and aggregation of platelets. Together with fibrinogen it can act in a complementary and synergistic way in the development of a thrombus (i.e., the release of vWF causes platelets to stick to the capillary wall (Figure 21.7b)). Following that, other platelets stick to these immobilized platelets (Figure 21.7c), thus forming a plug. This thrombus is then stabilized by the activation of fibrinogen to fibrin, which acts like a glue between the platelets (Figure 21.7d). In one of our vascular models [45–48] we have shown that this thrombus formation following PDT is accompanied by some degree of vascular stricture that helps to anchor the thrombus. One may thus envisage the photodynamic angioocclusion, as shown in Figure 21.7.

Note that in contrast to the thermal laser photocoagulation process used occasionally for extrafoveal and juxtafoveal CNV in patients with rapidly progressing disease, whom are not treatable by alternative modalities, PDT of subfoveal CNV spares photoreceptors and other neighboring parts of the retina. Thus in PDT, in

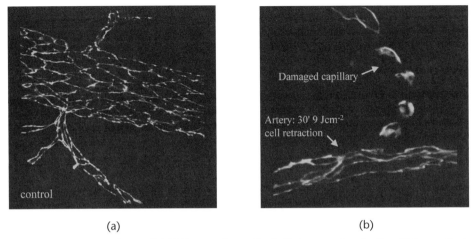

(a)   (b)

Figure 21.6   (a) Control eye. (b) PDT-treated eye. Occludin immunolocalization (flatmount) of endothelial cells of the retinal vein (adapted from Stepinac et al. [44]).

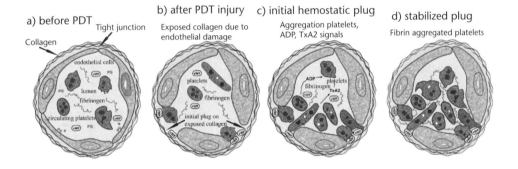

Figure 21.7   (a–d) Mechanism (simplified) of PDT leading to angiooclusion.

nearly all cases, retinal function is to a very large degree maintained (i.e., no scotoma).

Nevertheless, PDT appears to cause some damage to the endothelium of the normal choriocapillaries, as can be seen from the fluorescein (excitation 480, emission 520 nm) and indocyanine green (excitation and emission in the near infrared around 800 nm) angiographies reported in Figure 21.8. The dark areas shown in the early phase fluorescein angiography 1 week after PDT and in the late phase ICG angiography 1 week after PDT, indicate a large degree of nonselective closure of the normal choriocapillaries after PDT. This lack of selectivity appears to be somewhat improved when changing the fluence rate to 300 mW/cm^2 and the light dose consequently to 25 J/cm^2 [49].

21.6.4   PDT of CNV in AMD: Treatment Outcome

The selection of an optimal clinical treatment for neovascular AMD will depend, at least in the case of PDT (but not in several other modes of action discussed below),

Screening before PDT		One week after Visudyne® PDT	
Fluorescein	ICG	Fluorescein	ICG

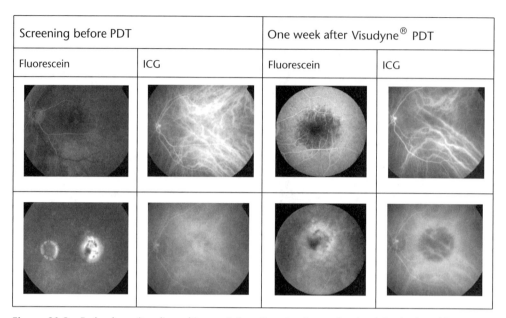

Figure 21.8 Early phase (top line of images) (less than 1 minute after i.v. injection) and late phase (bottom line of images) (more than 5 minutes after i.v. injection) of fluorescein and IGC angiograms obtained in clinical tests, before PDT and 1 week after PDT with Visudyne.

The "before PDT" pictures show early and late fluorescein and ICG angiograms of the retina of a patient before PDT with predominantly "classic" CNV, as demonstrated by the strong well-demarcated hyperfluorescent region near the center of the macula.

The right-hand side of the figure also shows the same eye 1 week after PDT with, in this case, 12 mg/m^2 of Visudyne, and 50 J/cm^2 of light at 689 nm given at 600 mW/cm^2 about 15 minutes after the start of the slow i.v. injection. The early phase fluorescein and the late phase ICG angiograms 1 week after PDT show the dark hypofluorescent spot, indicating that both the CNV and choriocapillaries remain closed on this time scale. The dark spot also helps to demonstrate that the retinal capillaries near the macula are still patent. The closure of the normal choriocapillaries invoked from the absence of fluorescein leakage has been confirmed by indocyanine green angiography.

on the classification of the lesion by fluorescence angiography, as indicated above. This classification will be, either as predominantly classic, minimally classic or occult. The efficacy of the PDT treatment will also depend on the size of the lesion (its greatest linear diameter), and the visual acuity of the patient at baseline. Other parameters and observations, such as can now be made by optical coherence tomography or OCT, may also provide to be useful in choosing the best treatment.

In the Treatment of AMD with PDT (TAP) study [50, 51], subfoveal CNV were treated that had some fraction of classic CNV. Other inclusion criteria in the study included a greatest linear diameter of less than or equal to 5.4 mm, and a visual acuity (VA) at baseline between 20/40 and 20/200. At the final measurement of the original study made 24 months after the baseline visit, PDT had decreased the probability of losing more than 3 lines in the EDTRS chart from 62% in the case of placebo (sham) treatment to 47% in the case of Visudyne PDT therapy (Figure 21.9).

The best results were obtained for the predominantly classic lesions, where 31% of the placebo group lost less than 3 lines, whereas 59% of the PDT treated eyes lost

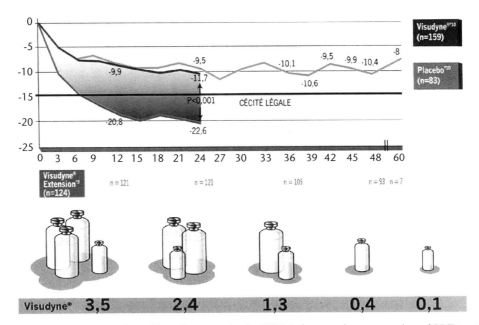

Figure 21.9 Mean number of lost characters in the ETDRS chart, and mean number of PDT treatments/year over these 5 years of followup (TAP study).

less than 3 lines. Large visual acuity losses (i.e., more than 6 lines or 30 letters) were relatively rare in the PDT-treated group as compared to more than one third of the patients (36%) in the placebo group. Improvement in VA by more than 3 lines was found in 9% of the PDT-treated patients at the end of this 2-year study, and was hardly observed at all in the placebo group.

In the Verteporfin In PDT (VIP) study [52–54], patients were enrolled with occult subfoveal lesions. Again, losses in VA were statistically significantly less in the PDT group as compared to the placebo group, with the best results obtained for the smaller lesions (≤4 MPS DA; i.e., less or equal to four Macular Photocoagulation Study disc areas). Outcome, in terms of letters/lines gained or lost, was also better for those patients with the worse VA at baseline.

In the most recent date obtained from a 3-year prolongation of the observation of a large fraction of the TAP patients (i.e., total period of observation = 60 months!) from both the placebo and PDT arms, safety and VA were both reported [55]. The main conclusions were that the mean change in VA from baseline was quite similar at 24 months (–1.5 lines) and at 60 months (–1.6 lines) (Figure 21.9 and Figure 21.10). No additional safety issues were found. The treatment rate (number of treatments/year), which was decided based on fluorescein angiography (i.e., leakage) was significantly lower in the third, fourth, and fifth years as compared to the first 2 years (bottom part of Figure 21.9).

In conclusion, PDT for treating CNV associated with AMD remains a standard therapy for patients with recent progression of wet AMD with subfoveal CNV. The lesions should be defined as either predominantly classic or occult and should be less than 4 MPS DA. The treatment is safe, has a proven long-term effect, and needs hardly any retreatments after the first few years. The latter sets PDT apart from the

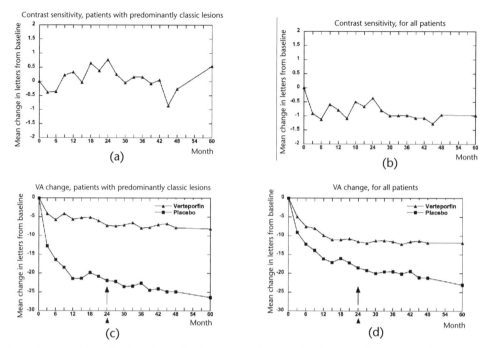

Figure 21.10   (a) patients with predominantly classic CNV; (b) the same figure for patients with all types of CNV; (c) the excellent results obtained in the contrast sensitivity for the verteporfin-treated patients with predominantly classic lesions; and (d) the same figure for all patients. Note that the placebo patients received PDT treatment after 24 months. (Data from TAP Report 8 [55].)

treatments discussed below that have as yet no proven long-term effect, and need very frequent retreatments.

21.7   Other Therapies for Managing Neovascular AMD

21.7.1   Anti-VEGF Therapies

When the choriocapillaries fails to supply enough oxygen to the macula, the cascade of events, including the release of hypoxia-inducible factor-1alpha (HIF-1∞) makes the retinal pigment epithelium (RPE) "sense" the hypoxia. Here VEGF-A gene expression is upregulated. The resulting increase in VEGF-A can restore the perfusion of the choriocapillaries and increases angiogenesis. Excessive VEGF-A may also increase the permeability of the blood vessels. The first drug in this class of substances to reach the market was pegabtanib sodium or Macugen®, an aptamer composed of ribonucleic acids that complexes specifically to VEGF-A 165. This drug was applied directly by injection in the vitreous every 6 weeks. Nevertheless, the results obtained in the VISION trial were somewhat disappointing, as can be seen in Figure 21.11.

The mean VA loss after 24 months was essentially 2 lines, leakage often persisted, and discontinuing the treatment resulted in further significant loss of VA. Overall the drug can be considered safe, but the results were not really better than PDT. It might be noted that the early results on the combination of Macugen with PDT were very encouraging [56].

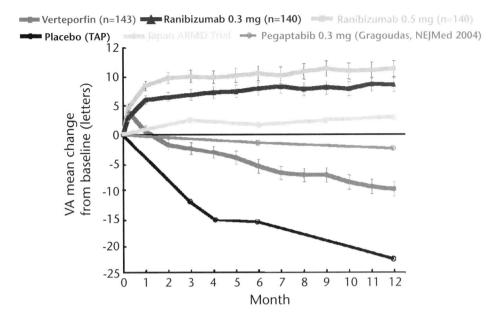

Figure 21.11   Comparison of VA mean change with different treatments.

Another development along the same lines (i.e., of blocking VEGF-A), was ranibizumab or Lucentis®. This is a "humanized" monoclonal antibody fragment (Fab) with enhanced binding to VEGF-A [57] (affinity maturation enhanced binding more than 100x). Lucentis was developed specifically for ocular application. It was hoped that being smaller than the full antibody, the fragment would penetrate better into tissue and possibly be eliminated more rapidly [58].

Lucentis binds to all active isoforms which consist of respectively 110, 121, 165, 189 and 206 amino-acids, and hence it inhibits VEGF-A's interaction with the VEGFR binding domain, which is at amino acids number 88-89. Whereas the larger VEGF-A 206 and 189 have an affinity for the extracellular matrix, the abundant VEGF-A 165 and VEGF-A 121, diffuse more freely, and are supposed to be the most bio-active. By preventing the binding of VEGF-A to VEGFR 1 and 2, the angiogenic cascade is inhibited so that progression of CNV is blocked. Furthermore, leakage is reduced.

In phase III Lucentis trials, patients were enrolled in the MARINA [59], ANCHOR [59–62], and PIER [59] trials. These were multicenter, randomized, double-masked, sham-controlled or active treatment controlled studies of, respectively, minimally classic or occult (no classic), predominantly classic, and primary or recurrent subfoveal CNV with and without classic CNV. In MARINA [62] with the higher 0.5 mg monthly dose of Lucentis, the rapid improvement in VA over 3 months was subsequently stabilized over 2 years, ending with +6.6 letters (5 letters/line) benefit, as compared to 14.9 letters (3 lines) loss in the sham patients. Thus, the total benefit of the treatment was nearly 4 lines! Retinal thickness, mostly due to edema, as measure by OCT, was also strongly reduced. In ANCHOR [60] the 12-month results showed +11.3 letters for the 0.5 mg/months injections of Lucentis in the vitreous, whereas Visudyne showed 9.5 letters loss (Figure 21.11).

Visudyne, either active or as sham, was applied every 3 months depending upon the leakage observed. Finally, the PIER study [59] demonstrated clear loss of the early Lucentis gains if injections were spaced at 3-month intervals. Nevertheless, on the average this trial showed that most patients maintained their baseline VA after 12 months [63]. The safety data showed that Lucentis is well tolerated up to 2 years, even with monthly intravitreal injections. Serious ocular adverse events are uncommon. Among these are endophthalmitis, which is an injection-related adverse event, uveitis or intraocular inflammation, and intraocular pressure increase.

Another drug used for blocking VEGF-A is bevacizumab or Avastin®, which is used extensively off-label. It is a full-length humanized antibody, which also binds to all VEGF isoforms. The binding affinity is not enhanced. Several reviews of the data on intravitreal Avastin showed a fast reduction of the retinal thickness, which often went hand in hand with VA improvement. One such article reported on 2 lines or even better improvement in nearly 50% of the patients, and most eyes demonstrated at least stable VA [64].

21.7.2 Anecortave Acetate (Retaane)

This is a substance with the angiostatic effect of a normal corticosteroid, but it has been chemically modified so as not to increase intraocular pressure or enhance cataract. The latter are side effects associated with certain corticosteroids. A phase III trial did not succeed in proving at least equal efficacy with PDT [65, 66].

21.7.3 VEGF-Trap

The VEGF-A binds specifically to the extracellular domains of the VEGFR-1 and VEGFR-2 receptors on the endothelial cells to trigger, among others, the stimulation of CNV. A combination of key ligand-binding domains of these two receptors has now been fused to a protein backbone that is human IgG Fc. VEGF-trap has a very high affinity for VEGF-A (i.e., it binds very tightly to it). Also, it is small and diffuses readily through the retina, and does not get stuck easily in extracellular matrix. The VEGF-trap also blocks placental growth factor, which may also be of use in slowing down CNV progression. A phase III trial is on its way where intravitreal Aflibercept is compared with versus IV infusion [67].

21.7.4 siRNA

Small interfering RNAs are bits of RNA consisting of 21 to 22 base pairs that can be introduced into a cell with, as a result, that an RNA silencing complex is formed that binds specifically to, and catalytically destroys, the messenger RNA that is coded in this specific case to produce VEGF. Note that the siRNA stops the increase in VEGF production but does not act on excess VEGF that is most likely already present in the CNV's surrounding. Thus it may act slower than an anti-VEGF, but may be, more efficient in the long term. In a phase I/II study bevasiranib was injected in the vitreous [68], on a milligram or submilligram scale. It switches off the gene that produces VEGF. Stabilization of the disease was observed after some time. In a similar approach Sirna-027 switches off the gene that produces the

VEGFR-1 receptor and this compound has also shown interesting results in a phase I-II study [69–71].

21.7.5 Inhibitors of Tyrosine Kinase Receptors

Rather than blocking the VEGFR binding domain on the VEGF-A molecules, one can alternatively inhibit the VEGF-A effects by blocking the receptors themselves. This blocking at the receptor level can be done by VEGFR tyrosine kinase inhibitors. These are potent small organic molecules that inhibit all VEGF receptors as well as other receptors such as PDGF-R (platelet-derived growth factor receptor), which also contributes to the cascades leading to CNV in the eye. In this class of molecules under development for AMD are Vatalanib (PTK-787, Novartis) as well as AG-013736 and AG-013958 (both from Pfizer) and AL-39324 from Alcon.

21.7.6 Squalamine

Evizon (squalamine lactate) blocks angiogenesis and is in phase III trials for the treatment of subfoveal CNV in AMD with GENEARA. This is a systemically administered small molecule. In fact it is an aminosterol (i.e., a steroid linked to an amino acid, which blocks VEGF as well as cytoskeleton and integrin expression). In phase I/II trials, nearly all patients were measured with stabilization of vision, and some patients even had an increase in VA of up to 8 lines [72, 73]!

21.8 Combination Therapy

We have discussed a number of monotherapies for CNV secondary to AMD together with part of what may be known about their mode of action. Possible synergies between these therapies and PDT might exist and suggestions for optimal combination therapies can be made [74, 75]. Many of the monotherapeutic treatments reported above represent significant advances in the treatment of CNV, in some cases even in the clinical context. Nevertheless further improvements are still required. The anti-VEGF therapies for instance still require intravitreal injection every 4 to 6 weeks. Furthermore, these treatments show reduced efficacy when the neovessels become more mature [76]. The latter may be the case in particular for idiopathic polypoidal choroidal vasculopathy (PCV), which is discussed in some detail below.

In combining two (or more) therapies for treating CNV in AMD, one may want to consider two strategies. First, in the case where one has a dominant vector for the disease, like VEGF, one may want to attack the VEGF biochemical pathway with multiple drugs, where one drug might be used at first to quickly stop the rapid proliferation of CNV and the leakage, whereas a second drug is used later on for maintaining the status quo in the disease progression attained with the first drug. Such an approach would be a particularly good choice if the second drug, which will have to be used over a much longer period in time, has significantly less side effects, or if it can be used at a much lower treatment frequency than the first drug.

A second approach to combination therapy is to gain efficacy by targeting multiple pathways at the same time. An example of this would be the blocking of the amino acid 88-89 positions on VEGF-A, which is then combined with the blocking of platelet-derived growth factor (PDGF-B). The latter is responsible for the maturing of CNV by, among others, recruiting pericites and smooth muscle cells. Because VEGF blockers do not work particularly well in mature vessels [77], the blocking of PDGF-B may consequently keep the CNV from maturing and make the VEGF blockers more efficient.

21.8.1 Combining PDT with VEGF Pathway Inhibition

Antiangiogenic therapy slows the leakage associated with CNV and decreases the growth of new CNV. Nevertheless, the CNV may persist. To solve the problem of the persisting CNV, PDT may thus be used to act synergistically with anti-VEGF, by inducing thrombosis in the CNV. One might in consequence expect a reduction in the retreatment frequency, as well as having more durable improvement/maintenance of VA as compared to anti-VEGF therapy alone. This combination of Lucentis and Visudyne therapies has been shown in the CAM model to be extremely synergistic for neovessel closure [78]. The same combination of PDT with Verteporfin and ranibizumab was also studied in Ryan's monkey model [79, 80]. Here the combination therapy was shown to be more effective than PDT monotherapy in reducing the leakage from the thermally induced CNV. In the same model, it was also demonstrated that there were no important adverse events in this particular combination of therapies.

Clinical trials along the same lines of combining PDT with anti-VEGF therapy have also been ongoing. They started with the phase I/II VISION trial (verteporfin PDT combined with pegabtanib), which showed a very encouraging improvement in VA by 3 lines in 60% of the treated patients [81]. In a second trial (FOCUS), the combination of ranibizumab with verteporfin PDT was compared with verteporfin PDT monotherapy [82]. At 24 months, nearly 25% of the patients treated with the combi-therapy gained 3 lines or more as compared to only 7 % of the verteporfin PDT monotherapy patients. The rate of PDT retreatments, which was based on fluorescein leakage measurements, was also significantly lower in the combi-therapy group. The mean change in VA over time was +4.6 letters at 24 months for the combi-therapy, and –7.8 letters for the Verteporfin PDT monotherapy.

The combi-treatment was found to be safe, especially after changing the formulation of the anti-VEGF compound [83–85]. In another phase II trial (PROTECT [86]), same-day administration of verteporfin PDT and intravitreal ranibizumab (liquid formulation now) was tested to measure the number of verteporfin retreatments after combi-therapy at baseline. In this trial, 90.6% of the patients needed a single retreatment or less at 9 months, two-thirds needed no retreatment at all, and less than 10% needed only two additional PDT. The reduction in mean retinal thickness was 164 μ, and the mean area of leakage decreased from 8.2 to 1.2 mm^2 at 9 months. The mean VA change was +2.4 letters relative to baseline for the 32 patients in this study. The latest trials in these series are the SUMMIT-DENALI and MONT BLANC trials [87]. Here the object is to demonstrate that Visudyne combi-therapy with Lucentis is not inferior to Lucentis monotherapy with respect to the mean change in VA. A second, and quite important, outcome of interest is the percentage of patients with a 3 months or more treatment free interval in the two arms of the study i.e. can one reduce the retreatment frequency without losing the gain (or maintenance) of VA [88].

21.8.2 Combining PDT with Triamcinolone or Anecortave Acetate

PDT has been shown to efficiently close CNV secondary to AMD, in particular for small classic lesions. But, one also observes some degree of closure of the normal choriocapillaries, and PDT induces supplementary VEGF as discussed above, and inflammation is also observed after PDT [89]. Thus steroids like triamcinolone and steroid derivatives like anecortave acetate have been suggested as being of interest to be used in combination with PDT. In the VERITAS trial, three arms were compared: verteporfin PDT + intravitreal pegabtanib 0.3 mg every 6 weeks; verteporfin PDT + intravitreal triamcinolone 1 mg every 3 months; and verteporfin + intravitreal triamcinolone 4 mg every 3 months. In data reported at ARVO in 2007, Augustin et.al. reported [90, 91] the following for the 307 eyes in the verteporfin PDT + steroid arm: rapid increase in VA of about 1 line relative to baseline in the first 3 months. This increase in VA was then essentially conserved for up to 85 weeks (~20 months) after baseline. The combination of verteporfin PDT with triamcinolone (1 and 4 mg) was more effective than the combination of verteporfin PDT with pegaptanib. The treatments were considered to be safe and well tolerated, but anatomically there was only a very modest decrease in lesion thickness as observed by OCT.

In the case of combination of verteporfin PDT with steroids in general, such a treatment might be considered for the long-term followup, although this needs still to be proven in proper clinical trials. The risk with some of the unmodified steroids remains increased risk of glaucoma and intraocular pressure increase. Verteporfin trials in combination with anecortave acetate, a steroidlike molecule that was modified to reduce side effects, are also under way. Many other combinations between PDT and various other anti-CNV in AMD strategies can be envisaged. Some of these will certainly be tried, but will have to wait for the outcome of the monotherapy trials in order to be considered. The prediction of the outcome of combination therapies, based on the relatively scarce information on the proteomics of the individual modes of action, will probably remain a somewhat difficult affair. Some examples of such arguments have been given above. Hence effective preclinical screening tests such as developed in the CAM model of the chicken embryo [45–48, 92–94], and at a later stage in Ryan's monkey model [79, 80], will probably dominate the early stages of future combi-therapy development.

21.9 Photodynamic Drug Delivery to the Eye

At extremely mild conditions of photodynamic action (i.e., low drug dose and/or low light dose), blood vessels that undergo photodynamic damage to their endothelium may start to leak significantly. The mechanism is essentially as described above, in the sense that endothelial cells have their cytoskeleton damaged and both shrink and round off. This causes rupture of the tight connections between the endothelial cells, which induces leakage. As under mild PDT conditions, especially in somewhat larger vessels, a complete thrombus is not formed and stabilized, this photodynamically induced leakage may last for some time. This leakage may now be used for drug dosing at the site of the photodynamic damage. We have recently demonstrated this possibility by selectively dosing i.v. injected FITC dextrans of varying size to specifically chosen sites in both the CAM and in an intravital microscopy mouse model. As the eye is particularly accessible to PDT, drug dosing to different compartments of the eye by low-dose PDT may well develop into an attractive possibility for systemically applied drugs. Finally, it should be mentioned that the problem of the repetitive injection of drugs into the vitreous mentioned above can be circumvented to a large extent by introducing slow release from nanoparticles or an implant [95].

21.10   PDT of Polypoidal Choroidal Vasculopathy (PCV)

So far we have discussed 2 forms of choroidal neovasculature. Polypoidal CNV, or PCV, is a third form of CNV, which is best distinguished using ICG angiography. PCV has two components, a network of vessels branching from the choriocapillaries downwards towards the sclera, which are combined with terminal aneurismal dilatations that can occasionally be observed as polypoidal vascular lesions. In pathology, PCV shows up as large thin-walled vessels, often lying below the RPE and the choriocapillaries. Although found in all races, there is a higher occurrence in the more pigmented persons. As detection depends to a large extent on ICG angiography, the presence of this disease is hard to estimate, but ranges from slightly less than 10% in AMD patients in Western countries to 60% of patients presenting with leaky macular detachment. 30% of the cases of neovascular AMD in elderly Asian patients represent PCV [96]. At present, PDT with Visudyne is the preferred therapy for PCV [96, 97]. Patients with this disease can be much younger than is the case for AMD. Verteporfin photodynamic therapy has been conducted in a number of these patients and been shown to be quite effective on the time scale of about 1 year, with about half the patients gaining one line, the other half remaining stable [98–101]. Because in PCV one may be dealing with more mature vasculature, PCV may be significantly less amenable to anti-VEGF therapies than CNV secondary to AMD. Nevertheless, anti-VEGF therapy has been shown to reduce the fluid leaking from PCV but appears to be ineffective in reducing the abnormal choroidal vascular changes [97]. It may well be that Visudyne therapy for angioocclusion of the polyps, combined with Lucentis therapy for the antipermeability effect, will lead to improved clinical outcome [97].

21.11   Conclusions

AMD can have a major impact on a person's quality of life. Important tasks like driving, recognizing money bills and faces of other people, as well as reading and writing, may be impaired, especially in the case of wet AMD in both eyes. Mobility is decreased, and risk of injury by falling increases. Dry AMD is generally accompanied by a slow decrease in visual acuity (VA) and is treated often by dietary supplements of vitamins and antioxidants. Such "mild" AMD has been associated with a 17% decrease in the quality of life [102–104]. In the severe, neovascular or wet form of AMD this may increase to a 60% reduction in the quality of life, part of which is caused by the increased dependence on others. PDT with Visudyne for subfoveal CNV offers an 8.1% quality of life improvement; intravitreal Lucentis shows a gain of 15.8%. The economic burden of AMD tends to be difficult to estimate, but for the United Kingdom, France, Italy, and Germany together (about 250 million people), the 2002 cost was 50 to 100 million Euros per year.

Verteporfin PDT reached the market in 2000; anti-VEGF therapy for the eye about half a decade later. PDT arrived at a time when only a very small percentage of the patients with wet AMD could be treated, and it offered a "stabilizing the VA" solution, tested now for over 60 months. Hundred of thousands of eyes have been saved. The cost-effectiveness of verteporfin PDT relative to placebo has been estimated as being reasonably good by pharmacoeconomic analysis. It can be defined as incremental costs relative to quality of life or vision years gained and will depend on VA, age, period of treatment, and perspective adopted. This aspect is discussed in detail by Brown et al. [105]. With arrival on the market of anti-VEGF therapies, tested for about 2 years, patients may now even hope for VA gain in a significant fraction of the cases. Six to eight weeks between the necessary intravitreal injections and difficulty in treating advanced disease with mature vessels points towards combination therapy as a possible optimal solution. The combination between PDT-induced angiooclusion and reduced leakage, may give optimal VA outcome together with reduced retreatment frequency. Early clinical tests for some of these modalities are encouraging; more definitive tests are under way. Novel combinations may be optimally and rapidly tested in the CAM and Ryan's model. Slower drug release is under investigation, also to reduce retreatment frequency. New data indicate that PDT may have a future as a drug delivery modality in the eye, both for AMD and other diseases. Finally, PDT for treating polypoidal choroidal vasculopathy (PCV) appears to be the best solution for dealing with this disease, which is very frequent in the Asian and other pigmented populations of our world.

References

[1] Bressler, N. M., Bressler, S. B., and Fine, S. L., "Age-related macular degeneration," *Surv Ophthalmol*, Vol. 32, 1988, pp. 375–413.

[2] Friedman, D. S., et al., "Prevalence of age-related macular degeneration in the United States," *Arch Ophthalmol*, Vol. 122, 2004, pp. 564–572.

[3] Mitchell, P., et al., "Prevalence of age-related maculopathy in Australia. The Blue Mountains Eye Study," *Ophthalmology*, Vol. 102, 1995, pp. 1450–1460.

[4] Vingerling, J. R., et al., "The prevalence of age-related maculopathy in the Rotterdam Study," *Ophthalmology*, Vol. 102, 1995, pp. 205–210.

[5] Bressler, S. B., et al., "Natural course of choroidal neovascular membranes within the foveal avascular zone in senile macular degeneration," *Am J Ophthalmol*, Vol. 93, 1982, pp. 157–163.

[6]   Ferris, F. L., 3rd, Fine, S. L., and Hyman, L., "Age-related macular degeneration and blindness due to neovascular maculopathy," *Arch Ophthalmol*, Vol. 102, 1984, pp. 1640–1642.

[7]   Roberts, J. E., "Ocular phototoxicity," *J Photochem Photobiol B*, Vol. 64, 2001, pp. 136–143.

[8]   Samiec, P. S., et al., "Glutathione in human plasma: decline in association with aging, age-related macular degeneration, and diabetes," *Free Radic Biol Med*, Vol. 24, 1998, pp. 699–704.

[9]   Sarna, T., "Properties and function of the ocular melanin—a photobiophysical view," *J Photochem Photobiol B*, Vol. 12, 1992, pp. 215–258.

[10] MPSG, "Krypton laser photocoagulation for neovascular lesions of age-related macular degeneration. Results of a randomized clinical trial. Macular Photocoagulation Study Group," *Arch Ophthalmol*, Vol. 108, 1990, pp. 816–824.

[11] MPSG, "Laser photocoagulation of subfoveal neovascular lesions of age-related macular degeneration. Updated findings from two clinical trials. Macular Photocoagulation Study Group," *Arch Ophthalmol*, Vol. 111, 1993, pp. 1200–1209.

[12] MPSG, "Visual outcome after laser photocoagulation for subfoveal choroidal neovascularization secondary to age-related macular degeneration. The influence of initial lesion size and initial visual acuity. Macular Photocoagulation Study Group," *Arch Ophthalmol*, Vol. 112, 1994, pp. 480–488.

[13] MPSG, "Laser photocoagulation for juxtafoveal choroidal neovascularization. Five-year results from randomized clinical trials. Macular Photocoagulation Study Group," *Arch Ophthalmol*, Vol. 112, 1994, pp. 500–509.

[14] Curcio, C. A., et al., "Human photoreceptor topography," *J Comp Neurol*, Vol. 292, 1990, pp. 497–523.

[15] Sarks, S. H., "Ageing and degeneration in the macular region: a clinico-pathological study," *Br J Ophthalmol*, Vol. 60, 1976, pp. 324–341.

[16] Sarks, J. P., Sarks, S. H., and Killingsworth, M. C., "Evolution of geographic atrophy of the retinal pigment epithelium," *Eye*, Vol. 2 (Pt 5), 1988, pp. 552–577.

[17] Shams, N., and Ianchulev, T., "Role of vascular endothelial growth factor in ocular angiogenesis," *Ophthalmol Clin North Am*, Vol. 19, 2006, pp. 335–344.

[18] Hera, R., et al., "Expression of VEGF and angiopoietins in subfoveal membranes from patients with age-related macular degeneration," *Am J Ophthalmol*, Vol. 139, 2005, pp. 589–596.

[19] Ida, H., et al., "RPE cells modulate subretinal neovascularization, but do not cause regression in mice with sustained expression of VEGF," *Invest Ophthalmol Vis Sci*, Vol. 44, 2003, pp. 5430–5437.

[20] Krussel, J. S., et al., "Vascular endothelial growth factor (VEGF) mRNA splice variants are differentially expressed in human blastocysts," *Mol Hum Reprod*, Vol. 7, 2001, pp. 57–63.

[21] Nagineni, C. N., et al., "Transforming growth factor-beta induces expression of vascular endothelial growth factor in human retinal pigment epithelial cells: involvement of mitogen-activated protein kinases," *J Cell Physiol*, Vol. 197, 2003, pp. 453–462.

[22] Bailey, I. L., and Lovie, J. E., "New design principles for visual acuity letter charts," *Am J Optom Physiol Opt*, Vol. 53, 1976, pp. 740–745.

[23] Ferris, F. L., 3rd, et al., "New visual acuity charts for clinical research," *Am J Ophthalmol*, Vol. 94, 1982, pp. 91–96.

[24] Hoeller, U., et al., "Results of radiotherapy of subfoveal neovascularization with 16 and 20 Gy," *Eye*, Vol. 19, 2005, pp. 1151–1156.

[25] Joseph, D. P., Uemura, A., and Thomas, M. A., "Subretinal surgery for juxtafoveal choroidal neovascularization," *Retina*, Vol. 23, 2003, pp. 463–468.

[26] Falkner, C. I., et al., "The end of submacular surgery for age-related macular degeneration? A meta-analysis," *Graefes Arch Clin Exp Ophthalmol*, Vol. 245, 2007, pp. 490–501.

[27] MPSG, "Subfoveal neovascular lesions in age-related macular degeneration. Guidelines for evaluation and treatment in the macular photocoagulation study. Macular Photocoagulation Study Group," *Arch Ophthalmol*, Vol. 109, 1991, pp. 1242–1257.

[28] MPSG, "The influence of treatment extent on the visual acuity of eyes treated with Krypton laser for juxtafoveal choroidal neovascularization. Macular Photocoagulation Study Group," *Arch Ophthalmol*, Vol. 113, 1995, pp. 190–194.

[29] Fenton, C., and Perry, C. M., "Verteporfin: a review of its use in the management of subfoveal choroidal neovascularisation," *Drugs Aging*, Vol. 23, 2006, pp. 421–445.

[30] Schmidt-Erfurth, U., and Hasan, T., "Mechanisms of action of photodynamic therapy with verteporfin for the treatment of age-related macular degeneration," *Surv Ophthalmol*, Vol. 45, 2000, pp. 195–214.

[31] van den Bergh, H., and Ballini, J. P. "Photodynamic Therapy for Age Related Macular Degeneration: Fundamentals, the Present Situation, and Future Developments," in E. S. Gragoudas, J. Miller, and L. Zographos (eds.), *Photodynamic Therapy of Ocular Diseases*, pp. 1–27. Lippincott William and Williams, 2002.

[32] van den Bergh, H., and Ballini, J. P. "Photodynamic Therapy: Basic Principles and Mechanisms," in F. Fankhauser and S. Kwasniewska (eds.), *Lasers in Ophthalmology—Surgical and Diagnostic Aspects*, pp. 1–23. The Hague: Kugler, 2002.

[33] Wormald, R., et al., "Photodynamic therapy for neovascular age-related macular degeneration," *Cochrane Database Syst Rev*, Vol., 2007, pp. CD002030.

[34] Chowdhary, R. K., Shariff, I., and Dolphin, D., "Drug release characteristics of lipid based benzoporphyrin derivative," *J Pharm Pharm Sci*, Vol. 6, 2003, pp. 13–19.

[35] Husain, D., et al., "Intravenous infusion of liposomal benzoporphyrin derivative for photodynamic therapy of experimental choroidal neovascularization," *Arch Ophthalmol*, Vol. 114, 1996, pp. 978–985.

[36] Kramer, M., et al., "Liposomal benzoporphyrin derivative verteporfin photodynamic therapy. Selective treatment of choroidal neovascularization in monkeys," *Ophthalmology*, Vol. 103, 1996, pp. 427–438.

[37] Richter, A. M., et al., "Liposomal delivery of a photosensitizer, benzoporphyrin derivative monoacid ring A (BPD), to tumor tissue in a mouse tumor model," *Photochem Photobiol*, Vol. 57, 1993, pp. 1000–1006.

[38] Renno, R. Z., et al., "Selective photodynamic therapy by targeted verteporfin delivery to experimental choroidal neovascularization mediated by a homing peptide to vascular endothelial growth factor receptor-2," *Arch Ophthalmol*, Vol. 122, 2004, pp. 1002–1011.

[39] Schmidt-Erfurth, U., et al., "Vascular Targeting in Photodynamic Occlusion of Subretinal Vessels," *Ophthalmology*, Vol. 101, 1994, pp. 1953–1961.

[40] Pournaras, C. J., "Retinal oxygen distribution. Its role in the physiopathology of vasoproliferative microangiopathies," *Retina*, Vol. 15, 1995, pp. 332–347.

[41] Fingar, V. H., "Vascular effects of photodynamic therapy," *J Clin Laser Med Surg*, Vol. 14, 1996, pp. 323–328.

[42] Henderson, B. W., and Dougherty, T. J., "How does photodynamic therapy work?" *Photochem Photobiol*, Vol. 55, 1992, pp. 145–157.

[43] Sporn, L. A., and Foster, T. H., "Photofrin and light induces microtubule depolymerization in cultured human endothelial cells," *Cancer Res*, Vol. 52, 1992, pp. 3443–3448.

[44] Stepinac, T. K., et al., "Light-induced retinal vascular damage by Pd-porphyrin luminescent oxygen probes," *Invest Ophthalmol Vis Sci*, Vol. 46, 2005, pp. 956–966.

[45] Debefve, E., et al., "Combination therapy using aspirin-enhanced photodynamic selective drug delivery," *Vascul Pharmacol*, Vol. 46, 2007, pp. 171–180.

[46] Pegaz, B., et al., "Photothrombic activity of m-THPC-loaded liposomal formulations: pre-clinical assessment on chick chorioallantoic membrane model," *Eur J Pharm Sci*, Vol. 28, 2006, pp. 134–140.

[47] Pegaz, B., et al., "Encapsulation of porphyrins and chlorins in biodegradable nanoparticles: the effect of dye lipophilicity on the extravasation and the photothrombic activity. A comparative study," *J Photochem Photobiol B*, Vol. 80, 2005, pp. 19–27.

[48] Pegaz, B., et al., "Preclinical evaluation of a novel water-soluble chlorin E6 derivative (BLC 1010) as photosensitizer for the closure of the neovessels," *Photochem Photobiol*, Vol. 81, 2005, pp. 1505–1510.

[49] Michels, S., et al., "Influence of treatment parameters on selectivity of verteporfin therapy," *Invest Ophthalmol Vis Sci*, Vol. 47, 2006, pp. 371–376.

[50] TAP Study Group, "Verteporfin therapy for subfoveal choroidal neovascularization in age-related macular degeneration. Three-year results of an open-label extension of 2 randomized clinical trials—TAP report 5," *Arch. Ophthalmol.*, Vol. 120, 2002, pp. 1307–1314.

[51] TAP Study Group, "Effects of verteporfin therapy on contrast on sensitivity: Results from the treatment of age-related macular degeneration with photodynamic therapy (TAP) investigation—TAP report No. 4," *Retina*, Vol. 22, 2002, pp. 536–544.

[52] VIP Study Group, "photodynamic therapy of subfoveal choroidal neovascularization in pathologic myopia with verteporfin. 1-year results of a randomized clinical trial—VIP report no. 1," *Ophthalmology*, Vol. 108, 2001, pp. 841–852.

[53] VIP Study Group, "Verteporfin therapy of subfoveal choroidal neovascularization in age-related macular degeneration: two-year results of a randomized clinical trial including lesions with occult with no classic choroidal neovascularization—verteporfin in photodynamic therapy report 2," *Am J Ophthalmol*, Vol. 131, 2001, pp. 541–560.

[54] VIP Study Group, "Verteporfin therapy of subfoveal choroidal neovascularization in pathologic myopia: 2-year results of a randomized clinical trial—VIP report no. 3," *Ophthalmology*, Vol. 110, 2003, pp. 667–673.

[55] Kaiser, P. K., "Verteporfin therapy of subfoveal choroidal neovascularization in age-related macular degeneration: 5-year results of two randomized clinical trials with an open-label extension: TAP report no. 8," *Graefes Arch Clin Exp Ophthalmol*, Vol. 244, 2006, pp. 1132–1142.

[56] Ng, E. W., et al., "Pegaptanib, a targeted anti-VEGF aptamer for ocular vascular disease," *Nat Rev Drug Discov*, Vol. 5, 2006, pp. 123–132.

[57] Chen, Y., et al., "Selection and analysis of an optimized anti-VEGF antibody: crystal structure of an affinity-matured Fab in complex with antigen," *J Mol Biol*, Vol. 293, 1999, pp. 865–881.

[58] Ferrara, N., et al., "Development of ranibizumab, an anti-vascular endothelial growth factor antigen binding fragment, as therapy for neovascular age-related macular degeneration," *Retina*, Vol. 26, 2006, pp. 859–870.

[59] Rosenfeld, P. J., Rich, R. M., and Lalwani, G. A., "Ranibizumab: Phase III clinical trial results," *Ophthalmol Clin North Am*, Vol. 19, 2006, pp. 361–372.

[60] Brown, D. M., et al., "Ranibizumab versus verteporfin for neovascular age-related macular degeneration," *N Engl J Med*, Vol. 355, 2006, pp. 1432–1444.

[61] Kaiser, P. K., et al., "Angiographic and optical coherence tomographic results of the MARINA study of ranibizumab in neovascular age-related macular degeneration," *Ophthalmology*, Vol. 114, 2007, pp. 1868–1875.

[62] Rosenfeld, P. J., et al., "Ranibizumab for neovascular age-related macular degeneration," *N Engl J Med*, Vol. 355, 2006, pp. 1419–1431.

[63] FDA Lucentis (ranibizumab injection), in FDA (ed.), 2006, Initial U.S. Approval: http://www.fda.gov/cder/foi/label/2006/125156lbl.pdf

[64] Spaide, R. F., et al., "Intravitreal bevacizumab treatment of choroidal neovascularization secondary to age-related macular degeneration," *Retina*, Vol. 26, 2006, pp. 383–390.

[65] Sharma, S., et al., "Drug pricing for a novel treatment for wet macular degeneration: using incremental cost-effectiveness ratios to ensure societal value," *Can J Ophthalmol*, Vol. 40, 2005, pp. 369–377.

[66] Slakter, J. S., et al., "Anecortave acetate (15 milligrams) versus photodynamic therapy for treatment of subfoveal neovascularization in age-related macular degeneration," *Ophthalmology*, Vol. 113, 2006, pp. 3–13.

[67] Saishin, Y., et al., "VEGF-TRAP(R1R2) suppresses choroidal neovascularization and VEGF-induced breakdown of the blood-retinal barrier," *J Cell Physiol*, Vol. 195, 2003, pp. 241–248.

[68] Reich, S. J., et al., "Small interfering RNA (siRNA) targeting VEGF effectively inhibits ocular neovascularization in a mouse model," *Mol Vis*, Vol. 9, 2003, pp. 210–216.

[69] Shen, J., et al., "Suppression of ocular neovascularization with siRNA targeting VEGF receptor 1," *Gene Ther*, Vol. 13, 2006, pp. 225–234.

[70] Tolentino, M. J., et al., "Intravitreal injection of vascular endothelial growth factor small interfering RNA inhibits growth and leakage in a nonhuman primate, laser-induced model of choroidal neovascularization," *Retina*, Vol. 24, 2004, pp. 132–138.

[71] Tolentino, M. J., et al., "Re: Intravitreal injection of vascular endothelial growth factor small interfering RNA inhibits growth and leakage in a nonhuman primate, laser-induced model of choroidal neovascularization," *Retina*, Vol. 24, 2004, p. 661.

[72] Connolly, B., et al., "Squalamine lactate for exudative age-related macular degeneration," *Ophthalmol Clin North Am*, Vol. 19, 2006, pp. 381–391, vi.

[73] Michels, S., Schmidt-Erfurth, U., and Rosenfeld, P. J., "Promising new treatments for neovascular age-related macular degeneration," *Expert Opin Investig Drugs*, Vol. 15, 2006, pp. 779–793.

[74] Ambati, J., et al., "Age-related macular degeneration: etiology, pathogenesis, and therapeutic strategies," *Surv Ophthalmol*, Vol. 48, 2003, pp. 257–293.

[75] Spaide, R. F., "Rationale for combination therapies for choroidal neovascularization," *Am J Ophthalmol*, Vol. 141, 2006, pp. 149–156.

[76] Jo, N., et al., "Inhibition of platelet-derived growth factor B signaling enhances the efficacy of anti-vascular endothelial growth factor therapy in multiple models of ocular neovascularization," *Am J Pathol*, Vol. 168, 2006, pp. 2036–2053.

[77] Gerhardt, H., and Betsholtz, C., "Endothelial-pericyte interactions in angiogenesis," *Cell Tissue Res*, Vol. 314, 2003, pp. 15–23.

[78] van den Bergh, H., et al. "Video monitoring of neovessel occlusion induced by photodynemic therapy in combination with anti-VEGF therapy," in Association for Research in Vision and Ophthalmology (ARVO), Fort Lauderdale, Florida, April 27–May 1, 2008.

[79] Husain, D., et al., "Safety and efficacy of intravitreal injection of ranibizumab in combination with verteporfin PDT on experimental choroidal neovascularization in the monkey," *Arch Ophthalmol*, Vol. 123, 2005, pp. 509–516.

[80] Kim, I. K., et al., "Effect of intravitreal injection of ranibizumab in combination with verteporfin PDT on normal primate retina and choroid," *Invest Ophthalmol Vis Sci*, Vol. 47, 2006, pp. 357–363.

[81] Gragoudas, E. S., et al., "Pegaptanib for neovascular age-related macular degeneration," *N Engl J Med*, Vol. 351, 2004, pp. 2805–2816.

[82] Heier, J. S., et al., "Ranibizumab combined with verteporfin photodynamic therapy in neovascular age-related macular degeneration: year 1 results of the FOCUS Study," *Arch Ophthalmol*, Vol. 124, 2006, pp. 1532–1542.

[83] Augustin, A. J., and Offermann, I., "Combination therapy for choroidal neovascularisation," *Drugs Aging*, Vol. 24, 2007, pp. 979–990.

[84] Kaiser, P. K., "Verteporfin photodynamic therapy and anti-angiogenic drugs: potential for combination therapy in exudative age-related macular degeneration," *Curr Med Res Opin*, Vol. 23, 2007, pp. 477–487.

[85] Kourlas, H., and Abrams, P., "Ranibizumab for the treatment of neovascular age-related macular degeneration: a review," *Clin Ther*, Vol. 29, 2007, pp. 1850–1861.

[86] Schmidt-Erfurth, U. "Preliminary results from an open-label, multicenter, phase II study assessing the effects of same-day administration of ranibizumab (Lucentis®) and verteporfin PDT (PROTECT Study), in Association for Research in Vision and Ophthalmology (ARVO), Fort Lauderdale, Florida, April 30–May 4, 2006.

[87] Lanzetta, P. "SUMMIT clinical programme," *7th International AMD Congress*, Marbella, Spain, October 18–20, 2007.

[88] Schmidt-Erfurth, U. M., et al., "Guidance for the treatment of neovascular age-related macular degeneration," *Acta Ophthalmol Scand*, Vol. 85, 2007, pp. 486–494.

[89] Tatar, O., et al., "Influence of verteporfin photodynamic therapy on inflammation in human choroidal neovascular membranes secondary to age-related macular degeneration," *Retina*, Vol. 27, 2007, pp. 713–723.

[90] Augustin, A. J., and Schmidt-Erfurth, U., "Verteporfin therapy combined with intravitreal triamcinolone in all types of choroidal neovascularization due to age-related macular degeneration," *Ophthalmology*, Vol. 113, 2006, pp. 14–22.

[91] Augustin, A. J., and Schmidt-Erfurth, U., "Verteporfin and intravitreal triamcinolone acetonide combination therapy for occult choroidal neovascularization in age-related macular degeneration," *Am J Ophthalmol*, Vol. 141, 2006, pp. 638–645.

[92] Lange, N., et al., "A new drug-screening procedure for photosensitizing agents used in photodynamic therapy for CNV," *Invest Ophthalmol Vis Sci*, Vol. 42, 2001, pp. 38–46.

[93] Pegaz, B., et al., "Effect of nanoparticle size on the extravasation and the photothrombic activity of meso(p-tetracarboxyphenyl)porphyrin," *J Photochem Photobiol B*, Vol. 85, 2006, pp. 216–222.

[94] Vargas, A., et al., "Improved photodynamic activity of porphyrin loaded into nanoparticles: an in vivo evaluation using chick embryos," *Int J Pharm*, Vol. 286, 2004, pp. 131–145.

[95] Bourges, J. L., et al., "Intraocular implants for extended drug delivery: therapeutic applications," *Adv Drug Deliv Rev*, Vol. 58, 2006, pp. 1182–1202.

[96] Chan, W. M. "Treatment guidelines: Asia-Pacific perspective," *7th International AMD Congress*, Marbella, Spain, October 18–20, 2007.

[97] Chan, W. M., "How to approach the management of polypoidal choroidal vasculopathy," *7th International AMD Congress*, Marbella, Spain, October 18–20, 2007.

[98] Spaide, R. F., et al., "Indocyanine green videoangiography of idiopathic polypoidal choroidal vasculopathy," *Retina*, Vol. 15, 1995, pp. 100–110.

[99] Uyama, M., et al., "Idiopathic polypoidal choroidal vasculopathy in Japanese patients," *Arch Ophthalmol*, Vol. 117, 1999, pp. 1035–1042.

[100] Yannuzzi, L. A., et al., "The expanding clinical spectrum of idiopathic polypoidal choroidal vasculopathy," *Arch Ophthalmol*, Vol. 115, 1997, pp. 478–485.

[101] Yannuzzi, L. A., et al., "Polypoidal choroidal vasculopathy and neovascularized age-related macular degeneration," *Arch Ophthalmol*, Vol. 117, 1999, pp. 1503–1510.

[102] Brown, G. C., et al., "Pharmacoeconomics and macular degeneration," *Curr Opin Ophthalmol*, Vol. 18, 2007, pp. 206–211.

[103] Brown, M. M., Brown, G. C., and Brown, H., "Value-based medicine and interventions for macular degeneration," *Curr Opin Ophthalmol*, Vol. 18, 2007, pp. 194–200.

[104] Gupta, O. P., Brown, G. C., and Brown, M. M., "Age-related macular degeneration: the costs to society and the patient," *Curr Opin Ophthalmol*, Vol. 18, 2007, pp. 201–205.

[105] Brown, G. C., et al., "The cost-utility of photodynamic therapy in eyes with neovascular macular degeneration—a value-based reappraisal with 5-year data," *Am J Ophthalmol*, Vol. 140, 2005, pp. 679–687.

CHAPTER 22

PDT in Dermatology

Amy Forman Taub

22.1 Introduction

Mainstream uses for PDT in dermatology include nonmelanoma skin cancer and its precursors, acne, photorejuvenation, and hidradenitis suppurativa. Many other dermatologic entities have been treated with PDT and published in the literature. These include psoriasis, cutaneous T-cell lymphoma, disseminated actinic porokeratosis (DSAP), localized scleroderma, vulval lichen sclerosus, bacterial infections, and verruca vulgaris. (Table 22.1).

22.2 Cutaneous Applications

The easy access of skin to light-based therapy has led dermatologists to apply PDT to cutaneous disorders [1]. A purified hematoporphyrin derivative (HPD, Photofrin) was used in combination with ultraviolet light to locate tumors, then in combination with visible light to treat tumors [2]. Although HPD has been used extensively as a photosensitizing agent, this drug accumulates in skin and clears slowly, resulting in cutaneous photosensitivity that may last several months. During this time, patients are at risk of phototoxic reactions [3].

Table 22.1 Chart of Dermatologic Conditions Treated by PDT

Nonmelanoma Skin Cancer	Inflammatory/ Immune Disorders	Infections Disorders	Miscellaneous	Other Neoplasia
Actinic keratosis	Acne	Human papillomavirus	Laser-assisted hair removal	Cutaneous T-cell lymphoma
Basal cell CA	Psoriasis	Methicillin-resistant Staph		
Bowen's disease	Lichen planus	Oral candidiasis		
Squamous cell CA	Lichen sclerosus	Molluscum contagiosum		
Actinic cheilitis	Scleroderma	Tinea rubrum		
DSAP	Alopecia areata			

22.2.1 Nonmelanoma Skin Cancer

22.2.1.1 Actinic Keratoses

Most frequently caused by long-term exposure to ultraviolet rays of the sun, AKs are probably a beginning stage of a biologic continuum leading to invasive squamous cell carcinoma (SCC) [4, 5]. The malignant potential of AKs is supported by studies showing that they have the same genetic tumor markers and mutations of tumor-suppressing p53 genes as SCCs in the dermis [6–9]. Which AKs will progress to SCC is not known, and conversion rates range from 0.1% to 20% [10–12]. One study showed that 97% of SCCs were associated with nearby AKs [13] and another showed that nearby AKs were found in 44% of cutaneous lesions that had metastasized [14]. The rate of death from nonmelanoma skin cancer is approximately one-fourth that of melanoma and 60% of these are due to metastatic SCC [15]. In 2002, 7,000 people died of melanoma in the United States [16]. One could then extrapolate that 1,050 people died from metastatic SCC. AKs should therefore be treated early to avoid malignancy and more extensive treatment [17].

22.2.1.2 Traditional AK Therapy

AKs have traditionally been treated with cryotherapy, curettage, and 5-fluorouracil (5-FU) [18, 19]. Choice of which modality depends on the number of lesions, tolerance, patient satisfaction, and compliance [19]. Standard procedures have some risk of pain, unsightliness, hypopigmentation, hyperpigmentation, and scarring [20]. With its 98% cure rate of individual lesions [21], cryosurgery is considered the standard of care for AK [18] when lesions are few in number [19]. When diffuse actinic damage and/or numerous AKs are present, therapies that address the entire affected cutaneous field have been more appropriate. Although 5-FU has been the gold standard of treatment for diffuse AKs, it is poorly tolerated by many patients due to significant crusting and discomfort that occurs over a period of weeks during and after treatment. Newer topical chemotherapeutic agents include imiquimod [22] and diclofenac [23]. Imiquimod can also cause significant crusting. Diclofenac has the advantage of being well tolerated by most patients but requires a longer therapeutic window. However, diclofenac is not as effective as 5-FU [24].

22.2.1.3 Early PDT Studies for AK

The use of PDT and its place among conventional treatments of AKs have been reviewed [12, 25]. Applying ALA to diffuse areas and capitalizing on its selective uptake by abnormally keratinized cells not only makes it more effective at treating diffuse diseases but also paves the way for PDT to be used for prevention of AKs by eradicating populations of abnormal cells before they become confluent and manifest as visible AKs. In addition, when AKs are extensive, as commonly occurs in the scalps of elderly bald men, standard treatments with topical 5-FU, cryotherapy, curettage, and cautery have limited benefit [26]. Markham et al., using broadband visible light (580–740 nm) at a low dose (20 J/cm^2) and dose rate (20 mW/cm^2), obtained complete responses (CRs) in 3 of 4 elderly men with diffuse, palpable scalp keratoses [26]. The fourth patient showed significant improvement. All patients were of skin type 1 and remission lasted 6 months. Pain during treatment, though significant, did not discourage patients from repeat treatments after 6 months.

In the early 1990s, reports appeared on the use of PDT with topically applied ALA for the treatment of both malignant and precancerous skin tumors, including AKs [3]. Kennedy et al. obtained a complete response (CR) with 9 of 10 AK lesions [3]. Wolf et al. [27], using 20% ALA, later reported a response in 9 of 9 AK lesions of three patients after PDT. Later reports [28, 29] led to a prospective clinical study to evaluate the effectiveness and tolerability of PDT in treating AKs [30].

In this clinical study, Szeimies et al. using 10% ALA, applied ALA-PDT once (under occlusion for 6 hours) to 36 AK lesions on the hands, arms, and heads of 10 patients. They irradiated the sites with red and infrared light (580–740 nm, 150 J/cm^2) and monitored the patients for 3 months. Twenty-eight days later, complete remission had occurred in 71% of the head lesions. None of the lesions on the hands and arms showed complete remission. Patients reported slight to moderate pain and itching during and after irradiation and the treated areas showed mild to moderate erythema. Cosmetic results were favorable in most cases. Subsequent studies explored different concentrations of topical ALA [31]; primary clinical response, long-term follow-up, and irradiation with different wave bands [32]; the use of laser [31] and nonlaser [33] light sources; substitution of green light for red light [34]; low doses (20 J/cm^2), and dose rates (20 mW/cm^2) of light for extensive AKs [26]; and blue light rather than red light [35] for photoactivation (Color Plate 26).

Mild stinging and burning during irradiation and localized edema and erythema were common adverse effects. Hypertrophic lesions did not respond well to treatment [31].

22.2.1.4 Topical ALA and Blue Light

In 2001, Jeffes et al. [36] reported the results of a phase II, 36-patient clinical trial of the safety and efficacy of PDT using a new topical ALA (20%, 14 to 18 hours without occlusive dressings) and blue light to treat AKs on the scalp and face. The investigators used a nonlaser source whose blue light more strongly activated PpIX than red light [36]. Although blue light penetrates less deeply into skin than red light, it has a much higher absorption peak for ALA than red light (Figure 22.1).

The treatment was effective against superficial AKs [36] with a light dose of 10 J/cm^2 and the investigators achieved complete clearance of 66% of AKs 8 weeks after a single treatment. One retreatment of 16 AK lesions at 8 weeks increased the CR rate to 85% at 16 weeks. Although patients experienced burning and stinging during treatment, these effects resolved within 1 week. Erythema appeared immediately after treatment in 96% of patients and disappeared within 4 weeks.

In phase III trials [37] of 243 patients with nonhypertrophic AKs, 83% of patients had CR after 8 weeks. Burning and stinging as well as erythema and edema occurred as in earlier studies. Cosmetic results were good to excellent in 92% of lesions. In a phase III study of 4-year efficacy and recurrence, Fowler et al. [19] reported that 69% of 32 AK lesions in four patients were still cleared, 9% were recurrent, and 22% were "uncertain." These results supported the FDA clearance of Levulan® Kerastick® and the BLU-U® Blue Light Photodynamic Therapy Illuminator (417 nm ±5 nm at 10 mW/cm^2) for the AK indication.

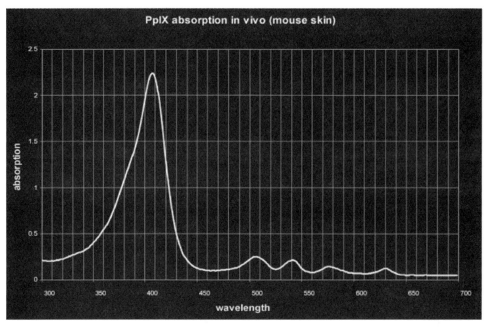

Figure 22.1   Absorption spectrum of protoporphyrin IX.

Most recently, a phase IV trial of 110 patients studied for AK treatment with 20% Levulan Kerastick revealed a clearance of 76%, with an increase to 86% with two treatments and an overall recurrence rate of 24% over a 1-year follow-up. All recurrent lesions were biopsied and 91% were confirmed as AKs, whereas 7% were SCC. One drawback of the study was that they used 14- to 17-hour incubation with ALA [38].

22.2.1.5   Methylaminolevulinate Photosensitizer and Red Light

In 2003, Freeman et al., in a prospective randomized study, compared the efficacy, safety, cosmetic outcome, and patient satisfaction of PDT using topical methylaminolevulinate (MAL, Metvix®, Photocure ASA, Norway) cream with cryotherapy in the treatment of AKs in 204 patients [39]. Response rates and cosmetic outcomes were statistically superior in the MAL-PDT group compared to cryotherapy and placebo PDT. In a smaller prospective, randomized, multicenter, placebo-controlled trial, Pariser et al. reported similar results in 80 patients with AKs [35]. MAL has an approvability letter from the FDA for the treatment of AK, but has not been marketed or released in the United States. Studies with MAL-PDT have been reviewed elsewhere (Table 22.2).

22.2.1.6   Practical Clinical Considerations for Treatment of AK with PDT

In the United States, ALA-PDT is performed with many light sources including blue, red, intense pulsed light, and pulsed dye laser for the treatment of AKs. The standard incubation time is 60 minutes based on two studies, one showing the equivalence of 14- to 3-hour incubation in terms of efficacy [40] and the other showing 1- and

Table 22.2   Summary of Reviewed Studies on Methyl Aminolaevulinate—Photodynamic Therapy (MAL-PDT) in Actinic Keratosis (AK)

Study Design	Comparator Group	Number of Patients Enrolled	Number Treated with MAL-PDT	Primary Aims	Key Results
U.S. multicenter randomized, double-blind study	Placebo	80	42	Efficacy, cosmetic outcome and patient satisfaction	High CR rate with MAL-PDT (89% vs. 38% with placebo, P < 0·001) Excellent or good cosmetic outcome in 97% (investigator assessed)/91% (patient assessed) of MAL-PDT-treated patients 73% of patients rated MAL-PDT more satisfactory than previous treatments
Open-label, prospective study. Two MAL-PDT sessions 1 week apart	Single MAL-PDT session	211	106	CR	Efficacy of MAL-PDT double application was similar to single application (89% vs. 93%, respectively) for thin lesions but less for thick lesions (84% vs. 70%)
European multicenter open, randomized study. One MAL-PDT application	Cryotherapy (double freeze-thaw)	202	102	CR, cosmetic outcome and patient satisfaction	CR for MAL-PDT was similar to cryotherapy (69% vs. 75%) following single application Superior cosmetic outcome with MAL-PDT (96% vs. 81%) Most patients preferred MAL-PDT to previous treatments
Multicenter, randomized, intraindividual (right-left) study. One MAL-PDT application	Cryotherapy (double freeze-thaw)	119	119	CR, cosmetic outcome and patient satisfaction	CR for MAL-PDT and cryotherapy was 83% and 72%, respectively at 3 months and 86% and 83%, respectively at 6 months. Percentage CR lesions at 6 months requiring retreatment at 3 months was 10% for MAL-PDT and 21% for cryotherapy Superior cosmetic outcome with MAL-PDT (77% vs. 50%)
Randomized, reference- and placebo-controlled, parallel-group multicenter study. Two MAL-PDT sessions 1 week apart	Cryotherapy (single freeze-thaw) or placebo-PDT	200	88	CR, cosmetic outcome	CR at 3 months for MAL-PDT was superior to cryotherapy or placebo-PDT (91% vs. 68% and 30%, P<0·001). Superior cosmetic outcome for MAL-PDT vs. cryotherapy (83% vs. 51%, P<0·001 investigator assessed/76% vs. 56%, P=0·013 patient assessed)

CR complete response. MAL was applied at 160 mg g1.
Source: Lehmann, P., "Methyl Aminolaevulinate–Photodynamic Therapy: A Review of Clinical Trials in the Treatment of Actinic Keratoses and Nonmelanoma Skin Cancer," British Journal of Dermatology, Vol. 156, No. 5, May 2007, pp. 793–801.

3-hour equivalence (a trial of short incubation, broad-area photodynamic therapy for facial actinic keratoses, and diffuse photodamage) [41]. It is generally recommended for optimal response to perform a microdermabrasion, acetone scrub, or other stratum corneum stripping technique prior to application of the ALA. The ALA should be incubated for 60 minutes for facial nonhyperkeratotic AKs, usually a dosage of 10 J with blue light, or with pulsed dye laser or IPL settings consistent with nonpurpuric fluences appropriate for skin type. Reexamination of lesions should be performed 1 to 3 months later for evaluation for possible retreatment and/or biopsy of any remaining lesions [42]. For more difficult to treat locations (arms, legs, chest), one may add either a topical 5-FU or a retinoid to the area for 1 to 2 weeks prior in order to increase the penetration of ALA and/or increase the time of incubation.

In Europe the standard is to undertake lesion preparation (gentle curettage of lesions) followed by incubation under occlusion of MAL for 3 hours. Light dosimetry is 37 J/cm^2 and posttreatment evaluation is 3 months [43].

While there are many options for the treatment of actinic keratoses, this author believes PDT comes the closest to being an ideal treatment, especially if cost were not a major consideration (Table 22.3) (Color Plate 27).

22.3 Basal Cell Carcinoma

Early attempts to treat BCC with PDT and non-ALA photosensitizers had limited success due to high lesion recurrence rates [44, 45].

In 1990, Kennedy et al. introduced ALA-induced PpIX PDT in the topical treatment of BCC, SCC (in situ or early invasive), AKs, and other conditions [3]. This report led to a series of studies in which (1) 20% ALA was topically applied for 3 to 8 hours to allow ALA to penetrate skin and be converted to PpIX, (2) lesions were verified by biopsy, and (3) results were evaluated after a single ALA-PDT treatment unless stated otherwise.

Investigators used ALA with nonlaser unfiltered visible light [27, 46], nonlaser filtered light [3, 27, 46–53] and lasers [28, 54–56]. Light doses ranged from 18 to 300 J/cm2 and dose rates from 15 to 250 mW/cm^2.

22.3.1 Superficial Basal Cell Carcinoma (sBCC)

In treating sBCC, reported CR rates with ALA-PDT have generally been high, ranging from 86% to 100% with follow-up times up to 45 months. Reported recurrence

Table 22.3 Comparison of Treatments for Actinic Keratoses with Multiple Variables

	5-FU	Imiquimod	Cryotherapy	Solaraze	PDT
Efficacy	+++	++	+++	+	+++
Tolerability	+	+	++	+++	+++
Cosmesis	++	++	+	+	+++
Cost	+++	++	++	++	+
Reimbursement	+	+	+++	+	++
Total	10	8	11	8	12

Source: Taub, A.F., "A Rational Approach to Contemporary AK Management," *Skin and Aging*, February 2007, pp. 39–44.
Range 1–3 with 1 being the least advantageous and 3 being the most.

rates often were higher when follow-up time was longer. In their 1990 report, Kennedy et al. reported a 90% response rate that decreased to 79% in a later report. Wolf et al. [27], after 7 months (median) had only one recurrence among 37 sBCC lesions cleared with ALA-PDT. In contrast, Cairnduff et al. [54] reported that half of 16 cleared lesions had returned within 17 months and suggested that the ALA may not have penetrated deeply enough into the tumors to prevent recurrence. Using desferrioxamine (an iron chelator) to stimulate ALA-driven photosensitization in deep regions, Fijan et al. [29] cleared 30 of 34 lesions with a single treatment and three more lesions with a second treatment. Only one lesion required surgical excision in this study. Lui et al. [48] found by histologic studies that tumor tissue persisted in 4 of 8 sites cleared of sBCC lesions 9 to 12 weeks earlier. Wennberg et al. [49] reported no recurrences of sBCC lesions among 144 that had cleared, whereas Fink-Puches et al. [46] reported a 44% recurrence rate 19 months after treatment. Soler et al. [56] used dimethylsulfoxide (DMSO) to enhance skin penetration of ALA in a study comparing CR rates with broadband light (570–740-nm continuous spectrum) and laser (630 nm). Two years after treatment, recurrence rates were 4% with laser and 5% with broadband light. Leman et al. [53] reported recurrence of 5 of 42 cleared sBCC lesions within 36 months after treatment. Morton et al. [51] reported four recurrences among 35 lesions cleared by 1 to 3 treatments and followed for 34 months. A recent international panel released guidelines for treatment of nonmelanoma skin cancers with MAL-PDT [43]. MAL-PDT was shown to be comparable to cryotherapy with respect to recurrence rates (22% for MAL-PDT vs. 19% for cryotherapy at 48 months), but with a superior cosmetic outcome in PDT. Recurrence rates are lower for lesions 1 cm or less in diameter (with a 36-month recurrence rate of only 6%) [57]. The conclusion of the international panel was that with recurrence rates comparable to alternative therapies for sBCC and the low risk of spread from these lesions, reduced cosmetic impairment is a valid reason to choose PDT over surgery.

22.3.2 Nodular Basal Cell Carcinoma (nBCC)

In numerous studies, clearance rates for nBCC were consistently lower than rates for sBCC [27–29, 49] possibly due to limited penetration of ALA [48], increasing thickness and pigmentation of lesions [28], or a combination of insufficient penetration of ALA and light [49]. Fijan et al. [29] obtained higher CR rates for nBCC when using desferrioxamine.

In September 2003, the Dermatologic and Ophthalmic Drugs Advisory Committee to the U.S. Food and Drug Administration did not recommend FDA approval of Metvix for the treatment of primary nodular BCC.

However, in the European Union, Australia, New Zealand, and Brazil, where PDT is approved for treatment of nBCC with a protocol of two treatments 1 week apart using lesion preparation, 3-hour incubation under occlusion with MAL-PDT and standard dosimetry of 37 J/cm^2 of red light, 3 months clearance rates are 91% with 5-year recurrence rate of 14% versus a 4% recurrence rate for surgery [58]. However, cosmetic outcome was superior for PDT over surgery [58]. At the present time, MAL-PDT can be recommended for the treatment of nBCC in these countries, particularly if the tumors are less than 2-mm thick [43] (Color Plate 28).

22.4   Bowen's Disease

Traditional treatments for Bowen's disease (cryotherapy, electrodessication, curettage, surgical excision, 5-FU, radiotherapy, topical chemotherapy) may be impractical when lesions are multiple, large, or located in anatomically difficult areas [59]. With cryotherapy, healing may be slow, scars may form, and nerve damage may occur [60, 61]. PDT with early photosensitizers (e.g., Photofrin) has been shown to be effective [59, 62, 63], but these agents remain in the body for up to 30 days, requiring patients to avoid sun exposure for 4 to 6 weeks [59].

ALA-PDT does not require patients to avoid sun exposure for more than 48 hours. Kennedy et al. [3], using PDT with ALA-induced PpIX, obtained CRs in six lesions with a diagnosis of either in situ SCC or early invasive SCC, although elevated lesions responded only partially. Cairnduff et al. [54] obtained a 97% CR 2 months after treatment, but three CRs were followed by relapse, reducing the single-treatment CR rate to 89% at 18 months (median). Lui et al. [48] noted three cleared lesions of in situ SCC; one was histologically positive for tumor after 12 weeks. Calzavara-Pinton et al. [28] treated nonmelanoma skin cancer lesions on alternate days until they cleared. Two treatments were typically required for clearance of six Bowen's lesions. After 29 months (median), no histologically apparent lesions had returned. Using desferrioxamine, Fijan et al. [29] obtained only a 30% CR rate after 20 months. Two lesions required retreatment at 1 and 4 months due to recurrence and five lesions failed to respond with repeated treatments.

Morton et al. [61], in a randomized trial comparing ALA-PDT with cryotherapy in the treatment of Bowen's lesions, showed that ALA-PDT with a nonlaser light source was more effective (75% CR) than cryotherapy (50% CR), than the current treatment of choice in Europe.

Ulceration, infection, and recurrent disease were reported in some lesions treated by cryotherapy, but not in ALA-PDT-treated lesions. Wennberg et al. [49], irradiating with a filtered gas discharge lamp, obtained a 78% CR 3 and 6 months after treating 18 Bowen's lesions. No recurrences occurred. Stables et al. [64], using intraepidermal injection of ALA before nonlaser irradiation, treated three very large patches of Bowen's disease with >90% CR 3 months after single treatment and 100% CR after a second treatment.

Morton et al. [50] compared the CR rates of red light (615–645 nm) and green light (525–555 nm) in the ALA-PDT treatment of Bowen's disease. Initial clearance rates were 94% for red light and 72% for green light. Recurrence rates at 12 months lowered CR rates to 88% for red light and to 48% for green light. The authors attributed the superiority of red light to its deeper penetration into tissue. Morton et al. [51] later showed high response rates for large and multiple patches of Bowen's disease after 1 to 3 treatments. Only 4 of 40 large patches and 4 of 45 (multiple) patches returned within 12 months of treatment.

Salim et al. [47] reported a 40-patient, randomized, two-center study comparing efficacy and adverse effects of ALA-PDT and topical 5-FU for the treatment of Bowen's disease. With use of a xenon lamp (615–645 nm), the CR rate for PDT was 88% initially and 82% after 12 months compared to 67% and 48%, respectively, for 5-FU. The difference in effectiveness was statistically significant. Although pain during treatment occurred with both modalities; severe eczematous reactions, ulceration, and erosions occurred only in lesions of patients treated with 5-FU. The authors concluded that ALA-PDT is superior to 5-FU in the treatment of Bowen's disease.

A reported 3% of Bowen's disease leads to invasive squamous cell carcinoma, yet this tumor often occurs on locations with poor wound healing characteristics such as the lower legs of patients with compromised vascular status [43]. For this reason, PDT, although associated with a higher recurrence rate than surgery (17% 64 months for PDT vs. 5% for surgery), is preferred by many patients due to its lack of invasiveness, preservation of tissue, and reduced need for prolonged eczematous reactions as that seen with 5-FU [65] (Color Plate 29).

22.5   Disseminated Superficial Actinic Porokeratosis (DSAP)

This condition is a clone of actinically damaged cells that have the potential to transform into squamous cell carcinoma. The general consensus anecdotally is that PDT is not effective for DSAP. However, only one paper treated three patients with topical PDT and failed to get a response [66]. The author has personally treated three patients with success for DSAP (unpublished observations). One patient is a 55-year-old woman with widespread DSAP (legs, arms, back) who had two lesions convert into histologically proven SCC. She had been treated with imiquimod and 5-flourouracil topically over many years, but developed systemic side effects from both. She responded well to multiple PDT sessions with 20% ALA solution. In the author's experience, DSAP can be treated with PDT successfully but multiple treatments are necessary at the highest light dosages.

22.6   Inflammatory/Immunologic Dermatologic Diseases

22.6.1   Acne

22.6.1.1   Red Light/Laser and ALA

In their 2000 landmark study, Hongcharu and colleagues [67] applied ALA-PDT with filtered red light (550–700-nm) to the treatment of mild to moderate acne, demonstrating that PpIX accumulates in pilosebaceous units [68,69] (Figure 22.2).

The authors reported statistically significant clearance (1) for 10 weeks after a single treatment and (2) for 20 weeks after four weekly treatments. The authors also suggested a mechanism of ALA-PDT by showing that after ALA-PDT, sebum excretion was decreased, bacterial fluorescence was decreased, and sebaceous glands were damaged (Figure 22.3).

Adverse effects included transient hyperpigmentation, superficial exfoliation, and crusting. The mechanism of ALA-PDT was further explored by Pollock and colleagues in their study of ALA-PDT with activation by laser-generated red light [70]. In their study of nine patients with mild to moderate acne, the authors found a reduction in lesion count (only at the ALA-PDT site) after the second of three weekly treatments, but no reduction in the population of skin surface P. acnes and no reduction in sebum excretion after ALA-PDT. The authors attributed the contrasting results to [67] to the difference between light sources.

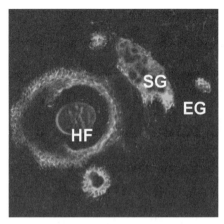

Figure 22.2 Fluorescence microscopy (Zeiss Axiophot, Carls Zeiss MicroImaging GmbH, Göttinger, Germany) of cross section of pig skin after 75 minutes of topical application of 20% ALA (water/alcohol solution), showing: hair follicle (HF), sebaceous glands (SG) and eccrine glands (EG) at 10x magnification. (Courtesy of Fernanda H. Sakamoto, MD—Wellman Center for Photomedicine, Massachusetts General Hospital, Boston, MA.)

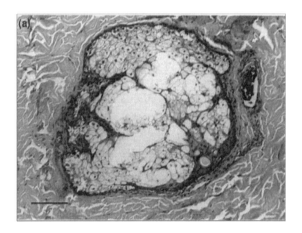
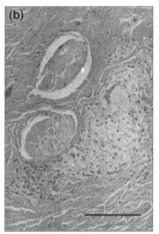

Figure 22.3 (a, b) Levulan PDT of the back—partially and completely destroyed sebaceous glands. (Photo reprinted from [67].)

22.6.1.2 Blue Light and ALA

In a controlled study, Goldman and Boyce [71] showed that ALA-PDT with blue light was more effective against acne than blue light alone and showed that short-contact ALA (<1 hour) provided efficacy and minimal adverse effects.

22.6.1.3 Long-Pulsed PDL

Alexiades-Armenakas showed that ALA-PDT with long-pulsed, pulsed dye laser activation was effective against a variety of acne lesion types with minimal adverse effects [72]. In an early study of ALA-PDT, Itoh and colleagues [73] used ALA-PDT to treat a single facial lesion of a patient with intractable acne. They allowed ALA to remain in contact with the lesion for 4 hours before irradiation with a 630-nm PDL.

The treated lesion was resolved with a single treatment and did not recur for at least 8 months. This study showed that a single treatment with polychromatic visible light activation was effective against intractable facial acne.

22.6.1.4   Intense Pulsed Light (IPL)

In a 15-patient study, Santos [74] showed that the formation of new acne lesions could be reduced by ALA-PDT with activation by IPL. Gold and colleagues [75] were the first to use IPL for ALA-PDT for acne and demonstrated its effectiveness (Color Plate 30).

In a subsequent randomized study of patients with moderate to severe acne, Taub compared IPL, blue light, and electrical optical synergy (elôs) devices as activators in ALA-PDT [76]. Acne grade and lesion count data showed approximately 70%, 50%, and 30% improvement associated with activation by IPL, elôs, and blue light, respectively, after three treatments and 3 months of follow-up (Color Plate 31).

22.6.1.5   Electrical Optical Synergy (elôs)

Taub [77] confirmed the efficacy of short-contact ALA for patients with moderate to severe refractory acne and showed that (elôs) technology was effective.

The results of these studies culminated in a consensus recommendation for the treatment of acne [85]. Consensus panel members agreed that ALA-PDT provides (1) the best results when used to treat inflammatory and cystic acne, and (2) modest clearance when used to treat comedonal acne (although recent data shows that ALA-PDT was effective against comedonal acne when the long-pulsed pulsed dye laser is used [72]). They also agreed that (1) acneiform flares may occur after any treatment, including ALA-PDT, and (2) although not supported by extensive documentation, PDL activation provides the best results in ALA-PDT for acne. One member (Dr. Nestor) stated that only PDL with ALA-PDT has maintained clearance of acne lesions for up to 2 years, even in patients resistant to other treatments. (To the author's knowledge, Dr. Nestor's data has not been published.) These comments came before Taub's study showing IPL as superior to blue, although PDL was not included in this study.

22.6.1.6   Red Light and MAL

Wiegell and Wulf reported MAL-PDT gave significant reductions in sebum excretion and bacterial indicators but no clinical efficacy [78].

22.6.1.7   Indocyanine Green and Diode Laser

The use of indocyanine green (ICG) in combination with an 803- to 810-nm diode laser has been reported by three groups [79, 80, 81]. ICG is a fluorescent dye used to evaluate hepatic function, blood volume, and cardiac output [80, 82]. In a complex, multifaceted study, Tuchin and colleagues reported that multiple treatments yielded more favorable results than a single treatment and attributed the efficacy to bacterial suppression [81, 82]. Lloyd and Mirkov [79] evaluated the effect of long pulse, 810-nm diode laser (Cynosure, Inc.) energy on enlarged sebaceous glands preloaded of a single patient with ICG. After confirming penetration of ICG into the enlarged gland, the authors performed a laser-tissue interaction analysis to determine the appropriate treatment parameters to selectively damage the enlarged ICG-loaded glands. After finding that laser energy of 810-nm, 50-ms pulse duration, 40-J/cm^2, and 4-mm spot size was required, they applied an ICG microemulsion to 10 sites on the backs of patients with active acne, covered the areas with occlusive dressing for 24 hours, cleansed the areas, and treated them with the laser. Fluorescence microscopy and histologic studies of the treated areas revealed selective necrosis of the targeted glands whereas clinical observations and serial photographs showed an improvement in acne at the treated area at 3, 6, and 10 months after the treatment. The authors concluded that the diode laser had selectively and safely damaged enlarged sebaceous glands.

In a similar study, Genina and colleagues [80] reported that the ICG-diode laser protocol provided the best results in patients with moderate to severe acne.

The consistent results of these studies support the conclusion that the ICG-diode laser is a valid option for the treatment of mild to severe acne.

22.6.1.8   Clinical Implications

Activating ALA for treatment of acne has a completely different set of priorities than that for AK. In treating AK, the main barrier is penetration of the ALA through the stratum corneum, requiring relatively long incubation times, occlusion, pretreatment with stratum corneum stripping techniques to increase penetration, and using a highly absorbed wavelength to increase yield of abnormal cells that contain high levels of PpIX. However, numerous papers have shown that extremely short incubation times (15–30 minutes) can be effective for acne. The author's hypothesis is that the follicle/sebaceous gland orifice represents a separate channel of absorption bypassing the stratum corneum and giving early absorption of ALA into glands followed over time by higher absorption into epidermis and therefore higher selectivity at shorter incubation times. One potential explanation of the seemingly superior efficacy of IPL over blue light for PDT for acne could be due to the pulsing as opposed to the continuous wave characteristics of the light. Red light would be thought to be a highly effective activator of ALA for acne, due to its deeper penetration. Yet almost all the studies with PDT utilizing red light in acne have had an unacceptably high rate of exfoliation, pain, and postinflammatory changes [78].

Is this due to too potent an activation that ruptures the gland, resulting in more inflammation? Or is it because there is so much epidermal absorption due to the cream form that then reacts with the light as well? Perhaps the pulsed light does modulate the response in ways we don't understand, given the success of both IPL and pulsed dye lasers for the treatment of acne.

A recent publication refutes the widely held concept that PDT for acne is effective due to destruction of oil glands and bacterial killing, by showing that despite clinical improvements in acne, no measurement of decreased sebum or reduced bacterial concentration have occurred [83].

The versatility of PDT and the emergence of short-acting photosensitizing agents that can be applied to skin before activation by light or laser devices has been one of the few truly new modalities for the treatment of acne vulgaris in the past 20 years [84].

The use of short (30–60-minute) incubation times and multiple treatment sessions provides optimal clinical efficacy and patient compliance, even in cases of recalcitrant acne and as an alternative to isotretinoin.

22.6.2 Hidradenitis Suppurativa (HS)

Hidradenitis suppurativa (HS) is a chronic, inflammatory disease of the apocrine gland-bearing skin, particularly the axilla, anogenital region, and breasts. It is thought that follicular occlusion is the inciting event followed by rupture of the follicle and an inflammatory reaction. The condition results in painful abscesses and sinus tract formation. HS can be progressive with marked morbidity related to chronic pain, draining sinuses, and scarring with restricted mobility. Complications of HS can lead to fistulas to the urethra, bladder, and rectum when the anogenital region is affected and limited mobility and lymph edema when the axilla are affected. Previous treatment options have included oral and topical antibiotics, antiandrogens, oral retinoids, immunosuppressive therapy, biologics, and surgery.

Despite the large amount of drainage, over 50% of HS lesions do not culture bacteria. The bacterial presence is variable in species and numbers and may change unpredictably. Therefore, approximately only 10% of HS patients have some benefit from oral and topical antibiotics [86], and a few cases have shown improvement with antiandrogens, probably due to the fact that apocrine glands are not androgen-sensitive. A few case studies have shown improvement in HS for patients on oral isotretinoin but tended to be patients who suffered from a combination of acne and HS [87]. Most patients who suffer from HS alone do not benefit from oral isotretinoin [89]. Cases have been shown that immunosuppressive therapy in the absence of bacteria can provide results for some HS patients [79]. Recent studies show improvement in HS with biologic therapy suggesting TNF in the pathogenesis of HS but is only little understood and needs to be studied further [90, 91]. One study suggests that even in mild HS, aggressive treatment by radical excision of all hair bearing areas and reconstruction with grafts or flaps is necessary for long-term improvement [92].

Because of the limitations of the aforementioned therapies, PDT has been studied as a treatment option for HS. Gold et al. studied four subjects with chronic HS unresponsive to previous therapies. They received three to four treatments at 1- to 2-week intervals consisting of 15 to 30 minutes of incubation of Levulan followed by blue light exposure. Three months after the final treatment, all subjects showed 75% to 100% clearance of their HS. The treatments were painless and no adverse events were reported [93]. This finding was supported by case studies of four subjects presented by DeVita and Taub [94]. All four subjects had moderate to severe HS and were unresponsive to previous therapies. Treatments were performed with either blue light or IPL after 30 to 60 minutes of incubation of Levulan. Treatments were performed at 2- to 4-week intervals and then followed with maintenance treatments every 1 to 2 months. Subjects achieved 50% to 75% clearance with the initial treatment series and were maintained or improved with further treatments during the maintenance phase. Subjects reported mild to no discomfort during treatments and no adverse events were reported. One study by Strauss et al., reported four subjects that received a maximum of three treatments at weekly intervals after 4-hour incubation with 20% ALA in unguentum and occlusion [95]. Three subjects received treatment with diode laser (633 nm) and one with red light. Two of the four subjects had significant improvement, one discontinued after the first treatment due to pain and one discontinued after two treatments due to worsening of HS. All subjects reported burning and stinging for several days posttreatment. Strauss concluded that PDT was not an effective treatment option for HS. It is possible that using ALA in unguentum vehicle under occlusion for 4 hours may have contributed to the poor results. Short contact incubation (30–60 minutes) may have yielded better results.

22.7 Photodynamic Photorejuvenation

PDT is associated with good cosmetic outcomes, and it was observed that not only did PDT eradicate precancerous and cancerous lesions, it also reduced mottled hyperpigmentation, mild rhytides, pore size, and overall texture and tone of photodamaged skin. Ruiz-Rodriquez coined the term "photodynamic photorejuvenation" to denote a cosmetic-based intent with treatment utilizing PDT [96]. He studied 17 patients with 38 AKs and diffuse photodamage by performing photodynamic treatment twice with 20% 5-ALA (4 hours occluded) and intense pulsed light. His results showed an 87% response with improvement in wrinkling, skin texture, pigmentation changes, telangiectasias, and AK.

This was followed by a 10-patient study by Gold [97] with full face application of 20% ALA for 15 to 30 minutes and the following parameters with IPL treatments: 550 to 570 nm, double pulsing, 3.5-msec pulse durations, and fluences of 20 to 34 J/cm^2. Three treatments were performed at 1-month intervals and follow-up was 1 month and 3 months posttreatment. The results showed that 90% had greater than 75% improvement compared to baseline (Color Plate 32).

There were no adverse serious events or downtime from daily activities, with 30% experiencing posttreatment erythema/edema for 24 to 48 hours. In 2004, Gold et al. [98] undertook a split-face study to try to determine if ALA gave additional benefit over IPL treatment itself. In this study, 13 patients had three treatments 4 weeks apart where half the face was treated with IPL alone and half with IPL plus ALA. The results were: (IPL with ALA vs. IPL alone) resolution of AK, 78% vs. 53.6%; crows feet, 55% vs. 28.5%; tactile roughness, 55% vs. 29.5%; hyperpigmentation, 60.3% vs. 37.2%; and erythema, 84.6% vs. 53.8%. A confirmation of these findings was found in the Dover et al. [99] study of 20 subjects split-face ALA-PDT IPL on one side and IPL alone on the other. They found a statistically significant difference in global photoaging, mottled hyperpigmentation, and fine lines on the PDT side, yet no difference in adverse events. Photodynamic photorejuvenation is useful for patients who have AKs or severe damage and are interested in cosmetic as well as medical improvement, who want fewer treatments, better and faster results than traditional photorejuvenation, and who are willing to stay indoors for 48 hours and have potential for downtime. In addition, it can be indicated for patients who have enlarged pores and/or desire skin cancer prevention.

22.8   Other Disorders

22.8.1   Psoriasis

There is a fair amount of literature devoted to the treatment of psoriasis with PDT decidedly mixed in its outlook or whether PDT is a practical or useful alternative for treatment.

The first hurdle was to demonstrate the mechanism of action of PDT or preferential uptake of a photosensitizer by psoriatic plaques. Bisonette et al. looked at the potential for specificity of oral ALA in dosages of 10, 20, and 30 mg as they thought using topical PDT would be too limiting [100]. They measured 12 patients with plaque psoriasis protoporphyrin IX (PpIX) fluorescence in the lesional and normal skin as well as in inflammatory cells. They found that there was a tenfold increase in fluorescence at 3 to 5 hours after administration of a single oral dose in the psoriasis over the normal skin, although they did note some fluorescence of noninvolved facial skin. They concluded that this was a modality that warranted potential study for clinical usage An earlier study [101] had established that PDT with red light caused a similar, although less potent, decrease in cytokine secretions (IL6, TNF alpha and IL-1beta) as PUVA therapy in mononuclear cells freshly isolated after irradiation with either modality. They also demonstrated progressive photobleaching corresponding to higher energy irradiations, establishing the specificity and dose dependency for PDT for psoriasis. A recent study showed that systemic PDT induces apoptosis in lesional T lymphocytes in psoriatic plaques, a feature that is supposed to predict a longer lasting therapeutic effect [102].

With some evidence of a mechanistic reason and proof of some specificity for psoriasis, small clinical trials were instituted to test the hypothesis of whether this was borne out in a clinical setting. Ten patients with plaque psoriasis [103] were treated multiple times at three times a week dosing with topical application of 5-aminolevulinic acid and broadband visible radiation at a dose of 8 J/cm². Eight out of 10 patients showed a clinical response, but only 1 of 45 sites cleared fully and five showed no improvement. More concerning was that fluorescence which was demonstrated by biopsy to remain in the epidermis, showed little consistency of uptake, even within the same plaque. Finally, there was so much discomfort with the treatments that the authors concluded this was not a practical therapy.

Three studies in 2005 shed new light on the clinical evaluation of PDT for psoriasis. Twelve patients (8 valuable) were studied for their response to topical 5-ALA 20% solution irradiated with red light weekly at 10 to 30 J/cm² [104]. There was a statistically significant improvement in the clinical presentation of the plaques but there was an average pain score of 7 out of 10, and 4 of 12 patients dropped out of the study due to pain during the treatments. A larger study was performed by the Regensberg, Germany, group composed of 29 psoriatics with chronic stable disease receiving 1% ALA after keratolytic treatment (10% salicylic acid in petrolatum for 2 weeks) in 3 plaques and either 5, 10, or 20 J/cm² light of a filtered metal halide light (Waldmann 1200 PDT, 600–740 nm) [105]. Although they demonstrated a clear decrease in the PSI in >95% of patients, the slow pace, pain during therapy and partial results were cited by the authors are reasons for the inadequacy of this form of PDT for psoriasis. They conclude that a more practical method might be oral ALA and blue light or verteporfin and red light. Finally, in a very recent study, eight patients with symmetric plaques were studied for clinical response and immunohistochemical markers in a randomized placebo controlled study where the patients' contralateral plaque served as control [106]. A 10% ALA ointment under occlusion was used on one plaque whereas the vehicle alone was used on the contralateral plaque; both were occluded for 4 hours and exposed to fractionated broadband light (Waldmann PDT 1200 L, 650–700 nm) at 2 J/cm² then 2 dark hours followed by 8 J/cm². The PDT-treated side exhibited a clinical improvement as well as a decrease in CD4+,CD8+, and CD45+RO cells as well as Ki67+ nuclei, with an increase in epidermal K10 expression These biologic changes were absent in the placebo-treated sides. Heterogeneity of plaques in fluorescent staining was still seen as an obstacle to practical therapy, and this despite use of a pretreatment with a salicylic acid-based cream to induce keratolysis.

Psoriasis treatment for PDT seems to be limited by pain, inconvenience, and mediocre results. Clearly it is not a first line therapy. However, there is good evidence that there is preferential uptake of photosensitizers in psoriatic plaques and confirmation by biological markers that specific antipsoriatic changes take place during PDT.

22.8.2 Lichen Planus

There is only one reference, a recent study in the use of PDT for the treatment of oral lichen planus (OLP). Twenty-six lesions of OLP were treated with gargling 5% methylene blue and subsequent irradiation with 632 nm at 120 J/cm². Significant symptoms and signs were decreased at both 1 and 12 weeks in 16 lesions and the author concluded that this was a promising treatment for control of OLP [107].

22.8.3 Lichen Sclerosus (LS)

This entity is mentioned twice in overviews of PDT and once by Polish authors who state they use it for both diagnosis and treatment of LS. However, the full text could not be obtained and there were no details in the abstract [108].

22.8.4 Scleroderma

Patients with localized scleroderma resistant to PUVA did respond well to PDT (109).

Cultured keratinocytes subjected to PDT produced increased IL-1, TNF, and MMP 1 and 3, postulated by the authors to be the mechanism responsible for the observed antisclerotic effect of PDT [110]. This observation would need to be repeated and is contrary to what is found clinically with photodynamic photorejuvenation in that fine wrinkles tend to get better and there has been no evidence of collagen breakdown. However, another study found a dosimetry range to reduce tissue contraction and reduce collagen density without damage to keratinocytes, which may prove helpful as an adjuvant treatment for keloids [111].

22.8.5   Alopecia Areata

Six patients with severe alopecia areata were treated with 5-ALA 15% solution twice weekly for 20 treatments with red light. Fluorescence microscopy revealed diffuse uptake in the epidermis and sebaceous glands, but not in hair follicles or the inflammatory infiltrate surrounding the epidermis. Also, a significant degree of erythema was noted in all ALA-treated sites but not in the control site, indicating that there was a clinical response to ALA. The authors conclude that PDT is not a successful therapy for alopecia areata [112].

22.8.6   Darier's Disease

A small pilot study of six patients who were also on systemic retinoids were treated with 5-ALA. One patient could not tolerate treatment. Of the other five, 4 out of 5 got an inflammatory response that lasted for 2 weeks but then was followed by improvement that lasted from 6 to 36 months. There was recurrence in one patient but in those who were clear, biopsy was negative after treatment [113].

22.8.7   Cutaneous T-Cell Lymphoma

Treatment of early cutaneous T-cell lymphoma has traditionally been accomplished with PUVA, electron beam radiation, nitrogen mustard, and even topical steroids. It seems a logical consequence that PDT might be effective for CTCL since it is effective in other neoplasias of skin. Many pilot studies and cases report positive findings although no large-scale studies have been reported. The first reported treatment of CTCL was in 1994 [114] when two plaque lesions were treated with 20% ALA in water-in-oil based cream, with incubation for 4 to 6 hours followed by laser irradiation. PpIX production was demonstrated by real-time laser-induced fluorescence to have a fivefold increase in lymphoma cells over normal cells. In 1995, Oseroff's group [115] hypothesized that activated lymphocytes (CD71+) would preferentially accumulate PpIX because of their lower intracellular iron levels and because of competition for iron between ALA-induced heme production and cellular growth processes. They demonstrated that application of ALA in patient with a Sezary syndrome's preferentially killed CD71+ lymphocytes over normal, unstimulated lymphocytes, indicating a possible mechanism for PDT as well as specificity for CTCL and potential for good clinical outcomes.

   In 1999, Eich et al. reported two cases, one of an uncommon type and location of CTCL (medium-large size pleiomorphic cells, CD8+, CD30-, ear) which had not responded to PUVA, interferon alpha, or retinoid therapy but achieved a histologically confirmed partial remission with PDT and subsequent complete remission (CR) with radiotherapy [116]. A second case had PDT to eyebrow and foot in combination with other modalities lead to CR. In 2000, Orenstein et al. presented two patients with stage I and III CTCL [117]. In stage I CTCL, lesions exhausted fluorescence 1 hour after irradiation and showed a good response with 170 J/cm^2. With the stage III lesion, fractionated dosages were necessary with a total dose required of 380 J/cm^2. All six lesions responded well. Other case reports include successful treatment of a patient with two isolated plaques [118] and of an

HIV-induced and infected CTCL patient with complete remission after two PDT treatment cycles [119].

In the largest study to date, Ros' group in Sweden examined 10 patients with 10 plaque and 2 tumor stage lesions [120]. They also looked at histological and immunohistochemical markers of the lesions The protocol was 20% ALA incubating for 6 hours followed with red light. Complete clinical remission was noted in 7 out of 10 plaques after a single treatment, with corresponding regression of infiltrate with markedly fewer proliferating cells and a decrease in Ki-67 and CD71. The tumor lesions did not respond. They concluded that there was good clinical and histological effect of PDT on local plaque CTCL.

In summary, the literature demonstrates a good response to PDT for localized plaque CTCL, stage I in case reports, and limited pilot studies, which were confirmed clinically, histologically, and via immunohistochemistry. A plausible mechanism for action and specificity has been postulated and partially demonstrated. Further large-scale studies are necessary to evaluated whether PDT will be useful in treating early CTCL, but would certainly be warranted if other modalities had failed or if other circumstances preclude patients from receiving other, more established, modalities.

22.9   Miscellaneous

22.9.1   Hair Removal

PDT was performed with ALA after cold wax epilation and a continuous-wave red laser. Hair removal was consistent with the amount of anagen hair present [121]. Alopecia presented as a side effect of ALA PDT in a case report of treatment of Bowen's disease with 5-ALA and red laser light on an upper posterior arm. The tumor was eradicated after a 2-year followup but complete alopecia of the treatment area also remained [122]. There is very little data to support the use of PDT as an adjunct to laser hair removal and there have been few reports of alopecia as a side effect of treatments. As noted previously [112], there has been no demonstration of specific uptake by hair follicle cells. This author has not found it useful anecdotally as an adjuvant for laser assisted hair removal.

22.10   Conclusions

PDT has found to be useful in nonmelanoma skin cancers, immunologic and inflammatory disorders, and neoplasias other than skin cancer and infections. The ability of this treatment to hone in on dysplastic epithelial and endothelial cells while retaining viability of surrounding tissue is its key feature, as this leads to specific tumor destruction with cosmesis and function of the target organ intact. The ability PDT to alter the course of immunologic and inflammatory diseases is still in an exploratory stage, but one which is exciting to behold and certainly well established for diseases of sebaceous glands and possibly apocrine glands. Finally, the demonstration that PDT is capable of killing various pathogens without induction of resistance could make PDT an important treatment for infections.

References

[1] Kalka, K., et al., "Photodynamic therapy in dermatology," *J Am Acad Dermatol*, 2000; 42:389–413.

[2] Mukhtar, H, et al., "Photodynamic therapy of murine skin tumors using Photofrin-II," *Photodermatol Photoimmunol Photomed 1991*, Aug; 8(4):169–75.

[3] Kennedy, J.C., et al., "Photodynamic therapy with endogenous protoporphyrin IX: basic principles and present clinical experience," *J Photochem Photobiol B 1990*; 6:143–148.

[4] Schwartz, R.A., "The actinic keratosis. A perspective and update," *Dermatol Surg*, 1997; 23:1009–1019.

[5] Salasche, S.J., "Epidemiology of actinic keratoses and squamous cell carcinoma," *J Am Acad Dermatol*, 2000; 42 (1 Pt 2):S4–S7.

[6] Ziegler, A., et al., "Sunburn and p53 in the onset of skin cancer," *Nature*, 1994; 372(6508):773–776.

[7] Leffell, D.J., "The scientific basis of skin cancer," *J Am Acad Dermatol*, 2000; 42 (1 Pt 2):18–22.

[8] Cockerell, C.J., "Histopathology of incipient intraepidermal squamous cell carcinoma ('actinic keratosis')," *J Am Acad Dermatol*, 2000; 42(1 Pt 2):11–17.

[9] Ortonne, J.P., "From actinic keratosis to squamous cell carcinoma," *Br J Dermatol*, 2002; 146 Suppl 61:20–23.

[10] Marks, R., et al., "Spontaneous remission of solar keratoses: the case for conservative management," *Br J Dermatol*, 1986; 115:649–655.

[11] Marks, R., et al., "Malignant transformation of solar keratoses to squamous cell carcinoma," *Lancet*, 1988; 1 (8589):795–797.

[12] Chamberlain, A.J., Kurwa, H.A., "Photodynamic therapy: is it a valuable treatment option for actinic keratoses?" *Am J Clin Dermatol*, 2003; 4:149–155.

[13] Hurwitz, R.M., Monger, L.E., "Solar keratosis: an evolving squamous cell carcinoma. Benign or malignant?" *Dermatol Surg*, 1995; 21:184.

[14] Dinehart, S.M., et al., "Metastatic cutaneous squamous cell carcinoma derived from actinic keratosis," *Cancer*, 1997; 79:920–923.

[15] Weinstock, M.A., et al., "Nonmelanoma skin cancer mortality. A population-based study," *Arch Dermatol*, 1991; 127:1194–1197.

[16] Geller, A.C., Annas, G.D., "Epidemiology of melanoma and nonmelanoma skin cancer," *Semin Oncol Nurs*, 2003; 19:2–11.

[17] Callen, J.P., "Statement on actinic keratoses," *J Am Acad Dermatol*, 2000; 42 (1 Pt 2):S1.

[18] Dinehart, S.M., "The treatment of actinic keratoses," *J Am Acad Dermatol*, 2000; 42 (1 Pt 2):S25–S28.

[19] Fowler, J.F., Jr., Zax, R.H., "Aminolevulinic acid hydrochloride with photodynamic therapy: efficacy outcomes and recurrence 4 years after treatment," *Cutis*, 2002; 69 (6 Suppl):2–7.

[20] Marcus, S.L., McIntire, W.R., "Photodynamic therapy systems and applications," *Expert Opin Emerging Drugs*, 2002; 7:319–331.

[21] Graham, G.F., "Advances in cryosurgery during the past decade," *Cutis*, 1993; 52:365–372.

[22] Salasche, S.J., et al.. "Cycle therapy of actinic keratoses of the face and scalp with 5% topical imiquimod cream: An open-label trial," *J Am Acad Dermatol*, 2002; 47:571–577.

[23] Wolf, J.E., Jr., et al., "Topical 3.0% diclofenac in 2.5% hyaluronan gel in the treatment of actinic keratoses," *Int J Dermatol*, 2001; 40:709-713.

[24] Fariba, I., et al., "Efficacy of 3% diclofenac gel for the treatment of actinic keratoses: a randomized, double-blind, placebo controlled study," *Indian J Dermatol Venereol Leprol*, 2006 Sep–Oct;72(5):346–349.

[25] Marcus, L., "Photodynamic therapy for actinic keratosis followed by 5-fluorouracil reaction," *Dermatol Surg*, 2003; 29:1061–4.

[26] Markham, T., Collins, P., "Topical 5-aminolaevulinic acid photodynamic therapy for extensive scalp actinic keratoses," *Br J Dermatol*, 2001; 145:502–504.

[27] Wolf, P., et al., "Topical photodynamic therapy with endogenous porphyrins after application of 5-aminolevulinic acid. An alternative treatment modality for solar keratoses, superficial squamous cell carcinomas, and basal cell carcinomas?" *J Am Acad Dermatol*, 1993; 28:17-21. Erratum in: *J Am Acad Dermatol* 1993; 29:41.

[28] Calzavara-Pinton, P.G., "Repetitive photodynamic therapy with topical delta-aminolaevulinic acid as an appropriate approach to the routine treatment of superficial non-melanoma skin tumours," *J Photochem Photobiol B*, 1995; 29:53–57.

[29] Fijan, S., et al., "Photodynamic therapy of epithelial skin tumours using delta-aminolaevulinic acid and desferrioxamine," *Br J Dermatol*, 1995; 133:282–288.

[30] Szeimies, R.M., et al., "Photodynamic therapy with topical application of 5-aminolevulinic acid in the treatment of actinic keratoses: an initial clinical study," *Dermatology*, 1996; 192:246–251.

[31] Jeffes, E.W., et al., "Photodynamic therapy of actinic keratosis with topical 5-aminolevulinic acid. A pilot dose-ranging study," *Arch Dermatol*, 1997; 133:727–732.

[32] Fink-Puches, R., et al., "Primary clinical response and long-term follow-up of solar keratoses treated with topically applied 5-aminolevulinic acid and irradiation by different wave bands of light," *J Photochem Photobiol B*, 1997; 41:145–151.

[33] Kurwa, H.A., et al., "A randomized paired comparison of photodynamic therapy and topical 5-fluorouracil in the treatment of actinic keratoses.," *J Am Acad Dermatol*, 1999; 41 (3 Pt 1):414–418.

[34] Fritsch, C., et al., "Green light is effective and less painful than red light in photodynamic therapy of facial solar keratoses" *Photodermatol Photoimmunol Photomed*, 1997; 13:181–185.

[35] Pariser, D.M., et al., "Photodynamic therapy with topical methyl aminolevulinate for actinic keratosis: results of a prospective randomized multicenter trial," *J Am Acad Dermatol*, 2003; 48:227–232.

[36] Jeffes, E.W., "Levulan: the first approved topical photosensitizer for the treatment of actinic keratosis," *J Dermatolog Treat*, 2002; 13 Suppl 1:S19–S23.

[37] Piacquadio, D.G., et al., "Photodynamic therapy with aminolevulinic acid topical solution and visible blue light in the treatment of multiple actinic keratoses of the face and scalp: investigator-blinded, phase 3, multicenter trials," *Arch Dermatol.*, 2004 Jan;140 (1):41–6.

[38] Tschen, E.H., et al., "Phase IV ALA-PDT Actinic Keratosis Study Group. Photodynamic therapy using aminolaevulinic acid for patients with nonhyperkeratotic actinic keratoses of the face and scalp: phase IV multicenter clinical trial with 12-month follow up," *Br J Dermatol*, 2006 Dec:155(6):1262–1269.

[39] Freeman, M., et al., "A comparison of photodynamic therapy using topical methyl aminolevulinate (Metvix) with single cycle cryotherapy in patients with actinic keratosis: a prospective, randomized study," *J Dermatolog Treat*, 2003; 14:99–106.

[40] Alexiades-Armenakas, M.R., Geronemus, R.G., "Laser-mediated photodynamic therapy of actinic keratoses," *Arch Dermatol*, 2003 Oct:139 (10):1313–20.

[41] Touma, D., et al., "A trial of short incubation, broad-area photodynamic therapy for facial actinic keratoses and diffuse photodamage," *Arch Dermatol*, 2004 Jan:140 (1):33–40.

[42] Nestor, M.S., et al., "The use of photodynamic therapy in dermatology: results of a consensus conference," *J Drugs Dermatol*, 2006 Feb: 5(2):140–154.

[43] Braathen, L.R., et al., "Guidelines on the use of photodynamic therapy for nonmelanoma skin cancer: an international consensus. International Society for Photodynamic Therapy in Dermatology, 2005," *J Am Acad Dermatol*, 2007 Jan; 56(1):125–43.

[44] Pennington, D.G., et al., "Photodynamic therapy for multiple skin cancers," *Plast Reconstr Surg*, 1988; 82:1067–1071.

[45] McCaughan, J.S., Jr., et al., "Photodynamic therapy for cutaneous and subcutaneous malignant neoplasms," *Arch Surg*, 1989; 124:211–216.

[46] Fink-Puches, R., et al., "Long-term follow-up and histological changes of superficial nonmelanoma skin cancers treated with topical delta-aminolevulinic acid photodynamic therapy," *Arch Dermatol*, 1998; 134:821–826.

[47] Salim, A., et al., "Randomized comparison of photodynamic therapy with topical 5-fluorouracil in Bowen's disease," *Br J Dermatol*, 2003; 148:539–543.

[48] Lui, H., et al., "Photodynamic therapy of nonmelanoma skin cancer with topical aminolevulinic acid: a clinical and histologic study," *Arch Dermatol*, 1995; 131:737–738.

[49] Wennberg, A.M., et al., "Treatment of superficial basal cell carcinomas using topically applied delta-aminolaevulinic acid and a filtered xenon lamp," *Arch Dermatol Res*, 1996; 288:561–564.

[50] Morton, C.A., et al., "Comparison of red and green light in the treatment of Bowen's disease by photodynamic therapy," *Br J Dermatol*, 2000; 143:767–772.

[51] Morton, C.A., et al., "Photodynamic therapy for large or multiple patches of Bowen disease and basal cell carcinoma," *Arch Dermatol*, 2001; 137:319–324.

[52] Soler, A.M., et al., "A follow-up study of recurrence and cosmesis in completely responding superficial and nodular basal cell carcinomas treated with methyl 5-aminolaevulinate-based photodynamic therapy alone and with prior curettage," *Br J Dermatol*, 2001; 145:467–471.

[53] Leman, J.A., et al., "Treatment of superficial basal cell carcinomaas with topical photodynamic therapy: recurrence rates and outcome," *Br J. Dermatol*, 2001; 145 (Suppl 59):17.

[54] Cairnduff, F., et al., "Superficial photodynamic therapy with topical 5-aminolaevulinic acid for superficial primary and secondary skin cancer," *Br J Cancer*, 1994; 69:605–608.

[55] Svanberg, K., et al., "Photodynamic therapy of non-melanoma malignant tumours of the skin using topical delta-amino levulinic acid sensitization and laser irradiation," *Br J Dermatol*, 1994; 130:743–751.

[56] Soler, A.M., et al., "Photodynamic therapy of superficial basal cell carcinoma with 5-aminolevulinic acid with dimethylsulfoxide and ethylendiaminetetraacetic acid: a comparison of two light sources," *Photochem Photobiol*, 2000; 71:724–729.

[57] Basset-Seguin, N., et al., "MAL-PDT versus cryotherapy in primary sBCC: results of 36 months follow-up," *J Eur Acad Dermatol Venereol*, 18 (2004) (Suppl 2), p. 412.

[58] Rhodes, L.E., et al., "Photodynamic therapy using topical methyl aminolevulinate vs surgery for nodular basal cell carcinoma: results of a multicenter randomized prospective trial," *Arch Dermatol 140*, 2004:17–23.

[59] Jones, C.M., et al., "Photodynamic therapy in the treatment of Bowen's disease," *J Am Acad Dermatol*, 1992; 27(6 Pt 1):979–982.

[60] Holt, P.J., "Cryotherapy for skin cancer: results over a 5-year period using liquid nitrogen spray cryosurgery," *Br J Dermatol*, 1988; 119:231–240.

[61] Morton, C.A., et al., "Comparison of photodynamic therapy with cryotherapy in the treatment of Bowen's disease," *Br J Dermatol*, 1996; 135:766–771.

[62] Waldow, S.M., et al., "Photodynamic therapy for treatment of malignant cutaneous lesions," *Lasers Surg Med*, 1987; 7:451–456.

[63] Robinson, P.J., et al., "Photodynamic therapy: a better treatment for widespread Bowen's disease," *Br J Dermatol*, 1988; 119:59–61.

[64] Morton, C.A., et al., "Development of an alternative light source to lasers for photodynamic therapy. 1. Clinical evaluation in the treatment of pre-malignant non-melanoma skin cancer," *Lasers Med Sci*, 1995; 10:165–171.

[65] Leman, J.A., Mackie, R.M., Morton, C.A., "Recurrence rates following aminolaevulinic acid-photodynamic therapy for intra-epidermal squamous cell carcinoma compare favour-

ably with outcome following conventional modalities," *Br J Dermatol 147*, 2002 (Suppl 62), p. 35.

[66] Nayeamuddin, F. A., et al., "Topical photodynamic therapy in disseminated superficial actinic porokeratosis," *Clin Exp Dermatol*, 2002 Nov; 27(8):703–706.

[67] Hongcharu, W., et al., "Topical ALA-photodynamic therapy for the treatment of acne vulgaris," *J Invest Dermatol*, 2000; 115:183–92.

[68] Kennedy, J., Pottier, R., "Endogenous protoporphyrin IX, a clinically useful photosensitizer for photodynamic therapy," *J Photochem Photobiol B: Biol*, 1992;14:275–292.

[69] Divaris, D., Kennedy, J., Pottier, R., "Phototoxic damage to sebaceous glands and hair follicles of mice after systemic administration of 5-aminolevulinic acid correlates with localized protoporphyrin IX fluorescence," *Am J Pathol*, 1990;136:891–897.

[70] Pollock, B., et al., "Topical aminolaevulinic acid-photodynamic therapy for the treatment of acne vulgaris: a study of clinical efficacy and mechanism of action," *Br J Dermatol*, 2004;151:616–622.

[71] Goldman, M., Boyce, S., "A single-center study of aminolevulinic acid and 417 NM photodynamic therapy in the treatment of moderate to severe acne vulgaris," *J Drugs Dermatol*, 2003; 2:393–396.

[72] Alexiades-Armenakas, M., "Long-pulsed dye laser-mediated photodynamic therapy combined with topical therapy for mild to severe comedonal, inflammatory, or cystic acne," *J Drugs Dermatol*, 2006; 5:45–55.

[73] Itoh, Y., Ninomiya, Y., Tajima, S., Ishibashi, A., "Photodynamic therapy of acne vulgaris with topical delta-aminolaevulinic acid and incoherent light in Japanese patients," *Br J Dermatol*, 2001;144:575–579.

[74] Santos, M., Belo, V., Santos, G., "Effectiveness of photodynamic therapy with topical 5-aminolevulinic acid and intense pulsed light versus intense pulsed light alone in the treatment of acne vulgaris: comparative study," *Dermatol Surg*, 2005; 31:910–15.

[75] Gold, M., et al., "The use of a novel intense pulsed light and heat source and ALA-PDT in the treatment of moderate to severe inflammatory acne vulgaris," *J Drugs Dermatol*, 2004;3 (6 Suppl):S15–19.

[76] Taub, A.F., "Procedural treatments for acne vulgaris," *Dermatol Surg*, 2007 Sep; 33(9):1005–1026.

[77] Taub, A., "Photodynamic therapy for the treatment of acne: a pilot study," *J Drugs Dermatol*, 2004;3 (6 Suppl):S10–S14.

[78] Wiegell, S.R., Wulf, H.C., "Photodynamic therapy of acne vulgaris using methyl aminolaevulinate: a blinded, randomized, controlled trial," *Br J Dermatol*, 2006;154:969–976.

[79] Lloyd, J., Mirkov, M., "Selective photothermolysis of the sebaceous glands for acne treatment," *Lasers Surg Med*, 2002; 31:115–120.

[80] Genina, E., et al., "Low-intensity indocyanine-green laser phototherapy of acne vulgaris: pilot study," *J Biomed Opt*, 2004; 9:828–834.

[81] Tuchin, V., et al., "A pilot study of ICG laser therapy of acne vulgaris: photodynamic and photothermolysis treatment," *Lasers Surg Med*, 2003; 33:296–310.

[82] Nouri, K., Ballard, C., "Laser therapy for acne," *Clin Dermatol*, 2006; 24:26–32.

[83] Horfelt, C., et al., "Photodynamic therapy for acne vulgaris: a pilot study of the dose-response and mechanism of action," *Acta Derm Venereol*, 2007; 87(4):325–329.

[84] Taub, A.F., "Procedural Treatments for Acne Vulgaris," *Dermatol Surg*, 2007; 33:1005–1026.

[85] Nestor, M.S., et al., "The use of photodynamic therapy in dermatology results of a consensus conference," *J Drugs Dermatol*, 2006 Feb; 5(2):140–154.

[86] Von der Werth, J.M., Williams, H.C., "The natural history of hidradenitis suppurativa," *J Eur Acad Dermatol Venereol*, 2000; 14:389–392.

[87] Harms, M., *Systemic Isotretinoin. A Unique Therapeutic Effect and Its Implications in the Pathogenesis of Acne*, Basel, Switzerland: Editiones Roche, 1994.

[88] Jermec, G.B.E., "Medical treatment of hidradenitis suppurativa," *Expert Opin Pharmacother*, 2004; 5:1767–1770.

[89] Rose, R.F., Goodfield, M.J.D., Clark, S.M., "Treatment of recalcitrant hidradenitis suppurativa with oral ciclosporin," *Clin Exp Dermatol*, 2005; 31:154–155.

[90] Katsanof, K.H., Christodoulou, D.K., Tsianos, E.V., "Axillary hidradenitis suppurativa successfully treated with infliximab in a Chron's disease patient," *Am J Gastroenterol*, 2002; 97:2155–2156.

[91] Wiseman, M.C., "Hidradenitis suppurativa; a review," *Dermatol Ther*, 2004; 17:50–54.

[92] Mandal, A., Watson, J.. "Experience with different treatment modules in hidradenitis suppurativa: a study of 106 cases," *Surgeon* 2005 Feb; 3(1):23–26.

[93] Gold, M., et al., "ALA-PDT and blue light therapy for hidradenitis suppurativa," *J Drugs Dermatol*, 2004 Jan–Feb; 3 (1 Suppl): S32–S53.

[94] DeVita, E., Taub, A.F., "Photodynamic Therapy for the Treatment of Hidradenitis Suppurativa," *Annual Meeting of the American Society of Laser Medicine and Surgery*, Grapevine, TX, Apr. 2007.

[95] Strauss, R.M., et al., "Photodynamic therapy using aminolaevulinic acid does not lead to clinical improvement in hidradenitis suppurativa," *Br J Dermatol*, 2005 Apr; 152(4): 803–804.

[96] Ruiz-Rodriguez, R., Sanz-Sánchez, T., Córdoba, S., "Photodynamic Photorejuvenation," *Dermatol Surgery*, 2002; 28 (8):742–744.

[97] Gold, M.H., "Intense pulsed light therapy for photorejuvenation enhanced with 20% aminolevulinic acid photodynamic therapy," *J Lasers Med Surg*, 2003; 15 (Suppl):47.

[98] Gold, et al., "Split-face comparison of photodynamic therapy with 5-aminolevulinic acid and intense pulsed light versus intense pulsed light alone for photodamage," *Dermatol Surg*, 2006 Jun; 32(6):795–801; discussion 801–803.

[99] Dover, J.S., et al., "Topical 5-aminolevulinic acid combined with intense pulsed light in the treatment of photoaging," *Arch Dermatol*, 2005 Oct;141(10):1247–1252.

[100] Bissonnette, R., et al., "Oral aminolevulinic acid induces protoporphyrin IX fluorescence in psoriatic plaques and peripheral blood cells," *Photochem Photobiol*, 2001 Aug; 74(2):339–345.

[101] Boehncke, W.H., et al., "Photodynamic therapy in psoriasis: suppression of cytokine production in vitro and recording of fluorescence modification during treatment in vivo," *Arch Dermatol Res*, 1994; 286(6):300–303.

[102] Bissonnette, R., et al., "Systemic photodynamic therapy with aminolevulinic acid induces apoptosis in lesional T lymphocytes of psoriatic plaques," *J Invest Dermatol*, 2002 Jul; 119(1):77–83.

[103] Robinson, D.J., et al., "Improved response of plaque psoriasis after multiple treatments with topical 5-aminolaevulinic acid photodynamic therapy," *Acta Derm Venereol*, 1999 Nov; 79(6):451–455.

[104] Fransson, J., Ros, A.M., "Clinical and immunohistochemical evaluation of psoriatic plaques treated with topical 5-aminolaevulinic acid photodynamic therapy," *Photodermatol Photoimmunol Photomed*, 2005; 21(6): 326–332.

[105] Radakovic-Fijan, S., et al. "Topical aminolaevulinic acid-based photodynamic therapy as a treatment option for psoriasis? Results of a randomized, observer-blinded study," *Br J Dermatol*, 2005 Feb;152(2):279–283.

[106] Smits, T., et al., "A placebo-controlled randomized study on the clinical effectiveness, immunohistochemical changes and protoporphyrin IX accumulation in fractionated 5-aminolaevulinic acid-photodynamic therapy in patients with psoriasis," *Br J Dermatol*, Online Early, doi:10.1111/j.1365-2133.2006.07290.

[107] Aghahosseini, F., et al., "Methylene blue-mediated photodynamic therapy: a possible alternative treatment for oral lichen planus," *Lasers Surg Med*, 2006 Jan; 38(1):33–38.

[108] Olejek, A., et al., "Photodynamic diagnosis and therapy in gynecology—current knowledge," [Article in Polish], *Ginekol Pol*, 2004 Mar; 75(3):228–234.

[109] Szeimies, R.M., Landthaler, M., Karrer, S., "Non-oncologic indications for ALA-PDT," *J Dermatolog Treat*, 2002;13 Suppl 1:S13–S18.

[110] Karrer, S., et al., "Keratinocyte-derived cytokines after photodynamic therapy and their paracrine induction of matrix metalloproteinases in fibroblasts," *Br J Dermatol*, 2004 Oct; 151(4):776–783.

[111] Chiu, L.L., et al., "Photodynamic therapy on keloid fibroblasts in tissue-engineered keratinocyte-fibroblast co-culture," *Lasers Surg Med*, 2005 Sept; 37(3):231–244.

[112] Bissonnette, R., et al., "Topical photodynamic therapy with 5-aminolaevulinic acid does not induce hair regrowth in patients with extensive alopecia areata," *Br J Dermatol*, 2000 Nov; 143(5):1032–1035.

[113] Exadaktylou, D., et al., "Treatment of Darier's disease with photodynamic therapy," *Br J Dermatol*, 2003 Sep; 149(3):606–610.

[114] Svanberg, K., et al., "Photodynamic therapy of non-melanoma malignant tumours of the skin using topical delta-amino levulinic acid sensitization and laser irradiation," *Br J Dermatol*, 1994 Jun; 130(6):743–751.

[115] Rittenhouse-Diakun, K., et al., "The role of transferrin receptor (CD71) in photodynamic therapy of activated and malignant lymphocytes using the heme precursor delta-aminolevulinic acid (ALA)," *Photochem Photobiol*, 1995 May; 61(5):523–528.

[116] Eich, D., et al., "Photodynamic therapy of cutaneous T-cell lymphoma at special sites," [Article in German], *Hautarzt*, 1999 Feb; 50(2):109–114.

[117] Orenstein, A., et al., "Photodynamic therapy of cutaneous lymphoma using 5-aminolevulinic acid topical application," *Dermatol Surg*, 2000 Aug; 26(8):765–769; discussion 769–770.

[118] Leman, J.A., Dick, D.C., Morton, C.A., "Topical 5-ALA photodynamic therapy for the treatment of cutaneous T-cell lymphoma," *Clin Exp Dermatol*, 2002 Sep; 27(6):516–518.

[119] Paech, V., et al., "Remission of cutaneous Mycosis fungoides after topical 5-ALA sensitization and photodynamic therapy in a patient with advanced HIV-infection," *Eur J Med Res*, 2002 Nov 25; 7(11):477–479.

[120] Edstrom, D.W., Porwit, A., Ros, A.M., "Photodynamic therapy with topical 5-aminolevulinic acid for mycosis fungoides: clinical and histological response," *Acta Derm Venereol*, 2001 Jun–Jul; 81(3):184–188.

[121] Grossman, M., Anderson, A., presented at 1996 ASLMS.

[122] Parlette, E.C., "Red light laser photodynamic therapy of Bowen's disease," *J Drugs Dermatol*, 2004; 3(6):S22–S24.

CHAPTER 23

Role of Photodynamic Therapy (PDT) in Lung Cancer

Keyvan Moghissi

23.1 Introduction

23.1.1 Definition

Lung cancer (bronchogenic carcinoma, carcinoma of the lung) is a generic term used for all malignant tumors of the lung, especially those arising from epithelial components of the bronchial tree. This definition applies to primary tumors that arise from broncho-pulmonary tissues.

23.1.2 Lung Cancer Development

It is generally acknowledged that lung cancer development is progressive whereby normal epithelial cells acquire characteristics of malignancy in a stepwise fashion. In this process carcinogenesis begins with intracellular, molecular, and genetic alterations, which initially show no apparent morphological abnormal features. A series of morphological alterations then develops that are collectively referred to as preneoplastic changes; these are metaplasia, varying grades of dysplasia, and carcinoma in situ that finally progresses to locally invasive and metastatic carcinoma [1, 2]. It is now possible to visualize some of the morphological changes using fluorescence techniques.

23.1. 3 Classification

The many varieties of lung cancer have been classified in a number of different ways.

23.1.3.1 Histological Classification

The World Health Organization (WHO) histological classification of lung cancer (last reviewed in 1982) recognizes four principal types and eight subtypes [3]. The principal cell types are:

1. Squamous cell carcinoma (epidermal);
2. Small cell (oat cell);
3. Adenocarcinoma;
4. Large cell.

Clinicians divide all lung cancers into two categories: (1) nonsmall cell lung cancer (NSCLC), which comprises all varieties of squamous cell, adenocarcinoma, and large cell carcinoma, and (2) small cell lung cancer (SCLC), which comprises this and all of its subtypes.

23.1.3.2 Stage Classification

Staging is the evaluation of the extent of cancer in a patient. It takes account of local, regional, and general extent of tumor in the body. It provides a level of understanding amongs researchers and those involved in cancer treatment and is an essential measurement for therapeutic planning. Staging of lung cancer uses the TNM system of classification [4, 5], where T refers to the primary tumor whose extent (size) is represented by a numeric suffix from 1 to 4, N represents the regional and more distant lymph node involvement identified by a number from 1 to 3, and M portrays the extent of metastatic spread.

The importance of stage classification is its correlation with outcome and prognosis. Clinicians sometimes use additional or alternative terminology of stage classification, namely, early and advanced stage. Early stage disease implies that the tumor is localized and limited (≤3 cm in diameter) without lymphatic satellite invasion or distant metastases.

Occult cancer refers to a case in which cytological examination of the sputum or bronchial secretion shows evidence of malignant or atypical (cancer) cells but there is no radiological abnormality to be seen on chest X-ray/CT of the thorax.

23.1.3.3 Topographical Classification

The precise site of a lesion in the lung is usually indicated by reference to its position within the bronchopulmonary segments or lobes. A less precise but therapeutically more relevant topographical classification for clinicians is to divide lung cancer cases into two types: central and peripheral. Peripheral tumors are within the substance of the lung. Central tumors are placed within or around the root (hilum) of the lung. In bronchology reference is made to early central lung cancer. This is understood to be a superficial malignant tumor confined to bronchial mucosa, without infiltration of the pulmonary parenchyma, or, lymph node involvement, and with no distant metastases

When considering therapeutic endoscopic methods, such as bronchoscopic photodynamic therapy, it is important to bear in mind that peripheral tumors are not usually visible and accessible bronchoscopically for cytohistological sampling nor are they suitable for treatments that use interventional bronchoscopy methods. Central tumors are usually visible bronchoscopically and accessible both for biopsy and for therapy via the bronchoscope.

23.1.4 Lung Cancer: The Size of the Problem and Standard Treatment

23.1.4.1 Statistics

Lung cancer is the most common cancer in men in the industrial world and the most common cause of death for men and women in the United Kingdom, Europe, and the United States (Table 23.1). Advances in diagnostic and therapeutic methods in the past 20 years have not made significant impact on the 5-year survival rate, which remains between 6% to 15%.

23.1.4.2   Standard Treatment

The first pneumonectomy for cancer in 1933 [12] was a milestone in the history of surgery and was instrumental in placing surgical resection at the forefront of lung cancer treatment, a position it has occupied despite considerable advances in chemo/radiation therapy in the second half of the twentieth century.

For the past 50 years, surgery, radiotherapy, and chemotherapy have dominated methods of lung cancer treatment, with surgical operation the first option in clinically and oncologically suitable cases. Nevertheless, a number of new treatment methods have emerged. In this regard PDT, with its ability to target lesions with almost surgical precision, has become the focus of attention for many clinicians. Furthermore, in recent years, lifestyle changes and longevity, cancer recurrence after surgery and/or chemo/radiotherapy, along with unsuitability for surgical resection and refusal by patients to consent to operation have provided compelling stimuli to expand therapeutic possibilities beyond the conventional trio of surgery, radiation, and chemotherapy.

23.2   PDT in Lung Cancer

23.2.1   Historic Review

PDT for lung cancer treatment began in the early 1980s. In 1981, Hyata and colleagues carried out the first bronchoscopic PDT in a patient with early lung cancer who was suitable for surgery but declined surgical resection [13, 14]. This patient survived for over 4 years and died from an unrelated cause. Since then, over 2,000 lung cancer patients have been treated with PDT. During the 1980s and early 1990s, the efficacy and safety of PDT in bronchogenic carcinoma was evaluated through multicenter trials in patients with locally advanced stage disease [15–18].

23.2.2   Principle, Mechanisms, and Methods of PDT for Lung Cancer

The principle of PDT has been described throughout this book and its mechanism has also been detailed [see Chapter 3]. It is, nevertheless, important to present

Table 23.1   Lung cancer statistics in UK, Europe and the USA.

Region	Year	Number of Lung Cancers Diagnosed	Number of Lung Cancer Deaths	Reference
United Kingdom	2003	37,127	33,500	[6–9]
Europe	2006	386,300 (predicted)	334,800	[10]
United States	2007	213,380 (predicted)	160,390	[11]

aspects of PDT that are applicable to lung cancer and the way it is practiced in this specific clinical anatomical situation.

Historically and currently, nearly 90% of all PDT in lung cancer cases is carried out for patients with central lung cancer. It therefore follows that for all practical purposes PDT in bronchopulmonary cancer means systemic intravenous administration of the photosensitizer followed by bronchoscopic illumination. Therefore, bronchoscopic PDT will be described fully while PDT for peripheral lung cancer will be touched upon proportionately within the limits of the available experience.

PDT for lung cancer is carried out as a two-stage procedure: *photosensitization* and *illumination*.

23.2.3 Photosensitization

This is the first stage of the procedure and is achieved by intravenous administration of a suitable photosensitizing drug to the patient.

23.2.3.1 Photosensitizers

The first photosensitizer used for PDT in lung cancer was a hematoporphyrin derivative (HPD). This is well documented in publications of the 1980s by several groups in North America, Asia, and Europe using HPDs that were synthesized in different laboratories and had different compositions [14, 19, 20]. Towards the end of the 1980s, most clinical investigators used Photofrin II, also a porphyrin sensitizer, in their clinical trials. The same drug was later made available as porfimer sodium. This drug is a purified variation of HPD produced initially by QLT Pharmaceuticals of Canada and marketed under the name Photofrin®, which is now used extensively throughout the world. Photofrin is currently distributed by Axcan Pharma of Canada and it is authorized by the Food and Drug Administration (FDA) in the United States and the European Union (EU) licensing authorities for use in a number of conditions, including bronchoscopic PDT for lung cancer. The drug is administered at a recommended dose of 2mg/kg/bw and is activated by 630-nm light. Apart from Photofrin which, by virtue of the length of time it has been in use and its licensing approval, and is currently the photosensitizer of choice for PDT of lung cancer, there are other photosensitizers that have been used by some investigators:

1. Photosan, also HPD, is marketed by Seehof Laboratories, Wesselburenerkoog, Germany [19], and is used as a photosensitizer for PDT in lung cancer in some European countries. It was certified as a medical device for PDT in the European Union in 2002.
2. Meta-tetrahydroxy-phenyl-chorine (m-THPC) (Temoporfin, Foscan) has been used for bronchoscopic PDT of lung cancer by one group in a small number of patients. This drug could potentially be more effective than Photofrin because it is activated by a longer wavelength of light. However, the drug is attended by much more toxicity than Photofrin [21] and its dosage in the lung cancer situation has yet to be standardized.
3. The photosensitizing prodrug 5-aminolevulenic acid (5-ALA) has been used by one group in lung cancer in a small series of patients [22].

4. NPe6 (mono-L-aspartyl-chlorin e6/Taloporfin) has undergone extensive evaluation and phase II clinical trials in Japan for use in bronchoscopic PDT. This drug has an absorption band at 664 nm. A phase II clinical study has suggested a dose of 40mg/bw/m² and laser radiation 4 hours after administration [23, 24].

23.2.4   Illumination

In this second stage of PDT, the presensitized tumor is exposed to light of specific matching wavelength after a designated latent period (between drug administration and light exposure). In lung cancer treatment one or both methods of illumination are used, namely interstitial and surface illumination (Color Plate 33). In the former, a light diffuser is inserted into the tumor mass. In the latter, the exposure is over the surface of the tumor.

23.2.4.1   Light Sources and Delivery Systems

From the beginning of clinical PDT for lung cancer, the light source used was a laser, producing light within the red region of the spectrum at 630 nm to activate the porphyrin-based photosensitizers. This was initially provided by argon lamps with appropriate filters, then tunable dye lasers such as copper vapor dye lasers pumping 630 to 640 nm and, more recently, diode lasers [25].

Light, which is generated and emitted by a laser, is delivered to the tumor by an optical fiber with either a cylindrical diffusing tip or a microlens. Cylindrical diffusers distribute light circumferentially and are used for interstitial treatment; in this case the diffuser is placed within the tumor mass. However, the cylindrical diffuser can also be used for superficial application, in which case it is laid over the surface of the tumor. A microlens projects light in a forward direction and is used for surface application to treat superficial growth. In endoscopic PDT the delivery fiber for illumination is introduced via the biopsy channel of the fiber-optic endoscope. The light dose is calculated at the point of delivery to provide the required level of exposure and is expressed in joules, made up from milliwatts × time (in seconds).

23.3   Bronchoscopic PDT for Lung Cancer: Indications and Selection of Patients

Bronchoscopic PDT is carried out in patients with central lung cancer. They can be classified under two groups, each with defined indications and criteria of selection, as well as treatment objectives:

1. Group A. This concerns patients with locally advanced disease in whom PDT is used for symptom relief (palliation). In a very small proportion of cases with locally advanced disease, bronchoscopic PDT is used to downstage the tumor in order to convert an unresectable (inoperable) case to a resectable one.

2. Group E. Patients in this group are those with early central lung cancer (ECLC). They are oncologically and technically operable but are, for a variety of reasons, unsuitable for surgical resection. PDT in these patients is with curative intent.

23.3.1 Bronchoscopic PDT in Advanced Stage Disease (Group A) [15–18, 26–28]

The major indication of PDT in this group is in oncologically and locally advanced stage tumor in patients with significant related symptoms. Typically the tumor is exophytic within the main stem and/or lobar bronchi, producing total or partial pulmonary collapse (atelectasis) (Color Plate 34). Dyspnoea (breathlessness) proportional to the severity of the obstruction and the topography of the lesion, cough, hemoptysis, and pulmonary infection are the ensuing symptoms. All histological types respond to PDT [28, 29] and are eligible for inclusion in a treatment protocol for as long as the criteria of inclusion (see below) are met. The fact that in almost all published literature concerned with bronchoscopic PDT there is no mention of small cell lung cancer, relates to the specific pathological behavior of this particular cell type and the pattern of referral. In effect, small cell lung cancer is rarely endobronchial and exophytic, and only exceptionally are patients with such a tumor referred to the interventional bronchoscopist for PDT. Nonsmall cell lung cancer cases are usually referred for bronchoscopic PDT on account of inoperability and/or following local recurrence of endobronchial disease after surgical resection, radiotherapy, and, in some cases, chemotherapy.

Patients with lung cancer allocated to bronchoscopic PDT would have had standard workup. The selection criteria include:

1. Symptomatic patients (or those with expected impending symptoms) whose symptoms relate to endobronchial cancer;
2. Oncologically advanced stage, inoperable patients with any T or N factor in the TNM classification but without distant metastases [4, 5];
3. Endoluminal, exophytic tumors with >50% bronchial luminal obstruction;
4. Patients with good performance status (>50% Karnofsky scale or ≤3 WHO scale).

The advantage of PDT in this group of patients, compared with many other treatment modalities used for palliation, is that PDT is both specific and also target-orientated. This relates to an inherent property of PDT, due to a higher concentration of photosensitizer in the tumor compared with normal surrounding tissue. The practical implication of this is reduced collateral damage with a lesser risk of complications and adverse effects.

Major contraindications for PDT in advanced stage endobronchial lung cancer are:

 • Infiltrative bronchial cancer rather than the exophytic type;
 • Extraluminal obstruction of the bronchus by lymph nodes;

- Dyspnoea with minor bronchial obstruction due to COPD or interstitial lung cancer;
- Extrathoracic metastatic disease;
- Poor performance status.

It is important to note that previous surgical pulmonary resection and/or chemoradiation therapy does not constitute contraindication to bronchoscopic PDT provided that selection criteria are adhered to.

23.3.2   Bronchoscopic PDT in Early Stage Disease (Group E)

Reference has been made previously to early central lung cancer (ECLC). In the context of bronchoscopic PDT, the term "early" cancer is used to describe cases in which the tumor is superficial and limited in its extent to the bronchial lumen and wall. The chest radiograph of patients with ECLC shows no evidence of tumor and CT scan reveals no lymph node involvement. Diagnosis is made almost entirely at bronchoscopy. Some early intraepithelial cancer may even escape being diagnosed by the standard white light endoscopic instrumentation.

Two recently developed methods assist the bronchoscopic diagnosis of early cancer. First, fluorescence bronchoscopy (FB) uses a blue light with greater discriminative power of differential imaging than its white light counterpart. This more accurately displays mucosal abnormalities than white light bronchoscopy [30–32] and is of use both for pre-PDT diagnosis of early endobronchial cancer and for monitoring response to treatment. The second development is endobronchial ultrasonography (EBUS), which enables imaging and evaluation of the depth of bronchial wall involvement by the tumor [33–35].

It is generally agreed that surgical resection remains the treatment of choice for an ECLC provided that the cancer is surgically resectable, the patient's general and cardiorespiratory functions are adequate for the extent of the pulmonary resection, and he or she consents to undergo the operation.

At the time of writing, there is some consensus of opinion in respect of the indications for bronchoscopic PDT in early stage lung cancer. These are for patients:

- Whose tumor topography within the bronchial tree is not amenable to bronchoplastic parenchyma saving operation;
- Whose general condition puts them in such a high-risk category as to prohibit resectional surgery;
- With inadequate predicted postoperative (postresection) pulmonary function with the expectation of disabling and poor quality of life after operation;
- With multifocal endobronchial early cancer whose surgical resection is either technically impossible or would entail too extensive a loss of pulmonary parenchyma;
- Who present with early stage metachronous cancer following previous extensive surgical resection;
- Who decline surgical resection but consent to PDT.

Only some patients with early lung cancer are symptomatic with cough, blood-stained sputum, and dyspnoea [36]. The latter is not usually related to endobronchial tumors but associated with coexisting conditions such as chronic obstructive pulmonary disease (COPD). Therefore, selection of patients with ECLC for PDT is made on prognostication of survival benefit and/or on the basis of curative intent.

23.4   Technique of Bronchoscopic PDT in Lung Cancer

23.4.1   Anesthesia and Instrumentation

Bronchoscopic PDT for lung cancer can be carried out under general or topical (local) anesthesia [27, 37].

23.4.1.1   Anesthesia and Instrumentation in Patients with Advanced Stage Disease

In this group of patients, bronchoscopic PDT is preferably carried out under general anesthetic. This involves the use of both the rigid (tube) and flexible bronchoscope [17]. After suitable anesthesia, the rigid instrument is first introduced into the trachea, where it remains for the purpose of ventilation. Then the flexible fiberoptic bronchoscope (FFB) is passed through the rigid instrument into the bronchial lumina for inspection and visualization. The biopsy channel of the FFB provides a conduit for the laser fiber for illumination. The rigid bronchoscope permits ready access for ventilation (oxygenation) and cleaning of the bronchus and provides a wide channel for suction in patients with tenacious secretions or bleeding (Figure 23.1).

23.4.1.2   Anesthesia and Instrumentation for Patients with Early Lung Cancer

Bronchoscopic PDT for early lung cancer may be carried out under general anesthesia as above. Alternatively, such bronchoscopies can be done under topical anesthesia and sedation using a similar method to the one used for diagnostic bronchoscopy [37].

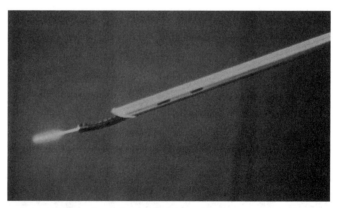

Figure 23.1   Instrumentation for bronchoscopic PDT under general anaesthesia. See Section 23.4.1.1.

Each method has its advantages and disadvantages. The use of general anesthetic necessitates the presence of an anesthetist and more elaborate equipment but provides a comfortable environment for the patient and facilitates the operative procedure. General anesthesia and use of the rigid instrument also allows the operator more time, better access to the lesion, and less risk of displacing the delivery fiber in patients with bulky tumors and/or multiple lesions. However, unifocal superficial lesions of early cancer which are limited in extent can easily be treated using the FFB under topical anesthesia. In my experience, use of the combined rigid and flexible instruments under GA should be considered for all patients with obstructive exophytic tumors of the major airway (trachea, main stem bronchi). In other cases the choice depends on the experience of the physician, patient preference, and available facilities.

Review of the literature concerned with bronchoscopic PDT indicates that many authors, whose series of patients predominantly had advanced stage disease and endoluminal obstruction of major airways, used GA and the associated instrumentation [16, 26, 28]. Authors treating early superficial lesions had mostly used topical anesthesia and FFB [29].

23.4.2   Bronchoscopic PDT Technique and Patient Management

The technique of bronchoscopic PDT is now well established and practiced using the method as described above with minor variation by different clinicians throughout the world.

The sequence of bronchoscopic PDT is shown diagrammatically (Figure 23.2) and follows the sequence:

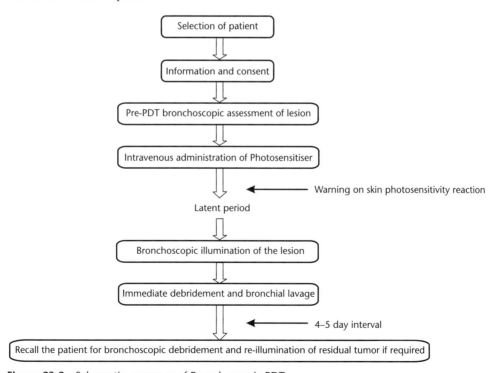

Figure 23.2   Schematic sequence of Bronchoscopic PDT.

1. After the standard workup and selection process, the patient has bronchoscopic assessment to evaluate and record the number, size, and extent of neoplastic lesions and their topography. In cases of advanced stage disease, the extent of luminal obstruction in terms of the percentage of total diameter (caliber) of the bronchial lumen is calculated. In early stage disease, autofluorescence bronchoscopy is carried out (if available) in addition to standard white light bronchoscopy.

2. Prior to intravenous administration of photosensitizer, the patient is fully counseled on all aspects of PDT, notably the possibility of photosensitivity skin reaction (skin burn).

3. Administration of photosensitizer is carried out. Photofrin is currently the photosensitizer of choice and is administered at a dose of 2mg/kg/bw. For other photosensitizers, there is, as yet, no standard dose for endobronchial lung cancer treatment.

4. After intravenous administration, a latent period is required (24–72 hours) for Photofrin PDT to distribute and to concentrate within the tumor.

5. Illumination of the presensitized tumor is carried out using devices appropriate to the tumor characteristics (bulky versus superficial flat tumors).

6. Post-PDT debridement and bronchial lavage is an important step. This is carried out in all cases after illumination is completed. In advanced cases with bulky endobronchial obstructive tumors, a further bronchoscopic debridement is necessary 4 to 5 days after bronchoscopic PDT, at which time reillumination of the residual tumor is also undertaken.

7. Discharge from hospital and follow-up. At the Yorkshire Laser Centre (YLC), all of our bronchoscopic PDT is carried out as a day-case procedure. The patients are regularly followed up with chest X-ray and bronchoscopy at 1 month and outpatient checks at 3 months, 6 months, and then every 6 months thereafter.

23.5   Results of Bronchoscopic PDT

Bronchoscopic PDT results are evaluated using the following parameters:

- Mortality and morbidity;
- Local pathological response to treatment;
- Patient satisfaction and clinical effect.

23.5.1   Mortality and Morbidity

There is no mortality associated with the bronchoscopic PDT procedure per se, and the 30-day mortality rate (empirically set for surgical operations) is less than 1%. A recent review article concerning 25 publications from the world literature and comprising 1,153 patients undergoing nearly 2,000 bronchoscopic PDT procedures for cancer confirms this [27].

The adverse reactions (complications) of bronchoscopic PDT are presented in Table 23.2. The most important of these relates to photosensitivity reaction of the skin when exposed to sunlight. Skin burn can be an important drawback and a prohibitive factor in the advancement of clinical PDT. Nevertheless, it should be emphasized that this is an avoidable complication and its incidence can be reduced considerably by thorough counseling. At the Yorkshire Laser Centre, with a total of nearly 500 PDTs using a systemically administered photosensitizer, the incidence of minor skin burn in different series has been consistently between 3.5% to 5.3% of patients [28, 38]. Furthermore, in the last 50 patients, no cases of skin burn have been recorded.

23.5.2   Local Pathological Response to Treatment

By convention, local response to treatment is described as:

- Complete response/remission (CR), when a treated area becomes macroscopically and microscopically (by cyto/histology) clear from tumor;
- Partial response/remission (PR), when after treatment the macroscopic extent of the tumor is reduced at least by 50% but cyto/histology demonstrates presence of malignancy;
- No response, when there is little (<50%) or no change in the macroscopic extent of the tumor and the histology remains unaffected.

It is important to note that CR and PR are not precise measurements but are nevertheless a useful concept both in terms of monitoring of treatment and also in relation to decision making for further management of the patient. It is also necessary to point out that response to treatment, be it CR or PR, becomes meaningful when it is further quantified by duration of response [36]:

- Patients with advanced stage disease. Pathologically, there is a partial response (PR) in all and complete response (CR) in some irrespective of histology.
- Patients with early stage cancer. CR is achieved in all patients for variable lengths of time. Note that monitoring response to treatment in early stage bronchial cancer is difficult without the aid of fluorescence bronchoscopy

Table 23.2   Mortality and Adverse Reactions (Complications) of Bronchoscopic PDT.

Series	Reference	Mortality		Complications				
		Operative	30-day	Skin burn	Hemorrhage	Respiratory	Other	
Personal series 160 pts (280 PDTs)	38	0	1 (0.6%)	4%	0%	8 (5%)	0	
Literature review 1,153 patients (nearly 2,000 PDTs)	27	0	10 (<0.9%)	5%–41%	2.4% Fatal: 0.3%	30 (29%)	1 Anaphylactic	

This is because localization of the treated area for sampling may prove impossible with the use of white light bronchoscopy alone. Also, without fluorescence endoscopy, newly developed early cancer adjacent to the treated area could either escape detection or be assumed to be at the previously treated area.

23.5.3 Patient Satisfaction, Clinical Effects and Survival

23.5.3.1 Patient Satisfaction

Patient level of satisfaction reflects the overall quality of care as well as subjective evaluation of the treatment. Therefore, it is important to constantly bear in mind that a treatment may objectively be judged as successful but, paradoxically, the patient may be dissatisfied due to lack of standard of care and understanding by the caregivers. In all clinical PDT patient satisfaction to treatment should be recorded. At the YLC this is recorded and shows total satisfaction of patients to treatment [28, 36].

23.5.3.2 Clinical Effects and Survival

Clinical effects include the relief of symptoms, which is the aim of PDT in patients with locally advance stage cancer (Group A) and can be achieved in almost all cases provided that the selection criteria are adhered to. This was evident from the review of the world literature involving 636 patients in 12 series (Moghissi et al., 2003 [27]). Dyspnoea, which is the outstanding symptom in such patients, is significantly improved following PDT. Objectively, this is closely matched by amelioration of ventilatory function, reflecting increased breathing capacity, radiological improvement shown on chest X-ray, and increase in percentage of bronchial luminal opening [18, 26–28]. A number of patients with ECLC may be totally asymptomatic. In those with symptoms dyspnoea cannot be attributed to ECLC. Cough and blood staining of the sputum, which usually are the other relevant symptoms, are alleviated in the majority of patients following PDT.

Survival is described as follows: In advanced stage group (A), generally survival is dependant on the stage of disease on admission for treatment. In addition, two subsets of patients have been shown to have survival benefit. First, those with a good performance status (≤ 2 WHO scale or >50 Karnofsky index) and second, patients without extrathoracic metastases [26, 28]. Histology per se does not appear to influence survival. While an overall majority of cases referred for and submitted to bronchoscopic PDT have NSCLC, patients with small cell cancer also benefit from the procedure provided that there is endoluminal tumor and the aforementioned criteria are fulfilled [28, 29]. In some such cases, bronchoscopic PDT has been carried out concomitantly with chemotherapy or following chemo/radiotherapy.

Patients with early cancer can achieve long survival amounting to cure of disease following single or repeated endoscopic PDT. The Tokyo Medical University has the largest experience of bronchoscopic PDT in early lung cancer and has shown nearly 60% overall 5-year survival and over 90% cancer-specific survival in such patients [24, 29]. Our results at the YLC, with a smaller series, echo this [36]. Review of 12 articles from world literature involving 650 patients undergoing bronchoscopic PDT for early cancer [27] shows that long survival of over 5 years is achieved in over 50% of cases. However, in some of these the selection process and the criteria of early cancer are not comparable or similar to the Tokyo Medical University or YLC series. Inconsistency of long-term response relates to difficulty in defining the "earliness" of the tumor.

It is important to note that the results of bronchoscopic PDT in lung cancer should reflect the objectives of treatment. In locally advanced disease results should be assessed by the quality of palliation and survival benefit as an added bonus.

As many patients with ECLC are asymptomatic at the time of treatment, assessment of the results in this subgroup should be based on pathological response and survival.

23.6   Miscellaneous Indications of Bronchoscopic PDT

PDT can be used adjunct to other forms of cancer therapy methods and within a multimodal protocol setting in order to enhance the overall treatment response results with better outcome.

23.6.1   Bronchoscopic PDT Prior to Surgical Resection [39–41]

The idea behind preoperative PDT in central-type lung cancer is to reduce the size of the tumor within the bronchial tree, with the goal of conversion from an unresectable to a resectable case to allow preservation of some healthy parenchyma that otherwise would be excised. The principle is to reduce unnecessary loss of parenchyma in cases where the bronchial involvement exceeds pulmonary parenchymal neoplastic disease. In practice a pneumonectomy can be avoided in favor of lobectomy after successful bronchoscopic PDT in a tumor affecting the lobe of a lung and main bronchial tree.

23.6.2   Sequential NdYAG Laser and PDT [42]

The principle is to debulk the tumor mass using NdYAG laser and then, 4 to 5 weeks later, to carry out bronchoscopic PDT. This allows expansion of the lung and elimination of infection prior to more manageable treatment by PDT.

23.6.3   Concomitant/Sequential Chemo/radiation and Endoscopic PDT

PDT can be used concomitant with chemotherapy in a small number of patients with small cell lung cancer. Kato and Moghissi have in fact used such a combination in the presence of endobronchial lesions [28, 29]. Many cases referred for PDT in locally advanced lung cancer are those who previously have had chemo/radiotherapy. In essence, there seems to be no incompatibility between PDT used concomitantly or sequentially. However, the clinician should consider the indications and benefits in individual cases.

23.6.4 Endoscopic PDT and Brachytherapy

This combination has been used both for advanced and early lung cancer with some benefit, particularly in early cancer cases [43].

23.7 PDT for Peripheral Lung Cancer

Compared with the number of endoscopic PDTs for central lung cancer, a relatively small proportion of PDTs have been performed for peripheral lung cancer. An important reason for this is the difficulty of access for illumination and difficulty of monitoring results. Also, since the development of minimal access pulmonary resection with the use of video-assisted thoracoscopic surgery (VATS), many small peripheral tumors can be treated by that method. PDT is only used to treat such peripheral lesions in certain cases. There are, however, two methods of access that have been used in a small number of cases:

1. Tokyo Medical University uses percutaneous radiologically (CT) guided method of illumination [44, 45];
2. The Yorkshire Laser Centre used thoracoscopic method and illumination under vision [46].

Localization and insertion of the probe may be difficult with both methods.

23.8 Conclusion

PDT is a powerful local method of therapy in lung cancer the potentials of which, as yet, have not been fully exploited. At the present time its role relates principally to bronchoscopic method in central lung cancer with two defined indications.

In advanced exophytic intraluminal tumors, PDT has a role for palliation of symptoms. There is substantial evidence that it can achieve this objective in all cases with survival benefit in some patients.

In early central lung cancer, PDT is used with curative intent. There is good evidence to suggest that long survival, amounting to cure, is achievable in an overall majority of cases. Fluorescence bronchoscopy is now an essential addition to white light bronchoscopy to diagnose the extent and the multifocality of early central lung cancer. More work is needed to determine with precision the true depth of infiltration of superficial tumors. There are good indications to forecast that with further development, better diagnostic methods, more appropriate photosensitizing drugs, and more advanced light source and delivery devices, PDT could take on the role of surgery in those ECLC cases in which parenchyma preservation needs serious consideration. Some such cases, currently at the borderline of inoperability, are already benefiting from bronchoscopic PDT (36).

PDT in lung cancer is a valid oncological treatment modality to be used alone or in conjunction with other available methods of therapy. This message needs advancing through education at all levels.

Acknowledgments

The author is particularly grateful to Kate Dixon and Elizabeth Binnington, who spent many hours reading and formatting the manuscript.

References

[1] Auerbach, O., Stout, A. P., and Hammond, E. C. et al., "Changes in bronchial epithelium in relation to cigarette smoking and in relation to lung cancer." *N Eng J Med*, Vol. 265. 1961; pp. 253–267.

[2] Saccomanno, G., Archer V. E., and Auerbach, O., et al. "Development of carcinoma of the lung as reflected in exfoliated cells." *Cancer*, Vol. 33 1974 pp. 256–270.

[3] World Health Organization International Histological Classification of Tumours: No 1 Histological typing of lung tumours, *2nd Ed. Am J Clin Pathol*, Vol. 77.

[4] Mountain, C F. "The new International staging for lung cancer. " *Surg Clin North Am*, Vol. 67, 1987, p. 925.

[5] Mountain, C. F. "Revision in the International system for staging of lung cancer." *Chest*, Vol. 111, 1997, pp. 1710–1717.

[6] Office for National Statistics, Cancer Statistics Registrations. "Registrations of cancer diagnosed in 2003." England, Series MB1 no 33. National Statistics, London.

[7] ISD online. 2005 Information and Statistics Division, NHS Scotland.

[8] Welsh Cancer Intelligence and Surveillance Unit. 2005.

[9] Northern Ireland Cancer Registry. Cancer Incidence and Mortality 2005.

[10] Ferlay, J., Autier, P., and Boniol, M., et al. Estimates of the cancer incidence and mortality in Europe in 2006. *Ann Oncol*, Vol. 18, 2007, pp. 581–592.

[11] Ries, L. A. G., Melbert, D., and Krapcho, M., et al. (eds.). *SEER Cancer Statistics Review 1975–2004*, National Cancer Institute. Bethesda, Maryland. http://seer.cancer.gov/csr/1975_2004 based on November 2006 SEER data submission, posted to the SEER website 2007.

[12] Graham, E. A., and Singer, J. J. "Successful removal of an entire lung for carcinoma of the bronchus." *JAMA*, Vol. 101, 1933, p. 1371.

[13] Hyata, Y., Kato, H., and Konoka, C., et al. "Haematoporphyrin derivative and laser photoradiation in the treatment of lung cancer." *Chest*, Vol. 81, 1982, pp. 264–277.

[14] Kessel, D. "Photodynamic Therapy from the beginning." *Photodiagnosis and Photodynamic Therapy*, Vol. 1, 2004, pp. 3–7.

[15] Balchum, O. J., Doiron, D. R., and Huth, G. C. "Photodynamic Therapy of endobronchial lung cancer employing the photodynamic action of the haematoporphyrin derivative." *Lasers Surg Med*, Vol. 14, 1984, pp. 13–30.

[16] McCaughan, J. S., Williams, T. E., and Bethel, B. H. "Photodynamic Therapy of endobronchial tumours." *Lasers Surg Med*, Vol. 6, 1986, pp. 336–345.

[17] Moghissi, K., Parsons, R. J., and Dixon, K. "Photodynamic Therapy for bronchial carcinoma with the use of rigid bronchoscope." *Lasers Med Sci*, Vol 7, 1991, pp. 381–385.

[18] Weinman, T. J., Diaz-Jiminez, J. P., and Moghissi, K. et al., "Photodynamic Therapy with Photofrin is effective in the palliation of obstructive endobronchial lung cancer: Results of 2 randomised trials," *Proceedings of the 34th Annual Meeting of the American Society of Clinical Oncology*, May 16–19, 1998, Los Angeles, California.

[19] Allison, R., Downie, G. H., and Cuenca, R., et al. "Photosensitisers in clinical photodynamic therapy." *Photodiagnosis and Photodynamic Therapy*, Vol. 1. 2004, pp. 27–42.

[20] Huang, Z. "PDT in China: over 25 years of unique clinical experience (part one: history & domestic photosensitisers)." *Photodiagnosis and Photodynamic Therapy*, Vol. 3, 2006, pp. 3–10.

[21] Radu, A., Grosjean, P., and Fontolliet, C. M. "Photodynamic therapy for 101 early cancers of the upper aerodigestive tract, the oesophagus and bronchus: a single institute experience." *Diagnostic Therapeutic Endoscop*, Vol 5, 1999, pp. 145–154.

[22] Maier, A., Tomaselli, F., and Matzi, V., et al. "Comparison of 5-aminolevulenic acid and porphyrin photosensitisation for photodynamic therapy of malignant bronchial stenosis: a clinical pilot study." *Laser Surg Med*, Vol. 30, 2002, pp. 12–17.

[23] Kato, H., Furukawa, K., and Sato, M. et al. "Phase II clinical study of photodynamic therapy using mono-L-aspartyl-chlorin e6 and diode laser for early superficial squamous cell carcinoma of the lung." *Lung Cancer*, Vol. 42, 2003, pp. 103–111.

[24] Kato, H., Harada, M., and Ichinose, S., et al. "Photodynamic therapy of lung cancer: experience of the Tokyo Medical University." *Photodiagnosis and Photodynamic Therapy*, Vol. 1, 2004, pp. 49–55.

[25] Mang, T. S. "Lasers and light sources for photodynamic therapy: Past, present and future." *Photodiagnosis and Photodynamic Therapy*, Vol. 1, 2004, pp. 43–48.

[26] McCaughan, J. S., and Williams, T. E. "Photodynamic Therapy for endobronchial malignant disease; a prospective 14 year study." *J Thorac Cardiovasc Surg*, Vol. 114, 1997, pp. 940–947.

[27] Moghissi, K., and Dixon, K. "Is bronchoscopic photodynamic therapy a therapeutic option in lung cancer?" *Eur Resp J*, Vol. 22, 2003, pp. 535–541.

[28] Moghissi, K., Dixon, K., and Stringer, M., et al. "The place of bronchoscopic photodynamic therapy in advanced unresectable lung cancer: Experience of 100 cases." *Eur J Cardiothorac Surg*, Vol. 15, 1999, pp. 1–6.

[29] Kato, H. "Photodynamic Therapy for lung cancer—A review of 19 years experience." *J Photochem Photobiol B*, Vol. 42, 1998, pp. 96–99.

[30] Hung, J., Lam, S., and Le Riche, J. C., et al. "Autofluorescence of normal and malignant bronchial tissue." *Lasers Surg Med*, Vol. 11, 1991, pp. 99–105.

[31] Lam, S., MacAulay, C., and Hung, J., et al. "Detection of dysplasia and carcinoma in situ with a lung imaging fluorescence endoscopy device." *J Thorac Cardiovasc Surg*, Vol 105, 1993, pp.1035–1040.

[32] Thiberville, L., Sutedja, T. G., and Vermijlen, P. "A multi centre European study using the light induced fluorescence endoscopy system to detect pre cancerous lesions in high-risk individuals." *Eur Resp J*, Vol. 14, 1999, pp. 2475.

[33] Iwamoto, Y., Miyazawa, T., and Kurimoto, N., et al. "Endobronchial ultrasonography in the assessment of centrally located early stage lung cancer before photodynamic therapy." *Am J Respir Crit Care Med*, Vol. 165, 2002, pp. 832–837.

[34] Herth, F., Becker, H. D., and LoCicero, J., et al. "Endobronchial ultrasound in therapeutic bronchoscopy." *Eur Respir J*, Vol. 1, 2002, pp. 118–121.

[35] Feller-Kopman, D., Lunn, W., and Ernst, A. "Autofluorescence bronchoscopy and endobronchial ultrasound: a practical review." *Ann Thorac Surg*, Vol. 80, 2005, pp. 2395–2401.

[36] Moghissi, K., Dixon, K., and Thorpe, J. A. C., et al. "Photodynamic Therapy in early central lung cancer: a treatment option for patients ineligible for surgical resection." *Thorax*, Vol. 65, 2007, pp. 391–395.

[37] Moghissi, K., and Thorpe, J. A. C. "Bronchoscopy," in *Moghissi's Essentials of Thoracic & Cardiac Surgery*, 2nd Edition. K. Moghissi, J. A. C. Thorpe, and F. Ciulli (eds.). Elsevier, 2003, pp. 17–23.

[38] Moghissi, K. Dixon, K., and Thorpe, J. A. C., et al. "Photodynamic therapy for lung cancer: The Yorkshire Laser Centre experience." *Photodiagnosis and Photodynamic Therapy*, Vol. 1, 2004, pp. 253–262.

[39] Kato, H., Konaka, C., and Ono, J., et al. "Preoperative laser photodynamic therapy in combination with operation in lung cancer." *J Thorac Cardiovasc Surg*, Vol. 90, 1985, pp. 420–429.

[40] Mortman, K. D., and Frankel, K. M. "Pulmonary resection after successful downstaging with photodynamic therapy." *Ann Thorac Surg*, Vol. 82, 2006, pp. 722–724.

[41] Ross, P. Jr., Grecula, J., and Bekaii-Saab, T., et al., "Incorporation of photodynamic therapy as an induction modality in non small cell lung cancer." *Lasers Surg Med*, Vol. 38, 2006, pp. 881–889.

[42] Moghissi, K., Dixon, K., and Hudson, E., et al., "Endoscopic laser therapy in malignant tracheobronchial obstruction using sequential NdYAG laser and photodynamic therapy." *Thorax*, Vol. 52, 1997, pp. 281–283.

[43] Freitag, L., Ernst, A., and Thomas, M., et al., "Sequential photodynamic therapy and high dose brachytherapy for endobronchial tumour control in patients with limited bronchogenic tumour." *Thorax*, Vol. 59, 2004, pp. 790–793.

[44] Okunaka, T., Kato, H., and Tsutsui, H., et al. "Photodynamic therapy for peripheral lung cancer." *Lung Cancer*, Vol. 43, 2004, pp. 77–82.

[45] Kato, H., Harada, M., and Ichinose, S., et al. "Photodynamic Therapy of lung cancer: experience of the Tokyo Medical University." *Photodiagnosis and Photodynamic Therapy*, Vol. 1, 2004, pp. 49–55.

[46] Moghissi, K., Dixon, K., and Thorpe, J. A. C. "A technique for video assisted thoracoscopic Photodynamic Therapy (PDT)." *Interactive Cardiovascular and Thoracic Surgery*, Vol. 2, 2003, pp. 373–375.

CHAPTER 24

Photodynamic Therapy of the Gastrointestinal Tract Beyond the Esophagus

Drew Schembre

24.1 Introduction

Photodynamic therapy can be applied to virtually every tissue that can be exposed to light. Because the GI tract is relatively accessible, these organs have become prime targets for PDT. Within the GI tract, the esophagus has been the most frequently targeted organ because of the ease of access and because Barrett's esophagus is a recognizable and potentially reversible precancerous condition. The principles that enable PDT to be effective in the esophagus remain the same throughout the GI tract. The three-pronged effect of direct tissue toxicity, microvascular thrombosis, and enhanced immune response to tumor cells as a result of PDT occurs in the stomach, duodenum, and colon as well as in the biliary tree and the pancreas. Although the experience in these areas is less extensive than in the esophagus, many early and more recent studies have demonstrated the potential for therapy in these locations. Availability of other treatments, such as mucosal resection, more precise thermal ablative therapies, and limited surgery have narrowed the scope of application for PDT in the stomach and colon; however, the paucity of other effective treatments has greatly increased the interest in PDT in the biliary system and in the pancreas.

This chapter explores the experience of PDT in the stomach, small bowel, bile ducts, pancreas, and colon.

24.2 Stomach

Each year, gastric cancer affects almost a million people worldwide and results in approximately 650,000 deaths. In the United States, over 20,000 individuals are diagnosed with the disease annually and over 11,000 are expected to die from it [1]. Survival has improved slightly as a result of declining incidence and significant advances in surgical therapy and adjuvant care. The overall five-year survival rate for all stages was 22% between 1996 and 2002, compared to 15% between 1975 and 1977 [2]. Surgery still offers the only reasonable chance for long-term survival for patients with localized, noninvasive disease. Chemotherapy or chemo-radiotherapy either before surgery or after probably improves survival [3]. Unfortunately, at the time of diagnosis, two-thirds of patients will have advanced disease. In contrast, in Japan, where gastric cancer is common, widespread screening programs have been initiated and this has resulted in a much higher rate of detection of gastric cancer at earlier and more treatable stages [4].

Curative approaches for gastric cancer have traditionally relied on surgery via either partial or total gastrectomy to remove all demonstrable disease. Further staging is done by inspecting and washing the peritoneum and harvesting lymph nodes in order to detect metastatic disease. Surgical mortality in the setting of gastric cancer ranges from 4% to 10% with morbidity ranging from 20% to 40% [5]. With improved imaging modalities such as high resolution, CT scanning, positron emission tomography, and endoscopic ultrasound, surgical staging alone is relied upon less commonly. Because detection of disease limited to the mucosa is rarely associated with lymph node or distant metastases [6], newer therapies for early stage disease has involved less radical surgery and more endoscopic therapy. Early enthusiasm for PDT in this setting has been eclipsed, at least in Japan, by the rapid application of endoscopic mucosal resection (EMR) and endoscopic submucosal dissection (ESD) techniques. Nevertheless, interest remains high for PDT to augment EMR/ESD and for use in areas of the stomach such as the cardia and proximal lesser curve not easily approachable by other endoscopic techniques.

Early clinical studies of PDT in the stomach suggested great promise but were marred by small numbers, limited follow-up, and variable outcome measures. For instance, one early study suggested a 100% response rate for gastric cancers treated with hematoporphyrin derivative (HPD) or dihematoporphyrin ethers and esters (DHE) but follow-up was only 2 to 19 months [7]. Another study reported using HPD 2.5 to 3 mg/kg followed by illumination at 628 nm with a pulsed gold vapor laser at 90 J/cm, resulting in a local cure of early gastric cancer in seven of eight patients [8]. Nakamura et al. also reported using DHE to treat seven patients with early gastric cancer, resulting in a complete response in all patients [9]. In a large study, also from Japan, 120 patients treated with a variety of protocols at seven hospitals, reportedly resulted in 100% response, although cancer recurred in 23% of patients within several months [10].

Uncertain pretreatment staging also plagued many early studies. Many patients in these series did not undergo pretreatment EUS and some may have harbored invasive or metastatic disease at the time of treatment. In addition, early photosensitizers and light sources may have resulted in undertreatment of a number of patients. For instance, Mimura et al., reported two groups of patients with early gastric cancer sensitized with either HPD or DHE but treated with different light sources. Those treated with an argon dye laser (ADL, Spectra-Physics, Mountain View, CA) achieved a cure in 13 of 23 (57%) of mucosal cancers, 10 of 19 (53%) submucosal cancers, and 0 of 2 cancers involving the muscularis propria. Among the group that was treated with an Excimer dye laser (EDL, Hamamatsu Photonics, Hamamatsu,

Japan), 15 of 15 (100%) superficial cancers, 9 of 12 (75%) submucosal cancers, and 1 of 5 (20%) T2 lesions were cured [11].

While cylindrical diffusing fibers are ideal in the esophagus and other tubular viscera, the stomach, with its greater size and variable shape, is more suited to treatment with a linear projecting microlens fiber that targets lesions much like a flashlight or a traditional thermal laser. These fibers have a fixed focal length, usually about 10 mm, and have a treatment diameter of about the same size. Because most lesions appropriate for PDT are relatively small, the target area may be encompassed by two or more overlapping treatment areas [12]. A shape-memory loop has been developed to mark a 2-cm diameter area of gastric mucosa, allowing the area to be treated with PDT in a more consistent manner. One small study suggested this approach yields better results [13].

Dosimetry and wavelength depend upon the photosensitizer used. Optimal treatment results in complete or nearly complete necrosis of the mucosal layer while delivering little additional energy to the submucosa, muscularis, and serosa. For porfimer sodium and amino leuvulinic acid, light doses of 200 to 300 J/cm^2 at 630 nm will usually cause complete mucosal destruction, while m-tetrahydroxyphenyl chlorin (mTHPC) requires only about 20 J/cm^2 at 652 nm to cause similar tissue damage [14]. Higher wavelengths are associated with deeper tissue penetration. While amino leuvulinic acid (ALA) may have an application for treating dysplastic mucosa in the esophagus, it appears to be less useful in the stomach. In one study of treatment of precancerous lesions in the stomach, a complete response was achieved in only 2 of 7 cases [15]. This may have been in part due to inadequate light exposure but highlights the difficulty of treating the stomach with its many contours and undulations, especially with a mild photosensitizer. At the other extreme, Ell et al. treated 22 patients with early gastric cancers with mTHPC at 0.075 mg/kg followed 96 hours later with illumination at 652 nm to provide 20 J/cm^2. This resulted in a complete remission in 16 of 22 patients (73%) that persisted at follow-up of 12 to 20 months. No severe reactions were reported, although skin photosensitivity was noted in 7 patients and 12 reported transient abdominal pain [16].

Palliation of gastric cancer with PDT has been less well studied. Limited proximal gastric cancers causing dysphagia can be treated much like esophageal cancers, with circumferential PDT via a cylindrical diffusing fiber. However, because established cancers of the stomach tend to infiltrate deeply and broadly, most palliative attempts with PDT in the stomach are likely to be minimally successful, if at all. Bulky obstructing lesions are probably better treated with expandable stents. The exception may be in the treatment of bleeding associated with bulky luminal tumors. Yanai et al. reported using a combination of PDT plus an infusion of activated autologous T lymphocytes to control aggressive oozing in two elderly patients with unresectable gastric cancers [17]. These patients went on to live for 14 and 32 months without significant further bleeding. At our own institution, we have used PDT to control chronic oozing in three individuals with gastric cardia, rectal, and duodenal cancers and eliminated the need for subsequent blood transfusions in each case (unpublished data).

24.3   Duodenum and Ampulla

Duodenal and other small bowel cancers are rare. New cases occur in fewer than 6,000 patients in the United States each year and lead to death in about half of these cases.

Despite the length of the small intestine, these malignancies account for only 2% of all gastrointestinal cancers, and less than 0.4% of all cancers in the United States [18]. Several conditions including Peutz-Jeghers syndrome, Gardner's syndrome and other familial polyposis syndromes, celiac disease, immunodeficiency states, Crohn's disease, and other autoimmune increase the risk of developing small bowel malignancies.

Risk factors for duodenal and other small bowel cancers are poorly characterized, but probably include dietary factors, cigarette smoking, alcohol intake, and obesity [19].

Unfortunately, most duodenal cancers present late with either bleeding, jaundice, or gastric outlet obstruction. At all but the most superficial stage, surgery offers the only chance of cure. In one study, patients with nonampullary carcinoma of the duodenum showed an overall 5-year survival rate of 54% [20]. Survival in stage I disease is close to 100% while in stage IV it is virtually 0%.

Palliative surgery by performing a gastrojejunal bypass as well as a biliary diversion or combined endoscopic biliary and duodenal stenting are common approaches to obstructive problems associated with late-stage disease. Palliative PDT, except for bleeding, has not been described in this setting and is unlikely to be successful. PDT for early duodenal and ampullary cancers and advanced adenomas has been described in a handful of case reports. Regula et al. reported using ALA PDT to identify and treat three duodenal adenomas and three ampullary carcinomas with at 50 to 100 J/cm^2 [21]. While ALA allowed identification of all lesions via photoporphyrin IX fluorescence, only minimal necrosis was seen. This was probably a result of the combination of the superficial effect of ALA sensitization plus low-light energy delivery. In another study, six patients with duodenal polyps treated with DHE, 2.5 mg/kg followed by illumination at 200 J/cm^2 led to the eradication of small (<3 mm) polyps, over half of flat polyps ranging from 4 to 10 mm but less than half of sessile polyps between 4 and 10 mm. Side effects included one case of pancreatitis and a transient elevation of liver function tests in five of six individuals [22].

About 60% of individuals with familial andenomatous polyposis syndromes (FAP) develop duodenal and ampullary polyps, and left untreated, many will progress to cancer. Duodenal and other small bowel cancers represent a leading cause of premature death in FAP patients who have undergone prophylactic colectomy [23]. Mlkvy et al. reported treating six patients with FAP and duodenal and rectal stump polyps with ALA or DHE PDT. Follow-up was short; however lesions treated with DHE PDT appeared to respond better [24]. Abulafi et al. treated 10 patients with ampullary cancers who were unfit for surgery with HPD at the high dose of 4 mg/kg followed by illumination at 630 nm to 50 to 200 J/cm^2 and repeated this at 3- to 6-month intervals, up to five times [25]. Three patients sustained a complete response while four patients had decreased tumor bulk and three showed no change. The only side effect noted was skin photosensitivity in three patients.

As in the stomach, endoscopic mucosal resection and endoscopic ampullectomy have been used increasingly to treat early-stage duodenal cancers and dysplastic adenomas. It is unclear whether PDT will have a large or lasting impact in the treatment of small bowel neoplasms or be relegated to footnote status, reserved primarily for multifocal disease of polyposis syndromes.

24.4 Biliary System

Cholangiocarcinoma (CCa) occurs rarely in the United States. With an incidence of about 1/100,000 it accounts for approximately 3% of all gastrointestinal malignancies [26]. These cancers arise from cholangiocytes, the cells that line the bile ducts and result in high mortality because they tend to present insidiously and late. Intrahepatic lesions may present with nonspecific symptoms such as weight loss, abdominal pain, or malaise while those with extrahepatic involvement typically present with jaundice. Tumors may spread widely in the biliary system before diagnosis and only about 20% to 30% of patients will be candidates for potentially curative surgery at presentation [27]. Median survival without treatment is only about 3 to 6 months, with death usually resulting from liver failure or cholangitis due to biliary obstruction (Figure 24.3). Unlike many other GI tumors, death often occurs in the setting of a relatively small tumor load, often well before the cancer spreads outside of the biliary system. Chemotherapy has historically been ineffective, although more recent, small series have suggested at least some benefit in selected patients [28]. Treatment is further limited by the liver's sensitivity to radiation. Liver transplantation has been curative in small series [29].

Risk factors for CCa include primary sclerosing cholangitis (PSC), which often occurs in conjunction with inflammatory bowel disease, especially ulcerative colitis, choledochal cysts, chronic intraductal stones, parasitic infections, and exposure to certain industrial chemicals. Chronic viral hepatitis, excessive alcohol use, and obesity may also increase risk [30]. Genetic predisposition may exist but has not been well characterized. Most patients who contract the disease have no obvious risk factors. Biliary tract cancers occur more frequently in older people, with most cases occurring in individuals between 50 and 70 years of age. Diagnosis depends on a high index of suspicion as cross-sectional imaging is often inconclusive. CT and MR scanning may demonstrate intrahepatic masses, but often fail to show extrahepatic malignant strictures, except by revealing upstream dilation. Biliary brushings and even intraductal biopsies obtained at endoscopic retrograde cholangiography are often non-diagnostic due to the inflammatory nature of the tumor [31]. Brush cytology alone has shown sensitivity of less than 25% [32], while adding intraductal pinch biopsy increases the yield to between 36% and 38% [33]. Per-oral cholangioscopy may further increase sensitivity to over 50%, but is limited to specialized centers. Targeting the primary lesion or suspicious local lymph nodes via endoscopic ultrasound-directed fine-needle aspiration may provide the highest yields with sensitivity reported between 43% and 86% [34].

Staging is described by the TMN system, but the older Bismuth-Corlette classification system is still widely used largely because it describes potential resectability (Figure 24.1). Surgical resection has been associated with perioperative mortality of

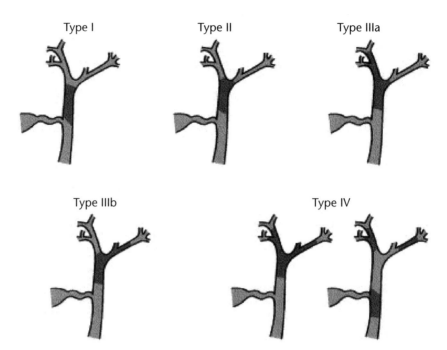

Figure 24.1   Bismuth-Corlette classification system.

5% to 10% and morbidity over 50% [35]. Even after resection with negative margins, survival after surgery for CCa has been reported at 69% after the first year and drops to between 19% and 47% at 5 years [36]. More recently, liver transplantation has been utilized in selected cases to treat unresectable CCa with 2- and 5-year survival rates of 48% and 23%, respectively [37].

Nonsurgical treatment has relied on establishing adequate biliary drainage. Endoscopic drainage has become the mainstay of minimally invasive therapy, although percutaneous drainage may be more widely available and is still occasionally required for some advanced lesions. Surgical drainage, while effective, has been associated with significant morbidity and mortality with survival only equivalent to less invasive methods [38]. The goal of drainage is palliative, but can relieve cholangitis, pruritis, and jaundice, preserve liver function, and ultimately prolong survival. It appears that expandable metal stents probably provide superior palliation than plastic stents because they tend to stay patent longer, migrate less frequently, and therefore require fewer repeat interventions [39]. It is less clear whether bilateral metal stents, provide better palliation in terms of liver function or length of survival than unilateral drainage [40].

Because early mortality from CCa often results from biliary obstruction (Color Plate 34) and not from tumor load, and because tumor-laden ducts are generally accessible via endoscopy or percutanous drainage (PTBD), PDT should offer a reasonable option for palliation for this disease.

Case reports of PDT for CCa began emerging in the 1990s [41], but it was not until Ortner et al. published their first experience with PDT versus endoscopic stenting alone for CCa in 1998 that the therapy received widespread attention [42]. In this uncontrolled, observational pilot study, nine patients with inoperable, Bismuth type III/IV CCa were treated with PDT endoscopically via a "mother-daughter scope" and were compared to three patients treated only by endoscopic stent drainage. Study endpoints were survival, resolution, of jaundice and quality of life. Photosensitization was achieved with porfimer sodium (Photofrin, Axcan Scandipharm, Mont Saint-Hilaire, Quebec, Canada), 2 mg/kg and red light at 630 nm was applied via endoscopically placed cylindrical diffusing fibers with 2.5 and 4 cm tips to deliver 180 J/cm^2 of energy. All patients received endoscopically placed plastic stents after treatment. At 2 months, serum bilirubin in the PDT group fell by 67% (318 ±72 to 103 ±35 nmol/L) and the Karnofsky performance index increased from 32% to 69% (p = 0.008). Median survival was 439 days in the PDT group compared with only 74 days in the control group (p<0.05). The PDT group demonstrated 0% 30-day mortality and 1-year survival was 78%. Side effects in the PDT group were limited to minor skin hyperpigmentation in all patients and fever and abdominal pain in one patient.

This study was followed 5 years later by the publication by the same authors of a multicenter, randomized controlled study of PDT plus stenting versus stenting alone for unresectable cholangiocarcinoma [43]. Seventy patients were enrolled in this study. Twenty were randomized to PDT via a treatment protocol identical to their initial study, porfimer sodium, 2 mg/kg, followed by 180 J/cm^2 delivered by an endoscopically or percutaneously placed light fiber at 630 nm, followed by bilateral plastic stenting. Nineteen were randomized to bilateral plastic stenting alone. Thirty-one patients who either refused consent to randomization or were otherwise excluded were followed in an open arm, consisting of PDT plus stenting. Patients underwent a mean of 1.5 PDT treatments (range: 1–4) and had bilateral, 15-cm plastic stents changed every 3 months. The results were dramatic. Median survival in the PDT+stenting group was 493 days compared to only 98 days in the stenting alone group (p<0.0001). The PDT+stenting group also experienced an increased quality of life based on Karnofsky performance scores and better biliary drainage. Further, survival in the open label group was similar to the PDT+stenting arm with median survival of 426 days. The study was terminated early due to the quickly apparent survival difference between the groups. There were no treatment-related deaths but cholangitis and skin photosensitivity were more frequent in the PDT group.

Other studies have shown similar, if less dramatic results. Witzigmann et al. treated 68 patients with sodium porfimer PDT followed by stenting and compared them to 56 patients treated with stenting alone [44]. Eight patients in the PDT group and six in the stenting group also received chemotherapy and/or radiotherapy. Median survival in the PDT group was 12 months, compared to 6.4 months in the stent alone group (p<0.01). Biliary drainage and Karnofsky performance scores were also significantly better among the PDT group. Interestingly, survival in the PDT group was statistically indistinguishable from 18 patients who underwent surgical therapy but were found to have incomplete resections histologically. Zoepf et al. conducted a randomized trial of 32 patients with cholangiocarcinoma, half of whom were treated with a newer hematoporphyrin derivative, Photosan-3®

(SeeLab, Wesselburenerkoog, Germany), 2 mg/kg followed by irradiation at 633 nm via diode laser at 200 J/cm^2, followed by plastic stenting versus stenting alone [45]. Among the PDT group, nine underwent a second course of treatment and one had a third PDT treatment. Stents were generally changed at 3-month intervals in all patients. Median survival for the PDT group was 21 months (3–31 months) compared to 7 months (1–24 months) for the control group (p = 0.01). Cholangitis was more common in the PDT group than in the control group (4 versus 1), which was successfully treated in all cases.

Other studies have followed. Pereira et al. treated 13 patients with malignant biliary obstructions (9 cholangiocarcinomas, 3 pancreatic cancers, and 1 gastric cancer) who already had indwelling metal stents with mTHPC PDT at 0.15 mg/kg followed by plastic stenting [46]. Stents opened in all patients and remained patent for a median of 7 months (range 1–43 months). Median survival in this late-stage treatment group was 8 months after treatment.

At our own institution, we have treated 23 CCa patients with porfimer sodium PDT in a protocol similar to that of Ortner. The difference has been that after treatment, we place metal stents instead of plastic stents (Color Plate 35). Mean survival has been 284 days, which compares favorably to historical controls at Virginia Mason Medical Center. Those who have undergone metal stenting alone have survived an average of 194 days (p = 0.19). However, when we compared PDT patients to those who underwent chemo or chemoradiotherapy, PDT appears less effective. The chemo/chemoradiotherapy group has demonstrated a mean survival of 401 days (p = 0.14). Ultimately, two patients died from treatment in the chemotherapy group while there were no major complications in the PDT group. Even though neither comparison reaches statistical significance—likely due to small numbers and possibly patient selection—the trends are compelling. We have now begun to use PDT+stenting in conjunction with chemotherapy and occasionally radiotherapy in suitable candidates with unresectable CCa with the belief that PDT will help control biliary drainage and maximal systemic therapy can then be given to patients who have preserved liver function. In the most recent large study from the United States, Kahaleh, et al. showed a significant survival benefit among 19 patients treated with porfimer sodium PDT plus plastic stents versus 29 who were treated with stents alone [47]. Interestingly, in this study, over half of the participants in each arm received chemo or chemo-radiotherapy as well. Mean and median survival were 16.2 months and 8 months in the PDT group compared to 7.4 and 5 months in the control group. Cholangitis occurred in over a third of patients in both arms, resulting in 2 deaths in the control arm. Additional studies and their results are shown in Table 24.1.

PDT represents one of the most promising palliative therapies for CCa available today. The debate over which photosensitizers, what type of stenting, and what additional therapy, if any, are needed, will continue. Hopefully, additional studies will help clarify some of these issues. However, the relative rarity of the cancer makes large, controlled studies difficult. Further, the lack of FDA approval for any photosensitizer for this indication limits patient options in the United States. Hopefully as awareness of the benefits of PDT for this disease grows, pressure will build to change this.

Table 24.1 Published Clinical Trials of PDT for Bile Duct Cancer.

Study and Year	Number of Patients	Number of Treatments	Stent Type	Dosimetry	Median Survival: Treatment (Days)	Median Survival: Control (Days)
Ortner et al. 1998	9	14	Plastic	180 J/cm^2	439	74
Berr et al. 2000	23	63	Plastic	242 J/cm^2	350	
Rumalla et al. 2001	6	14	Plastic	180 J/cm^2	199	
Dumoulin et al. 2003	24	24	Metal	200 J/cm^2	297	168*
Ortner et al. 2003	51	110	Plastic	180 J/cm^2	493	98
Wiedemann et al. 2004	23	73	Mixed	242 J/cm^2	288	
Schembre et al. 2007	23	25	Metal	180 J/cm^2	284	194*

*Historical at the same institution.

24.5 Pancreas

Pancreatic cancer remains a particularly lethal disease. Adenocarcinoma of the pancreas will affect about 34,000 individuals in the United States in 2007, and the vast majority of them will die from it [48]. Surgical resection affords the only real chance at cure, however only about 20% of newly diagnosed pancreas cancer patients can undergo definitive surgery. About 40% will have metastatic disease at presentation, and another 40% will have locally advanced unresectable tumors. Median survival is 8 to 12 months for those with locally advanced disease, and less for those with metastatic disease. Even among those who undergo successful surgery, 5-year survival is only 25% to 30% among patients with node negative disease and about 10% in those with positive nodes [49]. Only recently have positive results emerged in trials of chemo and chemoradiotherapy, and these have been modest, extending average survival by perhaps 6 months, often in exchange for the risk of significant toxicity [50].

For these reasons, interest has emerged for using PDT to ablate small pancreatic tumors or to debulk large ones. Early ex vivo studies suggested that PDT can have a toxic effect of pancreatic cancer cells [52]. In addition, PDT may initiate an immune response by the host to surviving cancer cells [51]. Regula et al. showed that hamsters with transplanted human pancreas tumors survived longer after ALA PDT than untreated hamsters [54]. Further, the photosensitizer HPD and others appear to accumulate preferentially in pancreatic cancer cells compared to the healthy pancreas [53]. The photosensitizer mTHPC when used in animals created large areas of necrosis but also appeared to affect viscera, leading to duodenal perforations [56]. Additional hamster studies showed that the photosensitizer verteporfin has properties similar to mTHPC. But when used at 2 mg/kg and combined with light does of 10, 25, and 50 J/cm^2, local areas of coagulative necrosis developed but the treatment was generally safe for liver, healthy pancreas, and colon [55]. Nevertheless, even with this treatment, focal areas of sealed duodenal perforations were encountered.

Unlike luminal tumors, the pancreas poses a special problem, as bulky tumors are often not approachable via the usual endoscopic means, even via pancreatoscopy. Bown et al. worked around this problem in the first phase I trial of PDT for pancreatic cancer in humans by approaching the tumors percutaneously [58]. This group implanted a series of 19-gauge needles under CT guidance into unresectable pancreatic cancers in 16 patients who had been sensitized with 0.15 mg/kg of mTHPC. Tumors were irradiated with 652-nm red light delivered through thin diffusing fibers with 3-mm tip exposure that had been passed through the probes. Total energy delivered was between 40J and 480J (median 240J). All patients demonstrated substantial tumor necrosis by CT scan at 2 weeks. Two patients experienced significant bleeds from the gastroduodenal artery as a result of local necrosis. Both of these bleeds were controlled nonsurgically, either endoscopically or angiographically. The maximum elevation in amylase was 2.8 times the upper limit of normal with no patient demonstrating clinical pancreatitis. Median survival was 9.5 months with 7 of 16 surviving over 1 year. These results have been encouraging. As it is often the case in gastroenterology, once a percutaneous technique has been described, it is not long before someone tries to do it endoscopically. Such was the case with Chan et al., who demonstrated successful light delivery and subsequent PDT to the pancreas as well as liver, kidney, and spleen via EUS-guided 19-gauge needles in pigs [57].

PDT for pancreatic cancer remains in its infancy. New photosensitizers will likely be developed with further specificity for pancreatic tumors and new targeting and delivery systems for light will undoubtedly be developed. Although the process may be long and difficult, the continued poor survival of most patients diagnosed with pancreatic cancer underscores the need for additional studies of PDT in this potentially very promising area.

24.6   Colon and Rectal Cancers

Despite the success of screening programs and public awareness that colon cancer can be cured and even prevented by colonoscopy, colon cancer still accounts for 10% of all cancer deaths in the United States [59]. About 150,000 new cases of colon cancer are diagnosed each year in the United States, of which about two-thirds arise in the colon and the remainder in the rectum. In 2007, more than 55,000 individuals were estimated to die of the disease, making it the second leading cause of cancer death after lung cancer and third both in frequency and cause of cancer death, behind prostate cancer in men and breast cancer in women. Risk factors include genetic factors such as polyposis syndromes such as familial adenomatous polyposis (FAP), Lynch syndrome and others, medical conditions such as inflammatory bowel disease, obesity, prior cholecystectomy, and diabetes and likely certain environmental factors such as alcohol, cigarette smoking, prior irradiation, low-fiber and high-fat diets. Although family history results in the greatest increases in risk, the majority of colon cancers are sporadic and occur in people with no obvious risk factors. Protective factors might include a low-fat, high-fiber diet, the use of aspirin or NSAIDs, as well as the use of statins and folic acid.

The idea of using PDT for curing early colon and rectal cancers and palliating advanced ones has been around for many years. Animal studies have shown that colon cancers can be readily sensitized for PDT and that the colon wall can withstand high levels of energy without perforation [60]. Despite this, the clinical application of PDT in the colon has been limited, perhaps due to the relative ease and reliability of polypectomy for large polyps, surgical resection for localized cancer, and endoluminal stenting for palliating advanced disease.

Numerous case reports and small studies, many from 20 years ago or more, have looked at using PDT to eradicate colon polyps as well as to palliate bulky colon and rectal cancers. Like many other small PDT studies, these suffer from a lack of consistent treatment and standard outcomes, small numbers, and short follow-up. Nevertheless, some valuable information can be gleaned from these reports.

Technical success in treating villous adenomas of the colon with PDT has been reported. In one of the first studies, McLaughen et al., treated eight patients with rectal cancers with dihematophorphyrin ether and reported an average survival of 16 months after treatment [61]. In another early study, HPD was used to treat nine villous adenomas in eight patients previously incompletely treated with Nd:YAG laser ablation [62]. Seven polyps were completely eradicated and there were no significant complications. Additional reports cited success from combining polypectomy with PDT in broad, flat polyps [63]. Two patients with FAP and extensive rectal polyps following subtotal colectomy underwent treatment with porfimer sodium PDT with reported clearance of the majority of polyps [64]. A Bulgarian case report describes a patient with an advanced colon cancer treated with HPD at 5 mg/kg then subjected to 350 J/cm^2 red light at 630 nm, which led to complete tumor ablation that persisted for 12 months [65]. In a U.K. study of 10 nonsurgical patients with colorectal cancers treated with HPD at 2.5 mg/kg, the two patients with small cancers had complete responses while those with bulky tumors did less well [66]. Patients with larger cancers experienced minor debulking but demonstrated persistent symptoms such as pain and urgency and one patient experienced posttreatment bleeding. In a French report of 21 patients with rectosigmoid cancers treated with HPD plus 200 J/cm^2, 50% demonstrated an initial complete response [67]. Similarly, Spinelli et al. reported technical success treating 27 patients with advanced or obstructing distal colon cancers, although follow-up was short and endpoints were not clearly defined [68].

Other studies have shown less positive results. Of 14 patients with residual or recurrent colorectal cancer in the pelvis treated with PDT with DHP, only two showed a prolonged complete response, although several others reported decreased pain and urgency [69]. In a large study of 93 patients with inoperable colon cancers, including 18 with large polyps, PDT using porfimer sodium was found to be less effective than Nd:YAG laser ablation for debulking large tumors [70].

PDT has also been used to try to reduce local recurrence of colon cancer by treating the operative field during surgery [71]. Unfortunately, there has been no clear improvement demonstrated in reduction of local recurrence or a difference in survival.

Novel therapies have been designed to treat colon cancer metastatic to the liver. In a report by Vogel et al., nine patients with liver metastases from colon cancer were treated with HPBC followed by percutaneous laser light illumination. This resulted in discrete, 1.5-cm areas of necrosis surrounding each treatment area, resulting in a complete response in five patients. The only side effects noted were two cases of cutaneous photosensitivity [72]. PDT has also been used to treat uncontrolled bleeding associated with rectal cancers. Four patients who had failed other therapies responded to dihematophorphyrin ether PDT [73]. HPD HPD PDT has also been used to treat bleeding associated with radiation proctitis [74].

As endoscopic techniques continue to improve and stent technology advances, PDT for colon and rectal cancer will likely be reserved for a few indications such as low rectal tumors associated with bleeding and urgency. This may change if newer, more potent, and more specific photosensitizers are developed. Animal studies have shown that photosensitizers can be linked to specific molecules such as carcinoembrionic antigen (CEA) and granulocyte stimulating factor in an attempt to further focus the phototoxic effects of treatment [75, 76]. Research in these areas as well as in new therapies for metastatic lesions may herald a resurgence for PDT in the lower gastrointestinal tract.

24.7　Conclusion

Effective PDT in the gastrointestinal system is clearly not limited to just the esophagus. While early enthusiasm for treatments in the stomach and colon has been eclipsed to some degree by new, aggressive endoscopic therapies, promising applications have emerged in the pacreaticobiliary system. Despite lack of regulatory approval, PDT for unresectable cholangiocarcinoma appears to be the most beneficial therapy currently available. Additional therapies for noncancer conditions of the alimentary tract are emerging as well. Continued research and further evolution of photosensitizers and illumination techniques will likely expand potential applications for PDT in the gastrointestinal tract.

References

[1] Jemal, A., et al., "Cancer Statistics," *CA Cancer J. Clin.*, Vol. 57, 2007, p. 43.

[2] Lau, M., A. Le, and H. B. El-Serag, "Noncardia Gastric Adenocarcinoma Remains an Important and Deadly Cancer in the United States: Secular Trends in Incidence and Survival," *Am. J. Gastroenterol*, Vol. 101, pp. 2485–2492.

[3] MacDonald, J. S., et al., "Chemoradiotherapy after surgery compared with surgery alone for adenocarcinoma of the stomach or gastroesophageal junction," *N. Engl. J. Med.*, Vol. 345, 2001, pp. 725–730.

[4] Yoshida, S., and Saito, D., "Gastric premalignancy and cancer screening in high-risk patients," *Am. J. Gastroenterol.*, Vol. 91, 1996, pp. 839–843.

[5] Bonenkamp, J. J., et al. "Randomised comparison of morbitity after D1 and D2 dissection for gasric cancer in 996 Dutch patients," *Lancet*, Vol. 345, 1995, pp.745–748.

[6] Baba, H, et al., "Lymph node metastasis and macroscopic features in early gastric cancer," *Gastroenterol. Hepatol.*, Vol. 41, 1994, pp. 380–383.

[7] Mimura S., "Photodynamic therapy for early gastric cancer," *5th International Photodynamic Association Biennial Meeting*, Amelia Island, Florida, 1994.

[8] Nakamura,T., et al., "Photodynamic therapy for early gastric cancer using a pulsed gold vapor laser," *J. Clin. Laser Med. Surg.*, Vol. 8, 1990, pp. 63–67.

[9] Nakamura, H., et al., "Experience with photodynamic therapy for the treatment of early gastric cancer," *Hepato-Gastroenterol.*, Vol. 48, 2001, pp. 1599–603.

[10] Kato, H., et al., "Photodynamic therapy in the early treatment of cancer," *Gan To Kagaku Ryoho*, Vol. 17, 1990, pp. 1833–1838.

[11] Mimura, S., et al., "Photodynamic therapy for gastric cancer," *Gan To Kagaku Ryoho*, Vol. 23, 1996, pp. 41–46.

[12] Gossner, L., and Ell, C., "Photodynamic therapy of gastric cancer," *Gastrointest. Clin. N. Am.*, Vol. 10, 2000, pp. 461–480.

[13] Nakamura, T., et al., "Shape-memory alloy loop snare for endoscopic photodynamic therapy of early gastric cancer," *Endoscopy*, Vol. 32, 2000, pp. 609–613.

[14] Gossner, L., and Ell, C., "Photodynamic therapy of gastric cancer," *Gastrointest. Clin. N. Am.*, Vol. 10, 2000, pp. 461–480.

[15] Smolka, J., et al., "In vivo fluorescence diagnostics and photodynamic therapy of gastrointestinal superficial polyps with aminolevulinic acid. A clinical and spectroscopic study," *Neoplasma*, Vol. 53, 2006, pp. 418–423.

[16] Ell, C., et al., "Photodynamic ablation of early cancers of the stomach by means of mTHPC and laser irradiation: preliminary clinical experience," *Gut*, Vol. 43, 1998, pp. 345–349.

[16] Yanai, H., et al., "The pilot experience of immunotherapy-combined photodynamic therapy for advanced gastric cancer in elderly patients," *Int. J. Gastrointest. Cancer*, Vol. 32, 2002, pp. 139–142.

[18] DiSario, J. A., et al., "Small bowel cancer: epidemiological and clinical characteristics from a population-based registry," *Am. J. Gastroenterol.*, Vol. 89, 1994, pp. 699–701.

[19] Neugut, A. I., et al., "The epidemiology of cancer of the small bowel," *Cancer Epidemiol. Biomarkers Prev.*, Vol. 7, 1998, pp. 243–251.

[20] Barnes, G. Jr., et al., "Primary adenocarcinoma of the duodenum: management and survival in 67 patients," *Ann. Surg. Oncol.*, Vol. 1, 1994, pp. 73–78.

[21] Regula, J., et al., "Photosensitization and photodynamic therapy of oesophageal, duodenal and colorectal tumours using 5 aminolaevulinic acid induced protoporphyrin IX—a pilot study," *Gut*, Vol. 36, 1995, pp. 67–75.

[22] Saurin, J. C., Chayvialle, J. A., and Ponchon, T., "Management of duodenal adenomas in familial adenomatous polyposi," *Endoscopy*, Vol. 31, 1999, pp. 472–478.

[23] Arvanitis, M.L., et al., "Mortality in patients with familial adenomatous polyposis," *Dis Colon & Rectum*, Vol. 33, 1990, pp.639–642

[24] Mlkvy, P., et al., "Photodynamic therapy for polyps in familial adenomatous polyposis—a pilot study," *Eur. J. Cancer*, Vol. 31A, 1995, pp.1160–1165.

[25] Abulafi, A. M., et al., "Photodynamic therapy for malignant tumours of the ampulla of Vater," *Gut*, Vol. 36, 1995, pp. 853–856.

[26] Jemal, A., et al., "Cancer statistics, 2006," *CA Cancer J. Clin.*, Vol. 56, 2006, p. 106.

[27] Nekeeb, A., et al.,"Cholangiocarcinoma: a spectrum of intrahepatic, perihilar, and disal tumors," *Ann. Surg.*, Vol. 224, 1996, pp. 463–73.

[28] Singh, P., and Patel, T., "Advances in the diagnosis, evaluation and management of cholangiocarcinoma," *Curr. Op. Gastroenterol*, Vol. 22, 2006, pp. 294–299.

[29] Malhi, H., and Gores, G. J., "The modern diagnosis and therapy of cholangiocarcinoma," *Alim. Pharm. Therapeut.*, Vol. 26, 2006, pp. 1287–1296

[30] Chapman, R.W., "Risk factors for biliary tract carcinogenesis," *Ann. Oncol.*, Vol. 10 (Suppl.), 1999, pp. 308–311.

[31] Henke, A. C., Jensen, C. S., and Cohen, M. B., "Cytologic diagnosis of adenocarcinoma in biliary and pancreatic duct brushings," *Adv. Anat. Pathol.*, Vol. 9, 2002, pp. 301–308.

[32] Baron, T. H., et al., "A prospective comparison of digital image analysis and routine cytology for the identification of malignancy in biliary tract strictures," *Clin. Gastroenterol. Hepatol.*, Vol. 2, 2004, pp. 214–219.

[33] Rosch, T., et al., "ERCP or EUS for tissue diagnosis of hiliar strictures? A prospective comparative study, " *Gastrointest. Endosc.*, Vol. 60, 2004, pp. 390–396.

[34] Eloubeidi, M. A., et al., "Endoscopic ultrasound-guided fine needle aspiration biopsy of suspected cholangiocarcinoma," *Clin. Gastroenterol. Hepatol.*, Vol. 2, 2004, pp. 209–213.

[35] Jarnagin, W. R., et al., "Staging, resectability, and outcome in 225 patients with hilar cholangiocarcinoma," *Ann. Surg.*, Vol. 235, 2001, pp. 507–517.

[36] Anderson, C. D., et al., "Diagnosis and treatment of cholangiocarcinoma," *Oncologist*, Vol. 9, 2004, pp. 43–57.

[37] Meyer, C. G., Penn, I., and James, L., "Liver transplantation for cholangiocarcinoma: results in 207 patients," *Transplantation*, Vol. 69, 2000, pp. 1633–1637.

[38] Smith, A. C., et al., "Randomized trial of endoscopic stenting versus surgical bypass in malignant low bile duct obstruction," *Lancet*, Vol. 344, 1994, pp. 1655–1660.

[39] Chahal, P., Baron, T. H., "Endoscopic palliation of cholangiocarcinoma," *Curr. Opin. Gastroenterol.*, Vol. 22, 2006, pp. 551–560.

[40] Chang, W. H., et al. "Outcome in patients with bifurcation tumors who undergo unilateral versus bilateral hepatic duct drainage," *Gastrointest. Endosc.*, Vol. 47, 1998, pp. 354–362.

[41] McCaughan, J. S., et al., "PDT to treat tumors of the extrahepatic biliary ducts," *Arch. Surg.*, Vol. 126, 1991, pp. 11–15.

[42] Ortner, M. E., et al., "Photodynamic therapy of nonresectable cholangioccarcinoma," *Gastroenterology*, Vol. 114, 1998, pp. 536–542.

[43] Orner, M. E., et al., "Successful photodynamic therapy for nonresectable cholangiocarcinoma: a randomized prospective study," *Gastroenterology*, Vol. 125, 2003, pp. 1355–1363.

[44] Witzigmann, J., et al., "Surgical and palliative management and outcome in 184 patients with hilar cholangiocarcinoma," *Ann. Surg.*, Vol. 244, 2006, pp. 230–239.

[45] Zoepf, T., et al., "Palliation of nonresectable bile duct cancer: improved survival after photodynamic therapy," *Am. J. Gastro.*, Vol. 100, 2005, pp. 2426–2430.

[46] Pereira, S. P., et al., "Photodynamic therapy of malignant biliary strictures using meso-tetrahydroxyphenylchlorin," *Eur. J. Gastro. Hep.*, Vol. 19, 2007, pp. 479–485.

[47] Khaleh M., et al., "Unresectable cholangiocarcinoma: Comparison of survival in biliary stenting versus stenting with photodynamic therapy," *Clin Gastro Hep*, Vol. 6, 2008, pp. 290–297.

[48] Jemal, A., et al., "Cancer statistics, 2007," *CA Cancer J. Clin.*, Vol. 57, 2007, p. 43.

[49] Trede, M., Schwall, G., and Saeger, H. D., "Survival after pancreatoduodenectomy. 118 consecutive resections without an operative mortality," *Ann. Surg.*, Vol. 211, 1990, pp. 447–458.

[50] Yeo, C. J., et al., "Pancreaticoduodenectomy for pancreatic adenocarcinoma: Postoperative adjuvant chemoradiation improves survival. A prospective, single-institution experience," *Ann. Surg.*, Vol. 225, 1997, pp. 621–636.

[51] Lui, C. D., et al., "Hypericin and photodynamic therapy decreases human pancreatic cancer in vitro and in vivo," *Br. Surg. Res.*, Vol. 93, 2000, pp. 137–143.

[52] Hajri, A., et al., "Human pancreatic carcinoma cells are sensitive to photodynamic therapy in vitro and vivo," *Br. J. Surg.*, Vol. 86, 1999, pp. 899–906.

[53] Regula, J., et al., "Photodynamic therapy using 5-aminolevulinic acid for experimental pancreatic cancer prolonged animal survival," *Br. J. Cancer*, Vol. 70, 1994, pp. 248–254.

[54] Schroder, T., et al., "Hematoporphyrin derivative uptake and photodynamic therapy in pancreatic carcinoma," *J. Surg. Oncol.*, Vol. 38, 1988, pp. 4–9.

[55] Mlky, P., et al., "Distribution and photodynamic effects of meso–tetrahydroxyphenylchlorin (mTHPC) in the pancreas and adjacent tissues in the Syrian golden hamster," *Br. J. Cancer*, Vol. 73, 1996, pp. 1473–1479.

[56] Ayaru, L., et al., "Photodynamic therapy using verteporfin photosensitiztion in the pancreas and surrounding tissues in the Syrian golden hamster," *Pancreatology*, Vol. 7, 2007, pp. 20–27.

[57] Bown, S. G., et al., "Photodynamic therapy for cancer of the pancreas," *Gut*, Vol. 50, 2002, pp. 549–557.

[58] Chan, H. H., et al., "EUS-guided photodynamic therapy of the pancreas: a pilot study," *Gastrointest. Endosc.*, Vol. 59, 2004, pp. 95–99.

[59] Jemal, A., et al., "Cancer statistics, 2006," *CA Cancer J. Clin.*, Vol. 56, 2006, p. 106.

[60] Fisher, D. G., et al. "Colonic mucosectomy using laser photodynamic therapy," *J. Surg. Research*, Vol. 46, 1989, pp. 579–583.

[61] McCaughan, J. S., Jr., "Miscellaneous treatments," in *Photodynamic Therapy for Malignancies: Clinical Manual*, J.S. McCaughan, Jr, (ed.) Austin, TX: *Landes*, 192, pp.135–144.

[62] Loh, C. S., et al., "Photodynamic therapy for villous adenomas of the colon and rectum," *Endosocopy*, Vol. 26, 1994, pp. 243–246.

[63] Nakamura, T., et al., "Photodynamic therapy with polypectomy for rectal cancer," *Gastrointest. Endosc.*, Vol. 57, 2003, pp. 266–269.

[64] Mlkvy, P., et al. "Photodynamic therapy for polyps in familial adenomatous polyposis—a pilot study," *Eur. J. Cancer*, Vol. 31A, 1995, pp. 1160–1165.

[65] Karanov, S., et al., "Photodynamic therapy in lung and gastrointestinal cancers," *J. Photochem. Photobiol. B*, Vol. 6, 1990, pp. 175–181.

[66] Barr, H., et al., "Photodynamic therapy for colorectal cancer: a quantitative pilot study," *Br. J. Surg.*, Vol. 77, 1990, pp. 93–96.

[67] Patrice, T., et al., "Endoscopic photodynamic therapy with haematoporphyrin derivative in gastroenterology," *J. Photochem. Photobiol. B*, Vol. 6, 1990, pp. 157–165.

[68] Spinelli, P., Mancini, A., and Dal Fante, M., "Endoscopic treatment of gastrointestinal tumors: indications and results of laser photocoagulation and photodynamic therapy," *Sem. Surg. Oncol.*, Vol. 11, 1995, pp. 307–318.

[69] Herrera-Ornelas, L., et al., "Photodynamic therapy in patients with colorectal cancer," *Cancer*, Vol. 57, 1986, pp. 677–684.

[70] Krasner, N., "Laser therapy in the management of benign and malignant tumours in the colon and rectum," *Int. J. Colorectal Dis.*, Vol. 4, 1989, pp. 2–5.

[71] Allardice, J. T., et al., "Adjuvant intraoperative photodynamic therapy for colorectal carcinoma: a clinical study," *Surg. Oncol.*, Vol. 3, 1994, pp. 1–10.

[72] Vogl, T., et al., "Interstitial photodynamic laser therapy in interventional oncology," *Eur. Radiol.*, Vol. 14, 2004, pp. 1063–1073.

[73] McCaughan, J. S., et al., "Photodynamic therapy to control life-threatening hemorrhage from hereditary hemorrhagic telangiectasia," *Lasers Surg. Med.*, Vol. 19, 1996, pp.492–494.

[74] Wong Kee Song, L. M., et al., "Photodynamic therapy for management of refractory hemorrhagic radiation proctitis" (abstract), *Gastrointest. Endosc.*, Vol. 47, 1998, p. AB106.

[75] Carcenac, M., et al., "Preparation, phototoxicity and biodistribution studies of anti-carcinoembryonic antigen monoclonal antibody-phthalocyanie conjugates," *Photochem. Photobiol.*, Vol. 70, 1999, pp. 930–936.

[76] Golab, J., et al., "Potentiation of the anti-tumour effects of photofrin-based photodynamic therapy by localized treatment with G-CSF," *Br. J. Cancer.*, Vol. 82, 2000, pp. 1485–1491.

CHAPTER 25

Photodynamic Therapy in the Esophagus

Seth A. Gross and Herbert C. Wolfsen

25.1 Introduction

The photochemical basis of the photodynamic reaction and photodynamic therapy has been reviewed elsewhere in this book. This chapter reviews the use of photodynamic therapy in the treatment of esophageal dysplasia and carcinoma. This work includes some of the best studied and earliest clinical photodynamic therapy (PDT) applications to receive regulatory approval. Initially, most of this work studied the use of porfimer sodium PDT in patients with advanced esophageal cancer [1–3] and led to regulatory approvals in Japan, North America, the United Kingdom, and Europe. Overholt later published the landmark multicenter study using porfimer sodium PDT in Barrett's esophagus patients with high grade dysplasia [4–6].This prospective, randomized, controlled international trial demonstrated significantly reduced rate of invasive carcinoma development in patients treated with porfimer sodium PDT. These studies, and many others, have established the importance of porfimer sodium PDT in the treatment of esophageal dysplasia and neoplasia and supported the development and clinical use of other photosensitizers [7–14].

In the review of clinical PDT studies, there are several issues to consider. First, it is important to remember the underlying disease state and stage of the patient population and the rigor of the diagnostic evaluation. For example, a study performed in patients with Barrett's metaplasia or low-grade dysplasia will be evaluated much differently that a study in patients with high-grade dysplasia or early carcinoma. The very meaning of the term "early esophageal cancer" has changed dramatically in the last decade as the use of endosonography with fine-needle aspiration of lymphadenopathy, endoscopic mucosal resection, high-resolution computed tomography, and positron emission tomography has become routine. Next, it is important to understand the methods used for PDT—the photosensitizer used and its dose and route of administration. Also, the light source and light dose can vary from lasers to filtered lamps or light-emitting diodes. The wavelength of light used is particularly important since red light at 630 nm penetrates the esophageal tissue more deeply than green light at 532 nm. Finally, it is critical to note what other methods of ablation were used in the study. While regulatory trials will only allow the use of PDT, clinical series frequently use "focal" ablation methods (such as radiofrequency energy or argon plasma coagulation) to remove small amounts of residual Barrett's disease that persist after the initial PDT procedure. Regardless of methods used, all PDT specialists agree that it is critically important to remove all

Barrett's glandular metaplasia and dysplasia to prevent the development or recurrence of invasive carcinoma.

25.2   Barrett's Esophagus with High-Grade Dysplasia and Early Cancer

The incidence of esophageal carcinoma, particularly in Western developed countries has continued to steadily increase over the past four decades [15–21]. Barrett's disease is known to be the most important risk factor in the development of dysplasia and progression to esophageal adenocarcinoma [4, 22–28]. Photodynamic therapy is an ideal therapy for esophageal disease including Barrett's esophagus as gastrointestinal endoscopy provides ready access to the target mucosa for laser light application. Depending on the photosensitizer selected and the wavelength and dose of light energy used, PDT permits deep mucosal penetration of light energy to drive the photodynamic reaction with little risk of perforation despite the relatively thin esophageal mucosa and its limited blood supply [29].

After the initial description of porphyrin-based PDT, the use of hematoporphyrin derivative (HpD), and dihematoporphyrin ether (DHE) activated with red light became the predominant form of PDT in the early clinical years [30]. Subsequently, these photosensitizers were better purified and characterized for commercial production in the form of porfimer sodium (Photofrin, Axcan Scandipharm, Mont-Saint-Hilaire, Quebec, Canada) [31]. Surgeons and gastrointestinal endoscopists have utilized the prolonged mucosal retention of porfimer sodium combined with red light activation for deep mucosal and submucosal necrosis in the palliative treatment of advanced, obstructing lesions as well as curative treatment of early cancers. Early clinical studies were performed in patients with advanced carcinoma compared with endoscopic palliation using stents or tumor ablation using thermal lasers. Improved endoscopic light delivery and dosimetry led to the use of porfimer sodium PDT in patients with esophageal dysplasia (squamous dysplasia and Barrett's esophagus with dysplasia). Porfimer sodium is a unique photosensitizer agent that is supported by extensive clinical experience, especially in North America, including a multicenter randomized controlled study using a centralized pathology laboratory with more than 5 years of follow-up data as well as numerous large single-center studies that have documented consistent and reproducible long-term treatment efficacy and safety.

Despite these advantages, porfimer sodium remains a first generation drug that is a relatively inefficient photosensitizer that produces prolonged photosensitivity, typically lasting 4 to 6 weeks. More recently developed photosensitizer agents include meta-tetrahydroxy-phenyl chlorin (mTHPC, temoporfin, Foscan, Biolitec AG, Jena, Germany), a potent photosensitizing agent that requires lower drug and light doses and induces only 2 to 3 weeks of cutaneous photosensitivity. However, previous studies using mTHPC have been associated with higher stricture formation or full-thickness tissue necrosis and perforation. Another photosensitizing agent, aminolevulinic acid (ALA), is converted within the gut mucosa to its active form protoporphyrin IX (PpIX), which is a specific mucosal photosensitizer [32]. Compared with porfimer sodium and mTHPC, ALA accumulates in the surface mucosa targeting ablation at the mucosal layer. This decreases the risk of stricture formation by sparing damage to the deeper esophageal wall and muscle layer [33]. Commercially available preparations of ALA include aminolevulinic acid (Levulan, DUSA Pharmaceuticals, Wilmington, Massachusetts, USA), delta-aminolevulinic acid (Medac Gmbh, Wedel, Germany), and methyl aminolevulinate (Metvix, Photocure ASA, Oslo, Norway). Clinical experience with ALA in the esophagus has produced varied results, particularly in controlled trials performed with other forms of thermal ablation. HPPH or Photochlor is an intriguing pheophorbide photosensitizer owned by the Roswell Park Cancer Institute that features only mild photosensitivity at antitumor doses but has not yet been widely tested in clinical studies [34]. A more complete listing of photosensitizers utilized in esophageal PDT may be found in Table 25.1.

Table 25.1 Types of Photosensitizers for Esophageal PDT

Class	Photosensitizer	Treatment Wavelength (λ nm)	Diagnostic Fluorescence Wavelength (λ nm)	Comments
Porphyrins	Porfimer sodium; also hematoporphyrin derivative (HpD); dihematoporphyrin ether (DHE)	630	665–690	Porfimer sodium excellent red light tissue penetration with risk of stricture and prolonged skin sensitivity (Photofrin); also Photosan
	5-aminolevulinie acid (5-ALA, a precursor of endogenous porphyrins)	630–635	525, 665–690	Limited tissue penetration ($\leq$2 mm); less photosensitivity (Levulan; Metvix)
Chlorins	Meso-tetrahydroxyphenyl chlorin (mTHPC; temoporfin);	650–660 (red) 514 (green)	525	Highly selective, potent 514 (green) compound suitable for less powerful light sources. Approved in EU, Norway, and Iceland (Foscan; biolitec pharma)
	Mono-L-aspartyl chlorin e6 (NPe6; talaporfin or LS11);			Phase III study using LS11 for hepatoma activated with LED, Light Sciences Oncology, Washington, USA
Phthalocyanine	Silicon phthalocyanine (Pc4); aluminum disulphonated phthalocyanine (AISPc); Chloroaluminum phthalocyanine tetrasulfonate (AIPcS4)	675	610	Limited phototoxicity and limited clinical information hydrophobic compounds that are difficult to purify. Selective tumor retention, minimal dark and cutaneous photosensitivity and excellent photodynamic activity are expected (Photosens)

Table 25.1 (continued)

Class	Photosensitizer	Treatment Wavelength (λ nm)	Diagnostic Fluorescence Wavelength (λ nm)	Comments
Benzoporphyrins	Benzoporphyrin derivative (BPD); benzoporphyrin derivative monoacid (BPDMA) Diethylene glycol benzoporphyrin derivative (Lemuteporfin)	690	690	Rapid tumor accumulation; transient limited skin photosensitivity and prominent vascular effects produced approval for use in macular degeneration (Visudyne); new diethylene glycol functionalized chlorin-type photosensitizer [95]
Porphyrin-like compounds	Motoxafin lutetium; lutetium texaphyrin	730–740	730–740	Rapid tissue uptake and clearance along with tissue penetration; used for photochemical angioplasty (Antrin, Lutrin, Lu-Tex)
Pheophorbides: (tetrapyriolea) chlorophyll derivatives	2-[1-hexyloxyethyl] 2-devinyt-pyropheophorhbide-a (HPPH)	680	680	Undergoing evaluations for use in esophageal, skin, and recurrent breast cancer (Photochlor)

25.3   Porfimer Sodium and Hematoporphyrin Derivative

Porfimer sodium is the most widely utilized photosensitizer in gastroenterologic PDT and its use is supported by the largest clinical experience. Porfimer sodium, a hematoporphyrin derivative first received regulatory approval in Canada (1994) and then the United States and Europe (1995) for the treatment of patients with advanced esophageal carcinoma [35]. Overholt et al. reported the use of porfimer sodium PDT in 84 patients with Barrett's esophagus with low-grade or high-grade dysplasia and 14 patients with T1 adenocarcinoma with a mean follow-up of 19 months. In order to obtain improved light dosimetry and more uniform light energy application, a balloon fiber centering device with mirrored caps was used to distend and flatten the esophageal mucosa. The idea was to prevent treatment overlap and reduce the risk of stricture formation. Overall results found that Barrett's esophagus and low-grade dysplasia was eliminated in 92% of patients and high-grade dysplasia was eliminated in 88% of patients. Complete elimination of Barrett's glandular mucosa was confirmed in 43% of patients. In the group of patients with early cancer, successful endoscopic ablation was confirmed in 10 out of 14 cancers. The most common post-PDT complication was stricture development in 34% of patients and this was often more common in those patients receiving more then one session of PDT. Over the 19 months mean follow-up of this study, in 6% of patients subsquamous epithelium was detected but dysplasia or cancer was not seen [36].

Several other centers subsequently reported large clinical series with similar results with emphasis on the diagnostic evaluation of patients with esophageal dysplasia, including the use of endoscopic mucosal resection and endoscopic ultrasound with fine-needle aspiration for lymphadenopathy [12, 37, 38]. Wolfsen et al. reviewed their experience treating 102 patients with PDT for Barrett's esophagus with high-grade dysplasia (n=69) or early cancer (n=33) over a mean follow-up of 1.6 years. In 56% of patients, complete ablation of Barrett's glandular epithelium was achieved with a single session of porfimer sodium PDT. Treatment failure was detected in four patients with persistent high-grade or carcinoma that required subsequent curative esophagectomy [39]. Prior reports included a combined Mayo Clinic study at two independent sites enrolled 142 patients (60 patients at Jacksonville, Florida, and 72 patients at Rochester, Minnesota) for treatment with porfimer sodium PDT and followed these patients for a mean of 19 months [40, 41]. Complete elimination of Barrett's disease was noted in 50% and 35%, respectively. A balloon centering device was not used during the treatment sessions and any residual disease after porfimer sodium PDT was treated with argon plasma coagulation (APC), resulting in elimination of high-grade dysplasia in 100% and 80% of patients, respectively. Post-PDT complication, stricture formation, was 20% and 27%, respectively, which was comparable to the rate previously reported by Overholt [36]. There was also a transient weight loss in patients who suffered from post-PDT chest discomfort or odynophagia [42]. The number of patients who reported experiencing cutaneous photosensitivity was similar in the Minnesota and Florida patients [43]. The rate of residual subsquamous epithelium was 0% and 4%, respectively and 4% (n=5) had residual dysplasia or neoplasm ultimately requiring curative esophagectomy. In an effort to reduce the rate of stricture formation, a group of 60 patients with BE HGD were treated with either PDT alone or PDT combined with oral prednisone, but this strategy did not impact the rate of stricture formation. In the PDT alone group the rate was 16% compared to 29% in the PDT and prednisone group [44]. Updated studies have compared the results of porfimer sodium PDT alone and combined with endoscopic mucosal resection as well as in a comparative cohort study with patients who have undergone esophagectomy with good results [45, 46]. Similar efficacy has been reported in patients with Barrett's high-grade dysplasia and esophageal carcinoma in reports from the General Infirmary at Leeds, United Kingdom, and the University of Pittsburgh Medical Center. Foroulis et al. retrospectively evaluated the effectiveness of porfimer sodium PDT in 31 patients with Barrett's high-grade dysplasia, 10 patients with intramucosal carcinoma, and six patients with endosonography stage T2 carcinoma over a median follow-up of 10 months. In patients with high-grade dysplasia or intramucosal cancer the treatment response was 80.9%. In patients with more advanced disease (T1b/T2), two of the six patients who were unfit for surgical resection had a complete response [47]. Keeley et al. reviewed their experience using porfimer sodium PDT in 50 patients treated for Barrett's high-grade dysplasia (13 patients) or locally advanced carcinoma with a mean follow-up of 28 months. Sixteen patients also received treatment with chemoradiation. At last follow-up, 16 patients were alive and disease-free while 15 patients were receiving additional treatment for persistent or recurrent disease. The study concluded that porfimer sodium PDT was potentially curative for patients with Barrett's high-grade dysplasia and superficial esophageal carcinomas but not more advanced disease [48].

The PHO-BAR trial was the first U.S. FDA approved multicenter randomized control trial to evaluate the utility of porfimer sodium PDT in patient with Barrett's esophagus and high-grade dysplasia. The study involved 30 sites, used an expert centralized pathology laboratory, and studied 208 patients randomized to PDT plus omeprazole or omeprazole alone (20 mg twice daily). After the initial treatment with porfimer sodium PDT at 12 months, 41% of patients had complete remission of Barrett's disease and 72% had complete elimination of Barrett's high-grade dysplasia, which was statistically significant compared to the group with omeprazole alone. Treatment with porfimer sodium PDT also decreased the rate of progression to adenocarcinoma from 28% in the drug-only group to less than 10% in the PDT plus omeprazole group. At 2 years follow-up, these results were maintained and resulted in the approval of porfimer sodium PDT for treatment of Barrett's esophagus with high-grade dysplasia in North America, United Kingdom, Europe, and Japan. Recently, Overholt et al. reported a 5-year follow-up of the original study with the persistent successful elimination of Barrett's high-grade dysplasia noted in significantly more patients in the porfimer sodium PDT plus omeprazole group (77%) compared with 39% of patients in the omeprazole alone group. The secondary outcome of progressing to cancer remained significantly lower (15%) in the PDT/omeprazole group compared to 29% in the omeprazole-alone group [5]. Based on these large single-center studies with long-term follow-up and the results of this randomized controlled trial, the use of porfimer sodium has become first-line therapy for treatment of Barrett's high-grade dysplasia and superficial carcinoma at many referral centers [49–51]. A recent study also compared pretreatment evaluation protocols, PDT light dosimetry, and follow-up evaluation protocols in 10 large PDT referral centers in the United States [7].

25.4   m-tetrahydroxyphenyl chlorin (mTHPC, Foscan)

The chlorin derivative, mTHPC, is an efficient photosensitizer that has been used in Europe mostly for the treatment of advanced head and neck cancer [52]. Unfortunately, a large U.S. trial performed in patients with head and neck squamous cell carcinoma was complicated with treatment-associated tissue necrosis, tissue breakdown, and stricture formation. This highly selective photosensitizer is associated with photosensitivity lasting only for 2 to 3 weeks after administration. Generally, mTHPC has been dosed intravenously at a dose of 0.15mg/kg with 652-nm light activation in a limited number of gastroenterologic studies [53]. Gossner et al. has used mTHPC as salvage therapy in a small number of patients with Barrett's high-grade dysplasia who had failed previous treatment with ALA PDT [54–56]. Javaid et al. treated four patients with Barrett's high-grade dysplasia using mTHPC with an argon-pump dye laser light of 652 nm and two patients using a xenon arc lamp (Patterson-Whitehurst lamp, 652 nm) with equivalent results demonstrating that efficient photosensitizers do not require high-power laser light sources for effective activation [57]. Etienne et al. used mTHPC with green light PDT in 12 patients with BE with HGD and seven patients with mucosal esophageal carcinoma. There was a mean follow-up of 34 months with only an 8% recurrence of disease [58]. Lovat et al. conducted a pilot study to assess the efficacy of mTHPC which included seven patients with BE and HGD and 12 patients with superficial esophageal cancer. Treatment results were variable but much better for patients treated with red light, including successful ablation in four out of six carcinoma patients and three out of four Barrett's high-grade dysplasia patients. None of the green light treated patients experienced successful disease eradication and reached long-term remission [59].

In summary, this limited experience demonstrates that while mTHPC is a very potent photosensitizer able to eliminate columnar epithelium in the esophagus and downgrade degree of dysplasia, the optimal light and drug dosimetry are not known. Further studies are required to determine ideal treatment parameters to avoid excessive tissue necrosis and high rates of stricture.

25.5 Aminolevulinic Acid (ALA)

As described above, aminolevulinic acid (ALA) is a prodrug that stimulates the endogenous production of protoporphyrin IX, mostly within the gut mucosa. ALA and Metvix brands have been used for several years mostly in Europe and Scandinavia. Levulan is a commercially available form of ALA that was recently granted orphan drug status by the U.S. Food and Drug Administration for the treatment of patients with Barrett's high-grade dysplasia. This unusual decision comes after recent approvals for treatment of Barrett's dysplasia using porfimer sodium PDT, radiofrequency energy ablation, and low-pressure liquid nitrogen cryotherapy ablation. Regardless, ALA has previously been used for PDT in the United Kingdom and Europe for Barrett's esophagus with dysplasia and superficial carcinoma. ALA is considered a second generation porphyrin-type photosensitizer that is activated using red light (635 nm) and offers several advantages including targeting the superficial mucosal layer and a shortened photosensitivity lasting only 24 to 48 hours [60–63]. The initial randomized double-blind placebo-controlled trial was done in the United Kingdom for patients with Barrett's low-grade dysplasia. ALA PDT was dosed at 30 mg/kg given orally and activated by a green light (514 nm) in order to enhance superficial mucosal damage and limit the risk of stricture formation [64, 65]. Patients were followed for a mean of 24 months and an endoscopic response was seen in 83% of patients. After ablation, surveillance endoscopy with biopsies demonstrated no dysplasia in 98% with only a single case of recurrent low-grade dysplasia over a 12 month follow-up. These encouraging results were also seen by other researchers treating BE with HGD [54, 56, 66, 67]. The group in Wiesbaden, Germany, has published several studies using ALA PDT in patients with Barrett's high-grade dysplasia and superficial carcinoma. These studies from the same group of authors presumably describe results in the same cohort of patients. Pech reported the treatment of 35 patients with Barrett's high-grade dysplasia using ALA PDT and noted a very high complete response rate in 97% of patients at a mean follow-up of 42 months [68]. In a follow-up study in 66 patients with Barrett's high-grade dysplasia (n=35) or and early adenocarcinoma (n=31) ALA was administered orally at a dose of 60 mg/kg 4 to 6 hours prior to endoscopy with laser light application using light between 630 to 635 nm with energy dose of 150J per square centimeter. Follow-up endoscopy procedures used argon beam coagulation or thermal KTP laser to destroy any residual glandular mucosa. An intensive endoscopic surveillance program schedule endoscopy at 1, 2, 3, 6, 9, and 12 months with procedures every 6 months thereafter for 5 years. During a follow-up period with a mean of 37 months patients with Barrett's high-grade dysplasia were said to have achieved a complete response 97% and 100% of early cancer patients. Yet, disease recurrence was detected in one patient with Barrett's high grade dysplasia (89% disease-free survival) and 10 carcinoma patients (68% disease free survival). However, there were no reported deaths related to Barrett's neoplasia [68, 69]. From the same group, Behrens and May have recently reported the combined use of endoscopic mucosal resection, ALA PDT, and argon beam coagulation in 44 and 49 patients, respectively [70, 71]. Unfortunately, PDT using orally administered ALA has been associated with adverse effects such as significant chest pain, elevated liver enzyme tests, acute neuropathy mimicking porphyria, and sudden death presumably related to cardiac dysrhythmia [72]. While considered by some to be only of minor importance, most ALA PDT treatment occurs in the hospital setting for safety reasons and pain control [73].

Ortner et al. attempted to avoid the risks of systemic ALA administration by using the drug topically with 15 or 60 mg/kg body weight in an 8.5% sodium bicarbonate solution in saline using a spray catheter during endoscopy in seven patients with Barrett's metaplasia and seven patients with Barrett's low-grade dysplasia [74]. While safe and effective in ablating low-grade dysplasia in all seven patients, a metaplasia patient progressed to high-grade dysplasia after this treatment. Complete ablation of all Barrett's disease was noted in only 21% of patients after the initial PDT and 20% after the second PDT. Topical administration of ALA, therefore, was not a reliable method of ablation in these patients. Several small randomized trials have been performed using ALA PDT in patients with Barrett's metaplasia or low-grade dysplasia. Generally, ALA PDT has performed poorly in studies that have compared its use with another endoscopic ablation treatment. Specifically, Ragunath et al. found that the use of argon beam coagulation was more effective, less expensive, and associated with fewer complications compared with ALA PDT in the treatment of 26 patients with Barrett's dysplasia (23 with low-grade, three with high-grade dysplasia) [75]. Similar disappointing results were reported in studies from Sheffield in 68 patients with Barrett's metaplasia and in Adelaide, South Australia, where 30 patients with Barrett's low-grade dysplasia were treated with 30 mg/kg of ALA compared with argon plasma coagulation [64, 76, 77]. The only positive randomized trial using 60 mg/kg ALA for PDT in 40 Barrett's patients (32 metaplasia; eight low-grade dysplasia) was performed in Rotterdam in comparison with argon plasma coagulation (APC). While successful reversal of Barrett's disease was achieved in more than two out of three patients in the study, multiple courses of therapy were required and one ALA PDT patient died of sudden death. The authors did not recommend either of those treatments for "prophylactic ablation of Barrett's esophagus" [77, 78]. Published the same year was a study in 20 patients with Barrett's high-grade dysplasia persistent after endoscopic mucosal resections were treated with ALA PDT (40 mg/kg) in Amsterdam [79]. The authors defined complete remission as the absence of Barrett's high-grade dysplasia in biopsies taken at two surveillance endoscopy procedures. After ALA PDT, all patients were found to have persistent Barrett's disease (median regression was 50%) and five out of 20 (25%) were found to have persistent high-grade dysplasia at surveillance examinations after PDT. Subsequent follow-up procedures found recurrence of high-grade dysplasia or carcinoma in another four patients, from 6 to 15 months after PDT. These findings suggest that ALA PDT may be unreliable for treatment of patients with advanced disease (high-grade dysplasia or carcinoma). Further, regardless of the initial therapy used, all Barrett's disease must be destroyed at follow-up endoscopy procedures in order to prevent the development or recurrence of carcinoma. An abstract form in May 2007 by Mackenzie et al. presented the results of a dosimetry study in 72 patients with Barrett's esophagus and high-grade dysplasia and compared the use of red or green light with varying doses of ALA. The main treatment outcome was the development of cancer after ALA PDT. In the patients treated using the higher doses of ALA (60 mg/kg) and higher energy red light (1,000 J/cm), only 3% of patients were subsequently diagnosed with invasive carcinoma at a follow-up of 36 months. However, in the other groups, a much higher rate of cancer development was noted (34%). These results, however encouraging, were found in a subset of patients participating in a study of varying drug and light energy doses where 14 patients overall (20%) progressed to cancer. In addition, there is no mention of concomitant acid blocker therapy, which is known to be critically important to successful ablation of Barrett's disease. Regardless, if this finally seems to be the ALA dose and the light dose and wavelength that is optimal, then it would seem high time for a randomized controlled trial of Levulan PDT in combination with acid blocker drugs versus drug therapy alone (as was done for porfimer sodium PDT and is currently being studied for radiofrequency ablation) [80].

25.6 Photodynamic Therapy and Light Dosimetry and Delivery Systems

Ultimately, the future of photodynamic therapy is often said to depend on the development of improved photosensitizers and light dosimetry. However, the enormous costs of drug discovery, clinical testing, and regulatory approval will likely impede the further development of photosensitizers in gastroenterology. So, if PDT is to be improved in order to remain a viable endoscopic mucosal ablation treatment option, improved light dosimetry is mandatory [81–84]. Currently, there are no means available to determine the ideal dose of light required for PDT in an individual patient. Less than ideal light dosimetry may lead to insufficient treatment with residual dysplasia or carcinoma. Alternatively, excessive light dosing may result in severe mucosal damage and stricture formation. To better target dysplastic tissue there is continued development of photosensitizers and optical devices such as lasers and arc lamps coupled to light delivery system. The light delivery system is often a quartz light diffuser or a specialized modified diffuser placed under fluoroscopy, which has been modified for the endoscopic usage. Due to the natural peristalsis of the esophagus and respiratory motion of the chest, it can be challenging to maintain central positioning of the fiber within the esophagus to achieve uniform light distribution [54]. Furthermore, the natural mucosal folds of the esophagus, in conjunction with esophageal peristalsis and respiratory movement, create areas of mucosa shielded from light exposure leading to incomplete mucosal ablation. This has lead to more advanced light systems to include an adaptable device to shape the esophagus using an elastic catheter balloon [85]. The balloon catheter allows for centering the fiber to provide an equal distribution to the treatment area by eliminating the "shadow phenomenon," the hill-and-valley effect a result of mucosal folds. Panjehpour et al. was able to flatten the esophageal mucosa using a nonelastic balloon stabilizing device [86]. It is important not to overdistend the wall of the esophagus, since decreased blood flow can lead to decreased effectiveness of PDT [85, 87]. Prasad et al. determined that a history of prior esophageal stricture, performance of endoscopic mucosal resection prior to PDT, and more than one PDT light application treatment were all risk factors for the development of stricture after PDT. Interestingly, the use a balloon centering device was not statistically significant in reducing the development of strictures [88]. The Swiss group in an effort to eliminate esophageal folds used a rigid large diameter light distributor greater then 18 mm, which also controlled esophageal peristalsis and respiratory motion [89]. In each patient the tissue drug level can vary, which makes it difficult to predict actual tissue damage. The use of advanced optical techniques such as fluorescence spectroscopy or optical coherence tomography may help assess drug levels at the level of the mucosa and the progression of the photodynamic reaction to improve PDT outcomes [90–92].

25.7 Conclusions

The summary of the photodynamic therapy for Barrett's dysplasia and carcinoma is presented in Table 25.2. Photodynamic therapy has been a critically important tool for the advancement of endoscopic therapy for esophageal dysplasia and superficial carcinoma. Based largely on the outcomes of large porfimer sodium PDT studies, endoscopic ablation therapy has been proven safe and reliable for the treatment of esophageal dysplasia to prevent the development of invasive carcinoma. Treatment results using all forms of PDT could be significantly improved with better photosensitizers and more sophisticated light dosimetry. However, there have been no such recent developments or improvements in esophageal PDT. Instead over the past 5 years there has been a rapid and progressive development of complimentary and competitive technologies that have severely diminished the role of PDT in the treatment of esophageal disease [93]. Techniques and technologies such as endoscopic mucosal resection, endoscopic submucosal dissection, and ablation using radiofrequency energy or low-pressure liquid nitrogen cryotherapy systems have steadily relegated the use of PDT to an increasingly smaller group of patients treated in an ever smaller number of PDT referral centers. As the currently available photosensitizers lurch steadily toward patent expiration, the future of PDT for esophageal disease remains in serious doubt and should serve as a stern lesson to those who do not remain committed to scientific innovation and clinical advancement.

Table 25.2 Photodynamic Therapy for Barrett's Dysplasia and Carcinoma

Author	Patients	Sensitizer	Route of Admin.	Dosage	Interval	Wave-length (nm)	Light Dosage	Complete Eradication Neoplasia	Buried Barrett's	Stenosis	Follow-up (Months)	Recurrence
Overholt [36]	100 (8 HGD, 9LGD, 3Ca)	Sodium porfimer	IV	2 mg/kg	48 hours	630	125–250 J/cm	88% HGD, 92% LGD, Ca 77%	5% (2 HGD, 1 Ca)	34%	19	23%
Wolfsen [39]	102 (69 HGD, 33 Ca)	Sodium porfimer	IV	2 mga/kg	48, 72 hours	630	150–225 J/cm	96%	4% (HGD)	20%	19	6%
Foroulis [47]	25 (15 HGD, Ca 10)	Sodium porfimer	IV	2 mg/kg	24 hours	630	200–250 J/cm	81%	20%	6%	14	18%
Keeley [48]	50 (19 HGD, Ca 31)	Sodium porfimer	IV	2 mg/kg	48 hours	630	300–400 J/cm	37% HGD	N/A	42%	28.1	31% HGD
Overholt [6]	138 HGD	Sodium porfimer	IV	2 mg/kg	40–50 hours	630	130 J/cm	77%	N/A	36%	43	13%
Overholt [5]	48 HGD	Sodium porfimer	IV	2 mg/kg	40–50 hours	630	130 J/cm + 50 J/cm	77%	N/A	2%	60	5%
Javid [57]	7 (6 HGD, Ca 1)	mTHPC	IV	0.15 mg/kg	96 hours	652	8–20 J/cm²	100%	N/A	29%	N/A	0%
Etienne [58]	14 (7HGD, Ca7)	mTHPC	IV	0.15 mg/kg	96 hours	514	75 J/cm²	100%	0%	29%	34	8%
Lovat [59]	19 (7 HGD, Ca 12)	mTHPC	IV	0.15 mg/kg	72 hours	511 or 652	7 J/cm2–75 J/cm2	42%	21%	11%	24	75%
Ackroyd [64]	18 LGD	5-ALA	Oral	30 mg/kg	4 hours	514	60 J/cm²	98%	0%	0%	24	N/A
Barr [66]	5 HGD	5-ALA	Oral	60 mg/kg	4 hours	630	50–150 J/cm²	100%	40%	0%	26-44	N/A
Pech [68]	51 (30 HGD, 21 Ca)	5-ALA	Oral	60 mg/kg	4–6 hours	635	150 J/cm²	100%	N/A	0%	38	24%
Gossner [56]	32 (10 HGD, Ca 22)	5-ALA	Oral	60 mg/kg	4–6 hours	635	150 J/cm²	84%	7%	0%	9.9	7%
Peters [79]	20 (18 HGD, Ca 2)	5-ALA	Oral	40 mg/kg	1.5–4 hours	630	100 J/cm²	75%	53%	0%	30	27%
Tan [96]	12 (2 HGD, Ca 10)	5-ALA	Oral	60 or 75 mg/kg	4–6 hours	630	100–200 J/cm²	16.6%	N/A	0%	N/A	N/A
Ortner [74]	7 LGD	5-ALA	Topical	15 mg/kg	1.5–2 hours	632	90 and 100 J/cm²	21%	N/A	0%	33	7%
Kelty [77]	25 NDBE	5-ALA	Oral	30 or 60 mg/kg	4–6 hours	635	85 J/cm²	0%	24%	0%	1	N/A
Kelty [76]	34 NDBE	5-ALA	Oral	30 mg/kg	4–6 hours	635	85 J/cm²	50%	24%	0%	12	N/A
Mackenzie [97]	24 HGD	5-ALA	Oral	60 mg/kg	3–5 hours	635	500–1,000 (x2) J/cm	38%	46%	0%	45 (1–78)	25% (Ca)
Ackroyd [98]	40 LGD	5-ALA	Oral	30 mg/kg	4 hours	514	60 J/cm²	97%	N/A	0%	53 (18–68)	3% (Ca)

HGD: high-grade dysplasia; LGD: low-grade dysplasia; Ca: Barrett's carcinoma; NDBE: nondysplastic Barrett's esophagus; ALA: amino-levulinic acid; mTHPC: m-tetrahydroxyphenylchlorin; IV: intravenous.

References

[1]   McCaughan, J. S., Jr., E. C. Ellison, J. T. Guy, et al., "Photodynamic therapy for esophageal malignancy: a prospective twelve-year study," *Ann Thorac Surg*, Vol. 62, 1996, pp. 1005–009.

[2]   Litle, V. R., J. D. Luketich, and N. A. Christie, et al., "Photodynamic Therapy as Palliation for Esophageal Cancer: Experience in 215 Patients," *Ann. Thorac. Surg.*, Vol. 76, 2003, pp. 1687-1692; discussion 1692–1683.

[3]   Lightdale, C. J., S. K. Heier, and N. E. Marcon, et al., "Photodynamic Therapy with Porfimer Sodium Versus Thermal Ablation Therapy with Nd:YAG Laser for Palliation of Esophageal Cancer: A Multicenter Randomized Trial," *Gastrointest. Endosc.*, Vol. 42, 1995, pp. 507–512.

[4]   Overholt, B. F., C. J. Lightdale, and K. K. Wang, et al., "International Multicenter Partially Binded Randomized Study of the Efficacy of Photodynamic Therapy (PDT) Using Portimer Sodium (POR) for Ablation of High-Grade Dysplasia (HGD) in Barrett's Esophagus (BE) and Results of 24 Month Follow Up," *Gastroenterology*, 2003, pp. A20 [Suppl. 21].

[5]   Overholt, B. F., K. K. Wang, J. S. Burdick, et al., "Five-Year Efficacy and Safety of Photodynamic Therapy with Photofrin in Barrett's High-Grade Dysplasia," *Gastrointest. Endosc.*, Vol. 66, 2007, pp. 460–468.

[6]   Overholt, B. F., C. J. Lightdale, and K. K. Wang, et al., "Photodynamic Therapy with Porfimer Sodium for Ablation of High-Grade Dysplasia in Barrett's Esophagus: International, Partially Blinded, Randomized Phase III Trial," *Gastrointest. Endosc.*, Vol. 62, 2005, pp. 488–498.

[7]   Wolfsen, H. C., "Endoluminal Therapy for Barrett's Esophagus," *Gastrointest. Endosc. Clin. N. Am.*, Vol. 17, 2007, pp. 59–82, vi–vii.

[8]   Wolfsen, H. C., "Present Status of Photodynamic Therapy for High-Grade Dysplasia in Barrett's Esophagus," *J. Clin. Gastroenterol.*, Vol. 39, 2005, pp. 189–202.

[9]   Wolfsen, H. C.,   "Carpe Luz ̃Seize the Light: Endoprevention of Esophageal Adenocarcinoma Using Photodynamic Therapy With Porfimer Sodium," *Gastrointest. Endosc.*, Vol. 62, 2005, pp. 499–503.

[10]   Wolfsen, H. C., "Endoprevention of Esophageal Cancer: Endoscopic Ablation of Barrett's Metaplasia and Dysplasia," *Expert Rev. Med. Devices*, Vol. 2, 2005, pp. 713–723.

[11]   Prosst, R. L., H. C. Wolfsen, and J. Gahlen, "Photodynamic Therapy for Esophageal Diseases: A Clinical Update," *Endoscopy*, Vol. 35, 2003, pp. 1059–1068.

[12]   Wang, K. K., "Current Status of Photodynamic Therapy of Barrett's Esophagus," *Gastrointest. Endosc.*, Vol. 49, 1999, pp. S20–23.

[13]   Overholt, B. F., M. Panjehpour, and D. L. Halberg, "Photodynamic Therapy for Barrett's Esophagus with Dysplasia or Early Stage Carcinoma: Long-Term Results," *Gastrointest. Endosc.*, Vol. 58, 2003, pp. 183–188.

[14]   Sampliner, R. E., "Prevention of Adenocarcinoma by Reversing Barrett's Esophagus with Mucosal Ablation," *World J. Surg.*, Vol. 27, 2003, pp. 1026–1029.

[15]   Falk, G. W., "Barrett's Esophagus," *Gastroenterology*, Vol. 122, 2002, pp. 1569–1591.

[16]   Cameron, A. J., A. R. Zinsmeister, and D. J. Ballard, et al., "Prevalence of Columnar-Lined (Barrett's) Esophagus. Comparison of Population-Based Clinical and Autopsy Findings," *Gastroenterology*, Vol. 99, 1990, pp. 918–922.

[17]   Cameron, A. J., B. J. Ott, and W. S. Payne, "The Incidence of Adenocarcinoma in Columnar-Lined (Barrett's) Esophagus," *N. Engl. J. Med.*, Vol. 313, 1985, pp. 857–859.

[18]   Reid, B. J., "Barrett's Esophagus and Esophageal Adenocarcinoma," *Gastroenterol. Clin. North Am.*, Vol. 20, 1991, pp. 817–834.

[19]   Ward, E. M., H. C. Wolfsen, and S. R. Achem, et al., "Barrett's Esophagus is Common in Older Men and Women Undergoing Screening Colonoscopy Regardless of Reflux Symptoms," *Am. J. Gastroenterol.*, Vol. 101, 2006, pp. 12–17.

[20] Conio, M., G. Lapertosa,and S. Blanchi, et al., "Barrett's Esophagus: An Update," *Crit. Rev. Oncol. Hematol.*, Vol. 46, 2003, pp. 187–206.

[21] Devesa, S. S., W. J. Blot, and J. F. Fraumeni, Jr., "Changing Patterns in the Incidence of Esophageal and Gastric Carcinoma in the United States," *Cancer*, Vol. 83, 1998, pp. 2049–2053.

[22] Montgomery, E., M. P. Bronner, and J. R. Goldblum, et al., "Reproducibility of the Diagnosis of Dysplasia in Barrett Esophagus: A Reaffirmation," *Hum. Pathol.*, Vol. 32, 2001, pp. 368–378.

[23] Buttar, N. S., K. K. Wang, and T. J. Sebo, et al., "Extent of High-Grade Dysplasia in Barrett's Esophagus Correlates with Risk of Adenocarcinoma," *Gastroenterology*, Vol. 120, 2001, pp. 1630–1639.

[24] Schnell, T. G., S. J. Sontag, and G. Chejfec, et al., "Long-Term Nonsurgical Management of Barrett's Esophagus with High-Grade Dysplasia," *Gastroenterology*, Vol. 120, 2001, pp. 1607–1619.

[25] Reid, B. J., D. S. Levine, and G. Longton, et al., "Predictors of Progression to Cancer in Barrett's Esophagus: Baseline Histology and Flow Cytometry Identify Low- and High-Risk Patient Subsets," *Am. J. Gastroenterol.*, Vol. 95, 2000, pp. 1669–1676.

[26] Weston, A. P., and P. Sharma, "Neodymium:Yttrium-Aluminum Garnet Contact Laser Ablation of Barrett's High Grade Dysplasia and Early Adenocarcinoma," *Am. J. Gastroenterol.*, Vol. 97, 2002, pp. 2998–3006.

[27] Hameeteman, W., G. N. Tytgat, and H. J. Houthoff, et al., "Barrett's Esophagus: Development of Dysplasia and Adenocarcinoma," *Gastroenterology*, Vol. 96, 1989, pp. 1249–1256.

[28] Zaninotto, G., F. Minnei, and E. Guirroli, et al., "The Veneto Region's Barrett's Oesophagus Registry: Aims, Methods, Preliminary Results," *Dig. Liver Dis.*, Vol. 39, 2007, pp. 18–25.

[29] Tokar, J. L., O. Haluszka, and D. S. Weinberg, "Endoscopic Therapy of Dysplasia and Early-Stage Cancers of the Esophagus," *Semin. Radiat. Oncol.*, Vol. 17, 2007, pp. 10–21.

[30] Dougherty, T. J., "An Update on Photodynamic Therapy Applications," *J. Clin. Laser Med. Surg.*, Vol. 20, 2002, pp. 3–7.

[31] Dougherty, T.J., C.J. Gomer, B.W. Hemderson, et al. "Photodynamic Therapy," *J. Natl. Cancer Inst.*, Vol. 90, 1998, pp. 889–905.

[32] Ackroyd, R., C. Kelty, and N. Brown, et al., "The History of Photodetection and Photodynamic Therapy," *Photochem. Photobiol.*, Vol. 74, 2001, pp. 656–669.

[33] Bown, S. G., and A. Z. Rogowska, "New Photosensitizers for Photodynamic Therapy in Gastroenterology," *Can. J. Gastroenterol.*, Vol. 13, 1999, pp. 389–392.

[34] Bellnier, D. A., W. R. Greco, and H. Nava, et al., "Mild Skin Photosensitivity in Cancer Patients Following Injection of Photochlor (2-[1-Hexyloxyethyl]-2-Devinyl Pyropheophorbide-A; HPPH) for Photodynamic Therapy," *Cancer Chemother. Pharmacol.*, Vol. 57, 2006, pp. 40–45.

[35] Overholt, B., M. Panjehpour, and E. Tefftellar, et al., "Photodynamic Therapy for Treatment of Early Adenocarcinoma in Barrett's Esophagus," *Gastrointest. Endosc.*, Vol. 39, 1993, pp. 73–76.

[36] Overholt, B. F., M. Panjehpour, and J. M. Haydek, "Photodynamic Therapy for Barrett's Esophagus: Follow-Up in 100 Patients," *Gastrointest. Endosc.*, Vol. 49, 1999, pp. 1–7.

[37] Wang, K. K., and J. Y. Kim, "Photodynamic Therapy in Barrett's Esophagus," *Gastrointest. Endosc. Clin. N. Am.*, Vol. 13, 2003, pp. 483–489, vii.

[38] Wolfsen, H. C., T. A. Woodward, and M. Raimondo, "Photodynamic Therapy for Dysplastic Barrett Esophagus and Early Esophageal Adenocarcinoma," *Mayo Clin. Proc.*, Vol. 77, 2002, pp. 1176–1181.

[39] Wolfsen, H. C., L. L. Hemminger, and M. B. Wallace, et al., "Clinical Experience of Patients Undergoing Photodynamic Therapy for Barrett's Dysplasia or Cancer," *Aliment. Pharmacol. Ther.*, Vol. 20, 2004, pp. 1125–1131.

[40] Wang, K. K., L. M. Wong Kee Song, and N. S. Buttar, et al., "Barrett's Esophagus After Photodynamic Therapy: Risk of Cancer Development During Long Term Follow Up [Abstract]," *Gastroenterology*, Vol. 126 (Suppl. 2), 2004, pp. A50.

[41] Wolfsen, H. C., and L. L. Hemminger, "Photodynamic Therapy for Dysplastic Barrett's Esophagus and Mucosal Adenocarcinoma (Abstract)," *Gastrointest. Endosc.*, Vol. 59, 2004, pp. AB251.

[42] Ukleja, A., J. S. Scolapio, and H. C. Wolfsen, "Nutritional Consequences Following Photodynamic Therapy," *Gastrotenterology*, Vol. 116, 1999, pp. A-582.

[43] Nijhawan, P. K., H. C. Wolfsen, and K. K. Wang, et al., "Cutaneous Photosensitivity After Photodynamic Therapy: Is It Really More Common in Sunny Climates? [Abstract]," *Gastroenterology*, Vol. 118, 2000, pp. A227.

[44] Panjehpour, M., B. F. Overholt, and J. M. Haydek, et al., "Results of Photodynamic Therapy for Ablation of Dysplasia and Early Cancer in Barrett's Esophagus and Effect of Oral Steroids on Stricture Formation," *Am. J. Gastroenterol.*, Vol. 95, 2000, pp. 2177–2184.

[45] Pacifico, R. J., K. K. Wang, and L. M. Wong Kee Song, et al., "Combined Endoscopic Mucosal Resection and Photodynamic Therapy Versus Esophagectomy for Management of Early Adenocarcinoma in Barrett's Esophagus," *Clin. Gastroenterol. Hepatol.*, Vol. 1, 2003, pp. 252–257.

[46] Prasad, G. A., K. K. Wang, and N. S. Buttar, et al., "Long-Term Survival Following Endoscopic and Surgical Treatment of High-Grade Dysplasia in Barrett's Esophagus," *Gastroenterology*, Vol. 132, 2007, pp. 1226–1233.

[47] Foroulis, C. N., and J. A. Thorpe, "Photodynamic Therapy (PDT) in Barrett's Esophagus with Dysplasia or Early Cancer," *Eur. J. Cardiothorac. Surg.*, Vol. 29, 2006, pp. 30–34.

[48] Keeley, S. B., A. Pennathur, and W. Gooding, et al., "Photodynamic Therapy with Curative Intent for Barrett's Esophagus with High Grade Dysplasia and Superficial Esophageal Cancer," *Ann. Surg. Oncol.*, Vol. 14, 2007, pp. 2406–2410.

[49] Hemminger, L. L., and H. C. Wolfsen, "Photodynamic Therapy for Barrett's Esophagus and High Grade Dysplasia: Results of a Patient Satisfaction Survey," *Gastroenterol. Nurs.*, Vol. 25, 2002, pp. 139–141.

[50] Hur, C., N. S. Nishioka, and G. S. Gazelle, "Cost-Effectiveness of Photodynamic Therapy for Treatment of Barrett's Esophagus with High Grade Dysplasia," *Dig. Dis. Sci.*, Vol. 48, 2003, pp. 1273–1283.

[51] Wolfsen, H. C., L. L. Hemminger, and K. R. DeVault, "Barrett's Dysplasia and Mucosal Carcinoma Patients Referred for Photodynamic Therapy—Do They Come from Surveillance Programs? (Abstract)," *Gastrointest. Endosc.*, Vol. 59, 2004, pp. AB265.

[52] Andrejevic-Blant, S., C. Hadjur, and J. P. Ballini, et al., "Photodynamic Therapy of Early Squamous Cell Carcinoma with Tetra(M-Hydroxyphenyl)Chlorin: Optimal Drug-Light Interval," *Br. J. Cancer*, Vol. 76, 1997, pp. 1021–1028.

[53] Andrejevic Blant, S., P. Grosjean, and J. P. Ballini, et al., "Localization of Tetra(m-Hydroxyphenyl)chlorin (Foscan) in Human Healthy Tissues and Squamous Cell Carcinomas of the Upper Aero-Digestive Tract, the Esophagus and the Bronchi: A Fluorescence Microscopy Study," *J. Photochem. Photobiol. B*, Vol. 61, 2001, pp. 1–9.

[54] Gossner, L., A. May, and R. Sroka, et al., "A New Long-Range Through-the-Scope Balloon Applicator for Photodynamic Therapy in the Esophagus and Cardia," *Endoscopy*, Vol. 31, 1999, pp. 370–376.

[55] Gossner, L., A. May, and R. Sroka, et al., "Photodynamic Destruction of High Grade Dysplasia and Early Carcinoma of the Esophagus after the Oral Administration of 5-Aminolevulinic Acid," *Cancer*, Vol. 86, 1999, pp. 1921–1928.

[56] Gossner, L., M. Stolte, and R. Sroka, et al., "Photodynamic Ablation of High-Grade Dysplasia and Early Cancer in Barrett's Esophagus by Means of 5-Aminolevulinic Acid," *Gastroenterology*, Vol. 114, 1998, pp. 448–455.

[57] Javaid, B., P. Watt, and N. Krasner, "Photodynamic Therapy (PDT) for Oesophageal Dysplasia and Early Carcinoma with mTHPC (M-Tetrahydroxyphenyl Chlorin): A Preliminary Study," *Lasers Med. Sci.*, Vol. 17, 2002, pp. 51–56.

[58] Etienne, J., N. Dorme, G. and Bourg-Heckly, et al., "Photodynamic Therapy with Green Light and M-Tetrahydroxyphenyl Chlorin for Intramucosal Adenocarcinoma and High-Grade Dysplasia in Barrett's Esophagus," *Gastrointest. Endosc.*, Vol. 59, 2004, pp. 880–889.

[59] Lovat, L. B., N. F. Jamieson, and M. R. Novelli, et al., "Photodynamic Therapy with m-Tetrahydroxyphenyl Chlorin for High-Grade Dysplasia and Early Cancer in Barrett's Columnar Lined Esophagus," *Gastrointest. Endosc.*, Vol. 62, 2005, pp. 617–623.

[60] Bedwell, J., A. J. MacRobert, and D. Phillips, et al., "Fluorescence Distribution and Photodynamic Effect of ALA-Induced PP IX in the DMH Rat Colonic Tumour Model," *Br. J. Cancer*, Vol. 65, 1992, pp. 818–824.

[61] Kennedy, J. C., and R. H. Pottier, "Endogenous Protoporphyrin IX, a Clinically Useful Photosensitizer for Photodynamic Therapy," *J. Photochem. Photobiol. B*, Vol. 14, 1992, pp. 275–292.

[62] Peng, Q., K. Berg, and J. Moan, et al., "5-Aminolevulinic Acid-Based Photodynamic Therapy: Principles and Experimental Research," *Photochem. Photobiol.*, Vol. 65, 1997, pp. 235–251.

[63] Webber, J., D. Kessel, and D. Fromm, "Side Effects and Photosensitization of Human Tissues after Aminolevulinic Acid," *J. Surg. Res.*, Vol. 68, 1997, pp. 31–37.

[64] Ackroyd, R., N. J. Brown, and M. F. Davis, et al., "Photodynamic Therapy for Dysplastic Barrett's Oesophagus: A Prospective, Double Blind, Randomised, Placebo Controlled Trial," *Gut*, Vol. 47, 2000, pp. 612–617.

[65] Ackroyd, R., N. J. Brown, and M. F. Davis, et al., "Aminolevulinic Acid-Induced Photodynamic Therapy: Safe and Effective Ablation of Dysplasia in Barrett's Esophagus," *Dis. Esophagus*, Vol. 13, 2000, pp. 18–22.

[66] Barr, H., N. A. Shepherd, and A. Dix, et al., "Eradication of High-Grade Dysplasia in Columnar-Lined (Barrett's) Oesophagus by Photodynamic Therapy with Endogenously Generated Protoporphyrin IX," *Lancet*, Vol. 348, 1996, pp. 584–585.

[67] Orth, K., A. Stanescu, and A. Ruck, et al., "Photodynamic Ablation and Argon-Plasma Coagulation of Premalignant and Early-Stage Malignant Lesions of the Oesophagus—An Alternative to Surgery?" *Chirurg.*, Vol. 70, 1999, pp. 431–438.

[68] Pech, O., L. Gossner, and A. May, et al., "Long Term Results of PDT for Early Neoplasia in Barrett's Esophagus," *Gastrointest. Endosc.*, Vol. 59, 2004, pp. W1567.

[69] Guelrud, M., I. Herrera, and H. Essenfeld, et al., "Enhanced Magnification Endoscopy: A New Technique to Identify Specialized Intestinal Metaplasia in Barrett's Esophagus," *Gastrointest. Endosc.*, Vol. 53, 2001, pp. 559–565.

[70] Behrens, A., A. May, and L. Gossner, et al., "Curative Treatment for High-Grade Intraepithelial Neoplasia in Barrett's Esophagus," *Endoscopy*, Vol. 37, 2005, pp. 999–1005.

[71] May, A., L. Gossner, and O. Pech, et al., "Intraepithelial High-Grade Neoplasia and Early Adenocarcinoma In Short-Segment Barrett's Esophagus (SSBE): Curative Treatment Using Local Endoscopic Treatment Techniques," *Endoscopy*, Vol. 34, 2002, pp. 604–610.

[72] Sylantiev, C., N. Schoenfeld, and R. Mamet, et al., "Acute Neuropathy Mimicking Porphyria Induced by Aminolevulinic Acid During Photodynamic Therapy," *Muscle Nerve*, Vol. 31, 2005, pp. 390–393.

[73] Siersema, P. D., "Photodynamic Therapy for Barrett's Esophagus: Not Yet Ready for the Premier League of Endoscopic Interventions," *Gastrointest. Endosc.*, Vol. 62, 2005, pp. 503–507.

[74] Ortner, M. A., K. Zumbusch, and J. Liebetruth, et al., "Is Topical Delta-Aminolevulinic Acid Adequate for Photodynamic Therapy in Barrett's Esophagus? A Pilot Study," *Endoscopy*, Vol. 34, 2002, pp. 611–616.

[75] Ragunath, K., N. Krasner, and V. S. Raman, et al., "Endoscopic Ablation of Dysplastic Barrett's Oesophagus Comparing Argon Plasma Coagulation and Photodynamic Therapy: A Randomized Prospective Trial Assessing Efficacy and Cost-Effectiveness," *Scand. J. Gastroenterol.*, Vol. 40, 2005, pp. 750–758.

[76] Kelty, C. J., R. Ackroyd, and N. J. Brown, et al., "Comparison of High- vs Low-Dose 5-Aminolevulinic Acid for Photodynamic Therapy of Barrett's Esophagus," *Surg. Endosc.*, Vol. 18, 2004, pp. 452–458.

[77] Kelty, C. J., R. Ackroyd, and N. J. Brown, et al., "Endoscopic Ablation of Barrett's Oesophagus: A Randomized-Controlled Trial of Photodynamic Therapy vs. Argon Plasma Coagulation," *Aliment. Pharmacol. Ther.*, Vol. 20, 2004, pp. 1289–1296.

[78] Hage, M., P. D. Siersema, and H. van Dekken, et al., "5-Aminolevulinic Acid Photodynamic Therapy Versus Argon Plasma Coagulation for Ablation of Barrett's Oesophagus: A Randomised Trial," *Gut*, Vol. 53, 2004, pp. 785–790.

[79] Peters, F., M. Kara, and W. Rosmolen, et al., "Poor Results of 5-Aminolevulinic Acid-Photodynamic Therapy for Residual High-Grade Dysplasia and Early Cancer in Barrett Esophagus after Endoscopic Resection," *Endoscopy*, Vol. 37, 2005, pp. 418–424.

[80] Mackenzie, G., C. Selvasekar, and N. Jamieson, et al., "Low Incidence of Esophageal Adenocarcinoma Following Optimal Regimen of ALA PDT for High Grade Dysplasia in Barrett's Esophagus (Abstract)," *Gastrointest. Endosc.*, Vol. 65, 2007, pp. AB132.

[81] Boere, I. A., D. J. Robinson, and H. S. de Bruijn, et al., "Monitoring In Situ Dosimetry and Protoporphyrin IX Fluorescence Photobleaching in the Normal Rat Esophagus During 5-Aminolevulinic Acid Photodynamic Therapy," *Photochem. Photobiol.*, Vol. 78, 2003, pp. 271–277.

[82] Cheung, R., M. Solonenko, and T. M. Busch, et al., "Correlation of In Vivo Photosensitizer Fluorescence and Photodynamic-Therapy-Induced Depth of Necrosis in a Murine Tumor Model," *J. Biomed. Opt.*, Vol. 8, 2003, pp. 248–252.

[83] Radu, A., R. Conde, and C. Fontolliet, et al., "Mucosal Ablation with Photodynamic Therapy in the Esophagus: Optimization of Light Dosimetry in the Sheep Model," *Gastrointest. Endosc.*, Vol. 57, 2003, pp. 897–905.

[84] Panjehpour, M., B. F. Overholt, M. and N. Phan, et al., "Optimization of Light Dosimetry for Photodynamic Therapy of Barrett's Esophagus: Efficacy vs. Incidence of Stricture after Treatment," *Gastrointest. Endosc.*, Vol. 61, 2005, pp. 13–18.

[85] van den Bergh, H., "On the Evolution of Some Endoscopic Light Delivery Systems for Photodynamic Therapy," *Endoscopy*, Vol. 30, 1998, pp. 392–407.

[86] Panjehpour, M., B. F. Overholt, and J. M. Haydek, "Light Sources and Delivery Devices for Photodynamic Therapy in the Gastrointestinal Tract," *Gastrointest. Endosc. Clin. N. Am.*, Vol. 10, 2000, pp. 513–532.

[87] Overholt, B. F., M. Panjehpour, and R. C. DeNovo, et al., "Balloon Photodynamic Therapy of Esophageal Cancer: Effect of Increasing Balloon Size," *Lasers Surg. Med.*, Vol. 18, 1996, pp. 248–252.

[88] Prasad, G. A., K. K. Wang, and N. S. Buttar, et al., "Predictors of Stricture Formation After Photodynamic Therapy for High-Grade Dysplasia in Barrett's Esophagus," *Gastrointest. Endosc.*, Vol. 65, 2007, pp. 60–66.

[89] Stepinac, T., P. Grosjean, and A. Woodtli, et al., "Optimization of the Diameter of a Radial Irradiation Device for Photodynamic Therapy in the Esophagus," *Endoscopy*, Vol. 34, 2002, pp. 411–415.

[90] Braichotte, D. R., J. F. Savary, and P. Monnier, et al., "Optimizing Light Dosimetry in Photodynamic Therapy of Early Stage Carcinomas of the Esophagus Using Fluorescence Spectroscopy," *Lasers Surg. Med.*, Vol. 19, 1996, pp. 340–346.

[91] Zellweger, M., P. Grosjean, and P. Monnier, et al., "Stability of the Fluorescence Measurement of Foscan in the Normal Human Oral Cavity as an Indicator of Its Content in Early Cancers of the Esophagus and the Bronchi," *Photochem. Photobiol.*, Vol. 69, 1999, pp. 605–610.

[92] Standish, B. A., V. X. Yang, and N. R. Munce, et al., "Doppler Optical Coherence Tomography Monitoring of Microvascular Tissue Response During Photodynamic Therapy in an Animal Model of Barrett's Esophagus," *Gastrointest. Endosc.*, Vol. 66, 2007, pp. 326–333.

[93] Ginsberg, G. G., E. E. Furth, and J. Ginsberg, et al., "Multi-Modal Endoluminal Eradication Therapy for Specialized Intestinal Metaplasia of the Esophagus and the Esophagogastric Junction with High-Grade Dysplasia and/or Intramucosal Carcinoma," Gastrointestinal Endoscopy Clinics of North America, Vol. 65, 2007, pp. AB154.

[94] Lustig, R. A., T. J. Vogl, and D. Fromm, et al., "A Multicenter Phase I Safety Study of Intratumoral Photoactivation of Talaporfin Sodium in Patients with Refractory Solid Tumors," *Cancer*, Vol. 98, 2003, pp. 1767–1771.

[95] Boch, R., A. J. Canaan, A. Cho, et al., "Cellular and Antitumor Activity of a New Diethylene Glycol Benzoporphyrin Derivative (Lemuteporfin)," *Photochemistry and Photobiology*, Vol. 82, 2006, pp. 219–224.

[96] Tan, W. C., C. Fulljames, and N. Stone, et al., "Photodynamic Therapy Using 5-Aminolaevulinic Acid for Esophageal Adenocarcinoma Associated with Barrett's Metaplasia," *J. Photochem. Photobiol. B*, Vol. 53, 1999, pp. 75–80.

[97] Mackenzie, G. D., N. F. Jamieson, and M. R. Novelli, et al., "How Light Dosimetry Influences the Efficacy of Photodynamic Therapy with 5-Aminolaevulinic Acid for Ablation of High-Grade Dysplasia in Barrett's Esophagus," *Lasers Med. Sci.*, Vol. 23, 2008, pp. 203–210.

[98] Ackroyd, R., C. J. Kelty, and N. J. Brown, et al., "Eradication of Dysplastic Barrett's Esophagus Using Photodynamic Therapy: Long-Term Follow-Up," *Endoscopy*, Vol. 35, 2003, pp. 496–501.

CHAPTER 26

PDT for Brain Cancer

M. Sam Eljamel

26.1 Introduction

Malignant brain tumors are diagnosed 5 to 10 times a year in every 100,000 of the population and are responsible for 3% of all cancer deaths worldwide. They are the second most common cause of cancer death among young people and the sixth most common cause of productive-years loss. They carry dismal prognosis and their presence in a patient's brain is comparable to a death sentence deferred by merely 36 weeks with no chance of pardon [1, 2]. One of the most common primary malignant brain tumors is high-grade glioma (HGG), comprising more than 40% of all intracranial tumors and consisting of glioblastoma multiforme (GBM 29%) and anaplastic astrocytoma (AA 11%). The standard treatment of GBM and AA is surgery followed by external beam radiotherapy (EBR) (4,000 cGy whole brain + 1,500 to 2,000 cGy to the tumor bed = 6,000 cGy to the tumor) [1]. Sadly, current standard management protocols offer a mean survival of less than 12 months to most patients and a 2-year survival rate of less than 7.5% [1]. Furthermore, patients above 65 years old have a mean survival of about 30 weeks regardless of recent advances in neuroimaging and surgical navigation technology. This is the main reason for pursuing new ways to treat these unpleasant cancers. Systemic chemotherapy has no more than 30% to 40% partial response rate in these tumors and in most circumstances a10% to 20% response rate [3]. Recent adjuvant therapies in the management of GBM include postoperative temazolamide (Temadol®) therapy and intracavity local carmusitine implants (Gliadel® wafers). Temazolamide offers a mere 26% 2-year survival compared to 10% in the placebo controls, 14.6 months median survival compared to 12.1 months in the placebo group, and a 7.2 months tumor-progression-free (TPF) survival compared to 5 months among the placebo controls [4]. On the other hand, carmustine implants prolong survival to 13.9 months compared to 11.9 months in the placebo group [5]. The poor outcome of these tumors is due to local invasion and local recurrence. The vast majority of these tumors recur locally and patients often succumb to and die from local recurrence, indicating that a more aggressive local therapy is required to eradicate the "weeds" of tumor that hide among the "flowers" of normal brain. However, complete radical surgical excision is hindered by the elusive nature of these tumors: a significant amount of tumor cells are invisible to the human eye even with the aid of the surgical microscope. The ability of these cancers to disguise themselves makes their identification at surgery almost impossible. Most of these tumors have invaded the brain widely by the time they manifest clinically, making a wider excision margin out of the question in most cases par polar lesions. What if we could one day discover a way to enhance our ability to visualize what is tumor and what is not? What if we could find a way to selectively kill residual tumor cells? Would that not be a method worth relentless pursuit? PD and PDT are the only techniques that have the potential answer to these questions.

26.2 Preclinical and Early PDT in Brain Cancers

PDT studies began in the 1970s in glioma cell cultures [6–14], glioma spheroids [15, 16], and animal models of gliomas and gliosacaromas [17–38]. These experimental laboratory studies have established that both photodetection (PD) and PDT have consistent encouraging antitumor effect and that glioma cells preferentially uptake and retain photosensitizers, making them potential aim for targeted PDT treatment. These experimental endeavors paved the way for phase I/II studies in brain tumors.

Perria et al. [39] reported one of the earliest attempts to photoirradiate postresection glioma cavity in humans and predicted that future refinement of the technique may produce better tissue penetration and more radical tumor kill.

Kaye et al. [40] reported a phase I/II trial involving 23 patients, of which there were 13 newly diagnosed GBM, six recurrent GBM, two newly diagnosed AA, and one recurrent AA. The authors used hematoporphyrin derivative (HPD) administered 24 hours before treatment at a dose of 5 mg/Kg body weight. PDT treatment was administered following maximum tumor removal. The tumor cavity was irradiated with 630-nm laser light without a diffuser. Two different lasers were used to deliver the light and the light-dose varied from 70 to 230 J/cm^2. Sixty-eight percent of their patients developed new tumors and underwent radiotherapy (20 Gy). Fifty-seven percent of the recurrent gliomas developed further recurrences 12 to 16 weeks after PDT and 13% of the newly diagnosed gliomas developed recurrences at 3 and 13 weeks from PDT. Fifteen patients had no recurrences at a mean follow-up of 7 months (1 to 16 months). The authors concluded that PDT can be used as an adjuvant therapy in these patients.

By 1988, more than 64 patients treated with PDT were reported in the literature and though some of the initial results in GBM were disappointing, most treated patients had a very low light dose and the patients were a very poor prognosis group who were unlikely to gain a benefit because of other adverse prognostic factors that determined their inevitable fatal outcome [41].

Kostron et al. [42] reported a series of 20 patients, including 18 GBM treated with a wavelength of 630 nm and 40-120J/cm^2. This was followed immediately by a single dose of radiation. Conventional radiotherapy followed in eight patients. The median survival of three recurrent GBM was 5 months and four of the newly diagnosed GBM died because of tumor recurrence with a median survival of 5 months. However, six of their patients were still alive 12 months after PDT and six patients were still alive at 22 months. This was a very encouraging outcome, considering that the mean survival of these patients at the time was less than 12 months and the 2-year survival was less than 7.5%.

Origitano and Reichman [43] reported their experience using image-guided computer assisted protocol to improve treatment volume coverage and pointed out that treatment failure is often due to lack of tumor coverage by the treatment and limited tissue penetration of the laser light. They have demonstrated that combining intracavity irradiation with peritumoral interstitial irradiation was possible and could achieve better tumor-volume coverage.

Muller and Wilson [44] reported 49 patients treated with PDT. These were young patients (mean age of 41) with a mean Karnofsky performance score (KPS) of 79, who had recurrent malignant gliomas. Thirty-two were GBM, 14 were AA, six were mixed, and four were malignant ependymomas. The total light dose in this series varied from 440 to 4500 J (median 1, 800J) and the energy density varied from 8 to 110 J/cm^2. The median survival of recurrent GBM was 30 weeks with a 1-year survival of 18%. The median survival of GBM from first diagnosis was 82% at 1 year and 57% at 2 years, which was significantly better than the 2-year survival of less than 7.5% following standard treatment. For recurrent AA, the median survival was 44 weeks and the 1-year and 2-year survival was 43% and 36%, respectively.

By 1996, over 310 patients with newly diagnosed or recurrent malignant gliomas were treated with PDT after tumor resection. Though there was wide variation in the light dose, the photosensitizer dose, the completeness of surgical resection, the patients' age, the KPS, the number of treatments received, and the number of recurrences, analysis of the data indicated that PDT significantly increased the survival of patients and the treatment was well tolerated.

The volume of residual tumor after surgical resection seems to be a significant adverse prognostic factor for recurrence of HGG. Therefore, complete tumor resection would seem to be the next logical step in the management of these unpleasant locally malignant cancers of the brain. However, the most limiting factor to achieve complete surgical resection safely is the inability of the surgeon to distinguish normal brain from tumor cells under normal surgical microscopy. Stummer et al. [45, 46] had reported the utilization of PD to achieve maximum tumor removal safely with 100% specificity and 85% sensitivity. In more than 60% of 52 consecutive patients in that study, the surgeon managed to completely excise the enhancing GBM on MRI scan [46]. Coupling this technology with the surgical microscope led to improved survival rates of patients with HGG.

PD and PDT was used not only in patients with very poor prognosis such as GBM and AA, but also in malignant ependymomas [44, 47], malignant meningioma [42], melanoma brain metastasis [42], lung brain metastasis [40], and recurrent pituitary adenomas [48]. The results of phase I/II PDT trials in the brain are summarized in Figure 26.1.

26.3   PD and PDT Techniques in Brain Cancer

The surgical techniques used in PD and PDT assisted surgical resection of intracranial tumors include the following steps.

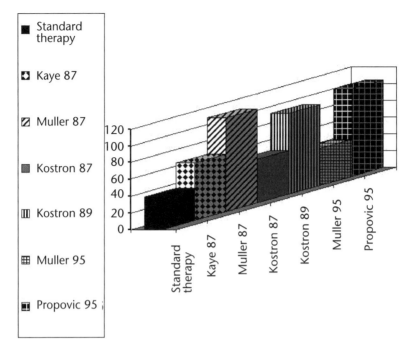

Figure 26.1 A bar graph representing the average survival of GBMs treated with PDT in phase I/II trials in the twentieth century compared to standard treatment.

26.3.1 Choice of Photosensitizer

Several photosensitizers have been used in brain cancers. These included hematoporphyrin derivative (HPD) [2, 40], porfimer sodium (Photofrin®) [2, 41, 44], 5-aminolevulinic acid (5-ALA) [2, 46] and m-tetrahydroxyphenylchlorin (mTHPC, Foscan®) [2, 42]. However, the most commonly used photosensitizers in brain tumors today are 5-ALA, Photofrin, and Foscan®. These photosensitizers are not licensed at the moment for treating brain tumors in most countries and their use in brain tumors is off-label on named patients' basis.

26.3.1.1 5-Aminolevulinic Acid (5-ALA)

5-ALA has been used in many fields to detect and treat precancer and cancerous lesions. It is a natural precursor for the heme synthesis in all living mammalian cells. Each cell metabolizes 5-ALA along a set pathway to heme, producing proto-porphyrin-IX (PpIX) along the way. However, conversion of PpIX to heme is blocked in cancer cells leading to accumulation of PpIX in the tumor. It can be applied topically or taken orally. In PD and PDT of brain tumors, it is given orally 3 to 4 hours before induction of anesthesia in a mixture of nonfizzy orange juice at 15 to 20 mg/Kg body weight. The active compound in the cells is PpIX, which can be activated by violet-blue light (375–440 nm) for PD and diode laser light (635 nm) for PDT, tissue depth penetration is 7 to 15 mm, the irradiation dose required for PDT is 100 J/cm^2, and skin photosensitivity continues for 7 to 10 days after ingestion.

26.3.1.2   Photofrin (Porfimer Sodium)

Photofrin is given intravenously at 2 mg/Kg body weight 48 to 96 hours before PDT. It is activated by diode laser light at 630-nm wavelength. The depth of tissue penetration is from 7 to 12 mm and the irradiation dose is 100 J/cm^2. Skin photosensitivity carries on for 30 days, after which it reduces significantly and by 90 days it is usually gone.

26.3.1.3   Foscan® (Temoporfin)

Foscan is given intravenously at a dose of 0.15 mg/Kg body weight about 90 to 110 hours before PDT. It is activated at 652-nm wavelength and its tissue penetration is 10 to 15 mm. The irradiation dose is 20 J/cm^2 and its skin photosensitivity continues for about 2 weeks.

Therefore, the photosensitizer is administered either orally (5-ALA) or intravenously (Photofrin and Foscan) 3 hours (5-ALA), 48 hours (Photofrin), or 96 hours (Foscan) before surgery to allow sufficient concentration of the photosensitizer in the tumor cells. Patients are counseled to take adequate protection from bright light and the sun to prevent skin and retinal damage.

26.3.2   Planning

The surgical approach and trajectories are planned usually on a workstation using preoperative MRI or CT images. The value of this step is precise localization of the tumor, minimally invasive craniotomy, and minimal collateral brain injury (Color Plate 35). For PD and particularly PDT, it is essential that the bulk of the tumor is removed and the postresection cavity is treated with PDT. This strategy will avoid raised intracranial pressure in the post-operative period [48].

26.3.3   Specific Brain PD and PDT Equipment

PD-assisted brain tumor resection can be performed using commercially available systems such as the Olympus® QTV55 and CLV-520 PD system attached to an endoscope with long pass observation filter [48] or the Zeiss™ OPMI® Pentero® or NC4 microscope with PD-system [46]. PDT, on the other hand, requires an inflatable diffuser filled with a mixture of Intralipid and normal saline (0.4 ml of Intralipid, 12.5 ml of normal saline, and 12.5 ml of radio-opaque dye) [46] and a diode laser that is capable of illuminating the postresection tumor cavity with the appropriate wavelength for the photosensitizer, such as the InGaAIP laser diode CW (630+/- 3 nm, Diomed, Cambridge, United Kingdom) for Photofrin PDT [46].

26.4   PD-Assisted Surgical Resection

The basic neurosurgical techniques utilized to excise the bulk of the tumor are implemented in the same way when using PD-assisted system. Once the tumor was localized using the neuronavigation technology, the tumor mass is reduced by removing tumor cells starting from the center and going out to the periphery. The ultrasonic dissector would be a useful tool to achieve this goal quickly. Once the bulk of tumor was removed, the remaining tumor margin is cleared using the PD-assisted technology. Once all fluorescent tumor cells were removed and hemostasis was secured, a balloon diffuser was inflated and placed in the tumor cavity and the craniotomy was closed in the usual fashion, leaving the catheter of the balloon diffuser exiting via one of the burr holes and through a separate stab incision in the scalp. It is of paramount importance that the catheter is not bent or kinked in any way to allow smooth insertion and extraction of the laser fiber. As the laser fiber is reusable, a disposable fiber sheet can be inserted in the balloon diffuser before inflation and placement (Color Plate 36).

26.5   PDT Dose Calculation and Administration

The PDT dose is dependent on the balloon-diffuser size, the laser fiber diffuser length, the prescribed dose of light, and the power output of the laser machine. For example, for a balloon-diffuser (tumor cavity) of 1 cm, laser fiber-diffuser of 1 cm, laser power of 400 mW, a dose of 100 J/cm^2, and irradiation of 127 mW/cm^2, a treatment duration of 785 seconds would be necessary (Table 26.1). In infratentorial and intrasellar tumors we gave a single shot of PDT treatment under the same anesthesia and the balloon diffuser was removed before closure of the operation (Color Plate 37). In supratentorial malignant tumors, we left the catheter in situ for treatment; the first treatment was given in the recovery and up to five subsequent treatments were given in the following days at the bedside (Color Plate 38).

26.6   PD and PDT in Brain Tumors: The Present

Phase I/II studies of PDT in brain tumors span over three decades. The Royal Melbourne Hospital's experience included 375 patients. There were 138 newly diagnosed GBMs, 140 recurrent GBMs, 41 newly diagnosed AAs, and 46 recurrent AAs.

Table 26.1 Dose Calculation and the Duration of Each PDT Treatment with Different Lesion and Fiber Diffuser Sizes

Lesion/balloon size (cm)	0.5	0.75	1	1.25	1.75
Laser fiber diffuser (cm)	1	1	1	1	1.5
Laser power (mW)	400	400	400	400	600
Dose (J/cm^2)	100	100	100	100	100
Irradiance (mW/cm^2)	509	226	127	81	85
PDT duration (sec)	196	442	785	1,227	1,178
Lesion/balloon size (cm)	1.75	2	2.25	2.5	3
Laser fiber diffuser (cm)	1.5	1.5	1.5	2.5	2.5
Laser power (mW)	600	600	600	1,000	1,000
Dose (J/cm^2)	100	100	100	100	100
Irradiance (mW/cm^2)	62	48	38	51	35
PDT duration (sec)	1,604	2,094	2,651	1,963	2,827

Long-term analysis was available for 145 patients: 31 newly diagnosed GBMs, 55 recurrent GBMs, 30 newly diagnosed AAs, and 29 recurrent AAs [49]. These patients received 5 mg HPD/Kg 24 hours before surgery and the light dose was 70 to 260 J/cm^2 using a bare fiber inserted in the middle of the tumor cavity without a balloon diffuser. 29% of these patients received adjuvant chemotherapy. The mean survival of newly diagnosed GBM was 14.3 months and 28% survived more than 2 years. The mean survival of newly diagnosed AA was 76.5 months and 73% survived more than 36 months. The mean survival of recurrent GBM was 14.9 months with 2- and 3-year survival of 41% and 37%, respectively. The mean survival of recurrent AA was 66.6 months and the 2- and 3-year survival was 61% and 57%, respectively. The complication rate was 1.4% cerebral infarction, 6.2% cerebral edema, and 1.4% sunburns. The HPD tumor uptake varied from 2 to 13 μg/gm of wet tissue. The HPD uptake correlated to GBM outcome (p<0.01) and the higher the dose of light, the better the outcome was (p<0.3). However, the Toronto group randomized patients between 40 and 120 J/cm^2 and found that the survival of the high-dose (48 patients) was 10 months compared to 9 months in the low-dose group (49 patients). This difference did not reach statistical significance at the 0.05 level. However, the light dose used in by the Toronto group was half the dose used by the Melbourne group, which would explain the difference in the response-dose relationship. In recent years three PD and PDT randomized controlled trials were completed in brain tumors. Stummer et al. (2006) [50] reported the results of the 5-ALA study group, a multicenter prospective randomized controlled trial in Germany. Muller et al. (2006) [51] reported the results of two center prospective randomized controlled trials using adjuvant Photofrin PDT in the study group. Eljamel et al. (2007) [52] reported a single center prospective randomized controlled study using 5-ALA and Photofrin. All three trials were performed in the most difficult tumor type to eradicate, GBM. The 5-ALA and PpIX-induced fluorescence technique led to complete removal of the enhancing tumor on MRI in 65% (90/139) of patients compared to 36% of the standard microscopic techniques (p<0.001) [50]. This trial demonstrated that time to tumor progression of the PD group was much better than that of the control group; 5.1 months in the PD group compared to 3.6 months in the controls (p<0.001). Although the PD group survived longer without tumor recurrence, the difference in the overall survival was not statistically significant; possibly due the fact that the trial was not designed to answer this particular question and there was no restriction on the additional adjuvant therapy after tumor recurrence in both the study and control groups [50]. The single Photofrin PDT treatment [50, 51] demonstrated that more patients survived for 12 months of the group who received adjuvant PDT (17/43, 39.5%) compared to those who did not have PDT (9/33, 27.3%). Sadly, the survival curves crossed over at 15 months. Nevertheless, the quality of survival in the treatment group was better than that in the controls. The last study [52] combining the techniques of 5-ALA induced fluorescence assisted surgical resection, PpIX spectroscopy, and fractionated Photofrin PDT up to 500 J/cm^2 divided in five fractions demonstrated that patients in the study group had significant survival, quality of life improvement, and time to tumor progression advantages compared to the control group (p<0.01). Therefore, the outcome of adjuvant PD and PDT techniques in GBM is in favor of PD/PDT (Figure 26.2).

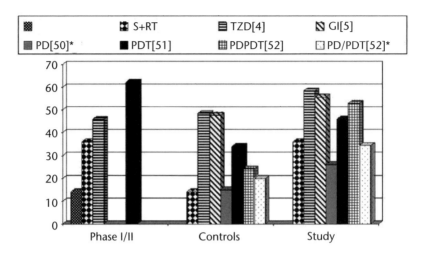

Figure 26.2 Comparison of recent treatment developments in GBM treatment with standard therapy (S=surgery alone, S+RT=surgery and radiotherapy, TZD= temazolamide treatment in addition to S and RT, Gl= Gliadel (carmustine) implants in addition to S+RT, PD= 5-ALA PD in addition to S and RT, PDT= Photofrin PDT in addition to S+RT, and PDPDT= 5-ALA and fractionated PDT in addition to S and RT). All bars represent percent of overall survival except those marked *, which represent tumor-free survival.

Two of the aforementioned prospective randomized controlled trials demonstrated that time to tumor progression/recurrence in GBM was significantly prolonged (p<0.01) with PD compared to standard neurosurgical resection under white light microsurgery [50–52]. Phase I/II studies on PDT in malignant brain tumors were in favor of PDT on the basis of prolonging survival. However, the results of PD/PDT randomized controlled trials in GBM were divided. The 5-ALA study group [50] was not designed to look ahead for the overall survival. The authors did not control for adjuvant therapy following recurrence such as chemotherapy and further surgery. The second trial, conducted in North America, demonstrated that the initial survival advantage with single fraction PDT was lost at 15 months. There were several reasons for this: a light dose of 120 J/cm^2 may not be sufficient, light dose distribution may not have been uniform, the use of KTP pumped dye laser with a wavelength of 532 nm (ideally for Photofrin a wavelength of 630 nm is required), and last, the Photofrin was injected 12 to 36 hours prior to surgery. All these factors may have contributed to the failure of this trial to demonstrate survival advantage in the study group despite all phase I/II trials having demonstrated significant survival advantages in both newly diagnosed and recurrent GBM. Although the last study demonstrated significant delay in the tumor recurrence in the study group and significant good quality survival in the study group, the critics pointed out that the study was single-center and used two photodynamic techniques and one cannot be sure which part of the technique (PD or PDT) was more significant. However, the fact that the study was performed in a single center was in fact a strength as the most difficult variable to control in any surgical trial is patient selection criteria and the surgical technique. It is less likely that there was significant variation in the equipoise for randomization or the surgical technique in a single-center study. The reason that the two techniques were tested together is important as the efficacy of PDT would be dependant on the amount of residual tumor left behind. PD and PDT therefore go hand in hand. PD has already been shown to help in removing the residual tumor in 65% compared to only 36% using conventional techniques [50] and therefore what this trial was testing is the addition of PDT to kill any remaining tumor cells.

26.7 Conclusion

Type A and type B scientific evidence for PD and PDT in brain cancer is accumulating rapidly, and as the technology becomes more widely available it will only be a matter of time before it becomes an accepted treatment in routine neurosurgical practice demanded by patients and accepted by healthcare providers.

References

[1] Obwegeser, A., et al., "Therapy of Glioblastoma Multiforme: A Cumulative Experience of 10 Years," *Acta Neurochir. (Wien)*, Vol. 137, 1995, pp. 29–33.

[2] Eljamel, S., "Photodynamic Assisted Surgical Resection and Treatment of Malignant Brain Tumors; Technique, Technology and Clinical Application," *Photodiag. Photodyn. Ther.*, Vol. 1, 2004, pp. 93–98.

[3] Komblith, P., "The Role of Cytotoxic Chemotherapy in the Treatment of Malignant Brain Tumors," *Surg. Neurol.*, Vol. 44, 1995, pp. 551–552.

[4] Taphoorn, M. J., et al., "Health-Related Quality of Life in Patients with Glioblastoma: A Randomised Controlled Trial," *Lancet Oncol.*, Vol. 6, 2005, pp. 937–944.

[5] Westphal, M., et al., "A Phase 3 Trial of Local Chemotherapy with Biodegradable Carmustine (BCNU) Wafers (Gliadel Wafers) in Patients with Primary Malignant Glioma," *Neuro. Oncol.*, Vol. 5, 2003, pp. 79–88.

[6] Tsai, J. C., et al., "Comparative Study on the ALA Photodynamic Effects of Human Glioma and Meningioma Cells," *Lasers Surg. Med.*, Vol. 24, 1999, pp. 296–305.

[7] Stummer, W., et al., "In Vitro and In Vivo Porphyrin Accumulation by C6 Glioma Cells after Exposure to 5-Aminolevulinic Acid," *J. Photochem. Photobiol. B*, Vol. 45, 1998, pp. 160–169.

[8] Sreenivasan, R., et al., "Binding of Monomeric and Oligomeric Porphyrins to Human Glioblastoma (U-87MG) Cells and Their Photosensitivity," *Cancer Lett.*, Vol. 120, 1997, pp. 45–51.

[9] Abernathey, C. D., et al., "Activity of Phthalocyanine Photosensitizers Against Human Glioblastoma In Vitro," *Neurosurgery*, Vol. 21, 1987, pp. 468–473.

[10] Eleouet, S., et al., "Heterogeneity of Delta-Aminolevulinic Acid-Induced Protoporphyrin IX Fluorescence in Human Glioma Cells and Leukemic Lymphocytes," *Neurol. Res.*, Vol. 22, 2000, pp. 361–368.

[11] Powers, S. K., et al., "Photosensitization of Human Glioma Cells by Chalcogenapyrylium Dyes," *J. Neurooncol.*, Vol. 7, 1989, pp. 179–188.

[12] Sharma, M., P. G. Joshi, and N. B. Joshi, "MC540 Induced Photosensitization of Glioma and Neuroblastoma Cells," *Indian J. Med. Res.*, Vol. 99, 1994, pp. 124–128.

[13] Leach, M. W., et al., "In Vitro Photodynamic Effects of Lysyl Chlorin P6: Cell Survival, Localization and Ultrastructural Changes," *Photochem. Photobiol.*, Vol. 58, 1993, pp. 653–660.

[14] Wharen, R. E., Jr., et al., "Hematoporphyrin Derivative Photocytotoxicity of Human Glioblastoma in Cell Culture," *Neurosurgery*, Vol. 19, 1986, pp. 495–501.

[15] Friesen, S. A., et al., "5-Aminolevulinic Acid-Based Photodynamic Detection and Therapy of Brain Tumors (Review)," *Int. J. Oncol.*, Vol. 21, 2002, pp. 577–582.

[16] Terzis, A. J., et al., "Effects of Photodynamic Therapy on Glioma Spheroids," *Br. J. Neurosurg.*, Vol. 11, 1997, pp. 196–205.

[17] Lobel, J., et al., "2-[1-Hexyloxyethyl]-2-Devinyl Pyropheophorbide-a (HPPH) in a Nude Rat Glioma Model: Implications for Photodynamic Therapy," *Lasers Surg. Med.*, Vol. 29, 2001, pp. 397–405.

[18] Schmidt, M. H., et al., "Preclinical Evaluation of Benzoporphyrin Derivative Combined with a Light-Emitting Diode Array for Photodynamic Therapy of Brain Tumors," *Pediatr. Neurosurg.*, Vol. 30, 1999, pp. 225–231.

[19] Obwegeser, A., R. Jakober, and H. Kostron, "Uptake and Kinetics of 14C-Labelled Meta-Tetrahydroxyphenylchlorin and 5-Aminolaevulinic Acid in the C6 Rat Glioma Model," *Br. J. Cancer*, Vol. 78, 1998, pp. 733–738.

[20] Lilge, L., and B. C. Wilson, "Photodynamic Therapy of Intracranial Tissues: A Preclinical Comparative Study of Four Different Photosensitizers," *J. Clin. Laser Med. Surg.*, Vol. 16, 1998, pp. 81–91.

[21] Chopp, M., et al., "Sensitivity of 9L Gliosarcomas to Photodynamic Therapy," *Radiat. Res.*, Vol. 146, 1996, pp. 461–465.

[22] Frisoli, J. K., et al., "Pharmacokinetics of a Fluorescent Drug Using Laser-Induced Fluorescence," *Cancer Res.*, Vol. 53, 1993, pp. 5954–5961.

[23] Lilge, L., et al., "The Sensitivity of Normal Brain and Intracranially Implanted VX2 Tumour to Interstitial Photodynamic Therapy," *Br. J. Cancer*, Vol. 73, 1996, pp. 332–343.

[24] Hebeda, K. M., et al., "5-Aminolevulinic Acid Induced Endogenous Porphyrin Fluorescence in 9L and C6 Brain Tumours and in the Normal Rat Brain," *Acta Neurochir. (Wien)*, Vol. 140, 1998, pp. 503-512; discussion 512–503.

[25] Olzowy, B., et al., "Photoirradiation Therapy of Experimental Malignant Glioma with 5-Aminolevulinic Acid," *J. Neurosurg.*, Vol. 97, 2002, pp. 970–976.

[26] Raffel, C., M. S. Edwards, and D. F. Deen, "The Effect of Bromodeoxyuridine and Ultraviolet Light on 9L Rat Brain Tumor Cells," *Radiat. Res.*, Vol. 118, 1989, pp. 409–419.

[27] Stummer, W., et al., "Photodynamic Therapy within Edematous Brain Tissue: Considerations on Sensitizer Dose and Time Point of Laser Irradiation," *J. Photochem. Photobiol. B*, Vol. 36, 1996, pp. 179–181.

[28] Whelan, H. T., et al., "The Role of Photodynamic Therapy in Posterior Fossa Brain Tumors. A Preclinical Study in a Canine Glioma Model," *J. Neurosurg.*, Vol. 79, 1993, pp. 562–568.

[29] Ji, Y., et al., "Improved Survival from Intracavitary Photodynamic Therapy of Rat Glioma," *Photochem. Photobiol.*, Vol. 56, 1992, pp. 385–390.

[30] Leach, M. W., et al., "Effectiveness of a Lysyl Chlorin p6/Chlorin p6 Mixture in Photodynamic Therapy of the Subcutaneous 9L Glioma in the Rat," *Cancer Res.*, Vol. 52, 1992, pp. 1235–1239.

[31] Fujishima, I., et al., "Photodynamic Therapy Using Pheophorbide a and Nd:YAG Laser," *Neurol. Med. Chir. (Tokyo)*, Vol. 31, 1991, pp. 257–263.

[32] Powers, S. K., et al., "Interstitial Laser Photochemotherapy of Rhodamine-123-Sensitized Rat Glioma," *J. Neurosurg.*, Vol. 67, 1987, pp. 889–894.

[33] Kostron, H., et al., "The Interaction of Hematoporphyrin Derivative, Light, and Ionizing Radiation in a Rat Glioma Model," *Cancer*, Vol. 57, 1986, pp. 964–970.

[34] Kaye, A. H., G. Morstyn, and R. G. Ashcroft, "Uptake and Retention of Hematoporphyrin Derivative in an In Vivo/In Vitro Model of Cerebral Glioma," *Neurosurgery*, Vol. 17, 1985, pp. 883–890.

[35] Sekimoto, T., et al., "Photoradiation Therapy of Experimental Brain Tumor," *No Shinkei Geka*, Vol. 13, 1985, pp. 991–996.

[36] Cheng, M. K., et al., "Photoradiation Therapy of 9L-Gliosarcoma in Rats: Hematoporphyrin Derivative (Types I and II) Followed by Laser Energy," *J. Neurooncol.*, Vol. 3, 1985, pp. 217–228.

[37] Rounds, D. E., et al., "Phototoxicity of Brain Tissue in Hematoporphyrin Derivative Treated Mice," *Prog. Clin. Biol. Res.*, Vol. 170, 1984, pp. 613–628.

[38] Boggan, J. E., et al., "Hematoporphyrin Derivative Photoradiation Therapy of the Rat 9L Gliosarcoma Brain Tumor Model," *Lasers Surg. Med.*, Vol. 4, 1984, pp. 99–105.

[39] Perria, C., et al., "Fast Attempts at the Photodynamic Treatment of Human Gliomas," *J. Neurosurg. Sci.*, Vol. 24, 1980, pp. 119–129.

[40] Kaye, A. H., G. Morstyn, and D. Brownbill, "Adjuvant High-Dose Photoradiation Therapy in the Treatment of Cerebral Glioma: A Phase 1-2 Study," *J. Neurosurg.*, Vol. 67, 1987, pp. 500–505.

[41] Muller, P., and B. Wilson, "Photodynamic Therapy of Brain Tumours—Post-Operative "Field Fractionation," *J. Photochem. Photobiol. B*, Vol. 9, 1991, pp. 117–119.

[42] Kostron, H., E. Fritsch, and V. Grunert, "Photodynamic Therapy of Malignant Brain Tumours: A Phase I/II Trial," *Br. J. Neurosurg.*, Vol. 2, 1988, pp. 241–248.

[43] Origitano, T. C., and O. H. Reichman, "Photodynamic Therapy for Intracranial Neoplasms: Development of an Image-Based Computer-Assisted Protocol for Photodynamic Therapy of Intracranial Neoplasms," *Neurosurgery*, Vol. 32, 1993, pp. 587-595; discussion 595–586.

[44] Muller, P. J., and B. C. Wilson, "Photodynamic Therapy for Recurrent Supratentorial Gliomas," *Semin. Surg. Oncol.*, Vol. 11, 1995, pp. 346–354.

[45] Stummer, W., et al., "Technical Principles for Protoporphyrin-IX-Fluorescence Guided Microsurgical Resection of Malignant Glioma Tissue," *Acta Neurochir.*, Vol. 140, 1998, pp. 995–1000.

[46] Stummer, W., et al., "Fluorescence-Guided Resection of Glioblastoma Multiforme by Using 5-Aminolevulinic Acid-Induced Porphyrins: A Prospective Study in 52 Consecutive Patients," *J. Neurosurg.*, Vol. 93, 2000, pp. 1003–1013.

[47] Krishnamurthy, S., et al., "Optimal Light Dose for Interstitial Photodynamic Therapy in Treatment for Malignant Brain Tumors," *Lasers Surg. Med.*, Vol. 27, 2000, pp. 224–234.

[48] Marks, P. V., et al., "Effect of Photodynamic Therapy on Recurrent Pituitary Adenomas: Clinical Phase I/II Trial—An Early Report," *Br. J. Neurosurg.*, Vol. 14, 2000, pp. 317–325.

[49] Stylli, S. S., et al., "Photodynamic Therapy of High Grade Glioma Long Term Survival," *J. Clin. Neurosci.*, Vol. 12, 2005, pp. 389–398.

[50] Stummer, W., et al., "Fluorescence-Guided Surgery with 5-Aminolevulinic Acid for Resection of Malignant Glioma: A Randomised Controlled Multicentre Phase III Trial," *Lancet Oncol.*, Vol. 7, 2006, pp. 392–401.

[51] Muller, P. J., and B. C. Wilson, "Photodynamic Therapy of Brain Tumors—A Work in Progress," *Lasers Surg. Med.*, Vol. 38, 2006, pp. 384–389.

[52] Eljamel, M. S., C. Goodman, and H. Moseley, "ALA and Photofrin Fluorescence-guided resection and repetitive PDT in glioblastoma multiforme: a single centre Phase III randomised controlled trial," *Lasers in Medical Science*, 2008.

CHAPTER 27

PDT for Pituitary Tumors

M. Sam Eljamel

27.1 Introduction

Pituitary adenomas (PAs) are benign tumors of the pituitary gland and represent about 12% of all intracranial tumors [1, 2]. They are classified according to their size and function into several groups (Table 27.1). If the PA is 10 mm or less, it is considered microadenoma. If the PA is hypersecreting one of the pituitary gland hormones, it is classified as hypersecreting PA. Hypersecreting PA may secret excess growth hormone, causing acromegaly, excess ACTH, causing Cushing's disease, or excess prolactin, causing hyperprolactinemia.

Nonsecreting PA tend to present late, and by the time they reveal themselves clinically they often have already compressed the optic chiasm [3–8] or invaded the cavernous sinus and surrounding structures [8, 9] (Figure 27.1).

Nonfunctioning PA represents 35% of PA. Prolactinomas account for 30%, acromegaly for 20%, and Cushing's disease for 15% [10]. Surgery is the best single therapy for PA that presents with acromegaly, Cushing's disease, and those that compress the optic chiasm. Some of PAs that present with hyperprolactinemia may also require surgery if medical therapy fails or the patient did not tolerate medical therapy because of side effects. The aims of surgery in pituitary adenomas are to remove the whole of the PA and preserve normal pituitary gland functions. The remission rate of acromegaly following surgery varies from 33% to 70% [10, 11],

Table 27.1 Classifications of PA

Scheme	Features
Size of microadenoma	=10 mm
Size of macroadenoma	> 10 mm
Nonfunctioning adenoma	These adenomas may have pituitary deficiency or slight hyperprolactinemia due to pituitary stalk pressure.
Functioning adenoma	These adenomas present with excess: • Growth hormone (acromegaly) • ACTH (Cushing's disease) • Prolactin (amenorrhea/ galactorrhea) • Thyroid-stimulating hormone • Gonadotrophic hormone • Mixed secretions

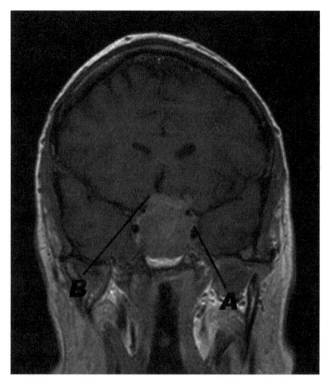

Figure 27.1   Coronal T1: MRI slice with gadolinium demonstrating a giant nonfunctioning pituitary adenoma invading the cavernous sinus (a) and the suprasellar region (b).

and for Cushing's disease from 85% to 90% [10, 12, 13]. In microprolactinomas, surgery is effective in only 84% to 87% [10, 14]. The remission rate after surgery in macroprolactinomas is only 56% [10]. One of the reasons why transsphenoidal surgery is not more successful in curing pituitary microadenomas is the difficulty in localizing the exact site of the microadenoma pre- and intraoperatively. One of the new and exciting applications of photodiagnosis (PD) is to pinpoint the exact location of the microadenoma. On the other hand, macroadenomas and giant pituitary adenomas cannot be cured by surgery due to their invasion of the cavernous sinus and other surrounding structures, leading to high failure rate of up to 73% in some series [15] (Table 27.2). A new and exciting application of photodynamic therapy (PDT) is to treat residual PA and improve the cure rate in invasive pituitary adenomas.

27.2   Preclinical and Early PDT in Pituitary Adenomas

In vivo studies using PDT in PA cells implanted subcutaneously in nude mice were studied in the 1990s [16, 17]. These studies not only proved the concept of PDT in PA but also demonstrated that PDT had produced significant microvascular changes, inflammatory reaction, and adenoma cell necrosis in the treatment group compared to the controls.

Table 27.2 Results of Surgery in Pituitary Adenomas

PA Type	Results of Surgery	
	Microadenoma	Macroadenoma
Growth hormone (acromegaly)	88%	57%
ACTH (Cushing's disease)	88%	65%
Prolactinoma	87%	56%
Nonfunctioning adenomas		82%
Giant pituitary adenomas		27%

27.3   PD and PDT Techniques in Pituitary Adenomas

The surgical techniques used in PD and PDT assisted surgical resection of PA include the following steps.

27.3.1   Choice of Photosensitizer

Because of the proximity of the cavernous sinus and the optic pathways (optic chiasm and optic nerves), the choice of photosensitizers is very important. Both porfimer sodium (Photofrin®) and 5-aminolevulinic acid (5-ALA) have been used in PD/PDT of PA. These photosensitizers are not licensed at the moment for treating PA in most countries and their use in PA is off-label on named patients' basis.

27.3.1.1   5-Aminolevulinic Acid (5-ALA)

5-ALA has been used in many fields to detect and treat precancer and cancerous lesions. Pituitary cells metabolize 5-ALA along a set pathway to heme, producing protoporphyrin-IX (PpIX) along the way. However, the conversion of PpIX to heme is blocked in PA cells, leading to accumulation of PpIX in these cells. In PD and PDT of PA, it is given orally 3 to 4 hours before induction of anesthesia in a mixture of nonfizzy orange juice at 20 mg/Kg body weight. The active compound in the cells is PpIX, which can be activated by violet-blue light (375–440 nm) for PD and diode laser light (635 nm) for PDT, tissue depth penetration is 7 to 15 mm, the irradiation dose required for PDT is 100 J/cm^2, and skin photosensitivity continues for 7 to 10 days after ingestion.

27.3.1.2   Photofrin (Porfimer Sodium)

Photofrin is given intravenously at 2 mg/Kg body weight 48 to 96 hours before PDT. It is activated by diode laser light at 630-nm wavelength. The depth of tissue penetration is from 7 to 12 mm and the irradiation dose is 100 J/cm^2. Skin photosensitivity carries on for 30 days, after which it reduces significantly and by 90 days it is usually gone.

Therefore, the photosensitizer is administered either orally (5-ALA) or intravenously (Photofrin and Foscan®) 3 hours (5-ALA) or 48 hours (Photofrin) before surgery to allow sufficient concentration of the photosensitizer in the adenoma cells.

Patients are counseled to take adequate protection from bright light and the sun to prevent skin and retinal damage.

27.3.2　Planning

The surgical approach and trajectories are usually planned on a workstation using preoperative MRI or CT images in the same way as any other pituitary surgery. The value of this step is precise localization of the adenoma (Color Plate 39).

27.4　Specific PD and PDT Equipment

PD-assisted adenoma resection can be performed using commercially available systems such as the Olympus® QTV55 and CLV-520 PD system attached to an endoscope with long-pass observation filter or the Zeiss™ OPMI® Pentero® or NC4 microscope with PD system. PDT, on the other hand, requires an inflatable balloon diffuser filled with 0.8% Intralipid solution made up by adding 0.4 ml of 20% Intralipid solution to 12.5 ml of normal saline and 12.5 ml of radio-opaque dye. A diode laser that is capable of illuminating the postresection tumor cavity with the appropriate wavelength for the photosensitizer, such as the InGaAIP Laser Diode CW (630 ± 3 nm, Diomed, Cambridge, United Kingdom) for Photofrin PDT.

27.5　Optical Intraoperative Localization of PA

One of the most exciting and interesting applications of PD in PA surgery is intraoperative localization of microadenomas. As surgery is the best single therapeutic modality for acromegaly, Cushing's disease, and nonfunctioning PA, it is paramount that the microadenomas responsible for these diseases are localized precisely to be able to remove them completely and save normal pituitary gland and its function. For years neuroendocrine teams did their best to improve preoperative microadenoma localization with some success. Although MRI had emerged as the imaging of choice for evaluating the pituitary, MRI cannot rule out a microadenoma if the MRI was normal and it cannot diagnose an adenoma if the MRI was abnormal, as incidental PA can be found in as high as 10% of people [18]. Dynamic MRI scanning has improved preoperative microadenoma localization and as high as 64% success rate was reported [19]. Bilateral inferior petrosal sinus sampling (BIPSS) has also improved the localization of the microadenoma in Cushing's disease. BIPSS can only lateralize microadenoma to the right or left half of the pituitary gland in Cushing's disease in up to 81% of cases [20]. Therefore, there is still a lot of room of maneuver to improve localization of microadenomas and improve their selective removal. Eljamel et al. [20] had reported a series of 17 newly diagnosed PAs localized by ALA-induced PpIX spectroscopy [20]. There were eight nonfunctioning PA, four acromegaly, three Cushing's disease, and two gonadotrophin-secreting PA. The specificity of the system was 100% and the sensitivity was 94%. The system had accurately located the site of the adenoma in 94% with no false positives. There was only one false negative in a patient who did not receive the accurate dose of 20 mg/kg body weight of 5-ALA 3 hours before surgery. There were seven microadenomas in this series and the false negative patient was in this group. All the growth hormone secreting PA (acromegaly) were accurately localized while two of the three ACTH secreting PA (Cushing's disease) were accurately localized. The optical localization system (Figure 27.2) consists of a gallium nitride laser emitting violet-blue light at 405 nm. The light wave is transmitted to fiber-optic probe that can be inserted within the pituitary gland under direct microscopic or endoscopic vision to detect PpIX spectrum at 632 nm. The spectroscopic signal from PpIX is carried back through the same fiber-optic probe and analyzed by a compact spectrometer. The output of the spectrometer is displayed in graphical form (Figure 27.3) on a laptop screen.

Once the location of the PA is detected, the PA is removed using either microscopic or endoscopic surgical techniques with the PD-assisted system. Most of PA can be removed using pituitary curettes and dissectors in the usual fashion. Once the bulk of the PA was removed, the remaining adenoma cells are removed using the PD-assisted technology.

27.6 PDT in PA

Once all fluorescent adenoma cells were removed and hemostasis was secured, a balloon-diffuser was placed and inflated in the sella turcica.

The PDT dose is dependant on the balloon-diffuser size, the laser fiber-diffuser length, the prescribed dose of light, and the power output of the laser machine. For example, for a balloon-diffuser (tumor cavity) of 1 cm, laser fiber-diffuser of 1 cm,

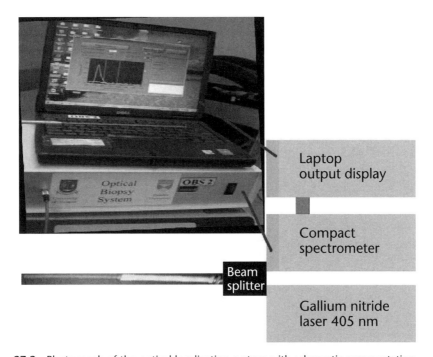

Figure 27.2 Photograph of the optical localization system with schematic representation.

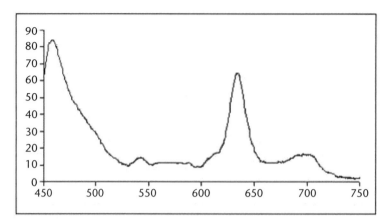

Figure 27.3 Graph of PpIX spectroscopy demonstrating the PpIX peak at 632 nm.

laser power of 400 mW, a dose of 100 J/cm^2 and irradiation of 127 mW/cm^2, a treatment duration of 785 seconds would be necessary (see Table 26.1).

Marks et al. reported a series of 12 recurrent PA treated with Photofrin-mediated PDT with a follow-up as long as 2 years in some cases [21]. The authors encountered one skin photosensitivity and one hemiparesis. The hemiparesis was not thought to be related to PDT. Both visual field deficits and hypersecretions improved in this series after PDT. They noted that initial swelling occurred by 22% at three days after PDT but PA shrinkage was noted at 3 months by 13% and thereafter by 34%, 40%, and 54% at 6 months, 18 months, and 2 years, respectively. Eljamel et al. [22] reported a series of 21 newly diagnosed consecutive pituitary lesions treated with PDT. These were 13 males and eight females with a mean age of 52.4 years. Eight were null cell adenomas, nine were secreting (four acromegaly, three Cushing's disease, two gonadotrphin), three were cystic (two Rathke-cleft, one Arachnoid), and one intraseller meningioma. The mean tumor volume was 12 cm^3. Out of the 14 PA, which underwent PDT, only one required further therapy due to tumor expansion after 10 months (7.1%) during a mean follow-up period of 27.1 months.

27. 7 Conclusion

PD offers a highly sensitive intraoperative localization method of PA that surpasses all other available pre- and intraoperative PA localization technology of today, and PDT in PA offers an excellent adjuvant therapy that enhances the outcome of surgery in invasive and secreting PA. The direction of travel in the management of PA is targeted therapy to the adenoma and preservation of normal pituitary gland. PD and PDT has this potential and further studies are awaited.

References

[1] Oruckaptan, H. H., et al., "Pituitary Adenomas: Results of 684 Surgically Treated Patients and Review of the Literature," *Surg. Neurol.*, Vol. 53, 2000, pp. 211–219.

[2]   Yildiz, F., et al., "Radiotherapy in the Management of Giant Pituitary Adenomas," *Radiother. Oncol.*, Vol. 52, 1999, pp. 233–237.

[3]   Amar, A. P., et al., "Invasive Pituitary Adenomas: Significance of Proliferation Parameters," *Pituitary*, Vol. 2, 1999, pp. 117–122.

[4]   Anson, J. A., et al., "Resection of Giant Invasive Pituitary Tumors Through a Transfacial Approach: Technical Case Report," *Neurosurgery*, Vol. 37, 1995, pp. 541–545; discussion 545–546.

[5]   Ebersold, M. J., et al., "Long-Term Results in Transsphenoidal Removal of Nonfunctionic Pituitary Adenomas," *J. Neurosurg.*, Vol. 64, 1984, pp. 713–719.

[6]   Majos, C., et al., "Imaging of Giant Pituitary Adenomas," *Neuroradiology*, Vol. 40, 1998, pp. 651–655.

[7]   Meij, B. P., et al., "The Long-Term Significance of Microscopic Dural Invasion in 354 Patients with Pituitary Adenomas Treated with Transsphenoidal Surgery," *J. Neurosurg.*, Vol. 96, 2002, pp. 195–208.

[8]   Scheithauer, B. W., et al., "Pathology of Excessive Production of Growth Hormone," *Clin. Endocrinol. Metab.*, Vol. 15, 1986, pp. 655–681.

[9]   Yokoyama, S., et al., "Are Nonfunctioning Pituitary Adenomas Extending into the Cavernous Sinus Aggressive and/or Invasive?" *Neurosurgery*, Vol. 49, 2001, pp. 857–862; discussion 862–853.

[10] Laws, E. R., and J. A. Jane, Jr., "Pituitary Tumors—Long-Term Outcomes and Expectations," *Clin. Neurosurg.*, Vol. 48, 2001, pp. 306–319.

[11] Jenkins, D., et al., "The Birmingham Pituitary Database: Auditing the Outcome of the Treatment of Acromegaly," *Clin. Endocrinol. (Oxf)*, Vol. 43, 1995, pp. 517–522.

[12] Kreutzer, J., et al., "Surgical Management of GH-Secreting Pituitary Adenomas: An Outcome Study Using Modern Remission Criteria," *J. Clin. Endocrinol. Metab.*, Vol. 86, 2001, pp. 4072–4077.

[13] Mampalam, T. J., J. B. Tyrrell, and C. B. Wilson, "Transsphenoidal Microsurgery for Cushing Disease. A Report of 216 Cases," *Ann. Intern. Med.*, Vol. 109, 1988, pp. 487–493.

[14] Buchfelder, M., et al., "Long-Term Follow-Up Results in Hormonally Active Pituitary Adenomas After Primary Successful Transsphenoidal Surgery," *Acta Neurochir. Suppl. (Wien)*, Vol. 53, 1991, pp. 72–76.

[15] Garibi, J., et al., "Giant Pituitary Adenomas: Clinical Characteristics and Surgical Results," *Br. J. Neurosurg.*, Vol. 16, 2002, pp. 133–139.

[16] Yano, T., et al., "Photodynamic Therapy for Rat Pituitary Tumor In Vitro and In Vivo Using Pheophorbide-A and White Light," *Lasers Surg. Med.*, Vol. 11, 1991, pp. 174–182.

[17] Kirollos, R. W., et al., "A Preliminary Experimental In Vivo Study of the Effect of Photodynamic Therapy on Human Pituitary Adenoma Implanted in Mice," *Br. J. Neurosurg.*, Vol. 12, 1998, pp. 140–145.

[18] Hall, W. A., et al., "Pituitary Magnetic Resonance Imaging in Normal Human Volunteers: Occult Adenomas in The General Population," *Ann. Intern. Med.*, Vol. 120, 1994, pp. 817–820.

[19] Batista, D., et al., "Detection of Adrenocorticotropin-Secreting Pituitary Adenomas by Magnetic Resonance Imaging in Children and Adolescents with Cushing Disease," *J. Clin. Endocrinol. Metab.*, Vol. 90, 2005, pp. 5134–5140.

[20] Eljamel, M. S., G. Leese, and H. Moseley, "Intraoperative Pituitary Adenoma Identification Using Intraoperative Spectroscopic System," *Skull Base*, Vol. 17, 2007, pp. 16–17.

[21] Marks, P. V., et al., "Effect of Photodynamic Therapy on Recurrent Pituitary Adenomas: Clinical Phase I/II Trial—An Early Report," *Br. J. Neurosurg.*, Vol. 14, 2000, pp. 317–325.

[22] Eljamel, M. S., et al., "Photodiagnosis and Photodynamic Therapy in Pituitary Adenomas.," *Skull Base*, Vol. 16, 2006, pp. 16–17.

CHAPTER 28

Photodynamic Therapy in the Head and Neck

Colin Hopper

28.1 Introduction: Oral Cavity Cancer

Worldwide oral cavity cancer constitutes 267,000 cases, amounting to 2.7% of all cancers [1]. While it is difficult to get accurate up-to-date figures, the most recent worldwide figures suggest there is little change. Global 2002 estimates were 274,289 [2].

The highest incidences of head and neck cancer are found in Singapore and India. In South East Asia and particularly in India, cancer of the oral cavity is the most common cancer, comprising 35% of all cancers in men and 18% of all cancers in women [3]. The high incidence in Southeast Asia is attributable to the local habit of chewing paan (a mixture of tobacco, areca nut, lime, and other substances wrapped in a betel leaf).

In the United States, American Cancer Society data suggests oral cavity cancer is the ninth most common cancer with 27,700 new cases per annum, accounting for 2% of all malignancies, with a death rate of 7,200. In 1997, new cases of cancer of the oral cavity were estimated at 22,000 [4] and deaths that year were estimated at 6,500. The incidence among the 38 countries in the United Nations defined area of Europe of oral cavity cancer was nearly 50,000 cases [5]. The mortality in 1990 was estimated at 19,200. Across the European Union there are wide variations in the incidence, with the incidence in France (approximately 50/100,000 men per year) being almost seven times that for Greece.

Within the oral cavity, the vast majority of tumors are squamous cell carcinomas of the mucosa, tongue, and lip. Most primary squamous cell carcinomas of the oral cavity are located in those areas of the oral mucosa that are exposed to saliva: the lateral border and under-surface of the tongue, and the floor of the mouth [3].

The most disappointing fact related to oral cancer is that age-adjusted death rates have remained unchanged over the past 30 years. Parker et al. [4] reported that overall 5-year relative survival rates for cancers of the oral cavity and pharynx have remained unchanged at around 55% since 1974 for Caucasians and have in fact declined slightly for African Americans (33%, down from 36%).

28.2   Treatment Options for Oral Cancer

Clinically, these tumors pose exceptional problems in management due to the poor prognosis in advanced cases and the intercurrent medical problems frequently experienced by patients. The proximity to vital structures in the head and neck region makes treatment difficult and often severely deforming, with a functional impact on speech and swallowing.

Surgical resection and radiotherapy, either singly or combined, are currently the main treatments for oral cancer. For small primary cancers (stages I and II, without regional spread), either technique on its own can provide good local control and long-term survival but often at the cost of functional or cosmetic impairment in the case of surgery, or short- and long-term side effects in the case of radiotherapy. What is more, there is an annual incidence of metachronous tumors of the upper aerodigestive tract [6]. When second primary tumors arise, treatment becomes increasingly difficult as there is only so much tissue that can be excised surgically and when the patient has been irradiated as part of the primary therapy, reirradiation is not usually possible.

Against this background there have been many attempts to find alternative therapeutic options for patients with oral cavity and other head and neck cancer.

28.3   Development of PDT in Head and Neck Cancer Management

The first of the recent treatments to be carried out was on a lip cancer by von Tappeiner and Jesionek about 100 years ago, and this started a long history of PDT for the treatment of oral cavity cancer (see Chapter 1 for details).

PDT has been successfully employed to treat early carcinomas of the oral cavity and larynx, preserving normal tissue and vital functions of speech and swallowing. Biel at al. reported 276 patients with early carcinomas of the oral cavity and larynx treated from 1990 to 2006. Among the treated lesions there were predominantly laryngeal, oral cavity, and pharynx squamous cell carcinomas (SCC), but also Kaposi sarcoma, melanoma, and SCC in other head and neck locations. The cure rates with a single treatment for early laryngeal and oral cancers were 91% and 94%, respectively [7]. The high yield of response among patients with early stage head and neck cancers have been confirmed in numerous other trials. Keller at al. [8] treated three patients for T1 and T2 oral cavity tumors with Photofrin-PDT and observed three complete cures. Others like Feyh et al. [9] treated 27 patients with carcinomas of the oral cavity and larynx. Of 15 patients with oral cancers, 13 obtained a complete response. One patient with recurrent disease occurred submucosally in the tongue. Of 12 patients with laryngeal cancers, 11 obtained a complete response (91%) [10]. Overall, more than 500 patients were subjected to Photofrin-based PDT for conditions, including T1 and T2 tumors of lip, oral cavity, larynx, and pharynx. Among this significant number of patients, around 450 responded completely to the treatment (~89%), while just over 50 responded with partial response (~10%), with only two without any response (~0.4%).

This high rate of cures was confirmed when researches used Foscan as a photosensitizer. In these studies they observed ~85% of complete responses with ~17% of partial responses and 0% of no responders.

The development of effective light sources (frequently lasers) and new powerful photosensitizing drugs has led to approved indications for treatment of head and neck cancer, at least in the EU. Early work in head and neck cancer was carried out with Photofrin in the early 1990s by Li [11], Gluckman [12], and Grant [13].

The results with a light-activating wavelength of 630 nm are encouraging, but the exact treatment parameters in the published works are variable and often impossible to compare. Typically, treatment parameters are drug light interval of 2 days with light dose of 50 to 100 J/cm^2. Initial studies using the drug were reported in advanced disease; however, it seems much more logical to use this treatment in early disease where the total volume of disease can be treated. Grant et al. [14] demonstrated that in the clinical setting, PDT damage could be inflicted on normal oral tissues with excellent healing, probably as a result of the preservation of collagen and elastin. Patients remain light sensitive for up to 6 to 8 weeks after sensitization and caution must be used with bright sunlight for up to 3 months.

A small amount of work has been done with 5-aminolevulinic acid, which has the advantage of only a brief period of photosensitivity (approximately 24 hours). This drug is activated at 635 nm with a drug light interval of 4 to 6 hours (depending on the exact route of administration) again at 100J/cm^3. Fan et al. [15] showed this could be useful in the treatment of dysplasia, but the depth of effect of about 1 mm was too superficial to be useful in the treatment of invasive disease. While the treatment effect can be increased by the introduction of treatment breaks and the use of adjunctive iron chelating agents, the main application of this therapy is currently in the treatment of skin cancer and Barrett's esophagus.

28.4 Foscan-PDT for Head and Neck Cancer

Most work over the last 10 years has been carried out using Foscan (m-tetrahydroxyphenylchlorin), a synthetic chlorin that produces necrosis to a depth of about 1 cm. The drug dose is 0.15 mg/kg, drug/light interval is 4 days and the activating wavelength is 652 nm, which is a little longer and penetrates deeper than the 630- and 635-nm doses used above. There are still problems of photosensitivity and controlled reexposure to light is required over a 2- to 3-week period. A series of prospective studies have been published that demonstrate a clear role for PDT in management of conditions of the head and neck.

The first study was on early oral cancer, where tumors up to 2.5 cm in diameter were treated [16]. There was clearly an inherent design flaw with the choice of lesion size, as 2 cm is the cutoff between T1 and T2 disease. This makes the interpretation of the results a little difficult. Also, some of the study centers only recruited one or two patients and their results were clearly not as good as centers who recruited 10 or more patients. However, complete response rate in the patients treated according to protocol was 85% (97 out of 114) at 12 weeks. Response rates were higher for smaller tumors (Table 28.1). Of the 17 patients not documented as

Table 28.1 Complete Response Rates by Tumor T-Stage

Tis	T1	T2	Overall	Confidence Intervals
3/3 (100%)	83/92 (90%)	11/19 (58%)	97/114 (85%)	77–91

having a complete response at 12 weeks, one was not assessed and one refused further treatment and died of extensive disease 1 year later. Two patients were initially lost to follow-up but were subsequently traced and found to be disease-free. The remaining 13 were partial responders who went on to receive other therapy. Of these, nine obtained a CR; four had disease progression and have since died. These results are very encouraging and clearly demonstrate that PDT can be used for thin disease.

In another study by Copper et al. [17], PDT has been used in the treatment of total of 27 patients with 42 second or multiple primary head and neck tumors. Cure rates for stage I or in situ disease were 85% versus 38% for stage II/III. This study clearly demonstrates the repeatability of this treatment and the value in the management of this particularly difficult disease.

Probably the most important study however was with advanced disease. One hundred twenty-eight patients with advanced head and neck cancer were treated with a single PDT session [18]. The patients treated had all failed or were unsuitable for conventional therapy and in fact all had been heavily pretreated (Table 28.2).

Overall, complete response rates were 13%, but interestingly, this figure rose to 30% WHO complete response rate when the total surface area of the tumor could be illuminated and the depth estimate was less than 1 cm. Not surprisingly, this group achieved a much better survival rate than partial responders.

From this, the concept has grown of identification of the tumor volume and light distribution within that volume to increase the chances of getting a complete response. The limitations here are the depth to which light can penetrate tissue is sufficient quantity to trigger the PDT effect. This means that either new, more powerful drugs need to be developed, or light has to be delivered directly into the tissues. This technique of interstitial PDT is one that is still being developed, but published data to date suggests a clear role for PDT in the treatment of advanced disease.

There are two main methods of delivering light—either point sources or diffuser fibers, and both techniques are in regular use. The tissue effects can be simulated using mathematical modeling—this can be quite useful in the calculation of light dis-

Table 28.2 Patient Details of Clinical Trial in [18]

Details of prior therapy (n=128)	n	%
Surgery, radiotherapy, and chemotherapy	30	23
Surgery and radiotherapy only	46	36
Surgery and chemotherapy only	4	3
Radiotherapy and chemotherapy only	16	13
Surgery only	8	6
Radiotherapy only	21	16
Chemotherapy only	0	0
No previous treatment	3	2

tribution and extent of treatment effects. There are limitations with these techniques that are related to the exact nature of tissue and the extent to which light can pass through that tissue. There is really no substitute for real-time monitoring of light distribution and this can be done in a number of ways. Isotropic fibers can be used and this technique has been advocated by Tan et al. A more innovative approach has been described by Gross [19], which uses BOLD MR as a marker of light distribution. None of this however is a substitute for histological confirmation of effect, although such evidence is hard to come by in human tissue.

Accurate evaluation of tumor extent is usually carried out using MRI, CT, ultrasound, and PET CT. These imaging techniques can also be used for real-time fiber placement, especially in sites deep within the head and neck that are close to sensitive structures. MR is particularly useful, although there are challenges of patient orientation within the scanner to ensure good visualization of titanium needles [20].

In the series of Lou et al. [21], 45 patients were treated after all other therapeutic options had been exhausted. All received 0.15 mg/kg Foscan and were illuminated at 652 nm using bare tip fibers delivering 20 J per fiber at 4 days. Thirty-three patients had at least a partial response with a median survival of 16 months. There were nine complete responders and at least two have survived 6 years, but what was most impressive was the symptomatic relief in terms of pain and bleeding that patients obtained. There were surprisingly few complications in terms of damage to nerves and blood vessels with the important exception of one fatal carotid blowout. Postmortem examination showed tumor on the internal surface of the vessel and while it is reassuring that the treatment had precipitated an inevitable event, it does make the case for prophylactic stenting of major vessels when there is a suspicion of tumor erosion.

The observation of the safety of this treatment around nerves and vessels was a very important one as it confers a significant advantage of PDT over surgery and reirradiation. Following on from these studies, interstitial PDT has been used in the treatment of difficult benign diseases of the head and neck such as neurofibroma, lymphangioma, and hemangioma. The study by Betz et al. [22] looked at 11 patients with lymphangioma and hemangioma and showed an impressive reduction in size of lesions. In this study there was no significant damage to skin or nerves, a great advantage over surgery especially when one considers that most treatments were carried out in close proximity to the facial and hypoglossal nerves. The other great advantage of this treatment is that it is repeatable and this makes it of particular value in management of benign diseases that have the potential to regrow.

The other area in the head and neck that PDT has much to offer is in the management of skin cancer. Much work has been done with ALA and this is a therapy that is widely available. However, there is a role for using more powerful sensitizers such as Photofrin and Foscan. The major problem is controlling the depth of effect and minimizing scar formation and this can be achieved by altering the treatment parameters. The studies performed by Triesscheijn et al. [23] suggest that skin cancers can be treated effectively using Foscan at a reduced drug dose of 0.01 mg/kg and treating with 10 J/cm^3 at 24 hours. The cosmetic results have been impressive and this technique certainly merits further evaluation.

28.5 Conclusions

The current position of PDT in the head and neck is that we have drugs that are licensed for use in advanced cancer, but it is disappointing that many of the wider applications are available in only a handful of centers. The problems of photosensitivity and lack of selectivity may well be addressed by the development of new drugs and antibody fragment targeting.

References

[1]   Parkin, D. M., et al., "Estimating the World Cancer Burden: Globocan 2000," *Int. J. Cancer*, Vol. 94, 2001, pp. 153–156.

[2]   Parkin, D. M., "Global Cancer Statistics in the Year 2000," *Lancet Oncol.*, Vol. 2, 2001, pp. 533–543.

[3]   Shah, J. P., M. J. Zelefsky, and B. B. O'Malley, "Squamous Cell Carcinoma of the Oral Cavity," in *Head and Neck Cancer—A Multidisciplinary Approach*, L. B. Harrison, et al. (eds.), Lippincott Williams & Wilkins, 1999, pp. 411–444.

[4]   Parker, S. L., et al., "Cancer Statistics," *CA Cancer J. Clin.*, Jan.–Feb., 1997, pp. 5–27.

[5]   Bray, F., et al., "Estimates of Cancer Incidence and Mortality in Europe in 1995," *Eur. J. Cancer*, Vol. 38, 2002, pp. 99–166.

[6]   Shibuya, H., et al., "Leukoplakia-Associated Multiple Carcinomas in Patients with Tongue Carcinoma," *Cancer*, Vol. 57, 1986, pp. 843–846.

[7]   Biel, M., "Advances in Photodynamic Therapy for the Treatment of Head and Neck Cancers," *Lasers Surg. Med.*, Vol. 38, 2006, pp. 349–355.

[8]   Keller, G. S., D. R. Doiron, and G. U. Fisher, "Photodynamic Therapy in Otolaryngology—Head and Neck Surgery," *Arch. Otolaryngol.*, Vol. 111, 1985, pp. 758–761.

[9]   Feyh, J., et al., "Photodynamic Therapy in Head and Neck Surgery," *J. Photochem. Photobiol. B*, Vol. 7, 1990, pp. 353–358.

[10] Feyh J, G. A., and A. Leunig, "A Photodynamic Therapy in Head and Neck Surgery," *Laryngo. Rhino. Otol.*, Vol. 73, 1993, pp. 273–278.

[11] Li, J. H., et al., "Photodynamic Therapy in the Treatment of Malignant Tumours: An Analysis of 540 Cases," *J. Photochem. Photobiol. B*, Vol. 6, 1990, pp. 149–155.

[12] Gluckman, J. L., "Photodynamic Therapy for Head and Neck Neoplasms," *Otolaryngol. Clin. North Am.*, Vol. 24, 1991, pp. 1559–1567.

[13] Grant, W. E., et al., "Photodynamic Therapy of Malignant and Premalignant Lesions in Patients with 'Field Cancerization' of the Oral Cavity," *J. Laryngol. Otol.*, Vol. 107, 1993, pp. 1140–1145.

[14] Grant, W. E., et al., "Photodynamic Therapy: An Effective, But Non-Selective Treatment for Superficial Cancers of the Oral Cavity," *Int. J. Cancer*, Vol. 71, 1997, pp. 937–942.

[15] Fan, K. F., et al., "Photodynamic Therapy Using 5-Aminolevulinic Acid for Premalignant and Malignant Lesions of the Oral Cavity," *Cancer*, Vol. 78, 1996, pp. 1374–1383.

[16] Hopper, C., et al., "mTHPC-Mediated Photodynamic Therapy for Early Oral Squamous Cell Carcinoma," *Int. J. Cancer*, Vol. 111, 2004, pp. 138–146.

[17] Copper, M. P., et al., "Photodynamic Therapy in the Treatment of Multiple Primary Tumours in the Head and Neck, Located to the Oral Cavity and Oropharynx," *Clin. Otolaryngol.*, Vol. 32, 2007, pp. 185–189.

[18] D'Cruz, A. K., M. H. Robinson, and M. A. Biel, "mTHPC-Mediated Photodynamic Therapy in Patients with Advanced, Incurable Head and Neck Cancer: A Multicenter Study of 128 Patients," *Head Neck*, Vol. 26, 2004, pp. 232–240.

[19] Gross, S., et al., "Monitoring Photodynamic Therapy of Solid Tumors Online by BOLD-Contrast MRI," *Natl. Med.*, Vol. 9, 2003, pp. 1327–1331.

[20] Jager, H. R., et al., "MR Imaging-Guided Interstitial Photodynamic Laser Therapy for Advanced Head and Neck Tumors," *AJNR Am. J. Neuroradiol.*, Vol. 26, 2005, pp. 1193–1200.

[21] Lou, P. J., et al., "Interstitial Photodynamic Therapy as Salvage Treatment for Recurrent Head and Neck Cancer," *Br. J. Cancer*, Vol. 91, 2004, pp. 441–446.

[22] Betz, C. S., et al., "Interstitial Photodynamic Therapy for a Symptom-Targeted Treatment of Complex Vascular Malformations in the Head and Neck Region," *Lasers Surg. Med.*, Vol. 39, 2007, pp. 571–582.

[23] Triesscheijn, M., et al., "Optimizing Meso-Tetra-Hydroxyphenyl-Chlorin-Mediated Photodynamic Therapy for Basal Cell Carcinoma," *Photochem Photobiol.*, Vol. 82, 2006, pp. 1686–1690.

CHAPTER 29

Intraperitoneal Photodynamic Therapy

Keith A. Cengel and Stephen M. Hahn

29.1 Introduction

The treatment of serosal surface malignancies, including recurrent peritoneal carcinomatosis resulting from ovarian cancer and gastrointestinal cancers and peritoneal sarcomatosis, is typically palliative in nature. Thus, the development of effective and safe novel therapies to address this pattern of cancer spread would be highly significant. One such therapy is PDT. The appeal of PDT in the treatment of peritoneal malignances is that PDT has the potential to combine selective destruction of cancerous tissue compared to normal tissue with the ability to treat and conform to relatively large surface areas. Moreover, the intrinsic, physical limitation in the depth of visible light penetration through tissue limits PDT damage to deeper structures, thereby providing additional potential for tumor cell selectivity. This is especially true after surgical debulking (cytoreduction) where the residual tumor is microscopic or less than 5 mm in depth. In combination with surgical debulking and systemic chemotherapy, intraperitoneal (IP) PDT has shown promise in phase I and II clinical trials of PDT using the first generation photosensitizer Photofrin. However, the toxicity of this treatment was not insignificant and this led to a suboptimal therapeutic index for IP PDT.

One reason for this may have to do with photosensitizer distribution. The tumor-to-normal-tissue ratio (TNTR) for Photofrin, when using relevant normal tissues such as bowel, was not as high as predicted by preclinical tumor models. Initial preclinical evidence suggested that some photosensitizers, including the first generation photosensitizer hematoporphyrin derivative (HPD), are retained in tumors to a far greater extent than in some normal tissues [1, 2]. In patients with peritoneal malignances, TNTRs were found to be generally between one and three [3, 4]. In addition, there was significant heterogeneity in Photofrin uptake in the tumor tissues examined in these studies. This combination likely explains the suboptimal therapeutic index for IP PDT with Photofrin.

One possible solution for this problem is to use a second generation photosensitizer that may have a higher TNTR than Photofrin. Unfortunately, preliminary human studies of photosensitizer distribution using motexafin lutetium show that the use of second generation photosensitizers may be insufficient to improve the therapeutic index of IP PDT [S. M. Hahn, unpublished observations]. Thus, alternative methods of improving the therapeutic index of IP PDT are needed, such as selectively altering the biological response of tumor cells to PDT or improving the tumor cell specificity of photosensitizer/light application.

Recent preclinical data indicates that altering survival signaling in tumor cells has the potential to biologically improve the therapeutic index of IP PDT [5]. This concept will be tested soon in humans in an upcoming clinical trial at the University of Pennsylvania. In addition, the creation of antitumor antibody-photosensitizer conjugates or tumor-targeted nanoparticles that encapsulate photosensitizer or facilitate light delivery may allow for better physical dose deposition in IP PDT [6].

Thus, PDT might be ideal for malignancies, such as ovarian, gastric, and colorectal cancers, that have the propensity to spread to peritoneal surfaces. However, for disseminated intraperitoneal malignancies, involvement of regional lymph nodes and other micrometastasic disease are clinical concerns. Therefore, a locoregional treatment such as intraperitoneal PDT is not likely to be successful as the sole modality of treatment for these cancers, but rather as a part of a multimodality treatment regimen that includes surgery and/or chemotherapy in addition to intraperitoneal PDT. Nevertheless, recent clinical trials of intraperitoneal PDT (see Section 29.3) and the emerging developments in the field of molecularly targeted PDT show that intraperitoneal PDT remains a highly exciting potential treatment for patients with disseminated intraperitoneal malignancy. In this chapter, the preclinical rationale, the clinical experience to date, and the prospects for future improvements in intraperitoneal PDT treatment outcomes will be presented.

29.2   Preclinical Studies of IP PDT

29.2.1   IP PDT Efficacy

The strong theoretical rational for intraperitoneal PDT was first tested in animal models by Douglass and colleagues [7]. In these experiments, rabbits with Brown-Pierce epithelioma implants in the serosa of the bowel, liver, pancreas, or bladder were treated with hematoporphyrin derivative (HPD)-mediated PDT (5 mg/kg HPD and 631-nm light). On days 5 to 7 following HPD-PDT, extensive tumor necrosis was reported. However, these experiments used a single focal spot of light at a very high fluence (300 J/cm^2) that most likely resulted in a combination of thermal and PDT-mediated tumor cell killing.

Tochner and colleagues carried out a series of experiments using ascites tumors in mice. In a mouse model of ovarian peritoneal carcinomatosis, they evaluated HPD-mediated PDT using 50 mg/kg HPD and 514-nm light [8]. Mice were injected intraperitoneally with ovarian embryonal cancer cells and then randomly assigned on day 9 following tumor inoculation to receive no treatment, treatment with HPD alone, treatment with light alone or treatment with HPD+light (HPD-PDT). The HPD and light (9.6 J delivered over 16 minutes) were both delivered intra-7peritoneally and the intraperitoneal tumor burden at the time of treatment was 2g to 4g. All of the untreated control animals as well as the HPD-only and light-only treated animals died of progressive disease between days 20 to 23 following tumor inoculation. The mice treated with a single treatment with HPD-PDT on day 9 showed prolonged survival, but only one animal (out of 16 total) survived past day

34. This animal survived >50 days and was presumably cured. However, a second group of mice that received two treatments with HPD-PDT on days 9 and 15 showed apparent cure of disease in six out of 16 animals. Note that in this tumor model, eradication of tumor is difficult to achieve with the administration of intraperitoneal chemotherapy. A 70% cure rate is observed with intraperitoneal doxorubicin but only if the agent is administered 2 days after tumor inoculation, when the tumor burden is low. If doxorubicin is administered on the same day as the PDT was given (day 9), a cure rate of less than 20% is observed, presumably because of a higher tumor burden [8, 9].

29.2.2 Fractionated IP PDT

Multifractionated HPD-PDT has also been studied using a murine ascitic malignant teratoma model. The mice in this study were treated with a total of four HPD-PDT treatments using 50-mg/kg HPD delivered intraperitoneally 2 hours prior to therapy and 514-nm light delivered to separate octants (each received 1.2J in 2 minutes) of the abdomen using a flat cut fiber [10]. One hundred percent of the HPD-PDT treated animals achieved a complete response and 85% showed no evidence of recurrence at necropsy. Taken together, this data suggests that multiple sequential treatments (fractionated PDT) might be necessary in order to achieve a high percentage of cures. These two preclinical studies by Tochner and colleagues provided the impetus for the development of the first phase I clinical trial of IP PDT at the National Cancer Institute (NCI) [11–13]. Fractionated IP PDT has also been studied by Veenhuizen and colleagues as a treatment for CC531 colon carcinoma implanted in the intraperitoneal fat pad of rats [14]. On day 7 after tumor implantation, rats were treated with porfimer sodium (5 mg/kg) and 628-nm light (25–75 J/cm^2). All animals treated with porfimer sodium-PDT showed significantly longer tumor regrowth time than untreated controls. However, animals treated with multiple fractions of porfimer sodium-PDT showed the most prolonged tumor regrowth delays and these results were comparable to or exceeded the results obtained with intraperitoneal cisplatin delivery.

In human trials, a single, intraoperative IP PDT treatment has been used due to the risk and morbidity of reoperation for delivery of a second IP PDT fraction. However, recent developments in nanotechnology have the potential to make multifraction PDT more feasible [15]. By using nanoparticles comprised of photosensitizer plus a crystal that is capable of upconverting infrared light to visible light, it may be possible to perform intraperitoneal PDT using an external infrared source. This external beam PDT technology would be more readily amenable to multifraction PDT and is now under evaluation and testing in the preclinical setting at several research centers [16, 17]

29.2.3 IP PDT Toxicity

Preclinical studies have not only helped to define the potential benefits of IP PDT, but also have aided in the prediction and evaluation of the potential toxicities of this treatment. Because of the depth of penetration that can be achieved in PDT is greater than the thickness of the bowel wall, toxicity to the bowel, especially bowel perforation, has always been a major concern. In addition to direct bowel toxicity from transmural light penetration, there is also a possibility that PDT could interfere with blood flow in the bowel and thereby indirectly lead to bowel damage through ischemic injury. There has been a suggestion that IP PDT with HPD interferes with jejunal blood flow [18]. However, others have found no significant damage to major blood vessels after intraperitoneal treatment [19]. Veenhuizen and colleagues found that the intestines of Wag/RijA rats were the most sensitive organs in a study evaluating intraperitoneal PDT with either porfimer sodium or meso-tetrahydroxyphenylchlorin (mTHPC) [20]. A steeper toxicity-dose response curve was reported for mTHPC compared to porfimer sodium but a similar spectrum of toxicities was observed. One bowel perforation in the mTHPC group was reported. The normal tissue toxicity of PDT in the peritoneum has also been studied using a dog model [21]. HPD (1.2 mg/kg) was administered intravenously and intraperitoneally. The entire peritoneal surface received 630-nm light 48 hours after IV injection and 2 hours after intraperitoneal injection of HPD. The doses of light ranged from 0.57 to 0.74 J/cm^2. Other than a reversible decrease in lymphocyte counts and a modest elevation of liver function tests, no significant toxicities were noted. A mild peritonitis was seen in biopsy specimens of the treated peritoneum. Mild reversible damage to the kidneys was seen on histologic analysis without functional impairment. Elevations in liver transaminases were also reported in animals treated with porfimer sodium. At high PDT doses, acute lethality caused by intraperitoneal PDT was reported to be the result of toxic shock and rhabdomyolysis leading to circulatory failure. As a consequence of these findings in the preclinical studies, human clinical trials started with treatment of the entire peritoneum using 514-nm light to reduce the depth of penetration, with a boost of more deeply penetrating 630-nm light given to high risk or suboptimally debulked sites of disease. In addition, liver and kidney functions were closely followed in the IP PDT patients.

Given the preclinical evidence that bowel toxicity might be the dose-limiting toxicity of intraperitoneal PDT, concerns were raised regarding the tolerance of bowel anastomoses [22]. Since the initial thoughts were to integrate intraperitoneal PDT with surgical debulking, it was likely that patients would require resection of small bowel as part of the surgical procedure. Small bowel anastomoses were created in New Zealand White rabbits followed by intraperitoneal PDT [22]. HPD was administered in doses of 1.5 to 2.5 mg/kg 24 hours prior to surgery and light doses of 0 to 20 J/cm^2 were evaluated. No adverse effects on the anastomoses were observed at these doses. Higher doses of HPD (10 mg/kg) administered with light doses of 20 J/cm^2 resulted in a high rate of anastomotic breakdown.

29.2.4 Preclinical Data with Second Generation Photosensitizers

Since the initiation of the phase I trial at the U.S. National Cancer institute (NCI), other researchers have investigated the preclinical efficacy of fractionated IP PDT. Molpus et al. studied PDT with BPD, a second generation photosensitizer, and 690-nm light in a xenograft murine model of the human ovarian cancer, NIH:OVCAR-5 [23]. The light was administered intraperitoneally using a dose of

20 J. Several multidose regimens were studied and all led to a reduction in tumor burden at necropsy and a median survival benefit. Despite these apparent benefits of multifraction intraperitoneal PDT in preclinical studies, this concept has yet to be tested in clinical trials, largely due to the inherent difficulty and increased risk of complications associated with repeated surgical procedures (see Section 29.3).

In addition to BPD, several other second generation photosensitizers have been evaluated in preclinical animal studies. 5-aminolevulinic acid (ALA) is converted in vivo into the photosensitizer protoporphyrin IX (PpIX). The ability of ovarian cancer micrometastases to convert ALA to PpIX has been tested in Fischer 344 rats [24]. In these studies, 60% to 70% of animals with peritoneal ovarian micrometastases showed fluorescence of PpIX on peritoneal surfaces as compared to 0% of the control (no tumor) animals following either intravenous or intraperitoneal ALA delivery. The conversion of ALA to PpIX in ovarian cancer micrometastases has been clinically tested in a study of 17 patients with 36 total biopsies taken from fluorescent and nonfluorescent tissues after intraperitoneal administration of ALA prior to second-look laparoscopy [25]. While the sample size is small, this preliminary study showed that for the detection of ovarian cancer micrometastases, the ALA→PpIX conversion has a specificity of 88%, a sensitivity of 100%, a negative predictive value of 100%, and a positive predictive value of 91%. However, while the toxicity of ALA-PDT has been evaluated [26], this method has not been tested for efficacy in either the preclinical or clinical setting. In addition, multiple groups have demonstrated that the efficiency of a tumor converting ALA→PpIX is inversely proportional to the degree of differentiation of the tumor cells [27–29]. Thus, it is possible that ALA-PDT would be far more effective at killing more highly differentiated intraperitoneal micrometastases and be less effective at killing more poorly differentiated, potentially biologically more aggressive, tumor cells. The potential mechanism for this effect is incompletely understood, but may be due to increased expression of efflux pumps such as ABCG2 on these cancer cells [30].

Motexafin lutetium (MLu) is another second generation photosensitizer that has an absorbance peak at 732 nm (near-infrared). This peak allows light delivery with less chance of interference from absorption of light by hemoglobin and also allows deeper tissue penetration of MLu-PDT. While this deeper penetration may increase the ability of PDT to treat a greater volume of residual disease, it also brings with it a greater potential for bowel toxicity. Therefore, the toxicity of MLu-PDT has been tested in canine models of intraperitoneal PDT [31]. In this study, 13 dogs were treated with 0.2–2 mg/kg MLu 3 hours prior to delivery of 0.5–2 J/cm^2 of 732-nm light at laparotomy. Overall this treatment was well tolerated and animals experienced only a mild, transient elevation in liver function tests, but no clinical evidence of significant hepatic or renal impairment. Bowel toxicity was assessed at a second laparotomy 7 to 10 days after MLu-PDT and histologic evidence of mild enteritis was found in both control and MLu-PDT treated animals. Importantly, in animals that underwent bowel resection at the first laparatomy, there were no anastomotic leaks or other increased bowel toxicities. In another study, similar results and minimal toxicities were observed in dogs undergoing low rectal stapled anastomosis followed by pelvic MLu-PDT [32].

29.3   Clinical Applications of Intraperitoneal PDT

29.3.1   Phase I Trial of IP Photofrin-Mediated PDT

A Phase I study of surgery and PDT with laser light and porfimer sodium was conducted by the Surgery and Radiation Oncology Branches of the NCI for disseminated intraperitoneal malignancies [11–13]. Seventy patients, mostly with recurrent ovarian cancer carcinomatosis or peritoneal sarcomatosis, were enrolled in the study. To be eligible for this trial, patients were required to have a workup that showed no evidence of disease in the liver parenchyma or outside the abdomen and had to be medically fit for surgery. Patients received porfimer sodium by IV injection prior to laparotomy and an attempt was made to resect all gross disease, where possible, or debulk residual tumor deposits to less than 5 mm in thickness. Any patient with >5-mm thick residual deposits did not continue on to receive light (PDT), since the effective tissue penetration of 630-nm light is only about 5 mm. Forty-six adequately debulked patients underwent light delivery to all peritoneal surfaces. Real-time light dosimetry was performed using flat photodiodes that were sewn into the right upper quadrant, left upper quadrant, right and left peritoneal gutters, and pelvis. These diodes, along with a mobile diode, measured only incident light and were connected to a computerized online dosimetry system. A flat cut fiber was used to illuminate the mesentery, the small bowel and then the large bowel, in that order. Next, the abdominal cavity was filled with dilute intralipid (0.02–0.05%) in order to better scatter the light and improve the homogeneity of light distribution to all areas of the peritoneum. Light to the peritoneal cavity was delivered with a light diffusing applicator that was comprised of an optical fiber enclosed in a modified endotracheal tube (Figure 29.1). This light diffusing applicator was moved over anatomic regions that were isolated to ensure uniform delivery of light (Figure 29.2).

In this phase I study, the PDT dose was sequentially escalated by increasing the sensitizer dose from 1.5 to 2.5 mg/kg, by shortening the drug-light interval, and by increasing the light dose. Initially, 630-nm red light alone was used but later a combination of 514-nm green light and 630-nm light was used. The reason for this change in wavelengths was that bowel toxicity was initially observed and because of

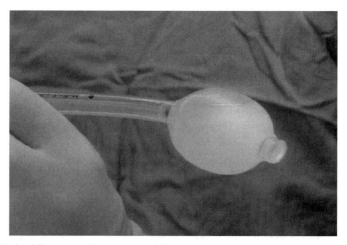

Figure 29.1   Light diffusing applicator for IP PDT.

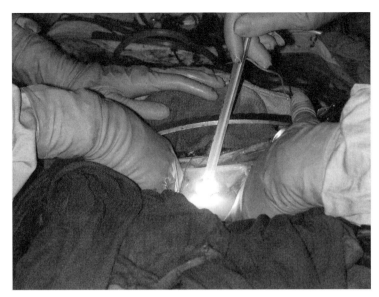

Figure 29.2 Light delivery during IP PDT.

the greater (and presumably transmural) penetration by red light, 514 nm-green light was substituted for illumination of the bowel and mesentery. Patients also received boost doses (10–15 J/cm^2) with 630-nm red light or 5 to 7.5 J/cm^2 with 514-nm green light to areas of gross disease on the diaphragms, gutters, and/or pelvis.

It should also be pointed out that the distinction between surgical and PDT-related complications was difficult to establish in this study. The patients had advanced refractory disease and often required extensive resections. Some of the complications described above are not atypical of debulking surgery in this patient population. However, most of the complications observed in patients treated on this trial were related to bowel toxicity, and bowel perforation was the PDT-dose limiting toxicity. Four patients developed intestinal fistulae and three patients developed a bowel perforation. One patient who suffered a colonic perforation died after multiple procedures and multiorgan failure. All patients who developed a bowel perforation received either 630-nm light to the bowel or a dose of 514-nm light to the bowel of 3.8 J/cm^2 or greater. Even at lower PDT doses, treatment of the entire peritoneum caused intra-abdominal fluid sequestration and small bowel edema that necessitated aggressive fluid resuscitation on the first postoperative day, although this problem was greatest in patients that required more extensive tumor resections or received higher total light doses. In addition to problems with bowel toxicity, seven patients who received light dose of 10 J/cm^2 to the diaphragms developed pleural effusions that caused respiratory compromise and required thoracentesis. Other major (but not dose-limiting) complications included postoperative hemorrhage, necrotizing pancreatitis, splenic rupture, and ureteral leak and urinoma. Sun sensitivity, thrombocytopenia, and asymptomatic liver function test abnormalities were also observed.

Based upon these observed toxicities, the maximally tolerated doses of photosensitizer and light were determined. The maximally tolerated porfimer sodium dose was 2.5 mg/kg, administered IV 48 hours prior to debulking surgery. The maximally tolerated green light (514-nm) dose to the mesentery and small and large intestine was 2.5 J/cm^2. The maximally tolerated red light (630-nm) dose was 5 J/cm^2 to the stomach, 7.5 J/cm^2 to the liver, spleen, omental bursa, and diaphragm, and 10 J/cm^2 to the retroperitoneal gutters and pelvis. A 15-J/cm^2 boost dose of 630-nm light to limited areas of gross disease in the pelvis, gutters, or diaphragms was also considered tolerable.

While designed to measure toxicity, data on patient outcome were also recorded. Pre-and postoperative peritoneal cytology was obtained in 17 patients. Thirteen of 17 patients with malignant peritoneal cytology were found to have negative follow-up cytologic analysis for an overall peritoneal cytologic response rate of 76%. The median survival of all patients that received PDT was 30 months and there were three long-term survivors in 25 patients with ovarian cancer. One of these patients died of lymphoma 28 months after treatment and one patient died of metastatic colon cancer 95 months after treatment. Both patients were free of ovarian cancer recurrence at the time of their deaths. It should be emphasized that these patients had no other treatment after surgical debulking and a single exposure to PDT.

29.3.2 Phase II Trial of IP Photofrin-Mediated PDT

Based upon the results of the phase I clinical trial, a phase II clinical trial of intraperitoneal PDT for disseminated intraperitoneal malignancies was initiated in 1997 at the University of Pennsylvania [3, 4, 33–40]. One hundred patients were enrolled, stratified according to cancer type (33 ovarian cancer patients, 37 gastrointestinal malignancy patients, and 30 sarcoma patients) and given doses of porfimer sodium and light at the maximally tolerated dose a defined in the NCI trial. Of these patients, 29 were not eligible because of the inability to confirm disease status on pathological examination (1 patient), presence of localized disease only (2 patients), or inability to adequately debulk the tumors to <5mm residual disease (26 patients). The primary objective was to define the efficacy of IP PDT in these three groups of patients and the secondary objectives were to report the toxicities of this treatment in each patient population and to assess photosensitizer uptake in tumor and normal tissues. A pathologic restaging of disease was also requested of all patients who were clinically free of disease 6 months after treatment with PDT.

As in the NCI trial, intraperitoneal PDT was associated with a postoperative capillary leak syndrome that necessitated massive fluid resuscitation in the immediate postoperative period [4, 35]. One patient died after suffering a perioperative myocardial infarction that was likely due to a low cardiac output state. A second patient died from sepsis after reoperation for a perioperative bleed. Grade 1 or 2 skin toxicities were observed in 20 patients as a result of skin photosensitization. The remainder of the complications experienced by patients treated on this trial included prolonged intubation secondary to adult respirator distress syndrome (4 patients), bowel fistulae/anastomotic leaks (4 patients), and poor wound healing/infection (4 patients) [4]. Other than the capillary leak syndrome and the skin photosensitivity, these complication rates are not atypical of the complication rates that are observed after similarly extensive surgery in the absence of PDT [41, 42].

With a 51-month median follow-up, the median failure-free survival and over-all survival for all enrolled patients by strata were: ovarian, 2.1 months and 20.1 months; gastrointestinal cancers, 1.8 months and 11.1 months; and sarcoma, 3.7 months and 21.9 months. For the patients that received PDT, the median fail-ure-free survival and overall survival were: ovarian, 3 months and 22 months; gas-trointestinal cancers, 3.3 months and 13.2 months; and sarcoma: 4 months and 21.9 months. At 6 months after therapy, the pathologic complete response rate was 3/33 (9.1%), 2/37 (5.4%), and 4/30 (13.3%) for the patients with ovarian cancer, gastrointestinal cancer, and sarcoma, respectively. Although most patients had dis-ease at early follow-up between 3 and 6 months, the median survival of almost 2 years in the ovarian patients and over 1 year in the gastrointestinal patients suggests some benefit from this treatment. In the patients with sarcoma, the prolonged over-all survival was primarily due to patients with sarcomatosis from gastrointestinal stromal tumors who were treated with Gleevec® when it became available. Analysis of the patterns of treatment failure in this study suggests that a significant percent-age of patients experienced treatment failure at sites not initially involved by gross disease [33]. Moreover, patients with gross residual disease (that received a PDT boost to these sites) showed similar recurrence kinetics as compared to patients without gross residual disease, suggesting a dose-response relationship in intraperitoneal PDT. However, given the presence of fairly significant toxicities at PDT doses that were not adequate to fully control local disease, the therapeutic win-dow for intraperitoneal PDT would appear to be quite narrow. Thus, undirected PDT dose escalation is unlikely to result in a significant improvement in treatment outcomes, at least when Photofrin is used as a photosensitizer.

29.3.3   TNTR for Photofrin in IP PDT

One of the reasons for this narrow therapeutic window appears to stem from the lower than expected tumor-to-normal-tissue ratio (TNTR) for porfimer sodium in these studies [3, 36]. In normal tissues, drug uptake significantly ($p<0.0001$) dif-fered as a function of seven different tissue types. In bowel, a toxicity-limiting organ for IP PDT, the mean Photofrin levels were 2.70 ng/mg and 3.42 ng/mg in full-thickness large and small bowel, respectively. In tumors, drug uptake signifi-cantly ($p=0.0015$) differed as a function of patient cohort: mean porfimer sodium level was 3.32 to 5.31 ng/mg among patients with ovarian, gastric, or small bowel cancer; 2.09 to 2.45 ng/mg among patients with sarcoma and appendiceal or colon cancer. Thus, ovarian, gastric, and small bowel cancers demonstrated significantly higher porfimer sodium uptake than full-thickness large and/or small bowel. How-ever, the ratio of mean drug level in tumor versus bowel was modest at 2.31. In addition, despite multiple analyses, there was no apparent relationship between clinical outcome on this trial and porfimer sodium uptake. This relatively low TNTR for photosensitizer binding are contrary to the expectations promoted by preclinical studies, but supported by similar results in a phase II trial of intrathoracic PDT using porfimer sodium [43]. Moreover, the absolute photosensitizer concen-trations measured compare favorably with those described in murine models [37]. It has been hypothesized that second generation photosensitizers might show even greater tumor selectivity than first generation photosensitizers such as porfimer sodium. Indeed, as noted above, ALA appears to concentrate well in peritoneal micrometastases from ovarian cancer, but this sensitizer has not yet been tested clinically in intraperitoneal PDT.

29.3.4 Physical Measurements of PDT Dose

One approach to explicitly estimate the tissue cytotoxic effects of PDT is to measure the tissue concentrations of oxygen and photosensitizer and combine these with measurements of the absorbed light dose. An estimate of tissue oxygen concentration can be determined using the difference in absorption spectra for oxy versus deoxy hemoglobin. In addition, it is also possible to estimate local photosensitizer tissue concentration using fluorescence and/or absorbance spectroscopy. The light dose that is delivered to an area can be quantitated using either incident or spherical dosimetry systems, combined with measurements of tissue optical properties.

In the processes of completing the phase II IP PDT trial, great strides were made in measurement of these highly relevant physical properties. A specialized broadband infrared spectroscopy system was evaluated for in vivo measurements of light penetration, blood oxygen saturation, hemoglobin concentration, and tissue photosensitizer concentration [40]. This trial also included a comparison of light dosimetry using incident light measurements (as in the NCI trial) with measurements made from a newer, spherical light dosimetry system that was developed by Starr and colleagues. This new system measures the total light dose, including both incident and scattered light [44, 45]. This spherical light dosimetry system permitted a more accurate measurement of the light dose delivered to superficial tissues [45].

In the phase II IP PDT trial, substantial intra- and interpatient heterogeneity of tissue optical properties was observed and these properties changed significantly over the course of light delivery. In addition, blood flow and tissue oxygenation can change dramatically within the course of PDT delivery and preclinical evidence indicates that these changes can be used to predict the overall efficacy of PDT [46]. Photosensitizer concentrations also change due to photobleaching during light exposure. Thus, for optimal measurement of physical parameters of PDT, these quantities should be measured in real time before, during, and after PDT. In principle, intentional inhomogeneities can be introduced into the light dose to compensate for inhomogeneities in photosensitizer or oxygen distribution. These concepts are being developed and implemented for future trials of IP PDT.

29.4 Enhancing the Therapeutic Index of IP PDT

The use of second generation photosensitizers and improvements in PDT delivery and dosimetry techniques alone may not sufficiently increase the therapeutic index of IP PDT to make this a feasible treatment option outside of a clinical trial. However, new data indicates that the therapeutic index of IP PDT may also be increased through manipulation of molecular targets involved in PDT survival signaling. Multiple lines of evidence have led to the hypothesis that PDT-stimulated signaling through EGFR and postreceptor molecules such as PI3K/AKT and MAPK pathways may lead to cellular resistance to PDT-mediated cytotoxicity. EGFR is a receptor tyrosine kinase that regulates important cellular functions including cell cycle progression and survival mediated through PI3K-AKT, proliferation through MAPK, and protection from apoptosis through STAT3 [47, 48]. The interactions between EGFR signaling and PDT are complex and may to some extent be dependent on the cell line, photosensitizer, or PDT dose. Some investigators have suggested that PDT-mediated EGFR activation is important for survival of cancer cells following PDT and that EGFR signaling is upregulated by PDT [49–51]. Others have found that PDT causes a temporary degradation/inactivation of cell surface receptors, including EGFR [52–54]. These observations may be related in that at lower PDT doses, EGFR and STAT3 are both activated/tyrosine phosphorylated and localize to the nucleus, possibly to signal cell survival [55]. At higher PDT doses, STAT3 forms nonfunctional oligomeric complexes that may be indicative of effective PDT treatment [54, 56].

In a recent preclinical study, the combination of the EGFR inhibitor cetuximab and BPD-mediated PDT led to a synergistic response in vivo [57]. In this study, the authors studied the effects of cetuximab-mediated EGFR inhibition on the response to BPD-PDT using a mouse model of ovarian carcinomatosis. Cetuximab was administered in four doses of cetuximab over 9 days (0.5 mg per dose), starting 1 day after the first treatment with BPD-PDT. An additional dose of BPD-PDT was delivered after completion of the cetuximab therapy. The combination of cetuximab + BPD-PDT led to the greatest in vivo tumor response (9.8% tumor burden vs. 38% for PDT alone). Median survival was also greatest in the combination group (80 days vs. 28 days). Importantly, no enhanced normal tissue toxicity was observed in the combination group compared to PDT or cetuximab alone. This study demonstrates that inhibition of the signal transduction cascade after PDT may improve the therapeutic index of this treatment. Preliminary experiments demonstrate that at least some of this effect likely stems from Cetuximab-mediated enhancement of direct cell killing by PDT [55]. Moreover, autocrine growth factor signaling networks involving the epidermal growth factor (EGF) receptors have been implicated in the development of malignant phenotype as well as the intraperitoneal spread of tumor in both gastrointestinal and ovarian cancers [58–60]. In this respect, cetuximab has the potential to reduce impact the efficacy of intraperitoneal PDT both by enhancing direct (and possibly indirect) PDT-mediated cancer cell killing and by inhibiting cancer cell survival signaling. The combination of cetuximab and BPD-PDT will be tested in an upcoming phase I/II trial of IP PDT.

Another potential mechanism for enhancing the efficacy of intraperitoneal PDT is through targeted photosensitizer delivery. In the phase II trial of intraperitoneal PDT conducted at the University of Pennsylvania, tumor hypoxia and photosensitizer uptake were poorly correlated with each other and neither correlated well with the size of tumor nodules [36]. There was also significant intra- and interpatient variability in photosensitizer uptake in both tumor and normal tissues. Along with the relatively narrow therapeutic window of intraperitoneal PDT, these factors suggest the strong clinical potential of molecularly targeted photosensitizers. Solban, Hasan, and colleagues have tested the efficacy of anti-EGFR antibody targeted PDT in a variety of settings [5]. In these experiments, an anti-EGFR antibody (OC125) or the F(ab')$_2$ binding portion of this antibody is linked covalently to chlorine6, a photosensitizer derived from chlorophyll. In one study, the efficacy and toxicity of cationic OC125 F(ab')$_2$ chlorine6 cationic conjugate-mediated PDT and free chlorine6-mediated PDT were compared using a mouse model of ovarian carcinomatosis [61]. Tumor treatment response was seen using both agents, but animals treated with OC125 F(ab')$_2$ chlorine6–mediated PDT showed significantly better initial tumor response to treatment, increased overall survival, and lower treatment toxicity than animals treated with chlorine6–mediated PDT. Another potential method to target photosensitizers would be to use nanoparticle technology. Early studies have demonstrated PDT-mediated cancer cell killing using ceramic or silica based nanoparticles as a delivery vehicles for photosensitizer [6, 16]. Theoretically, these nanoparticles could be targeted to cancer cells using a variety of ligands and could also be designed to release other toxic substances upon activation by light.

29.5   Summary and Conclusions

Peritoneal carcinomatosis and sarcomatosis are generally incurable problems for which there are few good treatment options. Intraperitoneal PDT is potentially an ideal therapy for peritoneal carcinomatosis because of its relatively superficial treatment effect. A phase II trial of IP PDT with the first generation photosensitizer, Photofrin, demonstrated that this treatment approach shows some clinical efficacy but is associated with substantial toxicity, suggesting a narrow therapeutic index. Remarkably, these responses were observed in heavily pretreated patients that are generally refractory to standard treatments. Correlative studies of photosensitizer uptake in human tumor and normal tissues show limited tumor selectivity. This lack of photosensitizer selectivity for tumor in combination with tumor hypoxia (as opposed to oxic normal tissues) is likely a major reason for the narrow therapeutic index of IP PDT. However, the advent of novel and potentially molecularly targeted photosensitizers, combined with enhancement of PDT cancer cell cytotoxicity through inhibition of growth factor signaling should greatly improve the therapeutic index of intraperitoneal PDT. In addition, other approaches, including the use of nanotechnology, may allow the administration of fractionated PDT, which may also improve the therapeutic index of this treatment. The clinical implementation of these technologies may allow for highly effective and well-tolerated treatment of IP malignancies with PDT.

References

[1]   Gomer, C. J., and T. J. Dougherty, "Determination of [3H]- and [14C]hematoporphyrin Derivative distribution in Malignant and Normal Tissue," *Cancer Res.*, Vol. 39, 1979, pp. 146–151.

[2]   Young, S. W., et al., "Lutetium Texaphyrin (PCI-0123): A Near-Infrared, Water-Soluble Photosensitizer," *Photochem. Photobiol.*, Vol. 63, 1996, pp. 892–897.

[3]   Hahn, S. M., et al., "Photofrin Uptake in the Tumor and Normal Tissues of Patients Receiving Intraperitoneal Photodynamic Therapy," *Clin. Cancer Res.*, Vol. 12, 2006, pp. 5464–5470.

[4]   Hahn, S. M., et al., "A Phase II Trial of Intraperitoneal Photodynamic Therapy for Patients with Peritoneal Carcinomatosis and Sarcomatosis," *Clin. Cancer Res.*, Vol. 12, 2006, pp. 2517–2525.

[5]   Solban, N., I. Rizvi, and T. Hasan, "Targeted Photodynamic Therapy," *Lasers Surg. Med.*, Vol. 38, 2006, pp. 522–531.

[6]   Roy, I., et al., "Ceramic-Based Nanoparticles Entrapping Water-Insoluble Photosensitizing Anticancer Drugs: A Novel Drug-Carrier System for Photodynamic Therapy," *J. Am. Chem. Soc.*, Vol. 125, 2003, pp. 7860–7865.

[7]   Douglass, H. O., Jr., et al., "Intra-Abdominal Applications of Hematoporphyrin Photoradiation Therapy," *Adv. Exp. Med. Biol.*, Vol. 160, 1983, pp. 15–21.

[8]   Tochner, Z., et al., "Treatment of Murine Intraperitoneal Ovarian Ascitic Tumor with Hematoporphyrin Derivative and Laser Light," *Cancer Res.*, Vol. 45, 1985, pp. 2983–2987.

[9]   Ozols, R. F., et al., "Chemotherapy for Murine Ovarian Cancer: A Rationale for Ip Therapy with Adriamycin," *Cancer Treat. Rep.*, Vol. 63, 1979, pp. 269–273.

[10] Tochner, Z., et al., "Photodynamic Therapy of Ascites Tumours Within the Peritoneal Cavity," *Br. J. Cancer*, Vol. 53, 1986, pp. 733–736.

[11] DeLaney, T. F., et al., "Phase I Study of Debulking Surgery and Photodynamic Therapy for Disseminated Intraperitoneal Tumors," *Int. J. Radiat. Oncol. Biol. Phys.*, Vol. 25, 1993, pp. 445–457.

[12] Sindelar, W., et al., "Intraperitoneal Photodynamic Therapy Shows Efficacy in Phase I Trial," *Proc. Am. Soc. Clin. Oncol.*, Vol. 14, 1995, pp. 447.

[13] Sindelar, W. F., et al., "Technique of Photodynamic Therapy for Disseminated Intraperitoneal Malignant Neoplasms. Phase I Study," *Arch. Surg.*, Vol. 126, 1991, pp. 318–324.

[14] Veenhuizen, R. B., et al., "Intraperitoneal Photodynamic Therapy of the Rat CC531 Adenocarcinoma," *Br. J. Cancer*, Vol. 73, 1996, pp. 1387–1392.

[15] Kapoor, R., et al., "Highly Efficient Infrared-to-Visible Energy Upconversion in Er3+:Y2O3," *Opt. Lett.*, Vol. 25, 2000, pp. 338.

[16] Kim, S., et al., "Organically Modified Silica Nanoparticles Co-Encapsulating Photosensitizing Drug and Aggregation-Enhanced Two-Photon Absorbing Fluorescent Dye Aggregates for Two-Photon Photodynamic Therapy," *J. Am. Chem. Soc.*, Vol. 129, 2007, pp. 2669–2675.

[17] Collins, J., et al., "Infrared Light Can Be Used for Photodynamic Therapy by Using Rare Earth Phosphors for Visible Light Generation," *SPIE—Photonics West Meeting*, January 20–25, 2007, Abstract # 6427-43.

[18] Selman, S. H., et al., "Jejunal Blood Flow after Exposure to Light in Rats Injected with Hematoporphyrin Derivative," *Cancer Res.*, Vol. 45, 1985, pp. 6425–6427.

[19] Suzuki, S., S. Nakamura, and S. Sakaguchi, "Experimental Study of Intra-Abdominal Photodynamic Therapy," *Lasers Med. Sci.*, Vol. 2, 1987, pp. 195–203.

[20] Veenhuizen, R. B., et al., "Intraperitoneal Photodynamic Therapy in the Rat: Comparison of Toxicity Profiles for Photofrin and MTHPC," *Int. J. Cancer*, Vol. 59, 1994, pp. 830–836.

[21] Tochner, Z., et al., "Photodynamic Therapy of the Canine Peritoneum: Normal Tissue Response to Intraperitoneal and Intravenous Photofrin Followed by 630 Nm Light," *Lasers Surg. Med.*, Vol. 11, 1991, pp. 158–164.

[22] DeLaney, T. F., et al., "Tolerance of Small Bowel Anastomoses in Rabbits to Photodynamic Therapy with Dihematoporphyrin Ethers and 630 Nm Red Light," *Lasers Surg. Med.*, Vol. 13, 1993, pp. 664–671.

[23] Molpus, K. L., et al., "Intraperitoneal Photodynamic Therapy of Human Epithelial Ovarian Carcinomatosis in a Xenograft Murine Model," *Cancer Res.*, Vol. 56, 1996, pp. 1075–1082.

[24] Major, A. L., et al., "In Vivo Fluorescence Detection of Ovarian Cancer in the Nutu-19 Epithelial Ovarian Cancer Animal Model Using 5-Aminolevulinic Acid (ALA)," *Gynecol. Oncol.*, Vol. 66, 1997, pp. 122–132.

[25] Loning, M. C., et al., "Fluorescence Staining of Human Ovarian Cancer Tissue Following Application of 5-Aminolevulinic Acid: Fluorescence Microscopy Studies," *Lasers Surg. Med.*, Vol. 38, 2006, pp. 549–554.

[26] Major, A. L., et al., "Intraperitoneal Photodynamic Therapy in the Fischer 344 Rat Using 5-Aminolevulinic Acid and Violet Laser Light: A Toxicity Study," *J. Photochem. Photobiol. B*, Vol. 66, 2002, pp. 107–114.

[27] Li, G., et al., "Effect of Mammalian Cell Differentiation on Response to Exogenous 5-Aminolevulinic Acid," *Photochem. Photobiol.*, Vol. 69, 1999, pp. 231–235.

[28] Ortel, B., et al., "Differentiation-Specific Increase in ALA-Induced Protoporphyrin IX Accumulation in Primary Mouse Keratinocytes," *Br. J. Cancer*, Vol. 77, 1998, pp. 1744-1751.

[29] Ortel, B., et al., "Differentiation Enhances Aminolevulinic Acid-Dependent Photodynamic Treatment of LNCaP Prostate Cancer Cells," *Br. J. Cancer*, Vol. 87, 2002, pp. 1321–1327.

[30] Liu, W., et al., "The Tyrosine Kinase Inhibitor Imatinib Mesylate Enhances the Efficacy of Photodynamic Therapy by Inhibiting ABCG2," *Clin. Cancer Res.*, Vol. 13, 2007, pp. 2463–2470.

[31] Griffin, G. M., et al., "Preclinical Evaluation of Motexafin Lutetium-Mediated Intraperitoneal Photodynamic Therapy in a Canine Model," *Clin. Cancer Res.*, Vol. 7, 2001, pp. 374–381.

[32] Ross, H. M., et al., "Photodynamic Therapy with Motexafin Lutetium for Rectal Cancer: A Preclinical Model in the Dog," *J. Surg. Res.*, Vol. 135, 2006, pp. 323–330.

[33] Wilson, J. J., et al., "Patterns of Recurrence in Patients Treated with Photodynamic Therapy for Intraperitoneal Carcinomatosis and Sarcomatosis," *Int. J. Oncol.*, Vol. 24, 2004, pp. 711–717.

[34] Hendren, S. K., et al. "Phase II Trial of Debulking Surgery and Photodynamic Therapy for Disseminated Intraperitoneal Tumors," *Ann. Surg. Oncol.*, Vol. 8, 2001, pp. 65–71.

[35] Canter, R. J., et al., "Intraperitoneal Photodynamic Therapy Causes a Capillary-Leak Syndrome," *Ann. Surg. Oncol.*, Vol. 10, 2003, pp. 514–524.

[36] Busch, T. M., et al., "Hypoxia and Photofrin Uptake in the Intraperitoneal Carcinomatosis and Sarcomatosis of Photodynamic Therapy Patients," *Clin. Cancer Res.*, Vol. 10, 2004, pp. 4630–4638.

[37] Menon, C., et al., "Vascularity and Uptake of Photosensitizer in Small Human Tumor Nodules: Implications for Intraperitoneal Photodynamic Therapy," *Clin. Cancer Res.*, Vol. 7, 2001, pp. 3904–3911.

[38] Bauer, T. W., et al., "Preliminary Report of Photodynamic Therapy for Intraperitoneal Sarcomatosis," *Ann. Surg. Oncol.*, Vol. 8, 2001, pp. 254–259.

[39] Dimofte, A., et al., "In Vivo Light Dosimetry for Motexafin Lutetium-Mediated PDT of Recurrent Breast Cancer," *Lasers Surg. Med.*, Vol. 31, 2002, pp. 305–312.

[40] Wang, H. W., et al., "Broadband Reflectance Measurements of Light Penetration, Blood Oxygenation, Hemoglobin Concentration, and Drug Concentration in Human Intraperitoneal Tissues Before and After Photodynamic Therapy," *J. Biomed. Opt.*, Vol. 10, 2005, pp. 14004.

[41] Rosen, S. A., et al., "Initial Presentation Wwith Stage IV Colorectal Cancer: How Aggressive Should We Be?," *Arch. Surg.*, Vol. 135, 2000, pp. 530–534; discussion 534–535.

[42] Sugarbaker, P. H., and K. A. Jablonski, "Prognostic Features of 51 Colorectal and 130 Appendiceal Cancer Patients with Peritoneal Carcinomatosis Treated by Cytoreductive Surgery and Intraperitoneal Chemotherapy," *Ann. Surg.*, Vol. 221, 1995, pp. 124–132.

[43] Friedberg, J. S., et al., "Phase II Trial of Pleural Photodynamic Therapy and Surgery for Patients with Non-Small-Cell Lung Cancer with Pleural Spread," *J. Clin. Oncol.*, Vol. 22, 2004, pp. 2192–2201.

[44] Van Staveren, H., et al., "Construction, Quality Control and Calibration of Spherical Iso-tropic Fibre-Optic Light Diffusers," *Lasers Med. Sci.*, Vol. 10, 1995, pp. 137–147.

[45] Vulcan, T. G., et al., "Comparison Between Isotropic and Nonisotropic Dosimetry Sys-tems During Intraperitoneal Photodynamic Therapy," *Lasers Surg. Med.*, Vol. 26, 2000, pp. 292–301.

[46] Wang, H. W., et al., "Treatment-Induced Changes in Tumor Oxygenation Predict Photodynamic Therapy Outcome," *Cancer Res.*, Vol. 64, 2004, pp. 7553–7561.

[47] Silva, C. M., "Role of STATs as Downstream Signal Transducers in Src Family Kinase-Mediated Tumorigenesis," *Oncogene*, Vol. 23, 2004, pp. 8017–8023.

[48] Hynes, N. E., and H. A. Lane, "ERBB Receptors and Cancer: The Complexity of Targeted Inhibitors," Natl. Rev. *Cancer*, Vol. 5, 2005, pp. 341–354.

[49] Fanuel-Barret, D., et al., "Influence of Epidermal Growth Factor on Photodynamic Ther-apy of Glioblastoma Cells In Vitro," *Res. Exp. Med. (Berl.)*, Vol. 197, 1997, pp. 219–233.

[50] Tong, Z., G. Singh, and A. J. Rainbow, "Sustained Activation of the Extracellular Sig-nal-Regulated Kinase Pathway Protects Cells from Photofrin-Mediated Photodynamic Therapy," *Cancer Res.*, Vol. 62, 2002, pp. 5528–5535.

[51] Moor, A., et al., "Photoimunotargeting of the Epidermal Growth Factor Receptor for the Treatment of Ovarian Cancer," *13th International Congress on Photobiology and 28th Annual Meeting ASP*, 2000, pp. 166.

[52] Ahmad, N., , K. Kalka, and H. Mukhtar, "In Vitro and In Vivo Inhibition of Epidermal Growth Factor Receptor-Tyrosine Kinase Pathway By Photodynamic Therapy," *Onco-gene*, Vol. 20, 2001, pp. 2314–2317.

[53] Wong, T. W., et al., "Photodynamic Therapy Mediates Immediate Loss of Cellular Responsiveness to Cytokines and Growth Factors," *Cancer Res.*, Vol. 63, 2003, pp. 3812–3818.

[54] Liu, W., A. R. Oseroff, and H. Baumann, "Photodynamic Therapy Causes Cross-Linking of Signal Transducer and Activator of Transcription Proteins and Attenuation of Interleukin-6 Cytokine Responsiveness in Epithelial Cells," *Cancer Res.*, Vol. 64, 2004, pp. 6579–6587.

[55] Cengel, K., et al., "Survival Signaling Through Nuclear Epidermal Growth Factor Recep-tor and STAT3 Mediates Photodynamic Therapy Resistance in Ovarian and Lung Cancer Cells," *Int. J. Radiat. Oncol. Biol. Phys.*, Vol. 69, No. 3, 2007, pp. S98–S99.

[56] Henderson, B. W., et al., "Cross-Linking of Signal Transducer and Activator of Transcrip-tion 3—A Molecular Marker for the Photodynamic Reaction in Cells and Tumors," *Clin. Cancer Res.*, Vol. 13, 2007, pp. 3156–3163.

[57] del Carmen, M. G., et al., "Synergism of Epidermal Growth Factor Receptor-Targeted Immunotherapy with Photodynamic Treatment of Ovarian Cancer In Vivo," *J. Natl. Can-cer Inst.*, Vol. 97, 2005, pp. 1516–1524.

[58] Mills, G. B., and W. H. Moolenaar, "The Emerging Role of Lysophosphatidic Acid in Can-cer," *Nat. Rev. Cancer*, Vol. 3, 2003, pp. 582–591.

[59] Agarwal, R., and S. B. Kaye, "Ovarian Cancer: Strategies for Overcoming Resistance to Chemotherapy," *Nat. Rev. Cancer*, Vol. 3, 2003, pp. 502–516.

[60] Yagi, H., et al., "Clinical Significance of Heparin-Binding Epidermal Growth Factor-Like Growth Factor in Peritoneal Fluid of Ovarian Cancer," *Br. J. Cancer*, Vol. 92, 2005, pp. 1737–1745.

[61] Molpus, K. L., et al., "Intraperitoneal Photoimmunotherapy of Ovarian Carcinoma Xenografts in Nude Mice Using Charged Photoimmunoconjugates," *Gynecol. Oncol.*, Vol. 76, 2000, pp. 397–404.

Conclusion: Photodynamic Therapy—The Next Hundred Years

Michael R. Hamblin and Paweł Mróz

The rate of increase in the progress being made in all of biomedical research and in research in PDT in particular is relentlessly exponential. Every year new journals are launched, and new meetings organized to discuss aspects of scientific research relevant to PDT, if not specifically about PDT itself. As mentioned in Chapter 1, PDT has been studied for more than a hundred years, but it has been only in the last 25 years that it has gained substantial interest among scientist and clinicians. The next hundred years will certainly reveal whether PDT matures into an accepted therapy for a wide variety of diseases or perhaps remains a "niche therapy" for a few indications.

Scientific efforts by chemists have been made to design, synthesize, and characterize an enormous variety of molecules that could act as photosensitizers. However, the effort necessary to fully test this large number of candidate compounds in suitable in vitro cell cultures and in vivo animal models of cancer and other diseases is immense. To some extent this has created a logjam when potentially very valuable photosensitizers remain on the shelf because the research manpower needed to test their capabilities is lacking. This problem is further exacerbated because many of the most active compounds are not water-soluble and need to be formulated in a drug delivery vehicle to make them biologically available. Again it is at present uncertain whether to look for a "universal photosensitizer" that will be applicable in any disease, or to tailor the PS structure, pharmacokinetics, and biodistribution for the particular disease to be treated.

The requirement for PDT light dosimetry measurements and treatment planning has evolved with the available light delivery technologies, and these developments have opened up new clinical applications of PDT. Today, the use of LEDs, fiber lasers, and conformal light delivery means the promise can only be properly achieved with simultaneous developments in PDT treatment planning.

This book has highlighted some new developments in PDT that may come to play a major role in the years to come. Elucidation of cellular mechanisms, signaling, and death pathways, together with new findings concerning processes that occur in tumors involving oxidative stress, inflammation, and dead cell disposal are active areas of research that may lead to insights into how the host response to PDT activates the immune system. Although the use of covalent photosensitizer conjugates to increase tumor and other tissue targeting is a very active area of preclinical research, there has been virtually no clinical applications of this technology up to now.

The application of PDT to a number of novel preclinical and clinical applications such as in bone, blood vessels, and for infections will increase the interest of the biomedical community in PDT as a whole. Photochemical internalization has the potential to be applied to a wide range of drug delivery problems.

In this collection of research advances in PDT there are unfortunately gaps for which the editors accept responsibility. We had hoped to cover photodynamic diagnosis using fluorescence imaging, PDT for arthritis, and applications of PDT in urology and gynecology. Nevertheless, we believe that this book has presented the most comprehensive coverage of PDT available thus far.

About the Editors

Michael Hamblin is a principal investigator at the Wellman Center for Photomedicine at Massachusetts General Hospital and an associate professor of dermatology at Harvard Medical School. He was trained as a synthetic organic chemist and received a Ph.D. from Trent University in England. His research interests lie in the areas of photodynamic therapy for infections, cancer, and heart disease. In particular, he has worked on covalent photosensitizer conjugates, induction of antitumor immunity by PDT, PDT for vulnerable atherosclerotic plaque, and antimicrobial photoinactivation. He is also interested in low-level light therapy for wound healing, arthritis, and hair regrowth. Dr. Hamblin has published over 150 book chapters, conference proceedings, and international abstracts; more than 85 peer-reviewed articles, and he holds 8 patents.

Paweł Mróz graduated in 2004 from the Medical University of Warsaw, Poland. While at the university he joined the student research group at the Department of Immunology, where under the supervision of Dr. Jakob Golab he participated in several research projects involving PDT. After graduation Dr. Mróz joined, as the International Union Against Cancer Fellow, the laboratory of Dr. Hava Avraham at BIDMC, Harvard Institutes of Medicine, where he worked on the molecular biology of human breast cancer. Since 2005, he has been working as a Research Fellow at the Wellman Center for Photomedicine at Massachusetts General Hospital. Under the supervision of Dr. Michael Hamblin, Dr. Mróz has been investigating the variety of antitumor immune responses after PDT as well as evaluating the applications of several new photosensitizers. He has received several awards for his research.

List of Contributors

Jean-Pierre Ballini, MD
Ecole Polytechnique Fédérale de Lausanne (EPFL)
Laboratory of Photomedicine
CH-1015 Lausanne, Switzerland
E-mail: Jean-Pierre.Ballini@epfl.ch

Kristian Berg, PhD
Department of Radiation Biology
Institute for Cancer Research
Rikshospitalet-Radiumhospitalet Medical Centre
Montebello
N-0310 Oslo 3, Norway
E-mail: kristian.berg@rr-research.no

Stuart K. Bisland, BSc(Hons), Phd
Associate Scientist IV
Department of BioImaging and Biophysics
University of Toronto
Princess Margaret Hospital
University Health Netowrk
610 Universtiy Avenue
Toronto, Ontario M5G 2M9
Canada
E-mail: sbisland@uhnres.utoronto.ca

Anette Bonsted, PhD
Department of Radiation Biology
Institute for Cancer Research
Rikshospitalet-Radiumhospitalet Medical Centre
Montebello
N-0310 Oslo 3, Norway
E-mail: anettbo@ulrik.uio.no

Stanley B. Brown, PhD
Director of the Centre for Photobiology and
Photodynamic Therapy
School of Biological Sciences
University of Leeds
Leeds, LS2 9JT, United Kingdom
E-mail: bmbsbb@bmb.leeds.ac.uk

Ana P Castano, MD
Renal Division
Brigham and Women's Hospital
Department of Medicine
Harvard Medical School
Boston MA 02115
E-mail: acastano@partners.org

Keith A. Cengel, MD, PhD
Assistant Professor and Director of
Photodynamic Therapy Program
Department of Radiation Oncology
University of Pennsylvania
3400 Spruce St.
2 Donner
Philadelphia, PA 19104
E-mail: Cengel@xrt.upenn.edu

Bin Chen, PhD
Department of Pharmaceutical Sciences
Philadelphia College of Pharmacy
University of the Sciences in Philadelphia
Department of Radiation Oncology
University of Pennsylvania
Philadelphia, PA 19104
E-mail: b.chen@usip.edu

Song-mao Chiu, PhD
Department of Radiation Oncology and the Case
Comprehensive Cancer Center
Case Western Reserve University
Cleveland, OH 44106
E-mail: song-mao.chiu@case.edu

Peter de Witte, PhD
Laboratory of Pharmaceutical Biology and
Phytopharmacology
Faculty of Pharmaceutical Sciences
Catholic University Leuven
B-3000 Leuven, Belgium
E-mail: peter.dewitte@pharm.kuleuven.be

Mahabeer P. Dobhal, PhD
Photodynamic Therapy Center
Department of Cell Stress Biology
Roswell Park Cancer Institute
Buffalo, NY 14263

M. Sam Eljamel, MD
Department of Neurosurgery
Ninewells Hospital and Medical School
The University of Dundee
Scotland, United Kingdom
E-mail: m.s.eljamel@dundee.ac.uk.

Manivannan Ethirajan, PhD
Photodynamic Therapy Center
Department of Cell Stress Biology
Roswell Park Cancer Institute
Buffalo, NY 14263
E-mail: man_ivan@yahoo.com

Jakub Golab, MD, PhD
Department of Immunology
Center of Biostructure Research
Medical University of Warsaw
1A Banacha Str., F building
02-097 Warsaw, Poland
E-mail: jgolab@ib.amwaw.edu.pl

Seth A. Gross, MD
Mayo Clinic College of Medicine
Rochester, Minnesota
Division of Gastroenterology & Hepatology
Mayo Clinic
4500 San Pablo Road
Jacksonville, FL 32224
E-mail: Sgross8900@aol.com

Anurag Gupta, PhD
Photodynamic Therapy Center
Department of Cell Stress Biology
Roswell Park Cancer Institute
Buffalo, NY 14263

Stephen M. Hahn, MD
Henry K. Pancoast Professor and Chair
Department of Radiation Oncology
University of Pennsylvania
3400 Spruce St.
2 Donner
Philadelphia, PA 19104
E-mail: hahn@xrt.upenn.edu

Michael R. Hamblin, PhD
Associate Professor
Department of Dermatology
Harvard Medical School
Wellman Center for Photomedicine
Massachusetts General Hospital
40 Blossom Street
Boston, MA 02114
E-mail: hamblin@helix.mgh.harvard.edu

Tayyaba Hasan, PhD
Professor
Department of Dermatology
Harvard Medical School
Wellman Center for Photomedicine
Massachusetts General Hospital
40 Blossom Street
Boston, MA 02114
E-mail: Thasan@partners.org

Chong He, PhD
Department of Pharmaceutical Sciences
Philadelphia College of Pharmacy
University of the Sciences in Philadelphia
Philadelphia, PA 19104

Anders Høgset, PhD
PCI Biotech AS
Hoffsvn. 48
N-0377 Oslo, Norway
E-mail: anders.hogset@pcibiotech.no

P. Jack Hoopes, DVM, PhD
Associate Professor of Surgery and Medicine
(Radiobiology)
Department of Surgery
Dartmouth Medical School
Lebanon, NH 03756
E-mail: Thayer.Receptionist@Dartmouth.edu

Colin Hopper, MD
Unit of Oral and Maxillofacial Surgery
Eastman Dental Institute and Hospital
University College London
256 Gray's Inn Road
London WC1X 8LD
United Kingdom
E-mail: c.hopper@ucl.ac.uk

Giulio Jori
Department of Biology
University of Padova
Via Ugo Bassi 58B
35121 Padova, Italy
E-mail: jori@bio.unipd.it

Asta Juzeniene, PhD, Postdoctoral Fellow
Department of Radiation Biology, Institute for
Cancer Research
Norwegian Radium Hospital
Rikshospitalet University Hospital
Montebello 0310
Oslo, Norway
E-mail: asta.juzeniene@rr-research.no

Mladen Korbelik, PhD
Department of Cancer Imaging
BC Cancer Research Centre
British Columbia Cancer Agency
675 West 10th Avenue
Vancouver, British Columbia V5Z 1L3
Canada
E-mail: mkorbelik@bccrc.ca

Mateusz Kwitniewski, MD
Department of Molecular Microbiology and Serology
National Salmonella Centre
Medical University of Gdansk
ul. Do Studzienki 38
80-227 Gdansk, Poland

Norbert Lange, PhD
Department of Pharmaceutics and Biopharmaceutics
School of Pharmaceutical Sciences
University of Geneva, University of Lausanne
Quai Ernest-Ansermet 30
1211 Geneva 4
Switzerland
E-mail: Norbert.Lange@pharm.unige.ch

Lothar Lilge, PhD
Staff Scientist
Division of Biophysics and Bioimaging
Ontario Cancer Institute
Associate Professor
Department of Medical Biophysics
University of Toronto
Toronto, Ontario, Canada
E-mail: llilge@uhnres.utoronto.ca

Michela Magaraggia, PhD, Postdoctoral Fellow
Research Unit for Medical and Environmental
Photobiology
Department of Biology
University of Padova
Via Ugo Bassi 58B
35121 Padova, Italy
E-mail:michela.magaraggia@unipd.it

Johan Moan, PhD
Professor, Researcher, Group Leader
Department of Radiation Biology, Institute for Cancer
Research
Norwegian Radium Hospital
Rikshospitalet University Hospital
Montebello 0310
and
Institute of Physics
University of Oslo
Blindern 0316
Oslo, Norway
E-mail: johan.moan@labmed.uio.no

Keyvan Moghissi, BSc., MD, FRCS, FETCS
Consultant Surgeon and Clinical Director
Yorkshire Laser Centre
Goole and District Hospital
Woodlands Avenue, Goole
E. Yorkshire, DN14 6RX
United Kingdom

Paweł Mróz
Department of Dermatology
Harvard Medical School
Wellman Center for Photomedicine
Massachusetts General Hospital
40 Blossom Street
Boston, MA 02114
E-mail: pmroz@partners.org

Anna-Liisa Nieminen, PhD
Associate Professor
Department of Pharmaceutical and Biomedical Sciences
and the Hollings Cancer Center
Medical University of South Carolina
QF218 Quadrangle Building
280 Calhoun Street, PO Box 250140
Charleston, SC 29425
E-mail: nieminen@musc.edu

Dominika Nowis, MD, PhD
Department of Immunology
Center of Biostructure Research
Medical University of Warsaw
1A Banacha Str., F building
02-097 Warsaw, Poland
E-mail: dnowis@ib.amwaw.edu.pl

Nancy L. Oleinick, PhD
Department of Radiation Oncology and the Case
Comprehensive Cancer Center
Case Western Reserve University
Cleveland, OH 44106
E-mail: nlo@po.cwru.edu

Ravindra K. Pandey, PhD
Photodynamic Therapy Center
Department of Cell Stress Biology
Roswell Park Cancer Institute
Buffalo, NY 14263
E-mail: ravindra.pandey@roswellpark.org

Brian W. Pogue, PhD
Associate Professor of Engineering
Thayer School of Engineering
Dartmouth College
Hanover, NH 03755
E-mail: brian.w.pogue@dartmouth.edu

Robert W Redmond, PhD
Department of Dermatology
Harvard Medical School
Wellman Center for Photomedicine
Massachusetts General Hospital
40 Blossom Street
Boston, MA 02114
E-mail: redmond@helix.mgh.harvard.edu

Courtney Saenz, PhD
Photodynamic Therapy Center
Department of Cell Stress Biology
Roswell Park Cancer Institute
Buffalo, NY 14263

Drew B Schembre, MD
Virginia Mason Medical Center
University of Washington School of Medicine
1100 9th Ave.,MS:C3
Seattle, WA, 98101
E-mail: drew.schembre@vmmc.org

Pål Kristian Selbo, PhD
Department of Radiation Biology
Institute for Cancer Research
Rikshospitalet-Radiumhospitalet Medical Centre
Montebello
N-0310 Oslo 3, Norway
E-mail: selbo@rr-research.no

Amy F. Taub, MD
Associate Clinical Professor
Department of Dermatology
Northwestern University Medical School
Chicago, IL
and
Medical Director
Advanced Dermatology
Skinfo, SKINQRI
275 Parkway Drive, Suite 521
Lincolnshire, IL 60069
E-mail: drtaub@skinfo.com

Robert Weersink, PhD
Division of Biophysics and Bioimaging
Ontario Cancer Institute
Toronto,Ontario, Canada
E-mail: weersink@uhnres.utoronto.ca

Anette Weyergang, PhD
Department of Radiation Biology
Institute for Cancer Research
Rikshospitalet-Radiumhospitalet Medical Centre
Montebello
N-0310 Oslo 3, Norway
E-mail: anette.weyergang@farmasi.uio.no

Brian C. Wilson, PhD
Division of Biophysics and Bioimaging,
Ontario Cancer Institute
and
Department of Medical Biophysics
University of Toronto
Toronto, Ontario M5G 2M9
Canada
E-mail: wilson@uhnres.utoronto.ca

Herbert C. Wolfsen , MD
Associate Professor of Medicine
Mayo Clinic College of Medicine
Rochester, Minnesota
Division of Gastroenterology & Hepatology
Mayo Clinic
4500 San Pablo Road
Jacksonville, FL 32224
E-mail: Wolfsen.Herbert@mayo.edu

Hubert van den Bergh, PhD
Ecole Polytechnique Fédérale de Lausanne (EPFL)
Laboratory of Photomedicine
CH-1015 Lausanne, Switzerland
E-mail: hubert.vandenbergh@epfl.ch

Index

Related Titles from Artech House

Biological Database Modeling, Jake Chen and Amandeep S. Sidhu, editors

Biomolecular Computation for Bionanotechnology, Jian-Qin Liu and Katsunori Shimohara

Electrotherapeutic Devices: Principles, Design, and Applications, George D. O'Clock

Fundamentals and Applications of Microfluidics, Second Edition, Nam-Trung and Steven T. Wereley

Genome Sequencing Technology and Algorithms, Sun Kim, Haixu Tang, and Elaine R. Mardis, editors

Life Science Automation Fundamentals and Applications, Mingjun Zhang, Bradley Nelson, and Robin Felder, editors

Matching Pursuit and Unification in EEG Analysis, Piotr Durka

Micro and Nano Manipulations for Biomedical Applications, Tachung C. Yih and Ilie Talpasanu, editors

Microfluidics for Biotechnology, Jean Berthier and Pascal Silberzan

Systems Bioinformatics: An Engineering Case-Based Approach, Gil Alterovitz and Marco F. Ramoni, editors

Text Mining for Biology and Biomedicine, Sophia Ananiadou and John McNaught, editors

For further information on these and other Artech House titles, including previously considered out-of-print books now available through our In-Print-Forever® (IPF®) program, contact:

Artech House	Artech House
685 Canton Street	46 Gillingham Street
Norwood, MA 02062	London SW1V 1AH UK
Phone: 781-769-9750	Phone: +44 (0)20 7596-8750
Fax: 781-769-6334	Fax: +44 (0)20 7630-0166
e-mail: artech@artechhouse.com	e-mail: artech-uk@artechhouse.com

Find us on the World Wide Web at: www.artechhouse.com